The Rehabilitation Specialist's Handbook

Second Edition

**Jules M. Rothstein,
PhD, PT, FAPTA**

Professor
Department of Physical Therapy
University of Illinois at Chicago and
University of Illinois Hospital
Chicago, Illinois

**Serge H. Roy,
ScD, PT**

Research Associate Professor
NeuroMuscular Research Center and
Sargent College of Health and
Rehabilitation Sciences
Boston University
Boston, Massachusetts

**Steven L. Wolf,
PhD, PT, FAPTA**

Professor and Director of Research
Department of Rehabilitation Medicine and
Associate Professor
Department of Anatomy and Cell Biology
Emory University School of Medicine
Atlanta, Georgia

F. A. DAVIS COMPANY ▪ Philadelphia

F. A. Davis Company
1915 Arch Street
Philadelphia, PA 19103

Printed in the United States of America

Last digit indicates print number: 10 9 8 7 6 5 4

Publisher: Jean-François Vilain
Developmental Editor: Crystal Spraggins
Production Editor: Rose Gabbay
Cover Designer: Louis J. Forgione

As new scientific information becomes available through basic and clinical research, recommended treatments and drug therapies undergo changes. The authors and publisher have done everything possible to make this book accurate, up to date, and in accord with accepted standards at the time of publication. The authors, editors, and publisher are not responsible for errors or omissions or for consequences from application of the book, and make no warranty, expressed or implied, in regard to the contents of the book. Any practice described in this book should be applied by the reader in accordance with professional standards of care used in regard to the unique circumstances that may apply in each situation. The reader is advised always to check product information (package inserts) for changes and new information regarding dose and contraindications before administering any drug. Caution is especially urged when using new or infrequently ordered drugs.

Library of Congress Cataloging-in-Publication Data

Rothstein, Jules M.
    The rehabilitation specialist's handbook / Jules M. Rothstein,
Serge H. Roy, Steven L. Wolf. — 2nd ed.
        p.   cm.
    Includes bibliographical references and index.
    ISBN 0-8036-0047-X (soft cover)
    1. Medical rehabilitation—Handbooks, manuals, etc.   I. Roy,
Serge H., 1949-   .   II. Wolf, Steven L.   III. Title.
    [DNLM: 1. Rehabilitation—handbooks.   2. Physical
Therapy—handbooks.   WB 39 R847r 1998]
    RM735.3.R68   1998
    617'.03—dc21
    DNLM/DLC
    for Library of Congress   97-18584
                                                                    CIP

Contributing Authors

Second Edition
David A. Scalzitti, PT, OCS
Instructor
University of Illinois at Chicago

First Edition
Thomas P. Mayhew, PhD, PT
Associate Professor
Medical College of Virginia

Dedication

A 10-year labor of love necessitates certain obsessive-compulsive behaviors, which, in our case, were directed toward the birth and nurturing of this book. As a result, we often ignored the callings of those who still, remarkably, love us to this day. For all the late dinners, broken promises, and unannounced sojourns, we are indebted to the unfaltering support and encouragement of our families. In the warmth of their caring about our obsession we found strength and sustenance.

We dedicate this book to our supportive wives: Marilyn Rothstein, Caroline Roy, and Lois Wolf; and to our children: Katherine and Jessica Rothstein; Lindsay and Renee Roy; and Josh and Adam Wolf. We pray that they will take as much pride in their husbands and fathers as we take in them and in this book, our newest baby.

Preface to the Second Edition

Completion of the first edition of this book required a remarkable team effort, and at times we wondered whether we would ever finish. With the help of our friends and the support of our families we managed to get the job done. Since the book first appeared there has never been a moment of regret. The reception of the first edition of *The Rehabilitation Specialist's Handbook* exceeded our expectations. Clinicians and students in many disciplines would often refer to us as "those guys who wrote the book that made our lives easier," and from our standpoint that was a very meaningful compliment. With such accolades, why even consider a second edition? After all, why mess with a good thing? We reflected on the labor needed to produce the more than 1,000 pages of the first edition, and we couldn't quite erase the memories of the all-night writing sessions, the hours checking details, and the enormous piles of manuscripts and proofs.

But times do change and, with them, the need for different, yet relevant, information. A new edition had to include materials that could assist practitioners to function in an outcomes-focused world in which pressures to be productive have become greater than ever. We had also promised our readers that we would take their needs and suggestions to heart if the time for a second edition were to arrive. With the assistance of our publisher, Jean-François Vilain, we conducted surveys to find out what people wanted added. In addition, we consulted with experts and reviewed the literature. Thanks to the remarkable persistence of Jean-François, and the promised tolerance of our families, we undertook the task of creating a second edition.

Initially we faced a serious obstacle. The first edition ended up being bigger than we had expected. How could we add material to the book and maintain its portability? After all, we didn't want to be responsible for ripping lab coat pickets throughout the world! Thanks to the folks at F. A. Davis, and particulary Director of Production Herb Powell, we came up with a solution. By changing the page size, we were able to enhance the portability of the book and add material primarily by reducing wasted space. As a result, the second edition is only several hundred pages longer than the first, but it contains at least one-third more material. Consequently, the second edition is virtually a new book. With new sections on the Americans with Disabilities Act, geriatrics, outcome measures, and pharmacology, the scope of the book has been expanded. Existing chapters have all been extensively revised, and once again as we write this preface we look back on the experience with more than a sigh of relief. We also want to thank David Scalzitti of the University of Illinois at Chicago, who joined our team as contributing author. His persistence and competence made completion of this second edition possible.

We offer the following suggestions to readers. We have color-coded tabs for each section and now begin each section with a brief guide about its contents. We hope this approach will assist readers in finding materials quickly, and we suggest readers use these same pages to write their own notes about where they can find material they need quickly.

We also want readers to understand the system we used to identify materials. Following sections you will often see one or more sources listed under the heading "For More Information." We spent considerable time choosing these listings. They are not necessarily the reference for the material we presented, but rather they are books and articles that we feel the reader can use to learn more about a topic than we have supplied in this book. Materials reproduced from other sources are noted with the word "From." Materials taken from a source and modified are denoted by "Based On."

We hope readers will find the book useful and will keep us informed about what they like and don't like. Although all three of us have busy careers and have authored other books, articles, and other types of materials, this handbook is very special. The feedback we have received has meant a lot to us. There is, however, an additional reward. We know firsthand about the wonderful things that our readers do for their clients and patients. If this book can make those efforts easier or more effective, we have accomplished our goal.

Jules M. Rothstein
Serge H. Roy
Steven L. Wolf

Preface to the First Edition

Most people sympathize with the plight of the female elephant who carries her young for a 1-year gestational period. We hope that they will be similarly sympathetic to the authors of this volume. For some of us, this book has been gestating for considerably more than a decade. This volume was conceived by two of us (JMR and SHR) shortly after we graduated from Physical Therapy School. We realized that there had to be a better way to carry around useful information than on an evergrowing collection of index cards. In our first year out of school we actually began to write some sample pages, some of which have even found their way into this final version. Professional and family obligations, however, soon made completion of the book impossible.

The manuscript pages lay on our shelves yellowing and collecting dust until the project was resurrected in early 1987. The third member of our writing team (SLW) heard of the idea and quickly joined our effort. He helped reshape our original outline and became a motivating force in bringing our idea into reality. The project then proceeded because of our collective belief that this book is needed. And it proceeded because of the extraordinary support of our publisher, F. A. Davis, and especially the tireless efforts of the unrelenting, brow-beating Allied Health Editor, and our friend, Jean-François Vilain. During later stages of development, the survival of the book was assured because of the nurturing of F. A. Davis's ever-patient production manager, Herb Powell.

Now that we have told you how this book came to be, we need to explain what this book is all about. The information needed by rehabilitation professionals is extraordinary. The diversity of information defies anyone's memory. Certainly chest physical therapists should know the positions for postural drainage, but if these techniques are hardly used, they may easily be forgotten. Similarly, someone who conducts electrodiagnostic testing should know normal and abnormal conduction values, but many of us do not routinely conduct such tests. Our understanding of such a report would be essentially impossible unless these values are known. This book is designed to provide the information clinicians need.

We have collected information and organized it so that the busy clinician has a quick source of information. The design of the book allows clinicians to carry the book with them so that it is always available. For example, we can imagine portability being particularly useful when someone needs to know how to communicate with a Spanish-speaking patient. Because clinicians can carry the book with them, all that is needed is to look up the table listing translations.

We have attempted to do more than just collect information and reprint it. We organized material into tables and figures to facilitate clinical practice. For example, by looking up the name of a muscle in the alphabetized listing you can read about the function of the muscle, the origin and insertion, and the innervation (both the nerve and the root). Or, if you want to know what muscles externally rotate the humerus you can look at the table that lists muscles by function and see in that same table the innervation (both the nerve and the root).

This book is not meant to replace reference books. We provide information that clinicians need in a succinct form. Because we recognize that clinicians may need additional information, we have listed references at the end of each section. These references are not necessarily the sources we have used for our material. The references are there because we believe they are useful resources that can be used to obtain more information. Because we wanted to guide readers to useful sources and not inundate them, we have kept the reference lists very small.

We have attempted to cover many areas in this book. There are some things that we have not attempted. We have walked a fine line in judging what to include. This is a quick reference volume, a compendium of useful and frequently used information. We have tried to present this information clearly and to present what readers will find useful, not just what we believe in or endorse. Realizing that we could not simply be passive conduits, we made some decisions. We have omitted treatment protocols and evaluation procedures that have yet to be validated. Whenever possible we make clear that we are conveying ideas from other sources, but we know that in choosing whose words we repeated we made decisions that we hope are good and responsible.

Only the reader can judge whether we have made clinical practice easier. We hope that we have. We also hope that by providing a source of information we have made it easier for clinicians to deliver a higher level of care. Every imaginable effort has been made to check the accuracy of our information and to organize it for efficient use. We hope we have kept errors to a minimum and have anticipated all the needs of clinicians. If your needs are not met, or if you find errors, please let us know. The content of future editions will be dictated by the responses and needs of our readers.

Jules M. Rothstein
Serge H. Roy
Steven L. Wolf

Contributors to the Second Edition

Many people assisted us in preparing this second edition. We will probably fail to recognize all of those who assisted us, and we want to apologize in advance for those omissions, but as you will note there were many people involved in the process and the second edition has been improved greatly because of their contributions.

The cardiopulmonary sections were revised thanks to the efforts of Cynthia Janulaitis, PT, of the University of Illinois Hospital, and we are grateful for all of her efforts. In addition, Mary Keehn, PT, of the University of Illinois Hospital and the entire physical therapy staff provided critical feedback as did Timothy J. Caruso, MBA, MS, PT, of Shriners Hospital, Chicago, Illinois. Thubi Kolobe, PhD, PT, and Suzann Campbell, PhD, PT, FAPTA, of the University of Illinois at Chicago; Susan Harris, PhD, PT, FAPTA, of the University of British Columbia; and Irene McEwen, PhD, PT, PCS, of the University of Oklahoma all provided important consultation in the area of pediatrics. Dan Riddle, PhD, PT, of the Medical College of Virginia helped in the area of orthopedics, while Alan Jette, PhD, PT, of Sargent College, Boston University, gave us feedback on the outcome section. Rebecca Craik, PhD, PT, FAPTA, of Beaver College assisted with the gait materials. In addition, many students at the University of Illinois read galleys and offered suggestions. Special thanks are due to Jacalyn Hennessey, Mary Johnson, Patrick Dziedzic, and Arthur Lubinski of the University of Illinois at Chicago's Physical Therapy Class of 1997 as well as to David Caby. Allane Storto and Angela Young of UIC facilitated our efforts by coordinating the movement of paperwork to and from the University.

Lynn Snyder-Mackler, ScD, PT, at the University of Delaware provided considerable assistance with our revisions in the area of modalities. Reginald L. Richard MS, PT, of Miami Valley Hospital, Dayton, Ohio, and Marlys J. Staley, MS, PT, of Shriners Burn Institute, Cincinnati, Ohio, provided input for the burn section, and we want to thank them. Michael Mueller, PhD, PT, of Washington University shared his expertise on amputations, prosthetics, and orthotics with us and also advised us on the gait section. Aimee B. Klein, MS, PT, OCS, of Massachusetts General Hopsital's Institute of Health Professions helped on the massage and soft-tissue techniques section. Scott Mackler, MD, reviewed and made suggestions on the general medical section, and we appreciate his assistance.

We wish to also thank Tom Pianta, PT, and Amelia Haselton, PT, at the Emory University Hospital, for their assistance with the material on organ transplants. The time provided by Lois Wolf, PT, to gather information about CNS tumor classification is also very much appreciated. We also appreciate Lue Dunagan, MSW; Diane Kirkpatrick, PT; Judy Hamby, OT; and Jill Tabone, OT, of the Emory University Center for Rehabilitation Medicine, who painstakingly assisted in refining terms and expressions commonly used in communicating with patients. Tony Stringer, PhD, Department of Rehabilitation Medicine, Emory University, was instrumental in restructuring our presentation of neuropsychological tests. We are indebted to Hattie Orel for assistance with the German phrases, Florence Blanc and Tony Roy for help with the French translations, and Giusi Bonato and Rosa L. Lo Conte for their efforts with the Italian phrases.

Contributors to the First Edition

Three authors are listed for this book, but in reality many people contributed. Nora Donohue, PT, developed the materials in the areas of cardiology and pulmonary care. In addition, she served as a consultant for many other areas. Dan L. Riddle, PT, developed some of the materials in orthopedics and consulted for other sections. Terrence Karselis, MT (ASCP) provided the section on instrumentation. Joan Edelstein, PT, developed most of the materials in the sections on prosthetics and orthotics. Thomas P. Mayhew, OT, PT, had the unenviable task of reading and commenting on the entire manuscript. He also contributed to various sections, particularly those containing anatomical and neuroanatomical information. The extraordinary efforts of these people made this book possible.

Contents

$\circledS \circledE \circledC \circledT \circledI \circledO \circledN$ ❶

Americans with Disabilities Act and Accessibility Issues (Including Wheelchair Information)

AMERICANS WITH DISABILITIES ACT (ADA)*

General Description: The ADA (Public Law 101-336) is a federal anti-discrimination statute designed to prohibit discrimination on the basis of disability. The ADA covers three primary areas: employment, public services, and public accommodations (Title I–III). There are two additional areas: one covers telecommunications, and the other contains miscellaneous provisions (Title IV–V).

Title I: Equal Employment Opportunity for Individuals with Disabilities

This part of the ADA seeks to ensure access to equal employment opportunities based on merit but does not guarantee equal results, establish quotas, or require preferences favoring individuals with disabilities over those without disabilities. When an individual's disability creates a barrier to employment opportunities, the ADA requires employers to consider whether reasonable accommodation could remove the barrier. Such accommodations usually take the form of adjustments to the way a job is customarily performed, or to the work environment itself. No specific form of accommodation is guaranteed for all individuals with a particular disability. Instead, an accommodation must be tailored on a case-by-case approach to match the needs of the disabled individual with the needs of the job's essential functions. The ADA establishes definitions to guide employers in considering how to take into account the disabling condition involved.

Title II: Nondiscrimination on the Basis of Disability in State and Local Government Services

This part of the ADA covers "public entities" which include any state or local government and any governmental departments, agencies or other instrumentalities (regardless of whether they receive federal funds). The regulations prohibit these public entities from refusing to allow a person with a disability to participate in a service, program, or activity simply because that person is disabled.

This title has prohibitions against discrimination in public transportation, specifying for example, that new buses, rapid transit or light rail vehicles purchased or leased by public agencies must be "readily accessible to and usable by the disabled." Special "paratransit services," such as door-to-door van service, must also be made available by public transportation agencies offering regularly scheduled bus or rail service. Title II also applies to any new facility built for transportation systems. Provisions governing Amtrak and intercity commuter rail lines differ from subway and rapid rail system requirements.

---

*From Americans with Disabilities Act Handbook. U.S. Equal Employment Opportunity Commission and the U.S. Department of Justice, Washington, DC, 1992.

Title III: Public Accommodations and Services Operated by Private Entities

This part of the ADA prohibits discrimination against individuals with disabilities in the "full and equal" enjoyment of the goods, services, facilities, privileges, advantages or accommodations of any place of public accommodation. Public accommodations are virtually all facilities open to the public, including but not limited to restaurants, hotels, stores, theaters, parks, etc. Private clubs and religious organizations are exempt. Public accommodations and services must be offered "in the most integrated setting appropriate to the needs of the individual." Removal of architectural barriers are required if it is "readily achievable" and would not impose undue burden. The "readily achievable" standard is a new and lesser standard than the "reasonable accommodation" standard which applies to employers. Auxiliary aids or services are also required by establishments providing that they do not impose an "undue burden." Before Title III there had been no federal laws to prevent private enterprises from discriminating against disabled individuals.

Title IV: Telecommunications

This part of the ADA requires that common carriers provide 24 hours a day interstate and intrastate telecommunications relay services to individuals who are hearing-impaired or speech-impaired. These relay services are conducted by a central bank of operators who make it possible for users of Telecommunications Device for the Deaf (TDD) or other non-voice terminal devices to communicate with non-users. Users will pay rates no greater than those paid for functionally equivalent voice communication services.

Title V: Miscellaneous Provisions

This part of the ADA includes numerous "cleanup" provisions not found in the other titles. Authorizes attorney fees in court or agency actions if the plaintiff prevails. It includes a provision authorizing alternative methods of resolving disputes and prohibits forms of coercion and provides a plan of technical assistance in implementing the Act. Addresses access to wilderness areas. States that being a transvestite is not a "disability" nor is being homosexual or bisexual. Also specifically precluded from being a disability are: forms of sexual deviance, compulsive gambling, kleptomania, pyromania or conditions resulting from the illegal use of drugs, including psychoactive drugs.

OVERVIEW OF THE AMERICANS WITH DISABILITIES ACT EFFECTIVE DATES, REGULATIONS, AND ENFORCEMENT POLICIES

	Effective Date	Overview of Regulations	Enforcement
Title I: Employment	7/26/91 for employers with 25 or more employees; 7/26/94 for employers with 15 or more employees	Applies to private employers, state and local governments, employment agencies, labor organizations, and labor-management committees. Prohibits employers from discriminating against "a qualified individual with a disability" in regards to job applications, hiring, advancements, discharge, or privilege of employment. Employers are required to make "reasonable accommodations" to the known physical or mental limitation of an otherwise qualified individual with a disability, unless to do so would impose an "undue hardship" (significant difficulty or expense).	Procedures and remedies identical to those under Title VII of the Civil Rights Act of 1964 (e.g., EEOC enforcement, private right of action, and relief including hiring, promotion, reinstatement, and back pay).

Title II: Public Services	In general, 1/26/92. For public transportation (excluding Amtrak and commuter rail) by 8/26/90 for new vehicles; one car per train by 7/26/95; new stations built after 1/26/92 must comply; retrofitting of stations by 7/26/93, with some exceptions to 7/26/2020. For Amtrak, same one-car-per-train rule and new stations as above. Existing stations retrofitted by 7/26/2010.	Prohibits discrimination against or excluding qualified individuals with disabilities from participating in services, programs, or activities of a "public entity." Public entities include any state or local government and any governmental department, agency, special purpose district or instrumentality and the National Railroad Passenger Corporation, and any commuter authority.	Remedies identical to those under the Rehabilitation Act of 1973, Section 505, which are private right of action, injunctive relief, and some damages.
Title III: Public Accommodations and Services Operated by Private Entities	Businesses and service providers: 1/26/92, generally; no lawsuit could be filed before 7/26/92 against businesses with 25 or fewer employees and	Prohibits discrimination against individuals with disabilities in full and equal enjoyment of the goods, services, facilities, privileges, advantages, or accommodations of any place of public accommodation	For individuals, remedies are identical to those in the Title II of the Civil Rights Act of 1964 (e.g., private right of action, injunctive relief). For *Continued on following page*

Continued on following page

OVERVIEW OF THE AMERICANS WITH DISABILITIES ACT
EFFECTIVE DATES, REGULATIONS, AND ENFORCEMENT POLICIES (Continued)

	Effective Date	Overview of Regulations	Enforcement
Title III: Public Accommodations and Services Operated by Private Entities	revenues of $1 million or less; or before 1/26/93, for businesses with 10 or fewer employees and revenues of $500,000 or less. New construction/alteration to public accommodations and commercial facilities: 1/26/92 for alterations; 1/26/93 for new construction.	requiring that these be offered "in the most integrated setting appropriate to the needs of the individual," except when the individual poses a direct threat to the health or safety of others.	Attorney General enforcement in pattern or practice cases or cases of general importance, with civil penalties and compensatory damages.
Title IV: Telecommunications	7/26/93, telecommunications relay services to operate 24 hours a day.	Requires that telephone companies provide "telecommunications relay services" through their service areas. Such services enable hearing-impaired individuals to communicate with hearing individuals through the use of Telecommunications Devices for the Deaf (TDD) or other nonvoice	Private right of action and FCC enforcement.

terminal devices by providing operators that relay messages between the TDD user and nonusers. Users will pay rates no greater than those paid for functionally equivalent voice communication services.

Title V: Miscellaneous Provisions

Authorizes attorney fees in court or agency actions if the plaintiff prevails. Provides a provision authorizing alternative methods of resolving disputes. Prohibits forms of coercion and provides a plan of technical assistance in implementing the Act. Addresses access to wilderness areas. States that being a transvestite is not a "disability" nor is being homosexual or bisexual. Also specifically precluded from being a disability are: forms of sexual

Continued on following page

	Effective Date	Overview of Regulations	Enforcement
Title V: Miscellaneous Provisions (Continued)		deviance, compulsive gambling, kleptomania, pyromania or conditions resulting from the illegal use of drugs, including psychoactive drugs.	

EEOC = Equal Employment Opportunity Commission; FCC = Federal Communications Commission.
From Americans with Disabilities Act Handbook. U.S. Equal Employment Opportunity Commission and the U.S. Department of Justice. Washington, DC, 1992.

8

TERMS USED TO DESCRIBE AMERICANS WITH DISABILITIES ACT ACCESSIBILITY REQUIREMENTS

General Terminology

comply with: Meet one or more specifications of these guidelines.

if, if . . . then: Denotes a specification that applies only when the conditions described are present.

may: Denotes an option or alternative.

shall: Denotes a mandatory specification or requirement.

should: Denotes an advisory specification or recommendation.

Definitions

access aisle: An accessible pedestrian space between elements, such as parking spaces, seating, and desks, that provides clearances appropriate for use of the elements.

accessible: A term that describes a site, building, facility, or portion thereof that complies with these guidelines.

accessible elements: An element specified by these guidelines (for example, telephone, controls, and the like).

accessible route: A continuous unobstructed path connecting all accessible elements and spaces of a building or facility. Interior accessible routes may include corridors, floors, ramps, elevators, lifts, and clear floor space at fixtures. Exterior accessible routes may include parking access aisles, curb ramps, crosswalks at vehicular ways, walks, ramps, and lifts.

accessible space: Space that complies with these guidelines.

adaptability: The ability of certain building spaces and elements, such as kitchen counters, sinks, and grab bars, to be added or altered so as to accommodate the needs of individuals with or without disabilities or to accommodate the needs of persons with different types or degrees of disability.

addition: An expansion, extension, or increase in the gross floor area of a building or facility.

administrative authority: A governmental agency that adopts or enforces regulations and guidelines for the design, construction, or alteration of buildings and facilities.

alteration: An alteration is a change to a building or facility made by, on behalf of, or for the use of a public accommodation or commercial facility that affects or could affect the usability of the building or facility or part thereof. Alterations include, but are not limited to, remodeling, renovation, rehabilitation, reconstruction, historic restoration, changes or rearrangement of the structural parts or elements, and changes or rearrangement in the plan configuration of walls and full-height partitions. Normal maintenance, reroofing, painting or wallpapering, or changes to mechanical and electrical systems are not alterations unless they affect the usability of the building or facility.

Continued on following page

area of rescue assistance: An area, which has direct access to an exit, where people who are unable to use stairs may remain temporarily in safety to await further instructions or assistance during emergency evacuation.

assembly area: A room or space accommodating a group of individuals for recreational, educational, political, social, or amusement purposes, or for the consumption of food and drink.

automatic door: A door equipped with a power-operated mechanism and controls that open and close the door automatically upon receipt of a momentary actuating signal. The switch that begins the automatic cycle may be a photoelectric device, floor mat, or manual switch (see *power-assisted door*).

building: Any structure used and intended for supporting or sheltering any use or occupancy.

circulation path: An exterior or interior way of passage from one place to another for pedestrians, including, but not limited to, walks, hallways, courtyards, stairways, and stair landings.

clear: Unobstructed.

clear floor space: The minimum unobstructed floor or ground space required to accommodate a single, stationary wheelchair and occupant.

closed-circuit telephone: A telephone with dedicated line(s) such as a house phone, courtesy phone, or phone that must be used to gain entrance to a facility.

common use: A term that refers to those interior and exterior rooms, spaces, or elements that are made available for the use of a restricted group of people (for example, occupants of a homeless shelter, the occupants of an office building, or the guests of such occupants).

cross slope: The slope that is perpendicular to the direction of travel (see *running slope*).

curb ramp: A short ramp cutting through a curb or built up to it.

detectable warning: A standardized surface feature built in or applied to walking surfaces or other elements to warn visually impaired people of hazards on a circulation path.

dwelling unit: A single unit which provides a kitchen or food preparation area, in addition to rooms and spaces for living, bathing, sleeping, and the like. Dwelling units include a single-family home or a townhouse used as a transient group home; an apartment building used as a shelter; guestrooms in a hotel that provide sleeping accommodations and food preparation areas; and other similar facilities used on a transient basis. For purposes of these guidelines, use of the term *dwelling unit* does not imply the unit is used as a residence.

egress, means of: A continuous and unobstructed way of exit travel from any point in a building or facility to a public way. A means of egress comprises vertical and horizontal travel and may include intervening room spaces, doorways, hallways, corridors, passageways, balconies, ramps, stairs, enclosures, lobbies, horizontal exits, courts, and yards. An accessible means of egress is one that complies with these guidelines and does not include stairs, steps, or escalators. Areas of rescue assistance or evacuation elevators may be included as part of accessible means of egress.

element: An architectural or mechanical component of a building, facility, space, or site (e.g., telephone, curb ramp, door, drinking fountain, seating, or water closet).

entrance: Any access point to a building or portion of a building or facility used for the purpose of entering. An entrance includes the approach walk, the vertical access leading to the entrance platform, the entrance platform itself, vestibules if provided, the entry door(s) or gate(s), and the hardware of the entry door(s) or gate(s).

facility: All or any portion of buildings, structures, site improvements, complexes, equipment, roads, walks, passageways, parking lots, or other real or personal property located on a site.

ground floor: Any occupiable floor less than one story above or below grade with direct access to grade. A building or facility always has at least one ground floor and may have more than one ground floor, as where a split level entrance has been provided or where a building is built into a hillside.

marked crossing: A crosswalk or other identified path intended for pedestrian use in crossing a vehicular way.

mezzanine or mezzanine floor: That portion of a story which is an intermediate floor level placed within the story and having occupiable space above and below its floor.

multifamily dwelling: Any building containing more than two dwelling units.

occupiable: A room or enclosed space designed for human occupancy in which individuals congregate for amusement, educational or similar purposes, or in which occupants are engaged at labor, and which is equipped with means of egress, light, and ventilation.

operable part: A part of a piece of equipment or appliance used to insert or withdraw objects, or to activate, deactivate, or adjust the equipment or appliance (e.g., coin slot, pushbutton, handle).

power-assisted door: A door used for human passage with a mechanism that helps to open the door, or relieves the opening resistance of a door, on the activation of a switch or a continued force applied to the door itself.

public use: Describes interior or exterior rooms or spaces that are made available to the general public. Public use may be provided at a building or facility that is privately or publicly owned.

ramp: A walking surface which has a running slope greater than 1:20.

running slope: The slope that is parallel to the direction of travel (see *cross slope*).

service entrance: An entrance intended primarily for delivery of goods or services.

signage: Displayed verbal, symbolic, tactile, and pictorial information.
Continued on following page

site: A parcel of land bounded by a property line or a designated portion of a public right-of-way.

site improvement: Landscaping, paving for pedestrian and vehicular ways, outdoor lighting, recreational facilities, and the like, added to a site.

sleeping accommodations: Rooms in which people sleep; for example, dormitory and hotel or motel guest rooms or suites.

space: A definable area (e.g., room, toilet room, hall, assembly area, entrance, storage room, alcove, courtyard, or lobby).

story: That portion of a building included between the upper surface of a floor and upper surface of a floor or roof next above. If such portion of a building does not include occupiable space, it is not considered a story for purposes of these guidelines. There may be more than one floor level within a story as in the case of a mezzanine or mezzanines.

structural frame: The structural frame shall be considered to be the columns and the girders, beams, trusses, and spandrels having direct connections to the columns and all other members that are essential to the stability of the building as a whole.

tactile: A term that describes an object that can be perceived using the sense of touch.

test telephone: Machinery or equipment that employs interactive graphic (i.e., typed) communications through the transmission of coded signals across the standard telephone network. Text telephones can include, for example, devices known as TDDs or computers.

transient lodging: A building, facility, or portion thereof, excluding inpatient medical care facilities, that contains one or more dwelling units or sleeping accommodations. Transient lodging may include, but is not limited to, resorts, group homes, hotels, motels, and dormitories.

vehicular way: A route intended for vehicular traffic, such as a street, driveway, or parking lot.

walk: An exterior pathway with a prepared surface intended for pedestrian use, including general pedestrian areas such as plazas and courts.

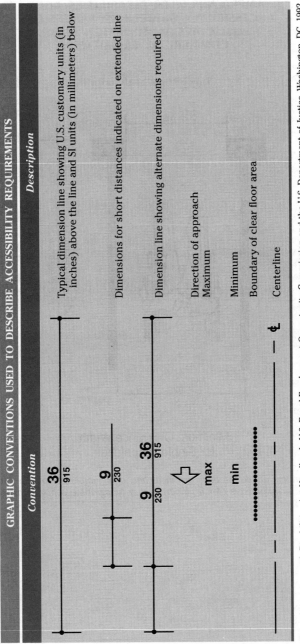

GRAPHIC CONVENTIONS USED TO DESCRIBE ACCESSIBILITY REQUIREMENTS

Convention	Description
36 / 915	Typical dimension line showing U.S. customary units (in inches) above the line and SI units (in millimeters) below
9 / 230	Dimensions for short distances indicated on extended line
9 36 / 230 915	Dimension line showing alternate dimensions required
⇩ max	Direction of approach Maximum
min	Minimum
••••••••••	Boundary of clear floor area
— ₵ —	Centerline

From Americans with Disabilities Act Handbook. U.S. Equal Employment Opportunity Commission and the U.S. Department of Justice. Washington, DC, 1992.

13

Space for Wheelchairs

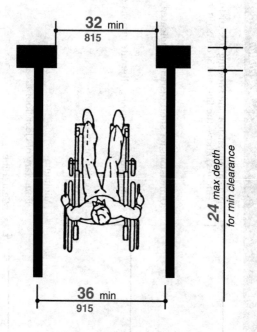

Minimum Clearance Width
for Single Wheelchair

Numbers above the lines are in inches, and numbers below the lines are in millimeters (for a guide to other typographic conventions, see p 13).

Space for Two Wheelchairs

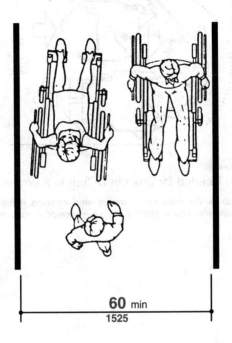

60 min
1525

Minimum Clearance Width
for Two Wheelchairs

*Numbers above the lines are in inches, and numbers below the lines
are in millimeters (for a guide to other typographic conventions, see
p 13).*

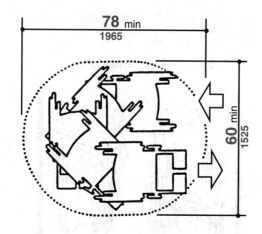

Space Needed for Smooth U-Turn in a Wheelchair

Numbers above the lines are in inches, and numbers below the lines are in millimeters (for a guide to other typographic conventions, see p 13).

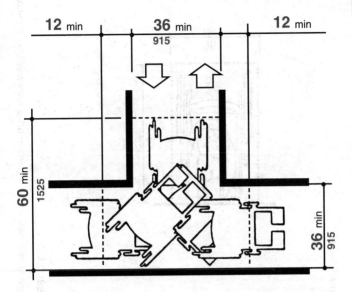

T-Shaped Space for 180° Turns

Numbers above the lines are in inches, and numbers below the lines are in millimeters (for a guide to other typographic conventions, see p 13).

Forward Reach

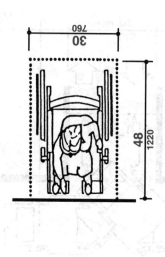

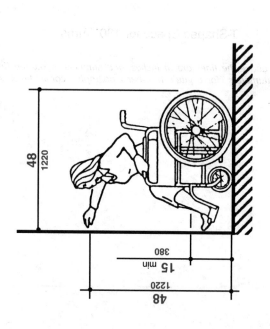

High Forward Reach Limit

Numbers above the lines are in inches, and numbers below the lines are in millimeters (for a guide to other typographic conventions, see p 13).

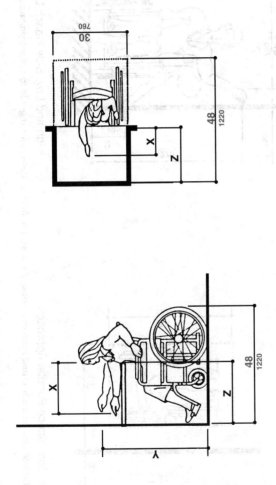

NOTE: x shall be ≤ 25 in (635); z shall be ≥ x. When x < 20 in (510 mm), then y shall be 48 in (1220 mm) maximum. When x is 20 to 25 in (510 to 635 mm), then y shall be 44 in (1120 mm) maximum.

Maximum Forward Reach over an Obstruction

Side Reach

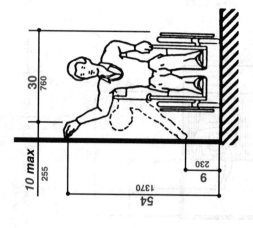

High and Low Side Reach Limits

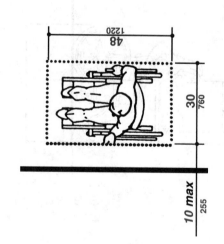

Clear Floor Space Parallel Approach

Numbers above the lines are in inches, and numbers below the lines are in millimeters (for a guide to other typographic conventions, see p 13).

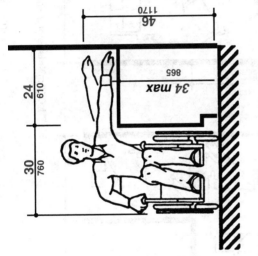

Maximum Side Reach over an Obstruction

Numbers above the lines are in inches, and numbers below the lines are in millimeters (for a guide to other typographic conventions, see p 13).

21

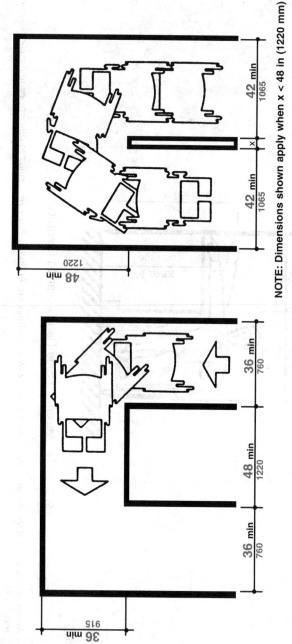

Turning Space for Wheelchairs

Turns Around an Obstruction

NOTE: Dimensions shown apply when x < 48 in (1220 mm)

42 min
1065

x

42 min
1065

48 min
1220

90° Turn

36 min
760

48 min
1220

36 min
760

36 min
915

22

Numbers above the lines are in inches, and numbers below the lines are in millimeters (for a guide to other typographic conventions, see p 13).

1

Changes in Levels

Changes in levels along an accessible route must be no greater than ½ in (13 mm). Changes greater than that level require a curb, ramp, elevator, or platform, as appropriate.

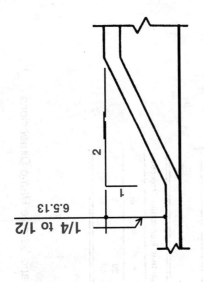

Changes in Level

Numbers above the lines are in inches, and numbers below the lines are in millimeters (for a guide to other typographic conventions, see p 13). Figure of changes in level continued on page 24.

Changes in Levels (Continued)

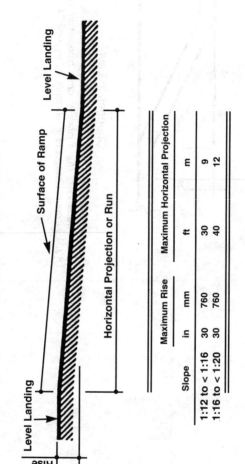

Slope	Maximum Rise		Maximum Horizontal Projection	
	in	mm	ft	m
1:12 to < 1:16	30	760	30	9
1:16 to < 1:20	30	760	40	12

Components of a Single Ramp Run and Sample Ramp Dimensions

Showers

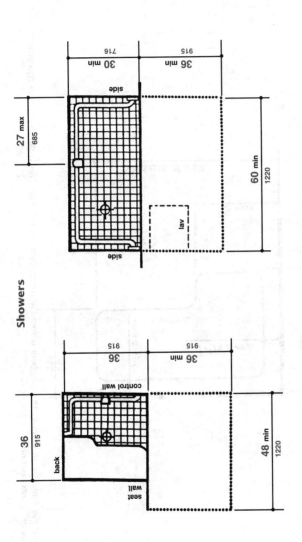

36 in by 36 in
(915 mm by 915 mm) Stall

30 in by 30 in
(760 mm by 1525 mm) Stall

Numbers above the lines are in inches, and numbers below the lines are in millimeters (for a guide to other typographic conventions, see p 13). Shower figures continued on pages 26–28.

25

Shower Stall

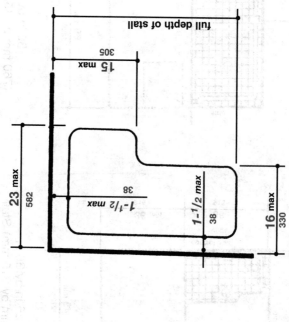

Numbers above the lines are in inches, and numbers below the lines are in millimeters (for a guide to other typographic conventions, see p 13). Shower figures continued on pages 27–28

Shower Seat Design

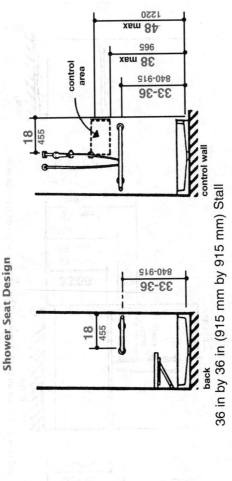

36 in by 36 in (915 mm by 915 mm) Stall

control area

control wall

back

18
455

33-36
840-915

38 max
965

48 max
1220

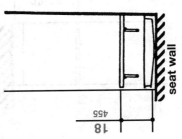

seat wall

18
455

Grab Bars at Shower Stalls

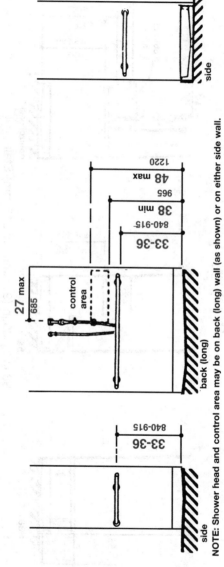

27 max / 685

control area

33-36 / 840-915

side

33-36 / 840-915
48 max / 1220
38 min / 965
back (long)

NOTE: Shower head and control area may be on back (long) wall (as shown) or on either side wall.

30 in by 60 in (760 mm by 1525 mm) Stall

28

Storage Shelves and Closets

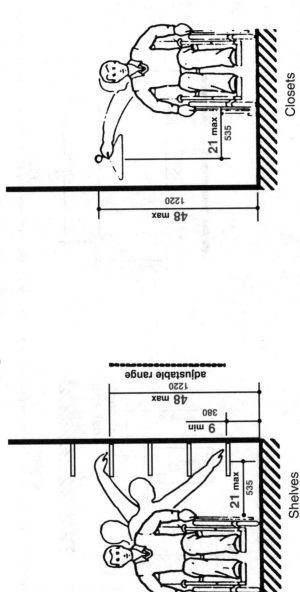

Shelves

Closets

Numbers above the lines are in inches, and numbers below the lines are in millimeters (for a guide to other typographic conventions, see p 13).

29

Telephones

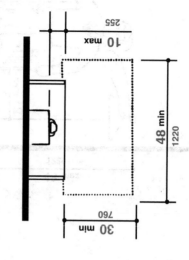

10 max / 255

48 min / 1220

30 min / 760

Plan

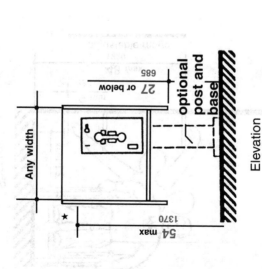

Any width

★

54 max / 1370

27 or below / 685

optional post and base

Elevation

Numbers above the lines are in inches, and numbers below the lines are in millimeters (for a guide to other typographic conventions, see p 13).

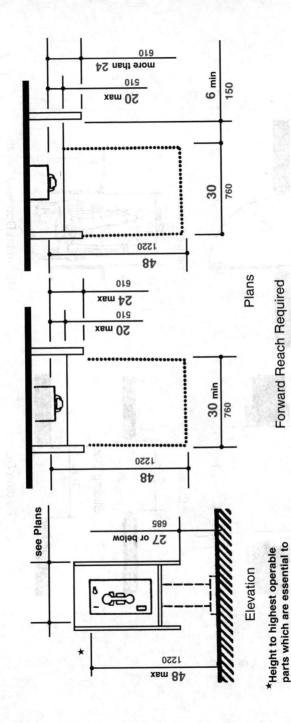

Forward Reach Required

Plans

510
20 max

610
24 max

510
20 max

610
more than 24

6 min
150

30
760

1220
48

30 min
760

1220
48

see Plans

685
27 or below

1220
48 max

Elevation

*Height to highest operable parts which are essential to basic operation of telephone

31

Doorways

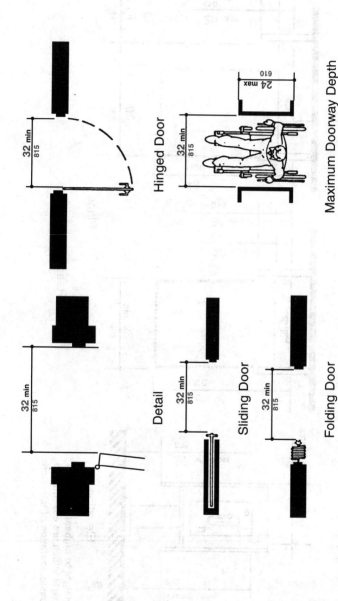

Detail

Hinged Door

Sliding Door

Folding Door

Maximum Doorway Depth

Numbers above the lines are in inches, and numbers below the lines are in millimeters (for a guide to other typographic conventions, see p 13). Doorway figures continued on pages 33–36.

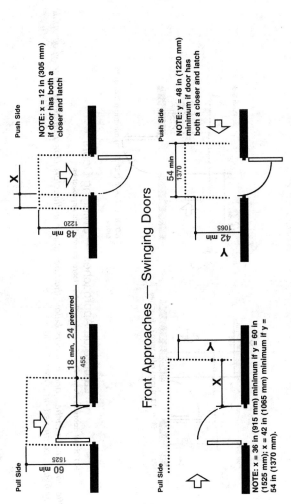

Push Side

NOTE: x = 12 in (305 mm) if door has both a closer and latch

X

48 min
1220

Pull Side

18 min, 24 preferred
455

60 min
1525

Front Approaches — Swinging Doors

Push Side

NOTE: y = 48 in (1220 mm) minimum if door has both a closer and latch

54 min
1370

42 min
1065

Y

Pull Side

Y

X

NOTE: x = 36 in (915 mm) minimum if y = 60 in (1525 mm); x = 42 in (1065 mm) minimum if y = 54 in (1370 mm).

Hinge Side Approaches — Swinging Doors

Numbers above the lines are in inches, and numbers below the lines are in millimeters (for a guide to other typographic conventions, see p 13). Doorway figures continued on pages 34–36.

34

Doorways (Continued)

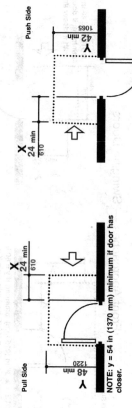

Pull Side

Y 48 min
1220

X 24 min
610

NOTE: y = 54 in (1370 mm) minimum if door has closer.

Push Side

Y 42 min
1065

X 24 min
610

NOTE: y = 48 in (1220 mm) minimum if door has closer.

Latch Side Approaches — Swinging Doors

NOTE: All doors in alcoves shall comply with the clearances for front approaches.

Numbers above the lines are in inches, and numbers below the lines are in millimeters (for a guide to other typographic conventions, see p 13). Doorway figures continued on pages 35–36.

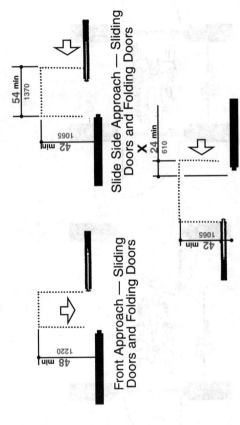

Front Approach — Sliding Doors and Folding Doors

48 min
1220

Slide Side Approach — Sliding Doors and Folding Doors

54 min
1370

42 min
1065

Latch Side Approach — Sliding Doors and Folding Doors

24 min
610

42 min
1065

X

NOTE: All doors in alcoves shall comply with the clearances for front approaches.

Numbers above the lines are in inches, and numbers below the lines are in millimeters (for a guide to other typographic conventions, see p 13). Doorway figures continued on pages 36.

Doorways (Continued)

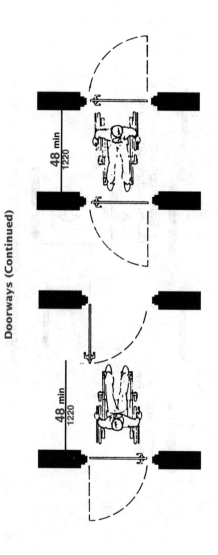

48 min
1220

48 min
1220

Drinking Fountains

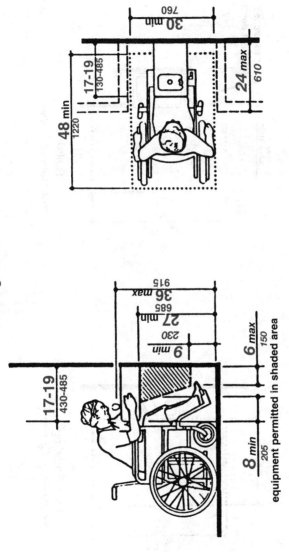

Spout Height and
Knee Clearance

Clear Floor Space

Numbers above the lines are in inches, and numbers below the lines are in millimeters (for a guide to other typographic conventions, see p 13). Figures of drinking fountains continued on page 38.

37

Drinking Fountains (Continued)

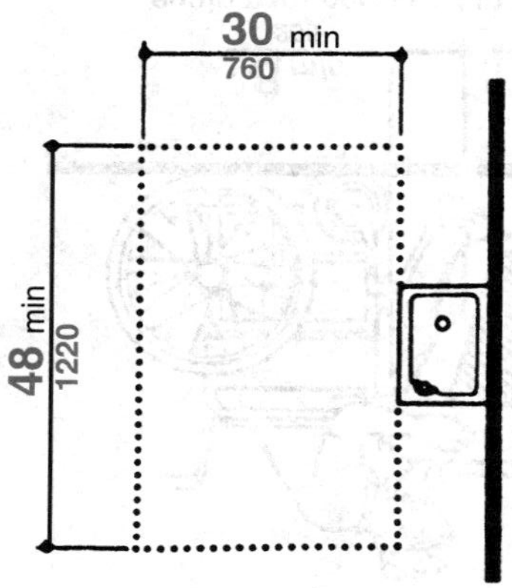

not to exceed fountain depth

30 min
760

48 min
1220

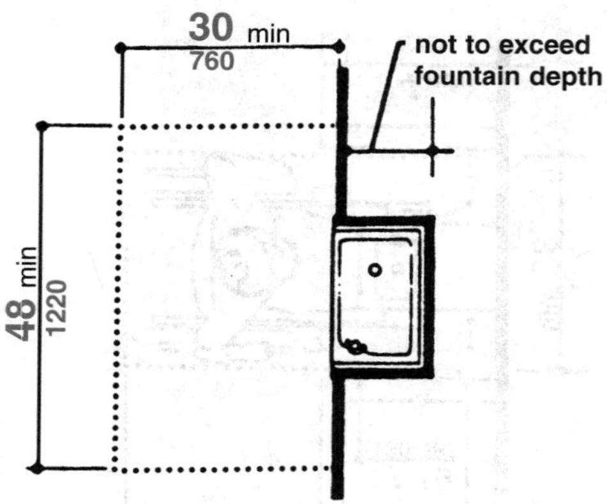

Built-In
Fountain or Cooler

30 min
760

48 min
1220

Free-Standing
Fountain or Cooler

Lavatories

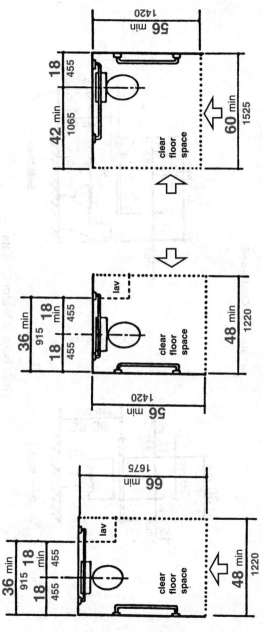

Numbers above the lines are in inches, and numbers below the lines are in millimeters (for a guide to other typographic conventions, see p 13). Figures of lavatories continued on page 40

39

Lavatories (Continued)

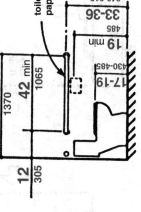

Grab Bars at Water Closets

Side Wall

toilet paper

54 min
1370

42 min
1065

12
305

19 min
485

33-36
840-915

17-19
430-485

Back Wall

36 min
915

36 min

12 min
305

12 min
305

33-36
840-915

40

Toilet Stalls

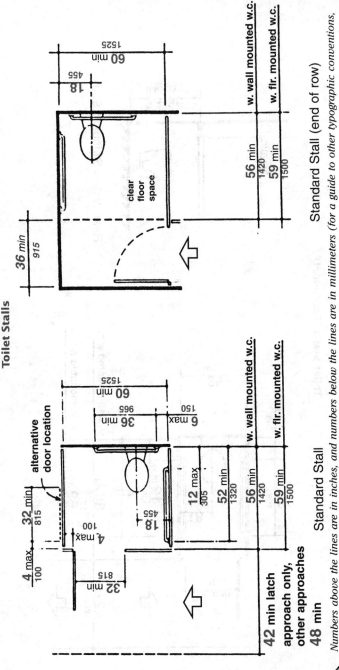

Standard Stall

Standard Stall (end of row)

42 min latch approach only, other approaches
48 min

Numbers above the lines are in inches, and numbers below the lines are in millimeters (for a guide to other typographic conventions, see p 13). Figures of toilet stalls continued on pages 42–43.

41

Toilet Stalls (Continued)

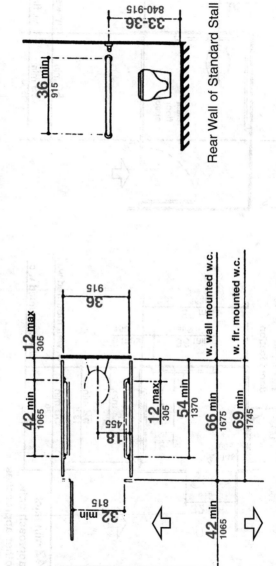

33-36
840-915

36 min
915

Rear Wall of Standard Stall

12 max
305

36
915

42 min
1065

12 max
305

54 min
1370

18
455

66 min
1675
w. wall mounted w.c.

69 min
1745
w. flr. mounted w.c.

32 min
815

42 min
1065

42

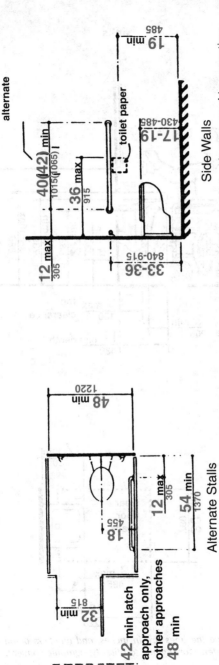

alternate

Side Walls

Alternate Stalls

Numbers above the lines are in inches, and numbers below the lines are in millimeters (for a guide to other typographic conventions, see p 13).

43

Sinks

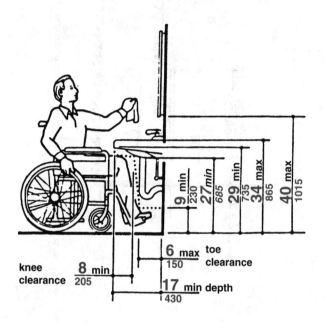

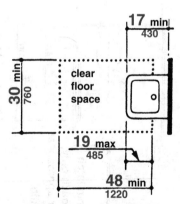

Numbers above the lines are in inches, and numbers below the lines are in millimeters (for a guide to other typographic conventions, see p 13).

Bathtubs

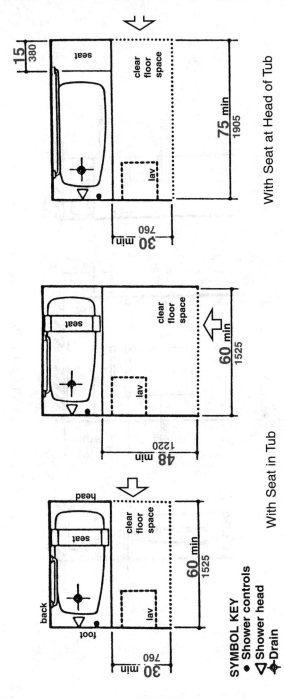

With Seat at Head of Tub

With Seat in Tub

15 / 380

75 min / 1905

seat

clear floor space

lav

30 min / 760

60 min / 1525

seat

clear floor space

lav

48 min / 1220

60 min / 1525

head

seat

back

foot

clear floor space

lav

30 min / 760

SYMBOL KEY
- ✛ Shower controls
- ▽ Shower head
- ⊕ Drain

Numbers above the lines are in inches, and numbers below the lines are in millimeters (for a guide to other typographic conventions, see p 13). Figures of bathtubs continued on pages 46–47.

Bathtubs (Continued)

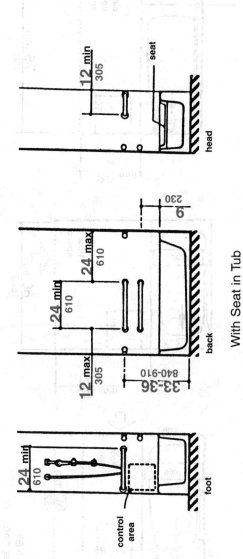

With Seat in Tub

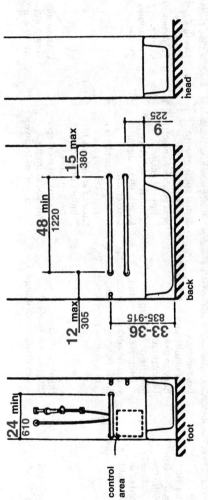

With Seat at Head of Tub

Grab Bars at Bathtubs

Numbers above the lines are in inches, and numbers below the lines are in millimeters (for a guide to other typographic conventions, see p 13).

ASSISTIVE LISTENING DEVICES

DESCRIPTIONS OF ASSISTIVE LISTENING DEVICES

System	Advantages	Disadvantages	Typical Applications
Induction Loop Transmitter: Transducer wired to induction loop around listening area. Receiver: Self-contained induction receiver or personal hearing aid with telecoil	Cost-effective. Low maintenance. Easy to use. Unobtrusive. May be possible to integrate into existing public address system. Some hearing aids can function as receivers.	Signal spills over to adjacent rooms. Susceptible to electrical interference. Limited portability. Inconsistent signal strength. Head position affects signal strength. Lack of standards for induction coil performance.	Meeting areas Theaters Churches and temples Conference rooms Classrooms TV viewing
FM Transmitter: Flashlight sized worn by speaker.	Highly portable. Different channels allow use by different groups	High cost of receivers. Equipment fragile. Equipment obtrusive.	Classrooms Tour groups Meeting areas

Receiver: With personal hearing aid via DAI or induction neck-loop and telecoil, or self-contained with earphone(s)	within the same room. High user mobility. Variable for large range of hearing losses.	High maintenance. Expensive to maintain. Custom fitting to individual user may be required.	Outdoor events One on one
Infrared Transmitter: Emitter in line of sight with receiver Receiver: Self-contained or with personal hearing aid via DAI or induction neck-loop and telecoil	Easy to use. Ensures privacy or confidentiality. Moderate cost. Can often be integrated into existing public address system.	Line of sight required between emitter and receiver. Ineffective outdoors. Limited portability. Requires installation.	Theaters Churches and temples Auditoriums Meetings requiring confidentiality TV viewing

DAI = Direct Audio Input.

From Rehab Brief, Vol. XII. no. 10. National Institute on Disability and Rehabilitation Research, Washington, DC, 1990.

REFERENCE GUIDE FOR U.S. GOVERNMENT AGENCIES PROVIDING ASSISTANCE WITH AMERICANS WITH DISABILITIES ACT

For Questions Pertaining to:	Consult These Government Agencies:
Employment (Title I)	Equal Employment Opportunity Commission (R,TA,E)
	President's Committee on Employment of People with Disabilities (TA)
	Small Business Administration (TA)
	National Institute on Disability and Rehabilitation Research (TA)
	Social Security Administration (P)
Public services (Title II)	Department of Justice (R,TA,E)
	Department of Transportation (R,TA,E
Public accommodations (Title III)	Department of Justice (R,TA,E)
	Department of Transportation (R,TA,E)
	Architectural and Transportation Barriers Compliance Board (G,TA)
Telecommunications (Title IV)	Federal Communications Commission (R,TA,E)
Rehabilitation and independent living services	Department of Education (P)
Accessibility	Architectural and Transportation Barriers Compliance Board (G,TA)
Tax law provisions	Department of Treasury (TA)

E = has enforcement authority, G = issue guidelines, P = administers programs relevant to successful implementation of the Act, R = issued regulations, TA = provides technical assistance on how to comply.

Addresses and Telephone Numbers for Government Agencies Dealing with ADA Issues

Architectural and Transportation Barriers Compliance Board
1331 F Street NW
Suite 1000
Washington, DC 20004-1111
(800) USA-ABLE
(800) USA-ABLE (TDD)

Department of Transportation
400 Seventh Street SW
Room 10424
Washington, DC 20590
(202) 366-9305
(202) 755-7687 (TDD)

Equal Employment Opportunity Commission
1801 L Street NW
Washington, DC 20507
(800) 669-EEOC (voice)
(800) 800-3302 (TDD)

Federal Communications Commission
1919 M Street NW
Washington, DC 20554
(800) 632-7260 (voice)
(800) 632-6999 (TDD)

Internal Revenue Service
U.S. Department of Treasury
1111 Constitution Avenue
Ben Franklin Station
Washington, DC 20224
(202) 566-3292 (voice only)
(800) 829-4059 (TDD)

National Institute on Disability and Rehabilitation Research
U.S. Department of Education
400 Maryland Avenue SW
Washington, DC 20202-2572
(202) 732-5801 (voice)
(202) 732-5316 (TDD)

Office on the Americans with Disabilities Act
Civil Rights Division
U.S. Department of Justice
PO Box 66118
Washington, DC 20035-6118
(202) 514-0301 (voice)
(202) 514-0383 (TDD)

President's Committee on Employment of People with Disabilities
1331 F Street NW
Third Floor
Washington, DC 20004

Continued on following page

(202) 376-6200 (voice)
(202) 376-6205 (TDD)

Rehabilitation Services Administration
U.S. Department of Education
Mary E. Switzer Building
Room 3028
330 C Street SW
Washington, DC 20202-2531
(202) 732-1406 (voice)
(202) 732-2848 (TDD)

Small Business Administration
Office of Advocacy
Office of Economic Research
409 Third Street NW
Fifth Floor
Washington, DC 20416
(202) 205-6751 (voice only)

Social Security Administration
Office of Disability
Room 545
Altimeyer Building
6401 Security Boulevard
Baltimore, MD 21235
(800) 772-1213 (voice only)

AMERICANS WITH DISABILITIES ACT

Publications

Americans with Disabilities Act

To obtain a copy of the ADA, call:
House Document Room (202) 225-3456 (voice only)
Senate Document Room (202) 224-7860 (voice) or
(202) 224-4300 (TDD)

Americans with Disabilities Act Handbook

This is a resource document containing annotated regulations for Titles I, II, and III, lists of resources for obtaining additional assistance, and an appendix with supplementary information related to the implementation of the ADA. This document is available in the following additional formats:
Braille
Large print
Audiotape
Electronic file on computer disk and electronic bulletin board
(202) 514-6193
To order:
From the **Equal Employment Opportunity Commission (EEOC):**
Call (800) 669-EEOC (voice)

(800) 800-3302 (TDD)
From the **Department of Justice (DOJ):**
Call (202) 514-0301 (voice)
(202) 514-0383 (TDD)

Americans with Disabilities Act Guidelines Checklist for Buildings and Facilities

This checklist has been prepared to assist individuals and entities with rights or duties under Title II and Title III of the ADA in applying the requirements of the ADA Accessibility Guidelines to buildings and facilities subject to the law. The checklist presents information in summary form on the Department of Transportation and the DOJ regulations for implementation of the ADA.

To order, write or call:

U.S. Architectural and Transportation Barriers Compliance Board
1331 F Street NW, Suite 1000
Washington, DC 20004-1111
(800) USA-ABLE

Americans with Disabilities Act Technical Assistance Manual

This two-volume manual offered by the EEOC addresses in part the implications of the ADA on workers' compensation and work-related injuries.

To order, call:
(800) 669-EEOC. Refer to Document number EEOC-M-1A.

The Americans with Disabilities Act: From Policy to Practice

This resource is published by the Milbank Memorial Fund (MMF) and edited by Jane West, PhD, who directed the nonprofit MMF ADA Implementation Project. It covers the effect of the ADA on employment, business, public accommodations, transportation, telecommunications, and public health.

The publication is available from the MMF by calling (212) 570-4800.

Telephone Numbers for Americans with Disabilities Act Information

American Foundation for the Blind	(202) 223-0101 (voice & TDD)
Architectural and Transportation Barriers Compliance Board	(800) 872-2253 (voice & TDD)
Association for Retarded Citizens of the United States	(800) 433-5255 (voice) (800) 855-1155 (TDD) (tell operator you would like to place a collect call to (817) 277-0553)
Association on Higher Education and Disability (AHEAD)	(800) 247-7752 (voice & TDD)
Disability Rights Education and Defense Fund	(800) 466-4232 (voice & TDD)

Continued on following page

**Equal Employment Opportunity
Commission**

For questions and documents: (800) 669-3362 (voice)
(800) 800-3302 (TDD)

Alternate number for ordering
documents (print and other
formats): (202) 663-4264 (voice)
(202) 663-7110 (TDD)

**Federal Communications
Commission**

For ADA documents and general
information: (202) 632-7260 (voice)
(202) 632-6999 (TDD)

Information Line: ADA Watch (301) 577-7814 (TDD)

Job Accommodation Network (800) 526-7234 (voice)
(800) 526-7234 (TDD)

Within West Virginia: (800) 526-4698 (voice & TDD)

**National Center for Law and
Deafness** (202) 651-5343 (voice & TDD)

National Council on Disability (800) 875-7814 (voice)

National Easter Seal Society (202) 347-3066 (voice)

National Federation of the Blind (410) 659-9314 (voice)
(410) 625-2867 (TDD)

**President's Committee on
Employment of People with
Disabilities Information Line:
ADA Work** (800) 232-9675 (voice & TDD)

**Project ACTION (Accessible
Community Transportation in
Our Nation)** (202) 347-7385 (TDD)

**The Foundation on Employment
and Disability (for California
residents only)** (800) 499-4232 (voice)
(800) 499-0559 (TDD)

U.S. Department of Justice (202) 514-0301 (voice)
(202) 514-0383 (TDD)

U.S. Department of Transportation

**Federal Transit Administration
(for ADA documents and
information)** (202) 366-1656 (voice)
(202) 366-2979 (TDD)

Office of the General Counsel
(for legal questions) (202) 366-9306 (voice)
(202) 755-7687 (TDD)

Federal Aviation Administration (202) 376-6406 (voice)

Rural Transit Assistance Program
(for information and assistance
on public transportation issues) (800) 527-8279 (voice & TDD)

Regional Disability and Business Technical
Assistance Centers

Toll-free number for reaching any
of the following centers: (800) 949-4232 (voice & TDD)

Region I (Maine, New Hampshire,
Vermont, Massachusetts,
Rhode Island, Connecticut) (207) 874-6535 (voice & TDD)

Region II (New York, New Jersey, Puerto Rico)	(609) 392-4004 (voice)
	(609) 392-7004 (TDD)
Region III (Pennsylvania, Delaware, Maryland, District of Columbia, Virginia, West Virginia)	(703) 525-3268 (voice & TDD)
Region IV (Kentucky, Tennessee, North Carolina, South Carolina, Georgia, Alabama, Mississippi, Florida)	(404) 888-0022 (voice)
	(404) 888-9098 (TDD)
Region V (Ohio, Indiana, Illinois, Michigan, Wisconsin, Minnesota)	(312) 413-7756 (voice & TDD)
Region VI (Arkansas, Louisiana, Oklahoma, Texas, New Mexico)	(713) 520-0232 (voice)
	(713) 520-5136 (TDD)
Region VII (Iowa, Missouri, Nebraska, Kansas)	(314) 882-3600 (voice & TDD)
Region VIII (North Dakota, South Dakota, Montana, Wyoming, Colorado, Utah)	(719) 444-0252 (voice & TDD)
Region IX (Arizona, Nevada, California, Hawaii, Pacific Basin)	(510) 465-7884 (voice)
	(510) 465-3172 (TDD)
Region X (Idaho, Oregon, Washington, Alaska)	(206) 438-3168 (voice)
	(206) 438-3167 (TDD)

FEDERAL DISABILITY LAWS IN ADDITION TO THE AMERICANS WITH DISABILITIES ACT

The following are descriptions of selected federal disability programs that relate to the purposes of ADA. The Department of Education publishes a booklet entitled *Summary of Existing Legislation Affecting Persons with Disabilities* that describes federal laws and programs that affect people with disabilities. To order, write or call: Clearinghouse on Disability Information, U.S. Department of Education, Room 3132 Switzer Building, Washington, DC 20202-2524, at (202) 732-1241 or (202) 732-1723 (both are voice and TDD numbers).

Programs Administered by the Rehabilitation Services Administration

Centers for Independent Living (Title VII, Part B of the Act): These centers are an excellent source of advice on an array of accessibility, attitudinal, and other issues of concern to people with disabilities. For information, contact: Independent Living Research Utilization Center, 2323 South Shephard Street, Suite 1000, Houston, TX 77019, (713) 520-0232 (voice) or (713) 520-5136 (TDD).

State Vocational Rehabilitation Agencies (Title I of the Act): These agencies operate in each state, territory, and the District of Columbia to provide vocational rehabilitation services to individuals with physical or mental disabilities. For information, contact: Rehabilitation Services Administration, Mary E. Switzer Building, Room 3028, 330 C Street, SW, Washington, DC 20202, (202) 732-1282 (voice) or (202) 732-1330 (TDD).

Projects with Industry (Title VI of the Act): This program provides a means of meeting local business people who have ex-

Continued on following page

perience in hiring, and a commitment to hiring, people with disabilities. For information, contact: Inter-National Association of Business, Industry and Rehabilitation at PO Box 15242, Washington, DC 20003, (202) 543-6535 (voice only).

Programs Administered by the National Institute on Disability and Rehabilitation Research

The National Institute on Disability and Rehabilitation Research (NIDRR) administers federal disability research programs, the Technology Related Assistance for Individuals with Disabilities Act, and regional ADA technical assistance centers.

National Rehabilitation Information Center (NARIC): NARIC is an information center and library on disability and rehabilitation. For information, contact: National Rehabilitation Information Center, 8455 Colesville Road, Suite 935, Silver Spring, MD 20910, (800) 346-2742 (voice or TDD) or (301) 588-9284 (voice or TDD).

Research and Training (R&T) Centers: R&T Centers conduct applied research directed towards producing new knowledge about disability and rehabilitation. For information, contact: National Institute on Disability and Rehabilitation Research, U.S. Department of Education, 400 Maryland Avenue, SW, Washington, DC 20202-2572, (202) 732-1134 (voice) or (202) 732-5079 (TDD).

Technical Assistance Programs to Facilitate the Implementation of the ADA: The following three major programs were funded under the NIDRR

> **Regional Disability and Business Accommodation Centers (RDBACs)**
> **National Peer Training Projects**
> **Materials Development Projects**

For information, contact: National Institute on Disability and Rehabilitation Research, U.S. Department of Education, 400 Maryland Avenue, SW, Washington, DC 20202-2572, (202) 732-1134 (voice) or (202) 732-5079 (TDD).

Technology Related Assistance for Individuals with Disabilities Act: This legislation provides technology-related assistance to persons with disabilities and training to service providers. For information, contact: National Institute on Disability and Rehabilitation Research, U.S. Department of Education, 400 Maryland Avenue, SW, Washington, DC 20202-2572 or at (202) 732-5066 (voice) or (202) 732-5079 (TDD).

Work Incentive Programs for People with Disabilities

These programs are intended to provide individuals with disabilities who are beneficiaries of SSDI and SSI programs support they may need to move from benefit dependency to self-sufficiency. For information, contact: Program Management Branch,

Social Security Administration, 3R1 Operations Building, 6401 Security Boulevard, Baltimore, MD 21235, (301) 965-9864 (voice only).

Protection and Advocacy (P&A) Program for Persons with Developmental Disabilities

Authorized under the Developmental Disabilities Assistance and Bill of Rights Act, P&A agencies are involved in protecting the rights of individuals with developmental disabilities covered under the ADA. For information, contact: Administration on Developmental Disabilities, Program Operations Division, 200 Independence Avenue SW, Room 39D, Washington, DC 20201, (202) 245-2897 (voice) or (202) 245-2890 (TDD).

Job Training Partnership Act

This legislation has been used to place persons with mild and moderate disabilities in community jobs. For information, contact: Office of Employment and Training Programs, Department of Labor, 200 Constitution Avenue NW, Room N4709, Washington, DC 20210, (202) 535-0580 (voice only).

Disability-Related Tax Provisions Applicable to Businesses

The three disability-related provisions in the Internal Revenue Code applicable to businesses are the:

Targeted Jobs Credit Tax (Title 26, Internal Revenue Code, Section 51)

Tax Deduction to Remove Architectural and Transportation Barriers to People with Disabilities and Elderly Individuals (Title 26, Internal Revenue Code, Section 190)

Disabled Access Tax Credit (Title 26, Internal Revenue Code, Section 44).

For information, contact: Internal Revenue Service, Office of the Chief Counsel, PO Box 7604, Ben Franklin Station, Washington, DC 20044, (202) 566-3292 (voice only).

WHEELCHAIR DIMENSIONS AND WHEELCHAIR PRESCRIPTIONS

Measurements Used for Wheelchair Prescriptions

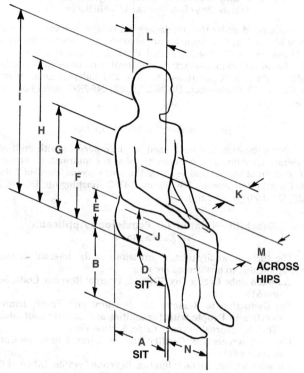

The following measurements are taken in the supine position:
Assist (right and left side): behind hips/popliteal fossa
B (right and left side): popliteal fossa/heel
D: knee flexion angle
E: sitting surface/pelvic crest
F: sitting surface/lower scapula
G: sitting surface/shoulder
H: sitting surface/occiput
I: sitting surface/crown of head
J: sitting surface/hanging elbow
K: width across trunk
L: depth of trunk
M: width across hips
N: heel/toe

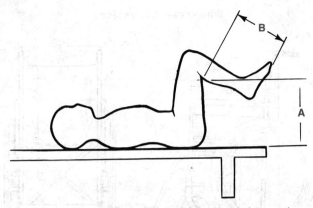

In the supine position with the hips and knees flexed, the examiner can measure the undersurface of the thigh from the popliteal fossa to a firm support surface (A) and the length from the popliteal fossa to the heel (B).

Wheelchair Dimensions

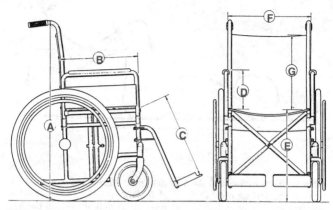

Dimension ranges for the basic adult wheelchairs from major US manufacturers. (A) Overall height: 36–37 in. (B) Seat depth: 16–17 in. (C) Footrest support (adjustment range): 16½–22 in. (D) Armrest height from seat rail (adjustment range): 5–12 in. (E) Seat height from floor: 19½–20½ in. (F) Seat and back width: 14–22 in. (G) Back height from seat rail: essentially as required.

Height (in.) from Floor	Width (in.)	Depth (in.)	Designation
19½	10	8	Preschool or tiny tot
19½	12	10–11½	Child's or tot's, high
16½	12	10–11½	Child's or tot's, low
21	14–14½	11½	Growing chair
17½–20½	14–16	11–13	Growing chair
18½	16*	14	Junior or slim adult
19½	16–16½	16–17	Narrow adult
19½–20½	18†	16	Adult
		17	Tall adult
19½–20½	20–22	16	Wide adult

*At least one manufacturer supplies 14 and 15 in as well.
†At least one manufacturer supplies 14, 15, 16, and 17 in as well.
From Department of Veterans Affairs: Choosing a wheelchair system. Journal of Rehabilitation Research and Development, Clinical Supplement #2, 1990.

Wheelchair Components

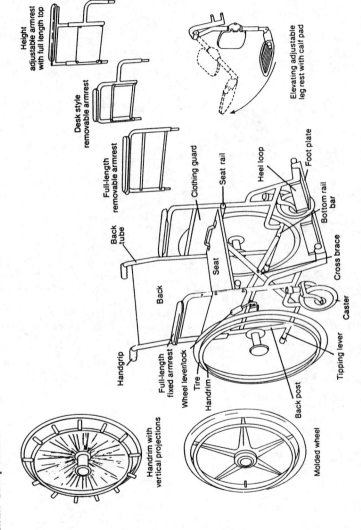

Height adjustable armrest with full length top

Desk style removable armrest

Full-length removable armrest

Elevating adjustable leg rest with calf pad

Clothing guard

Back tube

Seat rail

Heel loop

Foot plate

Bottom rail bar

Seat

Back

Cross brace

Caster

Handgrip

Full-length fixed armrest

Wheel lever/lock

Tire

Handrim

Back post

Tipping lever

Handrim with vertical projections

Molded wheel

Musculoskeletal Anatomy, Orthopedics, and Orthopedic Therapy

THE SKULL

Anterior (Frontal) View

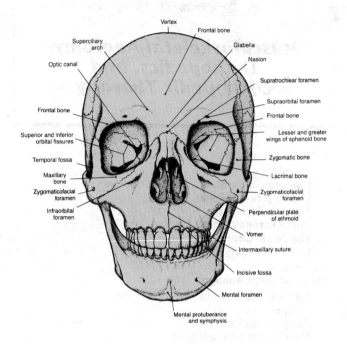

Vertex

Frontal bone

Superciliary arch

Glabella

Optic canal

Nasion

Supratrochlear foramen

Supraorbital foramen

Frontal bone

Frontal bone

Lesser and greater wings of sphenoid bone

Superior and inferior orbital fissures

Zygomatic bone

Temporal fossa

Lacrimal bone

Maxillary bone

Zygomaticofacial foramen

Zygomaticofacial foramen

Perpendicular plate of ethmoid

Infraorbital foramen

Vomer

Intermaxillary suture

Incisive fossa

Mental foramen

Mental protuberance and symphysis

Lateral View

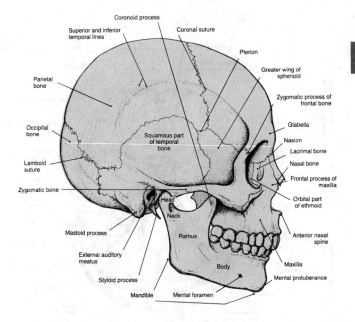

Coronoid process
Superior and inferior temporal lines
Coronal suture
Pterion
Greater wing of sphenoid
Parietal bone
Zygomatic process of frontal bone
Occipital bone
Glabella
Nasion
Squamous part of temporal bone
Lacrimal bone
Nasal bone
Lamboid suture
Frontal process of maxilla
Zygomatic bone
Orbital part of ethmoid
Head
Neck
Mastoid process
Ramus
Anterior nasal spine
External auditory meatus
Maxilla
Styloid process
Body
Mental protuberance
Mandible
Mental foramen

Interior View—Looking Laterally from the Midline

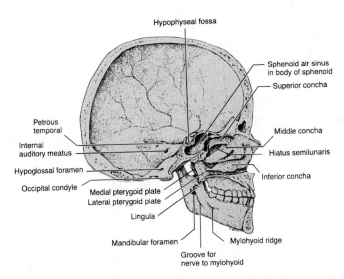

Hypophyseal fossa
Sphenoid air sinus in body of sphenoid
Superior concha
Petrous temporal
Middle concha
Internal auditory meatus
Hiatus semilunaris
Hypoglossal foramen
Inferior concha
Occipital condyle
Medial pterygoid plate
Lateral pterygoid plate
Lingula
Mandibular foramen
Mylohyoid ridge
Groove for nerve to mylohyoid

Interior View—Inferior Surface

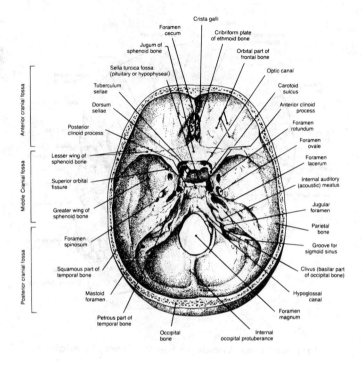

Anterior cranial fossa

Middle Cranial fossa

Posterior cranial fossa

Crista galli

Foramen cecum

Cribriform plate of ethmoid bone

Jugum of sphenoid bone

Orbital part of frontal bone

Sella turcica fossa (pituitary or hypophyseal)

Optic canal

Tuberculum sellae

Carotoid sulcus

Dorsum sellae

Anterior clinoid process

Posterior clinoid process

Foramen rotundum

Foramen ovale

Lesser wing of sphenoid bone

Foramen lacerum

Superior orbital fissure

Internal auditory (acoustic) meatus

Greater wing of sphenoid bone

Jugular foramen

Parietal bone

Foramen spinosum

Groove for sigmoid sinus

Squamous part of temporal bone

Clivus (basilar part of occipital bone)

Mastoid foramen

Hypoglossal canal

Foramen magnum

Petrous part of temporal bone

Occipital bone

Internal occipital protuberance

Exterior View

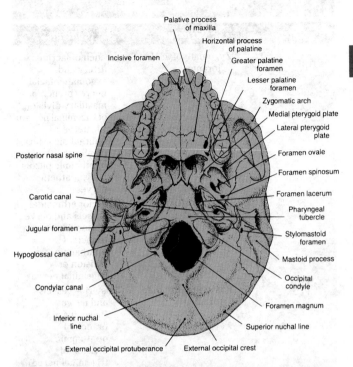

Palative process
of maxilla

Horizontal process
of palatine

Incisive foramen

Greater palatine
foramen

Lesser palatine
foramen

Zygomatic arch

Medial pterygoid plate

Lateral pterygoid
plate

Posterior nasal spine

Foramen ovale

Foramen spinosum

Carotid canal

Foramen lacerum

Pharyngeal
tubercle

Jugular foramen

Stylomastoid
foramen

Hypoglossal canal

Mastoid process

Condylar canal

Occipital
condyle

Foramen magnum

Inferior nuchal
line

Superior nuchal line

External occipital protuberance   External occipital crest

OPENINGS IN THE SKULL AND THEIR CONTENTS (by view)

View	Structure	Contents
Frontal	Supraorbital foramen	Supraorbital vessels, supraorbital nerve (frontal branch of ophthalmic division of trigeminal nerve)
	Supratrochlear foramen	Supratrochlear vessels and nerve
	Infraorbital foramen	Infraorbital vessels and nerve (branch of maxillary division of trigeminal nerve)

Continued on following page

OPENINGS IN THE SKULL AND THEIR CONTENTS (by view) (Continued)

View	Structure	Contents
Orbital	Zygomaticofacial foramen	Branch of lacrimal artery and zygomaticofacial nerve (branch of maxillary division of trigeminal nerve)
	Optic canal	Optic nerve, ophthalmic artery, meninges, ophthalmic plexus of sympathetic nerves
	Anterior ethmoidal foramen	Anterior ethmoidal vessels and nerve (nasociliary branch of ophthalmic division of trigeminal nerve)
	Posterior ethmoidal foramen	Posterior vessels and nerve (nasociliary branch of ophthalmic division of trigeminal nerve)
	Nasolacrimal canal	Nasolacrimal duct
	Infraorbital foramen	Infraorbital nerve and vessels
	Superior orbital fissure (lateral to origin of the lateral rectus muscle)	Lacrimal nerve, frontal nerve, trochlear nerve, meningeal branch of lacrimal artery, orbital branch of middle meningeal artery, sympathetic branches from the carotid plexus
	Superior orbital fissure (between the heads of the lateral rectus muscle)	Superior and inferior ophthalmic veins, oculomotor nerve, nasociliary nerve, abducens nerve

OPENINGS IN THE SKULL AND THEIR CONTENTS (by view)

View	Structure	Contents
Posterior	Mastoid foramen	Emissary vein connecting sigmoid sinus to the posterior auricular vein
Lateral	External auditory meatus	Air
	Tympanomastoid fissure	Auricular branch of vagus nerve
	Alveolar canals	Posterior superior alveolar nerves
	Infraorbital fissure	Infraorbital nerve and vessels
	Zygomaticofacial foramen	Branch of lacrimal artery and zygomaticofacial nerve (branch of maxillary division of trigeminal)
	Zygomaticotemporal foramen	Zygomaticotemporal nerve of the mandibular division of the trigeminal nerve
Inferolateral	Pterygomaxillary fissure	Maxillary artery to infratemporal fossa artery
Anterior wall	Inferior orbital fissure	Structure that connects with orbit
Inferior wall	Greater palatine canal	Structure that extends to posterior surface of hard palate
	Foramen rotundum	Structure that connects with middle cranial fossa and allows for passage of maxillary division of the trigeminal nerve

Continued on following page

View	Structure	Contents
Superior wall	Pterygoid canal	Structure that connects foramen lacerum via root of pterygoid process (vessel and nerve of pterygoid canal)
	Pharyngeal canal (palatinovaginal)	Structure that connects with posterior opening of nose
Medial wall	Sphenopalatine foramen	Structure that connects with superior meatus of nose
Inferior	Incisive foramen	Greater palatine artery, nasopalatine nerve
	Greater palatine foramen	Greater palatine artery and nerve
	Palatinovaginal canal	Pharyngeal branches of pterygopalatine (pharyngeal canal) ganglion and third portion of maxillary artery
	Foramen spinosum	Middle meningeal artery
	Foramen ovale	Mandibular division of trigeminal nerve, motor root of mandibular nerve, accessory meningeal artery, lesser superficial petrosal nerve, emissary veins connecting cavernous sinus to pterygoid venous plexus
	Foramen magnum	Spinal roots of accessory nerve, two vertebral

OPENINGS IN THE SKULL AND THEIR CONTENTS (by view)

View	Structure	Contents
		arteries, medulla oblongata, two posterior spinal arteries, one anterior spinal artery, sympathetic plexuses about vertebral arteries, tonsil of cerebellum
	Posterior condylar canal	Emissary vein connecting sigmoid sinus to suboccipital venous plexus
	Anterior condylar canal	Hypoglossal nerve, emissary veins connecting meningeal veins to pharyngeal venous plexus
	Stylomastoid foramen	Facial nerve
	Jugular foramen	
	Anterior compartment	Inferior petrosal sinus
	Middle compartment	Glossopharyngeal, vagus, and accessory nerves
	Posterior compartment	Sigmoid sinus to internal jugular vein
	Tympanic canaliculus	Tympanic branch of glossopharyngeal nerve
	Carotid canal	Internal carotid artery, sympathetic carotid plexus, emissary vein connecting cavernous sinus

Continued on following page

View	Structure	Contents
		to pharyngeal plexus
	Caroticotympanic canaliculi	Branches of carotid sympathetic plexus, tympanic branches of internal carotid artery
	Foramen lacerum	Meningeal branch of ascending pharyngeal artery, emissary vein connecting cavernous sinus to pharyngeal plexus, internal carotid artery, sympathetic plexus, deep petrosal nerve (from otic sympathetic plexus), greater petrosal nerve (parasympathetic from facial nerve)
	Canal for auditory tube (eustachian tube)	Temporal bone between tympanic plate and petrosal portion of temporal bone
	Petrotympanic fissure	Chorda tympani nerve of facial nerve
Internal		
Anterior cranial fossa	Foramen cecum	Emissary vein connecting superior sagittal sinus to veins of nose
	Cribriform plate of ethmoid bone	Filaments of olfactory nerve
Middle cranial fossa	Optic canal	Optic nerve, ophthalmic artery, meninges,

View	Structure	Contents
		ophthalmic plexus of sympathetic nerves
	Superior orbital fissure (lateral to origin of the lateral rectus muscle)	Lacrimal nerve, frontal nerve) trochlear nerve, meningeal branch of lacrimal artery, orbital branch of middle meningeal artery, sympathetic branches from the carotid plexus
	Superior orbital fissure (between the heads of the lateral rectus muscle)	Superior and inferior ophthalmic veins, oculomotor nerve, nasociliary nerve, abducens nerve
	Foramen rotundum	Structure that connects with middle cranial fossa and allows for passage of maxillary division of the trigeminal nerve
	Foramen ovale	Mandibular nerve of trigeminal nerve, motor root of mandibular division, accessory meningeal artery, lesser superficial petrosal nerve, emissary veins connecting cavernous sinus to pterygoid verous plexus
	Foramen spinosum	Middle meningeal artery

Continued on following page

2

View	Structure	Contents
	Foramen lacerum	Meningeal branch of ascending pharyngeal artery, emissary vein connecting cavernous sinus to pharyngeal plexus, internal carotid artery, sympathetic plexus, deep petrosal nerve (from otic sympathetic plexus), greater petrosal nerve (parasympathetic from facial nerve)
	Pterygoid canal	Nerve of pterygoid canal (formed by greater and deep petrosal nerves), artery of pterygoid canal (branch of maxillary artery)
Posterior cranial fossa	Foramen magnum	Spinal roots of accessory nerve, two vertebral arteries, medulla oblongata, two posterior spinal arteries, one anterior spinal artery, sympathetic plexuses about vertebral arteries, tonsil of cerebellum
	Anterior condylar canal	Hypoglossal nerve, emissary veins connecting meningeal veins to pharyngeal venous plexus

View	Structure	Contents
	Posterior condylar canal	Emissary vein connecting sigmoid sinus to suboccipital venous plexus
	Mastoid foramen	Emissary vein connecting sigmoid sinus to the posterior auricular vein
	Jugular foramen	
	Anterior compartment	Inferior petrosal sinus
	Middle compartment	Glossopharyngeal, vagus, and accessory nerves
	Internal auditory meatus	Motor and sensory roots of facial nerve, vestibulocochlear nerve
	Opening of aqueduct of vestibule	Endolymphatic duct
Mandible	Mandibular foramen	Inferior alveolar vessels and nerve (mandibular division of trigeminal)
	Mental foramen	Mental vessels and nerve (mandibular division of trigeminal)
	Mylohyoid groove	Mylohyoid vessels and mylohyoid nerve (mandibular division of trigeminal)
	Mandibular notch	Vessels to masseter muscle and nerve to masseter (mandibular division of trigeminal)

2

THE VERTEBRAL COLUMN
Lateral and Anterior Views

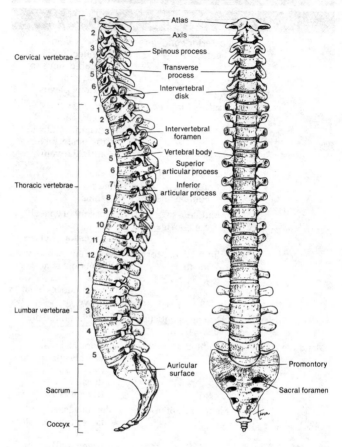

Cervical vertebrae

1 — Atlas
2 — Axis
3 — Spinous process
4
5 — Transverse process
6
7 — Intervertebral disk

Thoracic vertebrae

1
2
3 — Intervertebral foramen
4 — Vertebral body
5 — Superior articular process
6
7 — Inferior articular process
8
9
10
11
12

Lumbar vertebrae

1
2
3
4
5

Sacrum — Auricular surface

Coccyx

Promontory
Sacral foramen

CERVICAL VERTEBRAE
Superior Views

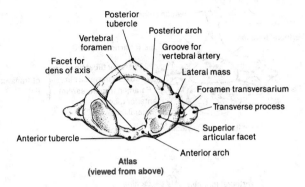

Posterior tubercle
Posterior arch
Vertebral foramen
Groove for vertebral artery
Facet for dens of axis
Lateral mass
Foramen transversarium
Transverse process
Superior articular facet
Anterior tubercle
Anterior arch

Atlas
(viewed from above)

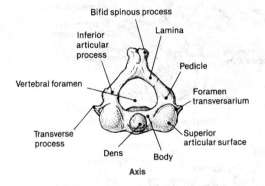

Bifid spinous process
Lamina
Inferior articular process
Pedicle
Vertebral foramen
Foramen transversarium
Transverse process
Superior articular surface
Dens
Body

Axis

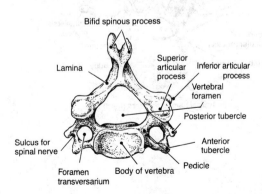

Bifid spinous process
Superior articular process
Inferior articular process
Lamina
Vertebral foramen
Posterior tubercle
Sulcus for spinal nerve
Anterior tubercle
Pedicle
Foramen transversarium
Body of vertebra

Typical cervical vertebra (fifth)

VERTEBRAE
Superior Views

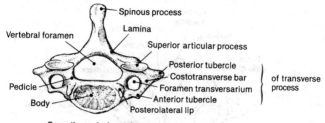

Spinous process

Vertebral foramen

Lamina

Superior articular process

Posterior tubercle

Costotransverse bar

Foramen transversarium

Anterior tubercle

} of transverse process

Pedicle

Body

Posterolateral lip

Seventh cervical vertebra

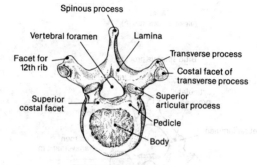

Spinous process

Vertebral foramen

Lamina

Facet for 12th rib

Transverse process

Costal facet of transverse process

Superior costal facet

Superior articular process

Pedicle

Body

Sixth thoracic vertebra

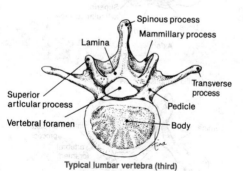

Spinous process

Mammillary process

Lamina

Transverse process

Superior articular process

Pedicle

Vertebral foramen

Body

Typical lumbar vertebra (third)

THE SACRUM AND COCCYX

Ventral and Dorsal Views

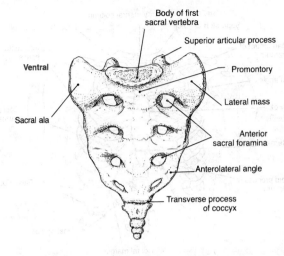

Ventral

- Body of first sacral vertebra
- Superior articular process
- Promontory
- Lateral mass
- Sacral ala
- Anterior sacral foramina
- Anterolateral angle
- Transverse process of coccyx

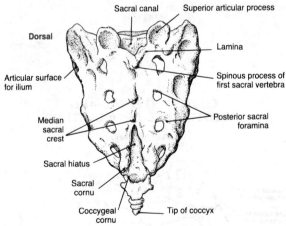

Dorsal

- Sacral canal
- Superior articular process
- Lamina
- Articular surface for ilium
- Spinous process of first sacral vertebra
- Median sacral crest
- Posterior sacral foramina
- Sacral hiatus
- Sacral cornu
- Coccygeal cornu
- Tip of coccyx

THE THORACIC CAGE
Anterior View

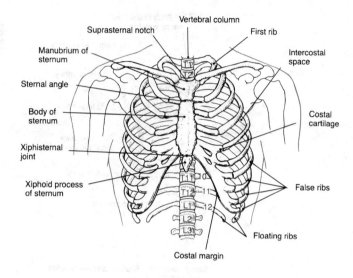

Vertebral column

Suprasternal notch

First rib

Manubrium of sternum

Intercostal space

Sternal angle

Body of sternum

Costal cartilage

Xiphisternal joint

Xiphoid process of sternum

False ribs

Floating ribs

Costal margin

COSTOVERTEBRAL AND COSTOSTERNAL ARTICULATIONS
Lateral View

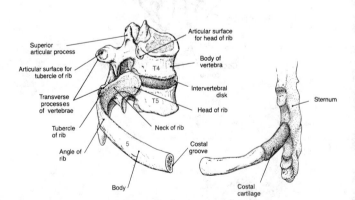

Superior articular process

Articular surface for head of rib

Articular surface for tubercle of rib

Body of vertebra

Transverse processes of vertebrae

Intervertebral disk

Tubercle of rib

Head of rib

Angle of rib

Neck of rib

Body

Costal groove

Sternum

Costal cartilage

THE CLAVICLE

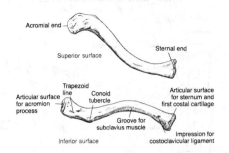

Acromial end

Superior surface

Sternal end

Trapezoid line

Conoid tubercle

Articular surface for acromion process

Articular surface for sternum and first costal cartilage

Groove for subclavius muscle

Impression for costoclavicular ligament

Inferior surface

THE SCAPULA
Costal and Dorsal Surfaces

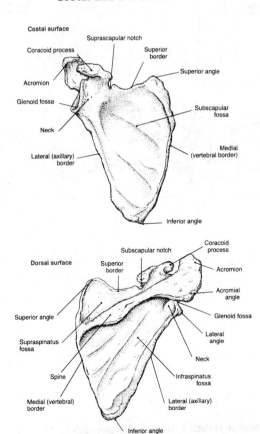

Costal surface

Suprascapular notch

Coracoid process

Superior border

Superior angle

Acromion

Glenoid fossa

Subscapular fossa

Neck

Lateral (axillary) border

Medial (vertebral border)

Inferior angle

Dorsal surface

Subscapular notch

Coracoid process

Superior border

Acromion

Acromial angle

Glenoid fossa

Superior angle

Lateral angle

Supraspinatus fossa

Neck

Spine

Infraspinatus fossa

Medial (vertebral) border

Lateral (axillary) border

Inferior angle

THE HUMERUS
Ventral and Dorsal Surfaces

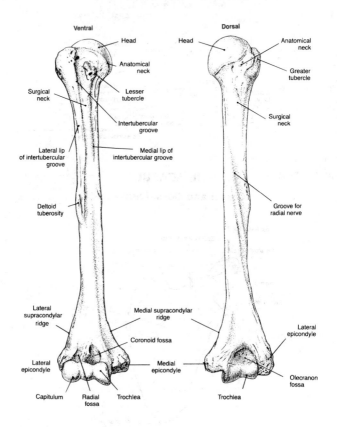

Ventral

Dorsal

Head

Anatomical neck

Lesser tubercle

Surgical neck

Intertubercular groove

Lateral lip of intertubercular groove

Medial lip of intertubercular groove

Deltoid tuberosity

Lateral supracondylar ridge

Medial supracondylar ridge

Coronoid fossa

Lateral epicondyle

Medial epicondyle

Capitulum

Radial fossa

Trochlea

Head

Anatomical neck

Greater tubercle

Surgical neck

Groove for radial nerve

Lateral epicondyle

Olecranon fossa

Trochlea

THE RADIUS AND ULNA
Ventral Surface

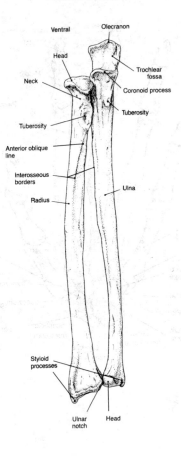

Ventral

Head

Neck

Tuberosity

Anterior oblique line

Interosseous borders

Radius

Olecranon

Trochlear fossa

Coronoid process

Tuberosity

Ulna

Styloid processes

Ulnar notch

Head

THE HAND
Palmar Surface

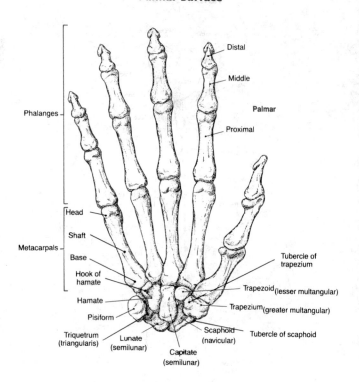

Phalanges
- Distal
- Middle
- Proximal

Palmar

Metacarpals
- Head
- Shaft
- Base

Hook of hamate

Hamate

Pisiform

Triquetrum (triangularis)

Lunate (semilunar)

Capitate (semilunar)

Scaphoid (navicular)

Tubercle of scaphoid

Trapezium (greater multangular)

Trapezoid (lesser multangular)

Tubercle of trapezium

ARTICULATIONS OF THE CARPAL BONES PROXIMAL ROW

Bone	Number of Articulations	Articulates With
Scaphoid (navicular)	Five	Radius, trapezium, trapezoid, capitate lunate
Lunate (semilunar)	Five	Radius, capitate, hamate, scaphoid, trapezium
Triquetrum (triangularis)	Three	Lunate, pisiform, hamate (separated from the ulna by the triangular articular disk)
Pisiform	One	Triquetrum

ARTICULATIONS OF THE CARPAL BONES DISTAL ROW

Bone	Number of Articulations	Articulates With
Trapezium (greater multangular)	Four	Scaphoid, first and second metacarpals, trapezoid
Trapezoid (lesser multangular)	Four	Scaphoid, second metacarpal, capitate, trapezium
Capitate	Seven	Scaphoid, lunate, second, third, and fourth metacarpals, trapezoid, hamate
Hamate	Five	Lunate, fourth and fifth metacarpals, triquetrum, capitate

ARTICULATIONS OF THE METACARPAL BONES

First: trapezium, proximal phalanx

Second: trapezium trapezoid, capitate, third metacarpal, proximal phalanx

Third: capitate, second and fourth metacarpals, proximal phalanx

Fourth: capitate, hamate, third and fifth metacarpals, proximal phalanx

Fifth: hamate, fourth metacarpal, proximal phalanx

THE PELVIC GIRDLE

Ventral Surfaces of the Female Pelvis and the Male Pelvis

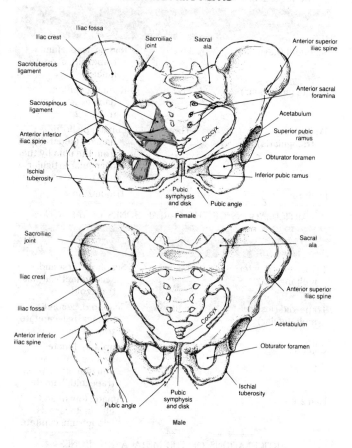

Female

Iliac fossa
Iliac crest
Sacroiliac joint
Sacral ala
Anterior superior iliac spine
Sacrotuberous ligament
Anterior sacral foramina
Sacrospinous ligament
Acetabulum
Coccyx
Superior pubic ramus
Anterior inferior iliac spine
Obturator foramen
Ischial tuberosity
Inferior pubic ramus
Pubic symphysis and disk
Pubic angle

Male

Sacroiliac joint
Sacral ala
Iliac crest
Anterior superior iliac spine
Iliac fossa
Coccyx
Acetabulum
Anterior inferior iliac spine
Obturator foramen
Ischial tuberosity
Pubic symphysis and disk
Pubic angle

COMPARISONS OF THE MALE AND FEMALE PELVISES

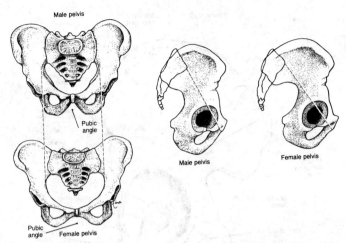

The female pelvic outlet is larger than the male pelvic outlet. The pubic angle on the female pelvis forms a more obtuse angle than does that of the male pelvis.

THE PELVIS
Lateral Surface

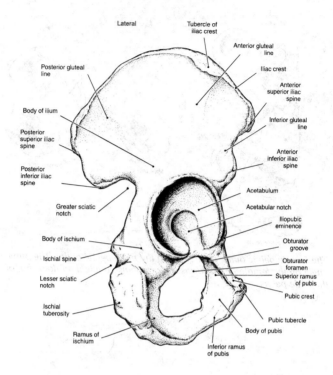

Lateral

Tubercle of iliac crest

Anterior gluteal line

Posterior gluteal line

Iliac crest

Body of ilium

Anterior superior iliac spine

Posterior superior iliac spine

Inferior gluteal line

Posterior inferior iliac spine

Anterior inferior iliac spine

Greater sciatic notch

Acetabulum

Acetabular notch

Iliopubic eminence

Body of ischium

Obturator groove

Ischial spine

Obturator foramen

Lesser sciatic notch

Superior ramus of pubis

Ischial tuberosity

Pubic crest

Pubic tubercle

Ramus of ischium

Body of pubis

Inferior ramus of pubis

THE PELVIS
Medial Surface

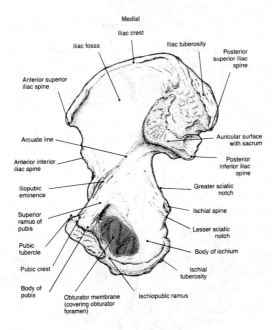

Medial

Iliac crest

Iliac fossa

Iliac tuberosity

Posterior superior iliac spine

Anterior superior iliac spine

Arcuate line

Auricular surface with sacrum

Anterior interior iliac spine

Posterior inferior iliac spine

Iliopubic eminence

Greater sciatic notch

Superior ramus of pubis

Ischial spine

Lesser sciatic notch

Pubic tubercle

Body of ischium

Pubic crest

Ischial tuberosity

Body of pubis

Obturator membrane (covering obturator foramen)

Ischiopubic ramus

THE FEMUR
Ventral Surface

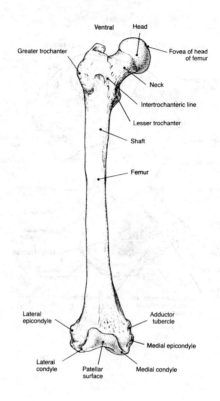

Ventral   Head

Greater trochanter

Fovea of head
of femur

Neck

Intertrochanteric line

Lesser trochanter

Shaft

Femur

Lateral
epicondyle

Adductor
tubercle

Medial epicondyle

Lateral
condyle   Patellar
surface

Medial condyle

THE FEMUR

Dorsal Surface

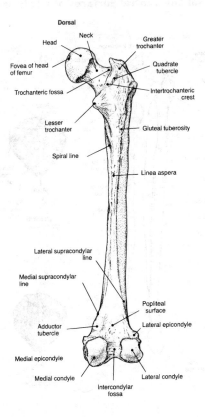

Dorsal

Head

Neck

Greater trochanter

Fovea of head of femur

Quadrate tubercle

Trochanteric fossa

Intertrochanteric crest

Lesser trochanter

Gluteal tuberosity

Spiral line

Linea aspera

Lateral supracondylar line

Medial supracondylar line

Popliteal surface

Adductor tubercle

Lateral epicondyle

Medial epicondyle

Medial condyle

Intercondylar fossa

Lateral condyle

THE LEG AND PATELLA

Ventral Surface of the Tibia and Fibula and Dorsal and Ventral Surfaces of a Left Patella

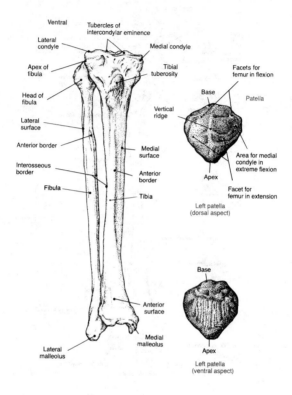

Ventral
Tubercles of intercondylar eminence
Lateral condyle
Medial condyle
Apex of fibula
Tibial tuberosity
Head of fibula
Base
Patella
Facets for femur in flexion
Lateral surface
Vertical ridge
Anterior border
Medial surface
Interosseous border
Anterior border
Area for medial condyle in extreme flexion
Fibula
Tibia
Apex
Facet for femur in extension

Left patella (dorsal aspect)

Anterior surface
Base
Medial malleolus
Lateral malleolus
Apex

Left patella (ventral aspect)

THE FOOT

Lateral and Medial Views

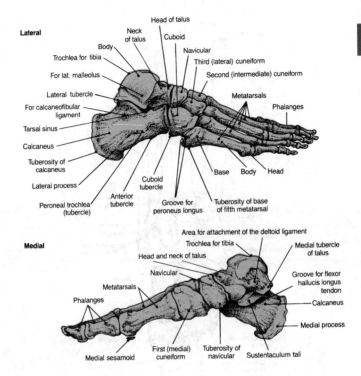

Lateral

- Head of talus
- Neck of talus
- Cuboid
- Body
- Navicular
- Trochlea for tibia
- Third (lateral) cuneiform
- For lat. malleolus
- Second (intermediate) cuneiform
- Lateral tubercle
- Metatarsals
- For calcaneofibular ligament
- Phalanges
- Tarsal sinus
- Calcaneus
- Tuberosity of calcaneus
- Base
- Body
- Head
- Lateral process
- Cuboid tubercle
- Peroneal trochlea (tubercle)
- Anterior tubercle
- Groove for peroneus longus
- Tuberosity of base of fifth metatarsal

Medial

- Area for attachment of the deltoid ligament
- Trochlea for tibia
- Medial tubercle of talus
- Head and neck of talus
- Navicular
- Groove for flexor hallucis longus tendon
- Metatarsals
- Calcaneus
- Phalanges
- Medial process
- Medial sesamoid
- First (medial) cuneiform
- Tuberosity of navicular
- Sustentaculum tali

See the table titled Articulations of the Foot, page 96.

THE FOOT
Superior View

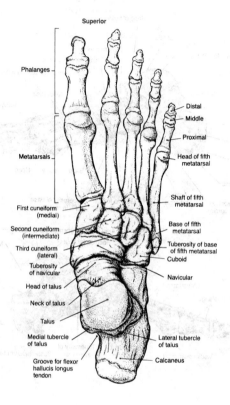

Superior

Phalanges

Distal

Middle

Proximal

Head of fifth
metatarsal

Metatarsals

Shaft of fifth
metatarsal

First cuneiform
(medial)

Base of fifth
metatarsal

Second cuneiform
(intermediate)

Tuberosity of base
of fifth metatarsal

Third cuneiform
(lateral)

Cuboid

Tuberosity
of navicular

Navicular

Head of talus

Neck of talus

Talus

Medial tubercle
of talus

Lateral tubercle
of talus

Groove for flexor
hallucis longus
tendon

Calcaneus

See the table titled Articulations of the Foot, page 96.

THE FOOT

Inferior View

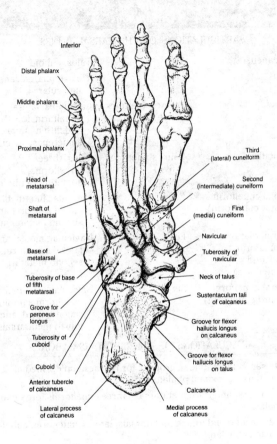

Inferior

Distal phalanx

Middle phalanx

Proximal phalanx

Head of
metatarsal

Shaft of
metatarsal

Base of
metatarsal

Tuberosity of base
of fifth
metatarsal

Groove for
peroneus
longus

Tuberosity of
cuboid

Cuboid

Anterior tubercle
of calcaneus

Lateral process
of calcaneus

Third
(lateral) cuneiform

Second
(intermediate) cuneiform

First
(medial) cuneiform

Navicular

Tuberosity of
navicular

Neck of talus

Sustentaculum tali
of calcaneus

Groove for flexor
hallucis longus
on calcaneus

Groove for flexor
hallucis longus
on talus

Calcaneus

Medial process
of calcaneus

See the table titled Articulations of the Foot, page 96.

ARTICULATIONS OF THE FOOT

Bone	Number of Articulations	Articulates with
ARTICULATIONS OF THE TARSAL BONES		
Calcaneus	Two	Talus, cuboid
Talus	Four	Tibia, fibula, calcaneus, navicular
Cuboid	Four (sometimes five)	Calcaneus, lateral cuneiform, fourth and fifth metatarsal, sometimes navicular
Navicular	Four (sometimes five)	Talus, three cuneiforms, sometimes cuboid
Medial cuneiform (first cuneiform)	Four	Navicular, intermediate cuneiform, first and second metatarsal
Intermediate cuneiform (second cuneiform)	Four	Navicular, medial and lateral cuneiforms, second metatarsal
Lateral cuneiform (third cuneiform)	Six	Navicular, intermediate cuneiform, cuboid, second, third, and fourth metatarsals

ARTICULATIONS OF THE METATARSAL BONES

First: second metatarsal, grooves for two sesamoids, medial cuneiform, proximal phalanx

Second: first and third metatarsals, three cuneiforms, proximal phalanx

Third: second and fourth metatarsals, lateral cuneiform, cuboid, proximal phalanx

Fourth: third and fourth metatarsals, lateral cuneiform, cuboid, proximal phalanx

Fifth: fourth metatarsal, cuboid, proximal phalanx

FRACTURE CLASSIFICATIONS
Salter's Fracture Classification

According to Salter, to describe a fracture completely, you must identify the site, extent, configuration, relationship of the fracture fragments to each other, the relationship of the fracture fragments to the external environment, and the presence or absence of complications.

Site

CLASSIFICATION. Diaphyseal, metaphyseal, epiphyseal, or intra-articular. A dislocation occurring in conjunction with a fracture is a fracture dislocation.

Extent

CLASSIFICATION. Complete or incomplete. Types of incomplete fractures are crack, hairline, buckle, and green-stick fractures.

Configuration

CLASSIFICATION. Complete fractures can have a transverse, oblique, or spiral arrangement. If there are more than two fragments, the fracture is a comminuted fracture.

Relationship of the Fracture Fragments to Each Other

CLASSIFICATION. Fragments can be either displaced or nondisplaced. When the fragments are displaced, they can be shifted sideways, angulated, rotated, distracted, overriding, or impacted.

Relationship of the Fracture Fragments to the External Environment

CLASSIFICATION. Closed or open. A closed fracture is one in which the skin in the area of the fracture is intact. An open fracture is one in which the skin in the area of the fracture is not intact. The fracture fragment may have penetrated the skin, or an object may have penetrated the skin to cause the fracture. Closed fractures are also called *simple fractures* and open fractures are also called *compound fractures*.

Complications

CLASSIFICATION. Complicated or uncomplicated. A complicated fracture is one that results in either a local or systemic complication due to the fracture or the treatment of the fracture. An uncomplicated fracture is one that does not immediately result in a local or systemic complication and heals uneventfully.

FROM

Salter, RB: Textbook of Disorders and Injuries of the Musculoskeletal System: An Introduction to Orthopaedics, Fractures, and Joint Injuries, Rheumatology, Metabolic Bone Disease and Rehabilitation, ed 2. Williams & Wilkins, Baltimore, 1983, with permission.

Orthopedic Trauma Association Classification of Long Bone Fractures

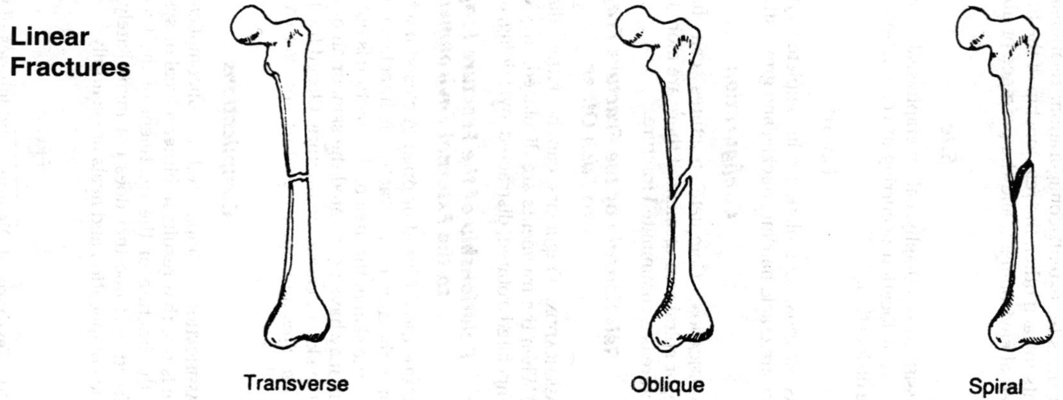

Spiral

Oblique

Transverse

Linear Fractures

Comminuted Fractures

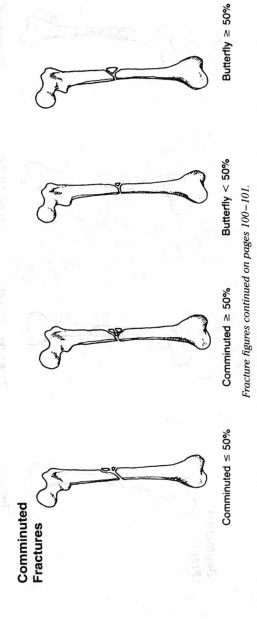

Comminuted ≤ 50%   Comminuted ≥ 50%   Butterfly < 50%   Butterfly ≥ 50%

Fracture figures continued on pages 100–101.

Orthopedic Trauma Association Classification of Long Bone Fractures (Continued)

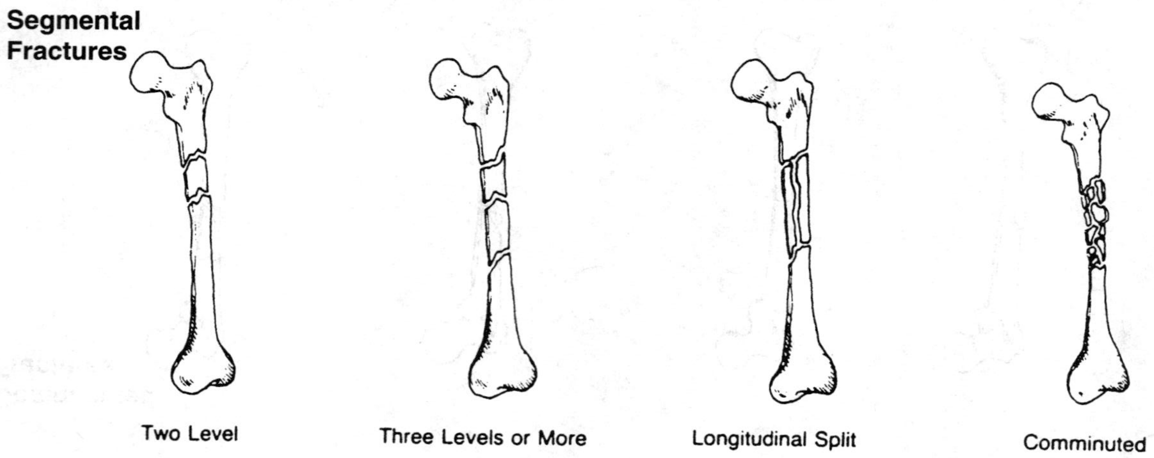

Segmental Fractures

Two Level

Three Levels or More

Longitudinal Split

Comminuted

**Boneloss
Fractures**

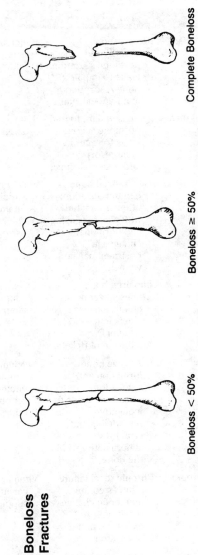

Boneloss < 50%   Boneloss ≥ 50%   Complete Boneloss

From Gustilo, RB: The Fracture Classification Manual. Mosby-Year Book, St. Louis, 1991, Fig. 22-1, with permission.

METABOLIC BONE DISEASES

EXAMPLES OF METABOLIC BONE DISEASES		
Disease	*Pathophysiology*	*Drug Treatment*
Hypoparathyroidism	Decreased parathyroid hormone secretion; leads to impaired bone resorption and hypocalcemia.	Calcium supplements, vitamin D.
Hyperparathyroidism	Increased parathyroid hormone secretion; leads to excessive bone resorption and hypercalcemia.	Usually treated surgically.
Osteoporosis	Generalized bone demineralization; often associated with effects of aging and hormonal changes in postmenopausal women.	Calcium supplements, vitamin D, calcitonin, estrogen.
Rickets	Impaired bone mineralization in children caused by a deficiency of vitamin D. Adult form of rickets.	Calcium supplements, vitamin D.
Osteomalacia Paget's disease	Excessive bone formation and resorption (turnover) leads to ineffective remodeling and structural abnormalities within the bone.	Calcium supplements, vitamin D. Calcitonin, etidronate.
Renal osteodystrophy	Chronic renal failure induces complex metabolic changes resulting in excessive bone resorption.	Vitamin D, calcium supplements.
Gaucher's disease	Excessive lipid storage in bone leads to impaired	No drugs are effective.

EXAMPLES OF METABOLIC BONE DISEASES		
Disease	*Pathophysiology*	*Drug Treatment*
	remodeling and excessive bone loss.	
Hypercalcemia of malignancy	Many forms of cancer accelerate bone resorption, leading to hypercalcemia.	Calcitonin, etidronate.

From Ciccone, CD: Pharmacology in Rehabilitation, ed 2. FA Davis, Philadelphia, 1996, p 471, with permission.

CLASSIFICATION SYSTEM USED FOR JOINTS

Fibrous

syndesmosis: A union via cordlike ligamentous fibers.

suture: Alignment of the growing edges of two bones with thin, fibrous tissue.

gomphosis: Tooth and periodontal membrane (membranous union).

Cartilaginous

synchondrosis: Residual cartilage plate between two bones.

symphysis: Two bones united by a coating of fibrocartilage and reinforced.

Synovial

Plane

arthrodial: Gliding articulations with flat surfaces.

amphiarthrodial: Bony articulating surfaces connected by cartilage.

synarthrodial: Skeletal articulations are maintained by a continuous intervening cartilage, fibrous tissue, or bone.

Uniaxial

ginglymus: Hinge.

trochoid: Pivot.

Biaxial

Allows circumduction.

    condyloid: Ball and socket without rotation.

    ellipsoid: Oval and socket.

Multiaxial

True ball and socket.

CLASSIFICATIONS OF THE JOINTS OF THE BODY
(in alphabetical order)

Joint	Classification
Acromioclavicular	Arthrodial
Ankle	Ginglymus
Atlantoaxial	Trochoid and arthrodial
Calcaneocuboid	Arthrodial
Capitate and hamate with scaphoid and lunate	Condyloid
Carpometacarpal	Condyloid
Cranial bones	Sutures
Distal carpal bones	Arthrodial
Elbow	Ginglymus
Hip	Multiaxial
Intercarpal joints	Arthrodial
Intermetatarsal	Arthrodial
Interphalangeal	Ginglymus
Knee	Ginglymus
Manubrium and sternum	Symphysis
Metacarpophalangeal	Condyloid
Metatarsophalangeal	Condyloid
Proximal carpal bones	Arthrodial
Pubic rami	Symphysis
Radioulnar (middle)	Syndesmosis
Radioulnar (proximal and distal)	Trochoid
Sacrococcygeal	Amphiarthrodial
Sacroiliac	Synchondrosis
Shoulder	Multiaxial
Sphenoid-ethmoid	Synchondrosis
Sternoclavicular	Double arthrodial
Sternocostal	Arthrodial
Subtalar	Arthrodial
Talocalcaneonavicular	Arthrodial
Tarsometatarsal	Arthrodial
Teeth and surrounding membrane	Gomphosis
Temporomandibular	Ginglymus and arthrodial
Tibiofibular	Arthrodial
Tibiofibular with interosseous membrane	Syndesmosis

CLASSIFICATIONS OF THE JOINTS OF THE BODY (in alphabetical order)	
Joint	*Classification*
Tubercles and necks of ribs	Arthrodial
Vertebral arches	Arthrodial and syndesmosis
Vertebral bodies	Amphiarthrodial
Vertebral column with cranium	Condyloid
Wrist (radiocarpal)	Condyloid

2

OSTEOLOGY AND ARTHROLOGY: JOINTS AND THEIR CLASSIFICATION

Anterior View

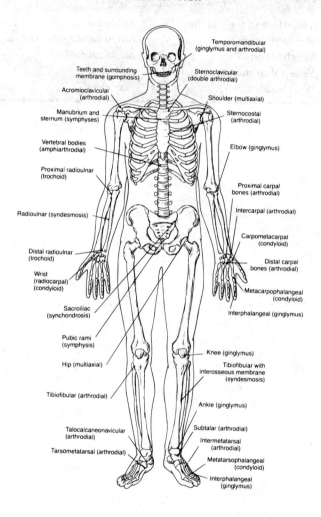

Temporomandibular (ginglymus and arthrodial)

Teeth and surrounding membrane (gomphosis)

Sternoclavicular (double arthrodial)

Acromioclavicular (arthrodial)

Shoulder (multiaxial)

Manubrium and sternum (symphyses)

Sternocostal (arthrodial)

Vertebral bodies (amphiarthrodial)

Elbow (ginglymus)

Proximal radioulnar (trochoid)

Proximal carpal bones (arthrodial)

Radioulnar (syndesmosis)

Intercarpal (arthrodial)

Carpometacarpal (condyloid)

Distal radioulnar (trochoid)

Distal carpal bones (arthrodial)

Wrist (radiocarpal) (condyloid)

Metacarpophalangeal (condyloid)

Sacroiliac (synchondrosis)

Interphalangeal (ginglymus)

Pubic rami (symphysis)

Hip (multiaxial)

Knee (ginglymus)

Tibiofibular with interosseous membrane (syndesmosis)

Tibiofibular (arthrodial)

Ankle (ginglymus)

Subtalar (arthrodial)

Talocalcaneonavicular (arthrodial)

Intermetatarsal (arthrodial)

Tarsometatarsal (arthrodial)

Metatarsophalangeal (condyloid)

Interphalangeal (ginglymus)

Posterior View

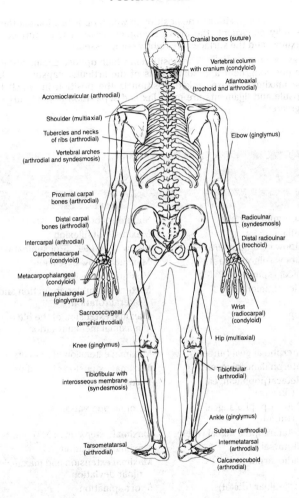

Cranial bones (suture)

Vertebral column with cranium (condyloid)

Atlantoaxial (trochoid and arthrodial)

Acromioclavicular (arthrodial)

Shoulder (multiaxial)

Tubercles and necks of ribs (arthrodial)

Vertebral arches (arthrodial and syndesmosis)

Elbow (ginglymus)

Proximal carpal bones (arthrodial)

Distal carpal bones (arthrodial)

Intercarpal (arthrodial)

Carpometacarpal (condyloid)

Metacarpophalangeal (condyloid)

Interphalangeal (ginglymus)

Radioulnar (syndesmosis)

Distal radioulnar (trochoid)

Sacrococcygeal (amphiarthrodial)

Wrist (radiocarpal) (condyloid)

Knee (ginglymus)

Hip (multiaxial)

Tibiofibular with interosseous membrane (syndesmosis)

Tibiofibular (arthrodial)

Ankle (ginglymus)

Subtalar (arthrodial)

Tarsometatarsal (arthrodial)

Intermetatarsal (arthrodial)

Calcaneocuboid (arthrodial)

CLOSE-PACKED AND LOOSE-PACKED POSITIONS FOR THE JOINTS

Definitions of Terms

close-packed position: The position in which opposing joint surfaces are fully congruent, the area of contact between joint surfaces is maximal, and the surfaces are tightly compressed.

loose-packed position: The position in which opposing joint surfaces are not congruent and some parts of the articular capsule are lax. The maximum loose-packed position is the position in which the capsule and ligaments are most lax and separation of joint surfaces is greatest.

CLOSE-PACKED POSITION OF JOINTS (in alphabetical order)	
Joint	*Close-Packed Position*
Acromioclavicular	Shoulder abducted to 30°
Ankle	Maximal dorsiflexion
Elbow (radiohumeral)	Elbow flexed 90°, 5° of supination
Elbow (ulnohumeral)	Maximal elbow extension
Facet (spine)	Maximal extension
Glenohumeral	Maximal shoulder abduction and lateral rotation
Hip	Maximal extension of the hip and maximal medial rotation of the hip
Interphalangeal (fingers)	Maximal extension of IP joints
Interphalangeal (toes)	Maximal extension of IP joints
Metacarpophalangeal (fingers)	Maximal flexion
Metacarpophalangeal (thumb)	Maximal opposition
Metatarsophalangeal (toes)	Maximal extension of MTP joints
Midtarsal	Maximal supination
Radiocarpal	Maximal extension and maximal ulnar deviation
Radioulnar (distal)	5° of supination
Radioulnar (proximal)	5° of supination
Sternoclavicular	Maximal shoulder elevation
Subtalar	Maximal supination
Tarsometatarsal	Maximal supination
Temporomandibular	Teeth clenched
Tibiofemoral	Maximal extension and maximal lateral rotation

MAXIMUM LOOSE-PACKED POSITIONS OF JOINTS
(in alphabetical order)

Joint	Loose-Packed Position
Acromioclavicular	Shoulder in anatomic position
Ankle	10° of plantar flexion
Carpometacarpal	Anatomic position of the wrist
Elbow (radiohumeral)	Anatomic position
Elbow (ulnohumeral)	70° of elbow flexion, 10° of supination
Facet (spine)	Midway between flexion and extension
Glenohumeral	55° of shoulder abduction, 30° of horizontal adduction
Hip	30° of hip flexion, 30° of hip abduction, and slight lateral rotation of the hip
Interphalangeal (fingers)	Slight flexion of IP joints
Interphalangeal (toes)	Slight flexion of IP joints
Metacarpophalangeal	Slight flexion of MCP joints
Metatarsophalangeal	Mid-range position
Midtarsal	Mid-range position
Radiocarpal	Anatomic position relative to flexion and extension with slight ulnar deviation
Radioulnar (distal)	10° of supination
Radioulnar (proximal)	70° of elbow flexion, 35° of supination
Sternoclavicular	Shoulder in anatomic position
Subtalar	Mid-range position
Tarsometatarsal	Mid-range position
Temporomandibular	Mouth slightly open
Tibiofemoral	25° of knee flexion

2

FOR MORE INFORMATION

Magee, DJ: Orthopedic Physical Assessment, ed 2. WB Saunders, Philadelphia, 1992.

Warwick, R and Williams, PL: Gray's Anatomy, ed 36. WB Saunders, Philadelphia, 1980.

MAJOR LIGAMENTS AND THEIR FUNCTIONS

UPPER EXTREMITY (proximal to distal)		
Joint	**Ligament**	**Function**
Shoulder girdle	Coracoclavicular	Binds the clavicle to the coracoid process
	Costoclavicular	Binds the clavicle to the costal cartilage of the first rib
Shoulder	Coracohumeral	Strengthens the upper portion of the joint capsule
	Glenohumeral	Reinforces the anterior aspect of the joint capsule
	Coracoacromial	Protects the superior aspect of the joint
Elbow	Annular	Holds the head of radius in position
	Ulnar collateral	Restricts medial displacement of the elbow joint
	Radial collateral	Restricts lateral displacement of the elbow joint
Wrist	Volar and dorsal radioulnar	Holds the distal ends of the radius and ulna in place
	Flexor and extensor retinacula	Holds tendons against fingers
	Interosseous	Binds the carpal bones together
	Dorsal and volar collateral	Connects articulations between the rows of carpal bones
Fingers	Volar and collateral interphalangeal	Prevents displacements of the interphalangeal joints

2

Joint	Ligament	Function
Ischium	Sacrospinous	Runs from sacrum to ischial spine to create the greater sciatic foramen
	Sacrotuberous	Runs from the sacrum to the ischial tuberosity and prevents the sacrum from tilting excessively; creates lesser sciatic foramen
Pubis	Transverse	Converts the acetabular notch into a foramen
	Superior pubic	Holds the pubic bones together
	Arcuate pubic	Holds the pubic bones together
Hip	Ligamentum teres	Carries nutrient vessels into the head of the femur
	Transverse	Holds the femoral head in place
	Iliofemoral	Limits extension of the hip joint
	Ischiofemoral	Limits anterior displacement of the hip joint
	Pubofemoral	Limits extension of the hip joint
Tibiofemoral	Medial collateral	Stabilizes the medial aspect of the knee joint (tibial-femoral articulation)
	Lateral collateral	Stabilizes the lateral aspect of the knee joint (tibial-femoral articulation)
	Medial and lateral menisci	Cartilages that provide stability and cushioning to

Continued on following page

Joint	Ligament	Function
		the tibial-femoral articulation
	Anterior cruciate	Prevents backward sliding of the femur and hyperextension of the knee
	Posterior cruciate	Prevents forward sliding of the femur
	Oblique and arcuate popliteal	Provides lateral and posterior support to the knee joint
Ankle	Deltoid	Provides stability between the medial malleolus, navicular, talus, and calcaneus
	Anterior and posterior talofibular	Secures the fibula to the talus
	Calcaneofibular	Secures the fibula to the calcaneus
Intertarsal	Long plantar	Provides a groove for the peroneus longus tendon and runs from the calcaneus to the metatarsals
	Calcaneonavicular	Supports the head of the talus between the navicular and the calcaneus
Tarsometatarsal	Dorsal and plantar interosseus	Limits movement of the tarsal bones
Intermetatarsal	Dorsal and plantar metatarsal	Limits movement of the metatarsal bones
Metatarsophalangeal	Plantar and transverse metatarsal	Holds the metatarsophalangeal joints in place

VERTEBRAL (caudal to cephalad)		
Joint	Ligament	Function
Vertebral column	Iliolumbar	Provides stability between L4–L5 and the iliac crest
	Interspinous	Limits movement between the spinous processes
	Lateral odontoid	Stabilizes the odontoid process of the axis with respect to the occipital condyles
	Lateral occipitoatlantal	Stabilizes the transverse process of the atlas and the jugular processes of the occipital bone
	Sacroiliac	Consists of two ligaments that hold the sacrum to the ilium
	Flava	Holds adjacent lamina together
	Nuchae	Runs from C7 to the occipital bone for reinforced neck stability; limits movement between cervical spinous processes
	Anterior and posterior longitudinal	Reinforces and strengthens the vertebral bodies and disks

2

GRADING OF LIGAMENTOUS SPRAINS

Grade I: Microscopic tearing of the ligament with no loss of function.

Grade II: Partial disruption or stretching of the ligament with some loss of function.

Grade III: Complete tearing of the ligament with complete loss of function.

FROM

Zarins, B and Boyle, J: Knee ligament injuries. In Nicholas, AJ and Hershman, EB (eds): The Lower Extremity and Spine in Sports Medicine, ed. 2. CV Mosby, St. Louis, 1995, with permission.

HUGHSTON CLASSIFICATION SYSTEM FOR QUANTIFYING KNEE JOINT LAXITY

1+: 0 to 5 mm of joint separation.

2+: 5 to 10 mm of joint separation.

3+: Greater than 10 mm of joint separation.

FROM

Hughston, JC, et al: Classification of knee ligament instabilities. Part 1: The medial compartment and cruciate ligaments. J Bone Joint Surg 58A: 159, 1976, with permission.

CLASSIFICATION OF KNEE LIGAMENT INJURIES ACCORDING TO O'DONOGHUE

mild (first degree): A few fibers of the ligament are damaged; there is no loss of the strength of the ligament. Little treatment is necessary. Treatment is only for relief of symptoms.

moderate (second degree): A definite tear in some component of the ligament with loss of strength of the ligament. There is no wide separation of the fibers. Treatment is primarily to protect the ligament.

severe (third degree): Ligament is torn completely and no longer functions. There is potentially a wide separation of fragments of the ligament. Treatment is to restore ligament continuity.

FROM

O'Donoghue, DH: Treatment of Injuries to Athletes, ed 4. WB Saunders, Philadelphia, 1984, with permission.

TERMS USED TO DESCRIBE POSITIONAL DEFORMITIES

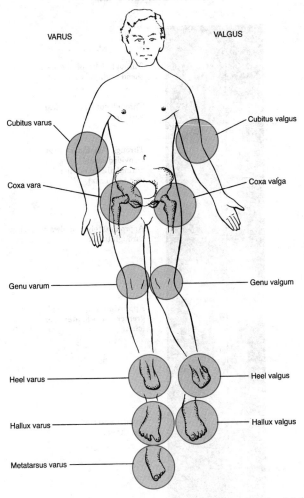

VARUS

VALGUS

Cubitus varus

Cubitus valgus

Coxa vara

Coxa valga

Genu varum

Genu valgum

Heel varus

Heel valgus

Hallux varus

Hallux valgus

Metatarsus varus

Varus deformities (on the left) and valgus deformities (on the right) as they occur at various limb segments.

IDEAL PLUMB LINE ALIGNMENT
ACCORDING TO KENDALL
Surface Landmarks

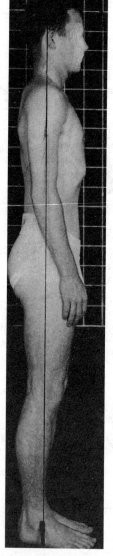

Through lobe of the ear (head is slightly forward)

Through bodies of cervical vertebrae

Through shoulder joint (provided arms hang in normal alignment in relation to thorax)

Approximately midway through trunk

Approximately through greater trochanter of femur

Slightly anterior to a mid-line through knee

Slightly anterior to lateral malleolus.

Surface landmarks that coincide with the plumb line.

Anatomic Structures

Slightly posterior to apex of coronal suture

Through external auditory meatus

Through odontoid process of axis

Through bodies of lumbar vertebrae

Through sacral promontory

Slightly posterior to center of hip joint

Slightly anterior to axis of knee joint

Through calcaneocuboid joint

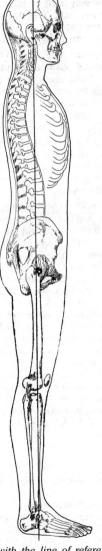

Anatomical structures that coincide with the line of reference. Pages 116 and 117 from Kendall, FP, McCreary, EK, and Provance, PG: Muscles: Testing and Function, ed 4. Williams & Wilkins, Baltimore, 1993, p 75, with permission.

SYSTEMS FOR NOTATING AND RECORDING ROM MEASUREMENTS

0 to 180 system: This system, first described by Silver, is probably the most widely used system of notating and recording range of motion measurements. The starting position (the anatomical position) for all movements except pronation and supination is considered to be 0. Movements then proceed toward 180 degrees.

180 to 0 system: According to Clark, who first described this system, the anatomical position is designated as the 180-degree position for all joints. Movements toward flexion approach 180-degrees, and movements toward extension or past the 180-degree or neutral position approach 0 degrees. Movements in the frontal plane also approach 0 degrees. External rotation movements approach 180 degrees, and internal rotation movements approach zero.

360-degree system: This system, first described by West, is similar to the 180- to 0-degree system in that the neutral starting position for most joints is designated as 180 degrees. Movements of flexion are toward 0 degrees, and movements beyond the neutral position are toward 360 degrees.

SFTR system of recording range of motion values: The SFTR (abbreviation for sagittal, frontal, transverse, and rotation) system combines the 0 to 180 method for notating range-of-motion (ROM) measurements with a systematic set of rules for recording these measurements. The following rules guide the use of the SFTR system. All joint motions are measured from the anatomical position. All joint motions and positions are recorded in the three basic planes (sagittal, frontal, and transverse). Motions of internal and external rotation are recorded as rotations.

All motions are recorded with three numbers. Motions leading away from the body are recorded first, and motions leading toward the body are recorded last. The starting position is recorded in the middle and is usually 0. For example, an elbow that can be hyperextended 10 degrees and flexed 140 degrees would be recorded as S 10-0-140. The S indicates motion in the sagittal plane. All fixed positions, such as ankyloses, are recorded with two numbers. For example, an elbow that is ankylosed at a position of 30 degrees of flexion would be recorded as S 0-30. Lateral bending and rotation of the spine to the left is recorded first and motions to the right are recorded last.

FROM

Clark, WA: A system of joint measurements. J Orthop Surg 2:687, 1920.

Gerhardt, JJ: Clinical measurements of joint motion and position in the neutral-zero method and SFTR recording: Basic principles. Int Rehab Med 5:161, 1983.

Gerhardt, JJ and Russe, OA: International SFTR Method of Measuring and Recording Joint Motion. Huber, Bern, 1975.

Silver, D: Measurement of the range of motion in joints. J Bone Joint Surg 21:569, 1923.

West, CC: Measurement of joint motion. Arch Phys Med 26:414, 1945.

CERVICAL SPINE RANGE OF MOTION FOR ADULTS
(in degrees)

Motion	AAOS*	AMA†	Capuano-Pucci et al.‡ ($N = 20$) Mean	Standard Deviation
Flexion	45	60	50.9	9
Extension	45	75	69.5	9.1
Left lateral flexion	45	45	43.7	8.3
Right lateral flexion	45	45		
Left rotation	60	80	70.8	5.3
Right rotation	60	80		

*Values were obtained using a universal goniometer.
†Values obtained using an inclinometer.
‡Values obtained using the CROM measurement device.
Data from American Academy of Orthopedic Surgeons: Joint Motion: Method of Measuring and Recording, AAOS, Chicago, 1965; American Medical Association: Guides to the Evaluation of Permanent Impairment, ed 3. AMA, Chicago, 1988; Capuano-Pucci, D et al: Intratester and intertester reliability of the cervical range of motion. Arch Phys Med Rehabil 72:338, 1991.

THORACOLUMBAR AND LUMBOSACRAL RANGE OF MOTION FOR ADULTS (in degrees)

Motion	AAOS (thoracolumbar)	AMA (lumbosacral)†
Flexion	80 (4 in)*	60
Extension	20–30	25
Right lateral flexion	35	25
Left lateral flexion	35	25
Right rotation	45	30
Left rotation	45	30

*Flexion measurement in inches was obtained with a tape measure using the spinous processes of C7 and S1 as reference points.
†Lumbosacral motion was measured from midsacrum to T12 using a two-inclinometer method.
Data from American Academy of Orthopedic Surgeons: Joint Motion: Method of Measuring and Recording, AAOS, Chicago, 1965; and American Medical Association: Guides to the Evaluation of Permanent Impairment, ed 3. AMA, Chicago, 1988.

RANGE OF MOTION FOR THE EXTREMITIES OF ADULTS ACCORDING TO VARIOUS AUTHORS (in degrees)

Joint	AAOS	AMA	Boone and Azen	Clark	CMA	Dorinson and Wagner	Esch and Lepley	Gerhardt and Russe	Hislop and Montgomery	Hoppenfeld	Kapandji	Kendall, McCreary, and Provance	Wiechec and Krusen
Shoulder													
Flexion	180	180	167	130	170	180	170	170	180	—	180	180	180
Extension	60	50	62	80	30	45	60	50	45	45	50	45	45
Abduction	180	180	184	180	170	180	170	170	180	180	180	180	180
Internal rotation	70	90*	69	90*	60*	90	80	80	80	55	95	70	90
External rotation	90	90*	104	40*	80*	90	90	90	60	45	80	90	90
Horizontal abduction	—	—	45	—	—	—	—	30	90	—	—	90	—
Horizontal adduction	135	—	140	—	—	—	—	135	130	—	—	40	—
Elbow													
Flexion	150	140	143	150	135	145	150	150	150	150	145	145	135
Radioulnar													
Pronation	80	80	76	50	75	80	90	80	80	90	85	90	90
Supination	80	80	82	90	85	70	90	90	80	90	90	90	90
Wrist													
Flexion	80	60	76	80	70	80	90	60	80	80	85	80	60
Extension	70	60	75	70	65	55	70	50	70	70	85	70	55
Radial deviation	20	20	22	15	20	20	20	20	—	20	15	20	35
Ulnar deviation	30	30	36	30	40	40	30	30	—	30	—	35	75
Hip													
Flexion	120	100	122	120	110	125	130	125	120	135	120	125	120
Extension	30	30	10	20	30	50	45	15	0	30	30	10	45

Abduction	45	40	46	55	50	45	45	45	45	50	30	45
Adduction	30	20	27	45	30	20	15	20	20	30	30	—
Internal rotation	45	40	47	20	35	30	33	45	45	35	30	—
External rotation	45	50	47	45	50	50	36	45	45	45	60	—
Knee												
Flexion	135	150	143	145	135	140	135	130	135	135	160	135
Ankle												
Plantar flexion	50	40	56	50	50	45	65	45	45	50	50	45
Dorsiflexion	20	20	13	15	15	20	10	20	20	20	30	30
Subtalar Joint												
Inversion	35	30	37	—	35	50	30	40	35	—	52	40
Eversion	15	20	26	—	20	20	15	20	25	—	30	20

*Measurements obtained with the shoulder in 0 degrees of abduction.

Data from American Academy of Orthopedic Surgeons: Joint Motion: Method of Measuring and Recording. AAOS, Chicago, 1965; American Medical Association: Guides to the Evaluation of Permanent Impairment, ed 3. AMA, Chicago, 1988; Boone, DC and Azen, SP: Normal range of motion in male subjects. J Bone Joint Surg 61A:756, 1979; Clark, WA: A system of joint measurement. J Orthop Surg 2:687, 1920; Commission of California Medical Association and the Industrial Accident Commission of the State of California: Evaluation of Industrial Disability. Oxford University Press, NY, 1960; Dorinson, SM and Wagner, ML: An exact technique for clinically measuring and recording joint motion. Arch Phys Med 29:468, 1948; Esch, D and Lepley, M: Evaluation of Joint Motion: Methods of Measurement and Recording. University of Minnesota Press, Minneapolis, 1974; Gerhardt, JJ and Russe, OA: International SFTR Method of Measuring and Recording Joint Motion. Huber, Bern, 1975; Hislop, HJ and Montgomery, J: Daniels and Worthingham's Muscle Testing: Techniques of Manual Examination, ed 6. WB Saunders, Philadelphia, 1995; Hoppenfeld, S: Physical Examination of the Spine and Extremities. Appleton-Century-Crofts, NY, 1976; Kapandji, IA: Physiology of the Joints, Vols 1 and 2, ed 2. Churchill Livingstone, London, 1982; Kendall, FP, McCreary, EK, and Provance, PG: Muscles: Testing and Function, ed 4. Williams & Wilkins, Baltimore, 1993; and Wiechec, FJ and Krusen, FH: A new method of joint measurement and a review of the literature. Am J Surg 43:659, 1939.

121

SUMMARY OF THE RELIABILITY OF GONIOMETRIC MEASUREMENTS AS OBTAINED IN A CLINICAL SETTING

The values can be interpreted as the percent agreement associated with multiple measurements; for instance, an intraclass correlation coefficient (ICC) of 0.95 means 95% agreement and 5% error associated with the measurement between or within therapists. Unless otherwise indicated the statistic used to calculate the ICC was formula (1,1) of Shrout and Fleiss. N indicates the number of subjects to obtain the ICC.

INTRATESTER RELIABILITY			
Joint	*Motion*	ICC	N
Shoulder	Flexion	0.98	100
	Extension	0.94	100
	Abduction	0.98	100
	Horizontal abduction	0.91	100
	Horizontal adduction	0.96	100
	External rotation	0.98	100
	Internal rotation	0.94	100
Elbow	Extension	0.95*	24
	Flexion	0.95*	24
Knee	Extension	0.95*	24
	Flexion	0.98*	24
Ankle	Subtalar neutral	0.77	100
	Inversion	0.74†	100
	Eversion	0.75†	100
	Dorsiflexion	0.90	100
	Plantarflexion	0.86	100

INTERTESTER RELIABILITY			
Joint	*Motion*	ICC	N
Shoulder	Flexion	0.88	50
	Extension	0.27	50
	Abduction	0.85	50
	Horizontal abduction	0.29	50
	Horizontal adduction	0.37	50
	External rotation	0.90	50
	Internal rotation	0.48	50
Elbow	Extension	0.94*	12
	Flexion	0.93*	12

INTERTESTER RELIABILITY			
Joint	**Motion**	**ICC**	**N**
Knee	Extension	0.70*	12
	Flexion	0.85*	12
Ankle	Subtalar neutral	0.25	50
	Inversion	0.32†	50
	Eversion	0.17†	50
	Dorsiflexion	0.50	50
	Plantar flexion	0.72	50

*These ICC values were calculated using a less conservative form of the ICC than the other ICC values listed in the table.

†These measurements were not referenced back to the subtalar position.

Data for Shoulder—Riddle, DL, Rothstein, JM, and Lamb, RL: Goniometric reliability in a clinical setting: Shoulder measurements. Phys Ther 67:668, 1987; Elbow and knee—Rothstein, JM, Miller, PJ, and Roettger, RF: Goniometric reliability in a clinical setting: Elbow and knee measurements. Phys Ther 63:1611, 1983; Foot and ankle—Elveru, R, et al: Goniometric reliability in a clinical setting: Subtalar and ankle measurements. Phys Ther 68:672, 1988; Shrout, PE, Fleiss, JL: Intraclass correlations: Uses in assessing rater reliability. Psychol Bull 86:420, 1979.

MUSCLES LISTED ALPHABETICALLY

The muscles of the body are listed in alphabetical order. The functions, secondary functions, origins, insertions, and innervations are listed for the major muscles.

abdominals: See *obliquus externus abdominis, obliquus internus abdominis, rectus abdominis,* and *transversus abdominis.*

abductor digiti minimi of the foot: *Function*—abducts the small toe; *origin*—medial and lateral processes of the calcaneal tuberosity, the plantar aponeurosis, and the intermuscular septum; *insertion*—the lateral side of the proximal phalanx of the fifth toe; *innervation*—lateral plantar nerve, S2–S3.

abductor digiti minimi of the hand: *Function*—abducts the fifth finger; *secondary function*—flexes the fifth finger; *origin*—the pisiform bone, the tendon of flexor carpi ulnaris; *insertion*—the ulnar side of the base of the proximal phalanx of the little finger; *innervation*—ulnar nerve, C8–T1.

abductor hallucis: *Function*—abducts and flexes the great toe; *origin*—the flexor retinaculum, the calcaneal tuberosity, the plantar aponeurosis, and the intermuscular septum; *insertion*—the medial side of the base of the proximal phalanx of the great toe; *innervation*—medial plantar nerve, L5–S1.

abductor pollicis brevis: *Function*—abducts the thumb; *origin*—the flexor retinaculum, the scaphoid, and the trapezium; *insertion*—the radial side of the proximal phalanx at the base of the thumb; *innervation*—median nerve, C8–T1.

Continued on following page

abductor pollicis longus: *Function*—abducts and extends the thumb; *secondary function*—abducts the wrist; *origin*—the middle third of the posterior surface of the radius, the posterior surface of the ulna, and the interosseous membrane; *insertion*—the radial side of the base of the first metacarpal bone; *innervation*—radial nerve, C6–C7.

adductor brevis: *Function*—adducts and flexes the thigh; *secondary function*—rotates the thigh medially; *origin*—the external aspect of the body and inferior ramus of the pubis; *insertion*—by an aponeurosis to the line from the greater trochanter to the linea aspera of the femur; *innervation*—obturator nerve, L2–L4.

adductor hallucis: *Function*—adducts the great toe; *origin*—the oblique head arises from the second, third, and fourth metatarsal bones, and the transverse head arises from the plantar ligaments of the third, fourth, and fifth toes; *insertion*—the lateral sesamoid bone and base of the first phalanx of the large toe; *innervation*—lateral plantar nerve, S2–S3.

adductor longus: *Function*—adducts and flexes the thigh; *secondary function*—rotates the thigh medially; *origin*—the pubic crest and symphysis; *insertion*—by an aponeurosis to the middle third of the linea aspera of the femur; *innervation*—obturator nerve, L2–L4.

adductor magnus: *Function*—adducts the thigh; *secondary function*—upper fibers flex and rotate the thigh medially, and lower fibers extend and rotate the thigh laterally; *origin*—the inferior ramus of the pubis, the ramus of ischium, and the inferolateral aspect of the ischial tuberosity; *insertion*—by an aponeurosis to the linea aspera and adductor tubercle of the femur; *innervation*—obturator nerve, L2–L4, and tibial portion of the sciatic nerve, L2–L4.

adductor pollicis: *Function*—adducts the thumb; *origin*—the oblique head arises from the capitate, bases of the second and third metacarpals, and the palmar carpal ligaments, and the transverse head arises from the distal two thirds of the palmar surface of the third metacarpal; *insertion*—fibers converge into a tendon containing a sesamoid bone that attaches to the ulnar side of the base of the proximal phalanx of the thumb; *innervation*—ulnar nerve, C8–T1.

anal sphincter (external): *Function*—closes the anal canal and orifice; *innervation*—S4 and inferior rectal branch of the pudendal nerve.

anal sphincter (internal): *Function*—assists external sphincter in an involuntary manner; *innervation*—sympathetic and sacral parasympathetic fibers by way of inferior mesenteric and hypogastric plexuses.

anconeus: *Function*—extends the forearm; *origin*—the posterior surface of the lateral epicondyle of the humerus; *insertion*—the lateral side of the olecranon and the proximal fourth of the posterior shaft of the ulna; *innervation*—radial nerve, C7–C8.

anterior deltoid: See *deltoid.*

articularis genus: *Function*—retracts the synovial membrane of the knee joint proximally (cephalad); *origin*—the anterior surface of the distal shaft of the femur; *insertion*—the upper part of the synovial membrane of the knee joint; *innervation*—femoral nerve, L3–L4.

aryepiglotticus: *Function*—closes the glottal opening; *innervation*— recurrent laryngeal branches of the vagus nerve.

arytenoid (arytenoideus): *Function*—closes glottal opening; *innervation*—recurrent branches of the vagus nerve.

auricularis anterior: *Function*—draws auricula forward and upward; *innervation*—temporal branches of the facial nerve.

auricularis posterior: *Function*—draws auricula backward; *innervation*—posterior auricular branches of the facial nerve.

auricularis superior: *Function*—draws auricula upward: *innervation*—temporal branches of the facial nerve.

biceps brachii: *Function*—flexes the arm (the long head), flexes the forearm (both heads), and supinates the forearm; *origin*—the short head arises from the coracoid process, and the long head arises from the supraglenoid tubercle at the apex of the glenoid cavity; *insertion*—the radial tuberosity of the radius; *innervation*—musculocutaneous nerve, C5–C6.

biceps femoris (long head): *Function*—flexes and laterally rotates the leg and extends and laterally rotates the thigh; *origin*—the ischial tuberosity and the sacrotuberous ligament; *insertion*—the head of the fibula and lateral condyle of the tibia; *innervation*—tibial portion of the sciatic nerve, S1–S3.

biceps femoris (short head): *Function*—flexes and laterally rotates the leg; *origin*—the lateral tip of the linea aspera of the femur; *insertion*—the head of the fibula and the lateral condyle of the tibia; *innervation*—peroneal portion of the sciatic nerve, L5–S2.

brachialis: *Function*—flexes the forearm; *origin*—the distal half of the anterior surface of the humerus; *insertion*—the tuberosity of the ulna and the coronoid process; *innervation*—musculocutaneous, C5–C6, and radial nerve (for sensory only).

brachioradialis: *Function*—flexes the forearm; *origin*—the proximal two thirds of the lateral supracondylar ridge of the humerus; *insertion*—the styloid process of the radius; *innervation*—radial nerve, C5–C6.

buccinator: *Function*—compresses the cheek (assists in mastication); *origin*—the alveolar process of the maxillary bone, the pterygomandibular raphe, and the buccinator ridge of the mandible; *insertion*—the orbicularis oris; *innervation*—buccal branches of the facial nerve.

bulbospongiosus (bulbocavernosus): *Function*—empties the canal of the urethra and in the female reduces the orifice of the vagina; *innervation*—perineal branch of pudendal nerve, S2–S4.

chondroglossus: See *hyoglossus.*

ciliaris: *Function*—draws the ciliary process centrally and relaxes the suspensory ligaments of the lens, changing the convexity of the lens; *innervation*—short ciliary nerves.

coccygeus: *Function*—brings the coccyx ventrally; *innervation*—pudendal plexus including S4–S5.

constrictor inferior: See *inferior constrictor.*

Continued on following page

constrictor medius: See *middle constrictor.*

constrictor superior: See *superior constrictor.*

coracobrachialis: *Function*—flexes and adducts the arm; *origin*—the coracoid process of the scapula; *insertion*—the middle of the medial surface of the humerus; *innervation*—musculocutaneous nerve, C6–C7.

corrugator supercilii: *Function*—draws the eyebrow down and medially; *origin*—the superciliary arch of the frontal bone; *insertion*—the skin over the middle third of the supraorbital margins; *innervation*—temporal and zygomatic branches of the facial nerve.

cremaster: *Function*—in the male draws testes up, and in the female draws labial folds up toward the superficial inguinal ring; *innervation*—genital branch of the genitofemoral nerve.

cricoarytenoideus lateralis: See *lateral cricoarytenoid.*

cricoarytenoideus posterior: See *posterior cricoarytenoid.*

cricothyroid (cricothyroideus): *Function*—tightens the vocal cords; *innervation*—internal laryngeal nerve of the vagus nerve.

deltoid: (see individual listings for anterior, middle, and posterior): *Function*—abducts the arm; *secondary function*—ventral fibers rotate the arm medially, and dorsal fibers rotate the arm laterally; *innervation*—axillary nerve, C5–C6.

deltoid (anterior): *Function*—flexes the arm; *origin*—the lateral third of the clavicle; *insertion*—the deltoid tuberosity of the lateral aspect of the humerus; *innervation*—axillary nerve, C5–C6.

deltoid (middle): *Function*—abducts the arm; *origin*—the superior surface of the acromion; *insertion*—the deltoid tuberosity of the lateral aspect of the humerus; *innervation*—axillary nerve, C5–C6.

deltoid (posterior): *Function*—extends the arm; *origin*—the spine of the scapula; *insertion*—the deltoid tuberosity of the lateral aspect of the humerus; *innervation*—axillary nerve, C5–C6.

depressor anguli oris: *Function*—Depresses the angle of mouth; *origin*—the oblique line of the mandible; *insertion*—the skin at the angle of the mouth; *innervation*—mandibular and buccal branches of the facial nerve.

depressor labii inferioris: *Function*—draws the lower lip down and back; *origin*—the oblique line of the mandible; *insertion*—the skin of the lower lip; *innervation*—mandibular and buccal branches of the facial nerve.

depressor septi: *Function*—draws the ala of the nose downward; *innervation*—buccal branches of the facial nerve.

diaphragm: *Function*—draws the central tendon downward and forward during inspiration to increase the volume and decrease the pressure within the thoracic cavity and also decreases the volume and increases the pressure within abdominal cavity; *origin*—the xiphoid process, the costal cartilages of the lower six ribs, and the lumbar vertebrae; *insertion*—the central tendon; *innervation*—phrenic nerve, C3–C5.

digastricus (anterior belly): *Function*—brings hyoid bone forward; *innervation*—mylohyoid nerve from the inferior alveolar branch of the mandibular division of the trigeminal nerve.

digastricus (posterior belly): *Function*—Brings hyoid bone backward; *innervation*—facial nerve.

dilator pupillae: *Function*—dilates the pupil; *innervation*—sympathetic efferents from the superior cervical ganglion.

dorsal interossei of the foot: See *interossei.*

dorsal interossei of the hand: See *interossei.*

extensor carpi radialis brevis: *Function*—extends the wrist; *secondary function*—abducts the wrist; *origin*—the lateral epicondyle of the humerus, the radial collateral ligament of the elbow and its covering aponeurosis; *insertion*—the dorsal surface of the base of the third metacarpal; *innervation*—radial nerve, C6–C7.

extensor carpi radialis longus: *Function*—extends and abducts the wrist; *origin*—the distal one third of the lateral supracondylar ridge of the humerus; *insertion*—the radial side of the base of the second metacarpal; *innervation*—radial nerve, C6–C8.

extensor carpi ulnaris: *Function*—extends and adducts the wrist; *origin*—the lateral epicondyle; *insertion*—the tubercle on the medial side of the base of the fifth metacarpal; *innervation*—radial nerve, C6–C8.

extensor digiti minimi: *Function*—extends the fifth finger; *origin*—the common extensor tendon; *insertion*—the extensor hood (dorsal digital expansion) of the fifth digit; *innervation*—radial nerve, C6–C8.

extensor digitorum: *Function*—extends the fingers; *secondary function*—extends the wrist; *origin*—the lateral epicondyle of the humerus by a common extensor tendon; *insertion*—the middle and distal phalanges of the second through fifth digits; *innervation*—radial nerve, C6–C8.

extensor digitorum brevis: *Function*—extends the proximal phalanges of the great toe and the adjacent three toes; *origin*—the superolateral surface of the calcaneus; *insertion*—the first phalanx of the great toe and the tendons of the extensor digitorum longus; *innervation*—deep peroneal nerve, L5–S1.

extensor digitorum longus: *Function*—extends the proximal phalanges of the four toes; *secondary function*—dorsiflexes, abducts, and everts the foot; *origin*—the lateral condyle of the tibia, the proximal three fourths of the anterior surface of the fibula, and the interosseous membrane; *insertion*—the middle and distal phalanges of the second through fifth digits; *innervation*—deep peroneal nerve, L4–S1.

extensor hallucis longus: *Function*—extends the proximal phalanx of the great toe; *secondary function*—dorsiflexes, adducts, and inverts the foot; *origin*—the middle two fourths of the medial surface of the fibula; *insertion*—the dorsal aspect of the base of the distal phalanx of the great toe; *innervation*—deep peroneal nerve, L4–S1.

Continued on following page

extensor indicis: *Function*—extends the index finger; *secondary function*—abducts the index finger; *origin*—the posterior surface of the ulna and the interosseous membrane; *insertion*—the extensor hood of the index finger; *innervation*—radial nerve, C6–C8.

extensor pollicis brevis: *Function*—extends the proximal phalanx of the thumb; *origin*—the posterior surface of the radius and interosseus membrane; *insertion*—the dorsal surface of the base of the proximal phalanx of the thumb; *innervation*—radial nerve, C6–C7.

extensor pollicis longus: *Function*—extends the second phalanx of the thumb; *origin*—the middle third of the posterior surface of the shaft of the ulna; *insertion*—the base of the distal phalanx of the thumb; *innervation*—radial nerve, C6–C8.

external intercostals: See *intercostales externi.*

external oblique: See *obliquus externus abdominis.*

extrinsic muscles of the eye: See *levator palpebrae superioris, obliquus inferior, obliquus superior, rectus inferior, rectus lateralis, rectus medialis,* and *rectus superior.*

flexor carpi radialis: *Function*—flexes and abducts the wrist; *origin*—the common flexor tendon from the medial epicondyle of the humerus; *insertion*—the palmar surface of the base of the second metacarpal; *innervation*—median nerve, C6–C7.

flexor carpi ulnaris: *Function*—flexes and adducts the wrist; *origin*—one head arises from the common flexor tendon of the medial epicondyle of the humerus, and the other head arises from the medial margins of the olecranon and the proximal two thirds of the posterior border of the ulna; *insertion*—the pisiform bone and the fifth metacarpal; *innervation*—ulnar nerve, C8–T1.

flexor digiti minimi brevis of the foot: *Function*—flexes the proximal phalanx of small toe; *origin*—the plantar surface of the base of the fifth metatarsal; *insertion*—the lateral side of the base of the proximal phalanx of the fifth toe; *innervation*—lateral plantar nerve, S2–S3.

flexor digiti minimi brevis of the hand: *Function*—flexes the fifth finger; *origin*—the hamulus (hook) of the hamate and the flexor retinaculum; *insertion*—the ulnar side of the base of the proximal phalanx of the little finger; *innervation*—ulnar nerve, C8–T1.

flexor digitorum accessorius: See *quadratus plantae.*

flexor digitorum brevis: *Function*—flexes the second phalanges of the four toes; *origin*—the medial process of the tuberosity of the calcaneus, the plantar aponeurosis, and the intermuscular septa; *insertion*—the tendons divide and attach to both sides of the middle phalanges of the second through fifth toes; *innervation*—medial plantar nerve, L5–S1.

flexor digitorum longus: *Function*—flexes the four toes; *secondary function*—plantar flexes the ankle and flexes, adducts, and inverts the foot; *origin*—the posterior surface of the tibia; *insertion*—the distal phalanges of the second through fifth toes; *innervation*—tibial nerve, L5–S1.

flexor digitorum profundus: *Function*—flexes the distal phalanx of each finger; *secondary function*—flexes the more proximal phalanges of each finger and flexes the wrist; *origin*—the proximal three fourths of the anterior and medial surfaces of the ulna, the interosseous membrane, and a depression on the medial side of the coronoid process; *insertion*—the palmar surface of the base of the distal phalanx of the second through fifth digits; *innervation*—median and ulnar nerves, C8–T1.

flexor digitorum superficialis: *Function*—flexes the second phalanx of each finger; *secondary function*—flexes the first phalanx of each finger and flexes the wrist; *origin*—the medial epicondyle of the humerus by the common flexor tendon, the intermuscular septa, the medial side of the coronoid process, and the anterior border of the radius from the radial tuberosity to the insertion of the pronator teres; *insertion*—tendons divide and insert into the sides of the shaft of the middle phalanx of the second through fifth digits; *innervation*—median nerve, C7–C8.

flexor hallucis brevis: *Function*—flexes the proximal phalanx of the great toe; *origin*—the medial part of the plantar surface of the cuboid, the lateral cuneiform, and the medial intermuscular septum; *insertion*—the tendon divides and attaches to the sides of the base of the proximal phalanx of the hallux (a sesamoid bone is usually in each of the attachments); *innervation*—medial plantar nerve, L5–S1.

flexor hallucis longus: *Function*—flexes the distal (second) phalanx of the great toe; *secondary function*—flexes, adducts, and inverts the foot; *origin*—the inferior two thirds of the posterior surface of the fibula, the distal part of the interosseous membrane, the posterior crural intermuscular septum, and the fascia; *insertion*—the plantar aspect of the base of the distal phalanx of the great toe; *innervation*—tibial nerve, L5–S2.

flexor pollicis brevis: *Function*—flexes the proximal phalanx of the thumb and adducts the thumb; *origin*—the superficial head arises from the distal border of the flexor retinaculum and the tubercle of the trapezium, and the deep head arises from the trapezoid and capitate; *insertion*—the superficial head attaches by a tendon containing a sesamoid bone to the radial side of the base of the proximal phalanx of the thumb, and the deep head attaches by a tendon that unites with the superficial head on the sesamoid bone and base of the first phalanx; *innervation*—superficial head: median nerve, C8–T1; deep head: ulnar nerve, C8–T1.

flexor pollicis longus: *Function*—Flexes the second phalanx of the thumb; *origin*—the grooved anterior surface of the radius, the interosseous membrane; *insertion*—the palmar surface of the base of the distal phalanx of the thumb; *innervation*—median nerve, C8–T1.

gastrocnemius: *Function*—plantar flexes the foot and flexes the leg; *origin*—the medial head arises from the posterior part of the medial femoral condyle, and the lateral head arises from the lateral surface of the lateral femoral condyle; *insertion*—both heads form a tendon that joins the tendon of the soleus to form the tendocalcaneus, which inserts on the posterior surface of the calcaneus; *innervation*—tibial nerve, S1–S2.

Continued on following page

gemelli (superior and inferior): *Function*—laterally rotates the extended thigh and abducts the flexed thigh; *origin*—the superior gemellus arises from the dorsal surface of the spine of the ischium, and the inferior gemellus arises from the upper part of the tuberosity of the ischium; *insertion*—both the superior and inferior gemelli attach to the medial surface of the greater trochanter; *innervation*—superior gemellus: nerve to obturator internus, L5–S2; inferior gemellus: nerve to quadratus femoris, L4–S1.

genioglossus: *Function*—protrudes or retracts the tongue and elevates the hyoid bone; *innervation*—hypoglossal nerve.

geniohyoid: *Function*—brings the hyoid bone anteriorly; *innervation*—branch of first cervical nerve via the hypoglossal nerve.

gluteus maximus: *Function*—extends and laterally rotates the thigh; *origin*—the posterior gluteal line of the ilium, the iliac crest, the aponeurosis of the erector spinae, the dorsal surface of the lower part of the sacrum, the side of the coccyx, the sacrotuberous ligament, and the intermuscular fascia; *insertion*—the iliotibial tract of the fascia lata and the gluteal tuberosity of the femur; *innervation*—inferior gluteal nerve, L5–S2.

gluteus medius: *Function*—abducts and medially rotates the thigh; *secondary function*—the anterior portion flexes the thigh, and the posterior portion extends the thigh; *origin*—the outer surface of the ilium between the iliac crest and the posterior gluteal line, the anterior gluteal line, and the fascia; *insertion*—the lateral surface of the greater trochanter; *innervation*—superior gluteal nerve, L4–S1.

gluteus minimus: *Function*—abducts and medially rotates the thigh; *origin*—the outer surface of the ilium between the anterior and inferior gluteal lines, and the margin of the greater sciatic notch; *insertion*—the ridge laterally situated on the anterior surface of the greater trochanter; *innervation*—superior gluteal nerve, L4–S1.

gracilis: *Function*—adducts the thigh; *secondary function*—flexes the leg and rotates the tibia medially; *origin*—the thin aponeurosis from the medial margins of the lower half of the body of the pubis and the whole of the inferior ramus; *insertion*—the proximal part of the medial surface of the tibia, below the tibial condyle and just proximal to the tendon of the semitendinosus; *innervation*—obturator nerve, L2–L3.

hamstrings muscles: See *biceps femoris, semitendinosus,* and *semimembranosus.*

hyoglossus and chondroglossus: *Function*—depresses the side of tongue and retracts the tongue; *innervation*—hypoglossal nerve.

iliacus: *Function*—flexes the thigh; *origin*—the superior two thirds of the iliac fossa and the upper surface of the lateral part of the sacrum; *insertion*—fibers converge with tendon of the psoas major; *innervation*—femoral nerve, L2–L3.

iliocostalis (cervicis, thoracis, lumborum): See individual muscles.

iliocostalis cervicis: *Function*—extends the vertebral column and bends it to one side; *origin*—angles of the third through sixth ribs; *insertion*—posterior tubercles of the transverse processes of the fourth, fifth, and sixth cervical vertebrae; *innervation*—dorsal primary divisions of the spinal nerves.

iliocostalis lumborum: *Function*—extends the vertebral column and bends it to one side and draws the ribs down; *origin*—the broad erector spinae tendon from the median sacral crest; the spines of the lumbar and lower thoracic vertebrae, and the iliac crest; *insertion*—lumbar borders of the angles of the lower six or seven ribs; *innervation*—dorsal primary divisions of the spinal nerves.

iliocostalis thoracis: *Function*—extends the vertebral column, bends it to one side, and draws the ribs down; *origin*—upper borders of the angles of the lower six ribs; *insertion*—upper borders of the angles of the upper six ribs; *innervation*—dorsal primary divisions of the spinal nerves.

inferior constrictor: *Function*—narrows the pharynx for swallowing; *innervation*—pharyngeal plexus and external laryngeal and recurrent nerves.

inferior gemellus: See *gemelli.*

inferior oblique: See *obliquus inferior.*

inferior rectus: See *rectus inferior.*

infraspinatus: *Function*—laterally rotates the arm; *secondary function*—the upper fibers abduct and the lower fibers adduct the arm; *origin*—the medial two thirds of the infraspinatus fossa; *insertion*—the middle impression (facet) on the greater tubercle of the humerus; *innervation*—suprascapular nerve, C5–C6.

intercostal muscles: See *intercostales externi* and *intercostales interni.*

intercostales externi: *Function*—elevates the ribs to increase the volume of the thoracic cavity; *origin*—the inferior border of the rib above; *insertion*—the superior border of the rib below; *innervation*—intercostal nerves.

intercostales interni: *Function*—elevates the ribs to decrease the volume of the thoracic cavity; *origin*—the floor of the costal grooves; *insertion*—the upper border of the rib below; *innervation*—intercostal nerves.

internal intercostals: See *intercostales interni.*

internal oblique: See *obliquus internus abdominis.*

interossei of the foot (dorsal): *Function*—abducts the toes; *secondary function*—flexes the proximal phalanges and extends the distal phalanges; *origin*—the dorsal interossei arise via two heads from the adjacent sides of two metatarsal bones; *insertion*—bases of the proximal phalanges and to the dorsal digital expansions, the first reaching the medial side of the second toe and the other three passing to the lateral sides of the second, third, and fourth toes; *innervation*—lateral plantar nerve, S2–S3.

interossei of the foot (plantar): *Function*—adduct the third through fifth digits; *secondary function*—flexes proximal phalanges and extends the distal phalanges; *origin*—bases and medial sides of the third, fourth, and fifth metatarsal bones; *insertion*—medial sides of the bases of the proximal phalanges of the same toes and into their dorsal digital expansions; *innervation*—lateral plantar nerve, S2–S3.

Continued on following page

interossei of the hand (dorsal): *Function*—abducts the fingers; *secondary function*—flexes the metacarpophalangeal joints and extends the interphalangeal joints; *origin*—adjacent sides of two metacarpal bones; *insertion*—bases of the proximal phalanges and extensor hoods (dorsal digital expansions), the first interosseus is attached to the radial side of the proximal phalanx of the index finger; the second and third interossei are attached to the middle finger, the second to the radial side and the third to the ulnar side; and the fourth interosseus attaches to the dorsal digital expansion of the ring finger; *innervation*—ulnar nerve, C8–T1.

interossei of the hand (palmar): *Function*—adducts fingers; *secondary function*—flexes the metacarpophalangeal joints and extends the interphalangeal joints; *origin*—with the exception of the first, each of the four arises from the entire length of the metacarpal bone of one finger, and the first interosseus arises from the ulnar side of the palmar surface of the base of the first metacarpal bone; *insertion*—the first interosseus inserts into a sesamoid bone on the ulnar side of the proximal phalanx of the thumb and into the thumb's dorsal digital expansion, and the remaining three interossei pass to the dorsal digital expansion of the same digit; *innervation*—ulnar nerve, C8–T1.

intertransversarii: *Function*—bends the vertebral column laterally; *origin*—transverse processes of the vertebrae; *insertion*—adjacent transverse processes; *innervation*—anterior, lateral, and posterior branches of the ventral primary divisions of the spinal nerves.

ischiocavernosus: *Function*—in the male compresses the crus of the penis and in the female compresses the crus of the clitoris; *innervation*—perineal branch of the pudendal nerve, S2–S4.

lateral cricoarytenoid: *Function*—narrows the glottis; *innervation*—recurrent laryngeal nerve of the vagus nerve.

lateral pterygoid: *Function*—opens the jaw, protrudes the mandible, and moves the mandible from side to side; *origin*—the upper head arises from the infratemporal surface and infratemporal crest of the greater wing of the sphenoid bone, and the lower head arises from the lateral surface of the lateral pterygoid plate; *insertion*—a depression on the front of the neck of the mandible, the articular capsule, and the disk of the temporomandibular joint; *innervation*—lateral pterygoid nerve of the mandibular division of the trigeminal nerve.

lateral rectus: See *rectus lateralis*.

latissimus dorsi: *Function*—adducts, extends, and medially rotates the arm; *origin*—spines of the lower six thoracic vertebrae, the posterior layer of the thoracolumbar fascia, and the posterior part of the crest of the ilium; *insertion*—the bottom of the intertubercular sulcus of the humerus; *innervation*—thoracodorsal nerve, C6–C8.

levator anguli oris: *Function*—raises the angle of the upper lip; *innervation*—buccal branches of the facial nerve.

levator ani iliococcygeus: *Function*—supports and raises the pelvic floor and resists any increase in intra-abdominal pressure; *innervation*—pudendal plexus, including S3–S5.

levator ani pubococcygeus: *Function*—brings the anus toward the pubis and constricts it; *innervation*—pudendal plexus, including S3–S5.

levator labii superioris: *Function*—elevates the upper lip; *innervation*—buccal branches of the facial nerve.

levator labii superioris alaeque nasi: *Function*—elevates the upper lip and dilates the naris; *innervation*—buccal branches of the facial nerve.

levator palpebrae superioris: *Function*—raises the upper eyelid; *innervation*—oculomotor nerve.

levator scapulae: *Function*—elevates the scapula; *secondary function*—rotates the scapula downward; *origin*—transverse processes of the atlas and axis and posterior tubercles of the transverse processes of the third and fourth cervical vertebrae; *insertion*—medial border of the scapula between the superior angle and the spine; *innervation*—C3–C4 and frequently the dorsal scapular nerve, C5.

levator veli palatini: *Function*—elevates the soft palate; *innervation*—pharyngeal plexus.

levatores costarum: *Function*—raises the ribs to increase the thoracic cavity and extends the vertebral column, bending it laterally with slight rotation to opposite side; *origin*—ends of the transverse processes of the seventh cervical and first to eleventh thoracic vertebrae; *insertion*—the upper edge and external surfaces of the rib immediately below the vertebrae, from which it takes origin between the tubercle and the angle; *innervation*—intercostal nerves.

longissimus capitis: *Function*—extends the head and bends it to the same side, rotating the face to that side; *origin*—transverse processes of the upper four or five thoracic vertebrae; *insertion*—the posterior margin of the mastoid process; *innervation*—dorsal primary divisions of spinal nerves.

longissimus cervicis: *Function*—extends the vertebral column and bends it to one side while drawing the ribs down; *origin*—transverse process of the upper four or five thoracic vertebrae; *insertion*—posterior tubercles of the transverse processes of C2–C6; *innervation*—dorsal primary divisions of spinal nerves.

longissimus thoracis: *Function*—extends the vertebral column and bends it to one side while drawing the ribs down; *origin*—the whole length of the posterior surfaces of the transverse processes of the lumbar vertebrae; *insertion*—to the tips of the transverse processes of all the thoracic vertebrae and lower 9 or 10 ribs; *innervation*—dorsal primary divisions of spinal nerves.

longus capitis: *Function*—flexes head; *origin*—the anterior tubercles of the transverse processes of the third, fourth, fifth, and sixth cervical vertebrae; *insertion*—the inferior surface of the basilar part of the occipital bone; *innervation*—branches of spinal nerves C1–C3.

longus colli: *Function*—flexes the neck with slight cervical rotation; *origin*—the superior oblique portion arises from the anterior tubercles of the transverse processes of the third, fourth, and fifth cervical vertebrae, the inferior oblique portion arises from the anterior surfaces of the first two thoracic vertebrae, and the vertical portion arises from the anterolateral surface of the bodies of the first three thoracic and last three cervical vertebrae; *insertion*—the superior
Continued on following page

oblique portion inserts on the tubercle of the atlas, the inferior oblique portion inserts on the anterior tubercles of the transverse processes of the fifth and sixth cervical vertebrae, and the vertical portion inserts into the anterior surface of the bodies of the second through fourth cervical vertebrae; *innervation*—ventral branches of the C2–C6 spinal nerves.

lower trapezius: See *trapezius.*

lumbricals of the foot: *Function*—flexes the proximal phalanges and extends the distal phalanges of the four toes; *origin*—tendons of the flexor digitorum longus; *insertion*—the extensor hoods (dorsal digital expansions) on the proximal phalanges of the second through fifth digits; *innervation*—first lumbrical is by the medial plantar nerve, L5–S1, and second through fourth lumbricals by the lateral plantar nerve, S2–S3.

lumbricals of the hand: *Function*—flexes the metacarphalangeal joints and extends the interphalangeal joints; *origin*—tendons of the flexor digitorum profundus; *insertion*—lateral margins of the extensor hoods (dorsal digital expansions) of the second through fifth digits; *innervation*—first and second lumbricals by the median nerve, C8–T1, and third and fourth lumbricals by the ulnar nerve, C8–T1.

masseter: *Function*—closes the jaw; *origin*—the zygomatic process of the maxilla and from the anterior two thirds of the lower border of the zygomatic arch; *insertion*—the angle and ramus of the mandible; *innervation*—masseteric branch of the mandibular division of the trigeminal nerve.

medial pterygoid: *Function*—closes the jaw; *origin*—the medial surface of the lateral pterygoid plate and the pyramidal process of the palatine bone; *insertion*—the posterior part of the medial surfaces of the ramus and angle of the mandible; *innervation*—medial pterygoid branch of the mandibular division of the trigeminal nerve.

medial rectus: See *rectus medialis.*

mentalis: *Function*—raises and protrudes the lower lip and wrinkles the chin; *origin*—the incisive fossa of the mandible; *insertion*—the skin of the chin; *innervation*—mandibular and buccal branches of the facial nerve.

middle constrictor: *Function*—narrows the pharynx for swallowing; *innervation*—pharyngeal plexus.

middle deltoid: See *deltoid.*

multifidus: *Function*—extends the vertebral column and rotates it toward opposite side; *origin*—the sacral portion arises from the posterior superior iliac spine and the dorsal sacroiliac ligaments, the lumbar portion arises from the mamillary processes, the thoracic portion arises from all thoracic transverse processes, and the cervical portion arises from the articular processes of the lower four vertebrae; *insertion*—the whole length of the spine of the vertebrae above; *innervation*—dorsal primary divisions of the spinal nerves.

musculus uvulae: *Function*—elevates the uvula; *innervation*—pharyngeal plexus of the accessory nerve.

mylohyoid: *Function*—raises the hyoid bone and tongue; *innervation*—mylohyoid nerve of the mandibular division of the trigeminal nerve.

nasalis: *Function*—enlarges the opening of nares; *innervation*—buccal branches of the facial nerve.

obliques: See *obliquus externus abdominis* and *obliquus internus abdominis*.

obliquus capitis inferior: *Function*—rotates the atlas and turns the head to the same side; *origin*—the spine of the axis; *insertion*—the transverse process of the atlas; *innervation*—dorsal primary ramus of the suboccipital nerve.

obliquus capitis superior: *Function*—extends and bends the head laterally; *origin*—the transverse process of the atlas; *insertion*—the occipital bone between the superior and inferior nuchal lines; *innervation*—dorsal primary ramus of the suboccipital nerve.

obliquus externus abdominis: *Function*—compresses the abdominal contents, flexes the vertebral column, and rotates the column to bring forward the shoulder on the same side as the active muscle; *origin*—inferior borders of the lower eight ribs; *insertion*—the iliac crest, the aponeurosis; *innervation*—intercostal nerves, T7–T12.

obliquus inferior: *Function*—elevates, abducts, and rotates the eye laterally; *innervation*—oculomotor nerve.

obliquus internus abdominis: *Function*—compresses abdominal contents, flexes the vertebral column, and rotates the column to bring the shoulder forward on the side opposite from the active muscle; *origin*—the lateral two thirds of the upper surface of the inguinal ligament, the iliac crest, and the thoracolumbar fascia; *insertion*—posterior fibers pass upward and laterally to the inferior borders of the lower three or four ribs, the inguinal ligament fibers attach to the crest of the pubis, and the remainder of the fibers end in an aponeurosis that forms the linea alba; *innervation*—branches of the intercostal nerves from T8–T12 and the iliohypogastric and ilioinguinal branches of L1.

obliquus superior: *Function*—depresses, abducts, and rotates the eye laterally; *innervation*—trochlear nerve.

obturator externus: *Function*—laterally rotates the thigh; *origin*—rami of the pubis, the ramus of the ischium, and the medial two thirds of the outer surface of the obturator membrane; *insertion*—the trochanteric fossa of the femur; *innervation*—obturator nerve, L3–L4.

obturator internus: *Function*—laterally rotates the thigh; *secondary function*—abducts when the thigh is flexed; *origin*—the internal surface of the anterolateral wall of the pelvis and the obturator membrane; *insertion*—the medial surface of the greater trochanter; *innervation*—nerve to obturator internus, L5–S2.

occipitofrontalis: *Function*—draws scalp back to raise the eyebrows and wrinkles forehead; *origin*—the superior nuchal line of the occipital bone and intermuscular attachments with the orbicularis oculi; *insertion*—the galea aponeurotica; *innervation*—temporal and posterior auricular branches of the facial nerve.

Continued on following page

omohyoid: *Function*—draws the hyoid bone downward; *innervation*—ansa cervicalis containing fibers of C1–C3.

opponens digiti minimi: *Function*—abducts, flexes, and laterally rotates the fifth finger; *origin*—the hamulus (hook) of the hamate bone and the flexor retinaculum; *insertion*—the whole length of the ulnar margin and the fifth metacarpal bone; *innervation*—ulnar nerve, T1.

opponens pollicis: *Function*—abducts, flexes, and medially rotates the thumb; *origin*—the ridge of the trapezium and the flexor retinaculum; *insertion*—the whole length of the lateral border of the metacarpal bone of the thumb; *innervation*—median nerve (sometimes by branch of the ulnar nerve), C8–T1.

orbicularis oculi: *Function*—closes the eyelids; *innervation*—temporal and zygomatic branches of the facial nerve.

orbicularis oris: *Function*—closes the lips; *innervation*—buccal branches of the facial nerve.

palatoglossus: *Function*—elevates the posterior tongue and constricts the fauces; *innervation*—pharyngeal plexus of the accessory nerve.

palatopharyngeus: *Function*—constricts the fauces and closes off the nasopharynx; *innervation*—pharyngeal plexus.

palmar interossei of the foot: See *interossei.*

palmar interossei of the hand: See *interossei.*

palmaris brevis: *Function*—wrinkles the skin of the ulnar side of the palm; *origin*—the flexor retinaculum and the palmar aponeurosis; *insertion*—the dermis on the ulnar border of the hand; *innervation*—ulnar nerve, C8–T1.

palmaris longus: *Function*—flexes the hand; *origin*—the palmar longus arises from the common flexor tendon on the medial epicondyle of the humerus; *insertion*—the palmar aponeurosis; *innervation*—median nerve, C6–C7.

pectineus: *Function*—flexes and adducts the thigh; *secondary function*—rotates the thigh medially; *origin*—the pecten of the pubis; *insertion*—along a line leading from the lesser trochanter to the linea aspera; *innervation*—femoral, obturator, or accessory obturator nerves, L2–L4.

pectoralis major: *Function*—flexes and adducts the arm; *secondary function*—rotates the arm medially; *origin*—the anterior surface of the sternal half of the clavicle, the anterior surface of the sternum as low as the attachment of the cartilage of the sixth rib, from the cartilages of all true ribs, and from the aponeurosis of the obliquus externus abdominis; *insertion*—the lateral lip of the intertubercular sulcus of the humerus; *innervation*—medial and lateral pectoral nerves, C5–T1.

pectoralis minor: *Function*—rotates the scapula downward and forward; *secondary function*—raises third, fourth, and fifth ribs; *origin*—third, fourth, and fifth ribs; *insertion*—the medial border of the coracoid process; *innervation*—medial pectoral nerve, C8–T1.

peroneus brevis: *Function*—everts and abducts the foot; *secondary function*—plantar flexes the foot; *origin*—the distal two thirds of the lateral surface of the fibula and the crural intermuscular septa; *insertion*—the tubercle on the base of the fifth metatarsal bone on its lateral side; *innervation*—superficial peroneal nerve, L4–S1.

peroneus longus: *Function*—everts and abducts the foot; *secondary function*—plantar flexes the foot; *origin*—the head and the proximal two thirds of the lateral surface of the fibula and the crural intermuscular septa; *insertion*—lateral side of the base of the first metatarsal bone and the medial cuneiform; *innervation*—superficial peroneal nerve, L4–S1.

peroneus tertius: *Function*—abducts, dorsiflexes, and everts the foot; *origin*—the lower (distal) third of the anterior surface of the fibula and the crural intermuscular septum; *insertion*—the dorsal surface of the base of the fifth metatarsal bone; *innervation*—deep peroneal nerve, L5–S1.

piriformis: *Function*—laterally rotates and abducts thigh; *origin*—anterior sacrum, the gluteal surface of the ilium, the capsule of the sacroiliac joint, and the sacrotuberus ligament; *insertion*—the upper border of the greater trochanter of the femur; *innervation*—sacral plexus, S1.

plantar interossei: See *interossei.*

plantaris: *Function*—flexes the leg; plantar flexes the foot; *origin*—the distal linea aspera (lower part of the lateral supracondylar line) and from the oblique popliteal ligament; *insertion*—inserts with the tendocalcaneus into the calcaneus; *innervation*—tibial nerve, L4–S1.

platysma: *Function*—retracts and depresses the angle of the mouth; *innervation*—cervical branch of the facial nerve.

popliteus: *Function*—flexes the leg, rotates the leg (tibia) medially; *origin*—the lateral condyle of the femur and the arcuate popliteal ligament; *insertion*—the medial two thirds of the triangular area above the soleal line on the posterior surface of the tibia; *innervation*—tibial nerve, L4–S1.

posterior cricoarytenoid: *Function*—opens the glottis; *innervation*—recurrent laryngeal nerve of the vagus nerve.

posterior deltoid: See *deltoid.*

procerus: *Function*—wrinkles the nose and draws the medial eyebrow downward; *origin*—the fascia covering the lower part of the nasal bone; *insertion*—the skin over the lower part of the forehead between the eyebrows; *innervation*—buccal branches of the facial nerve.

pronator quadratus: *Function*—pronates the forearm; *origin*—the oblique ridge on the distal part of the anterior surface of the shaft of the ulna; *insertion*—the distal fourth of the anterior border and the surface of the shaft of the radius; *innervation*—median nerve, C8–T1.

pronator teres: *Function*—pronates the forearm; *origin*—the humeral head arises from the common flexor tendon on the medial epicondyle of the humerus, and the ulnar head arises from the me-

Continued on following page

dial side of the coronoid process of the ulna; *insertion*—the rough area midway along the lateral surface of the radial shaft; *innervation*—median nerve, C6–C7.

psoas major: *Function*—flexes the thigh; *secondary function*—flexes the lumbar vertebrae and bends them laterally; *origin*—transverse processes of all the lumbar vertebrae, bodies and intervertebral disks of the lumbar vertebrae; *insertion*—lesser trochanter of the femur; *innervation*—lumbar plexus, L2–L3.

psoas minor: *Function*—flexes the pelvis and the lumbar vertebrae; *origin*—sides of the bodies of the 12th thoracic and 1st lumbar vertebrae and from the disk between them; *insertion*—the pecten pubis (pectineal line) and iliopectineal eminence; *innervation*—lumbar plexus, L1.

pyramidalis: *Function*—tightens the linea alba; *origin*—the pubic crest; *insertion*—linea alba; *innervation*—branch of 12th thoracic nerve.

quadratus femoris: *Function*—rotates the thigh laterally; *origin*—the ischial tuberosity; *insertion*—the quadrate tubercle of the femur; *innervation*—nerve to quadratus femoris, L4–S1.

quadratus lumborum: *Function*—laterally flexes the lumbar vertebral column; *origin*—the iliolumbar ligament and the iliac crest; *insertion*—the inferior border of the last rib and the transverse processes of the first four lumbar vertebrae; *innervation*—T12–L3 (or L4).

quadratus plantae (flexor digitorum accessorius): *Function*—flexes the distal phalanges of the third through fifth digits; *origin*—a medial head arises from the medial concave surface of the calcaneus, and a lateral head arises from the lateral border of the calcaneus and long plantar ligament; *insertion*—tendons of the flexor digitorum longus; *innervation*—lateral plantar nerve, S2–S3.

quadriceps femoris: See *rectus femoris, vastus lateralis, vastus intermedius,* and *vastus medialis.*

rectus abdominis: *Function*—flexes the vertebral column, tenses the anterior abdominal wall, and assists in compressing the abdominal contents; *origin*—the crest of the pubis; *insertion*—fifth, sixth, and seventh costal cartilages; *innervation*—T7–T12 and ilioinguinal (L1) and iliohypogastric nerves, (T12–L1).

rectus capitis anterior: *Function*—flexes the head; *origin*—the anterior surface of the lateral mass of the atlas; *insertion*—the basilar part of the occipital bone in front of the occipital condyle; *innervation*—fibers from cervical nerve of C1 and C2.

rectus capitis lateralis: *Function*—bends the head laterally; *origin*—the upper surface of the transverse process of the atlas; *insertion*—the inferior surface of the jugular process of the occipital bone; *innervation*—fibers from cervical nerves, C1–C2.

rectus capitis posterior major: *Function*—extends and rotates the head to the same side; *origin*—the spine of the axis; *insertion*—the lateral part of the inferior nuchal line of the occipital bone; *innervation*—dorsal ramus of C1 (suboccipital nerve).

rectus capitis posterior minor: *Function*—extends the head; *origin*—the tubercle on the posterior arch of the atlas; *insertion*—the medial part of the inferior nuchal line of the occipital bone; *innervation*—dorsal ramus of C1 (suboccipital nerve).

rectus femoris: *Function*—flexes the thigh and extends the leg; *origin*—by two heads, from the anterior inferior iliac spine, and a reflected head from the groove above the acetabulum; *insertion*—the base of the patella; *innervation*—femoral nerve, L2–L4.

rectus inferior: *Function*—depresses, adducts, and rotates the eye medially; *innervation*—oculomotor nerve.

rectus lateralis: *Function*—abducts the eye; *innervation*—abducens nerve.

rectus medialis: *Function*—adducts the eye; *innervation*—oculomotor nerve.

rectus superior: *Function*—elevates, adducts, and rotates the eye medially; *innervation*—oculomotor nerve.

rhomboid major: *Function*—adducts the scapula; *secondary function*—rotates the scapula down; *origin*—spines of the second through fifth thoracic vertebrae and supraspinous ligaments; *insertion*—medial border of the scapula between the root of the spine and the inferior angle; *innervation*—dorsal scapular nerve, C5.

rhomboid minor: *Function*—adducts the scapula; *secondary function*—rotates the scapula down; *origin*—the lower part of the ligamentum nuchae and from the spines of the seventh cervical and first thoracic vertebrae; *insertion*—the triangular smooth surface at the medial end of the spine of the scapula; *innervation*—dorsal scapular nerve, C5.

risorius: *Function*—retracts the angle of the mouth; *origin*—parotid fascia; *insertion*—the skin at the angle of the mouth; *innervation*—mandibular and buccal branches of the facial nerve.

rotatores: *Function*—extends vertebral column and rotates it toward the opposite side; *origin and insertion*—each of the rotatores connects the upper and posterior part of the transverse process of one vertebra to the lower border and lateral surface of the spine of the one or two vertebrae above; *innervation*—dorsal primary divisions of the spinal nerves.

salpingopharyngeus: *Function*—elevates the nasopharynx; *innervation*—pharyngeal plexus.

sartorius: *Function*—flexes, abducts, and laterally rotates the thigh, and also flexes and rotates the tibia medially; *origin*—the anterior superior iliac spine and the notch below the anterior superior iliac spine; *insertion*—the upper part of the medial surface of the tibia anterior to the gracilis; *innervation*—femoral nerve, L2–L3.

scalenus anterior: *Function*—raise the first rib; *origin*—anterior tubercles of the transverse processes of the third, fourth, fifth, and sixth cervical vertebrae; *insertion*—the scalene tubercle on the inner border of the first rib; *innervation*—branches from the anterior rami of C5–C6.

Continued on following page

scalenus medius: *Function*—raises the first rib; *origin*—the transverse process of the atlas and the posterior tubercles of the transverse processes of the lower six cervical vertebrae; *insertion*—the upper surface of the first rib; *innervation*—branches from the anterior rami of C3–C8.

scalenus posterior: *Function*—raises the second rib; *origin*—posterior tubercles of the transverse processes of the fourth, fifth, and sixth cervical vertebrae; *insertion*—the second rib; *innervation*—ventral primary rami of C6–C8.

semimembranosus: *Function*—flexes the leg and extends the thigh; *secondary function*—medially rotates the flexed leg; *origin*—the ischial tuberosity; *insertion*—medial tibial condyle; *innervation*—tibial portion of the sciatic nerve, L5–S2.

semispinalis capitis: *Function*—extends the head and rotates it toward opposite side; *origin*—transverse processes of the upper six or seven thoracic and the seventh cervical vertebrae; *insertion*—the medial part of the area between the superior and inferior nuchal lines of the occipital; *innervation*—dorsal primary divisions of cervical nerves.

semispinalis cervicis: *Function*—extends the vertebral column and rotates it toward opposite side; *origin*—transverse processes of the upper five or six thoracic vertebrae; *insertion*—spines of the cervical vertebrae; *innervation*—dorsal primary divisions of spinal nerves.

semispinalis thoracis: *Function*—extends the vertebral column and rotates it toward opposite side; *origin*—transverse processes of the 6th to 10th thoracic vertebrae; *insertion*—spines of the upper four thoracic and lower two cervical vertebrae; *innervation*—dorsal primary divisions of spinal nerves.

semitendinosus: *Function*—flexes the leg and extends the thigh; *secondary function*—medially rotates the flexed leg; *origin*—the ischial tuberosity; *insertion*—the upper part of the medial surface of the tibia behind the attachment of the sartorius and below that of the gracilis; *innervation*—tibial portion of the sciatic nerve, L5–S2.

serratus anterior: *Function*—rotates the scapula upward and abducts the scapula; *origin*—outer surfaces of the upper eight or nine ribs; *insertion*—the costal aspect of the medial border of the scapula; *innervation*—long thoracic nerve, C5–C7.

serratus posterior inferior: *Function*—draws the ribs down and out; *origin*—spines of the lower two thoracic and upper two lumbar vertebrae; *insertion*—inferior borders of the lower four ribs; *innervation*—ventral primary divisions of T9–T12.

serratus posterior superior: *Function*—raises the ribs to increase the size of the thoracic cavity; *origin*—the lower part of the ligamentum nuchae and the spines of the seventh cervical and the upper two thoracic vertebrae; *insertion*—upper borders of the second, third, fourth, and fifth ribs; *innervation*—ventral primary divisions of T1–T4.

soleus: *Function*—plantar flexes the foot; *origin*—the head and proximal third of the posterior surface of the fibula, and from the soleal line and middle third of the medial border of the tibia; *inser-*

tion—the soleus joins the tendon of gastrocnemius to form the tendocalcaneus inserting on the calcaneus; *innervation*—tibial nerve, S1–S2.

sphincter pupillae: *Function*—constricts the pupil; *innervation*—motor root of the ciliary ganglion from the oculomotor nerve.

sphincter urethrae: *Function*—compresses the urethra; *innervation*—perineal branch of the pudendal nerve, S2–S4.

spinalis (capitis, cervicis, thoracis): *Function*—extends the vertebral column; *origin*—arises from the spines of vertebrae in each region; *insertion*—on vertebral spines a few segments above; *innervation*—dorsal primary divisions of the spinal nerves.

splenius capitis: *Function*—brings the head and neck posteriorly and laterally with some rotation; *origin*—the lower half of the ligamentum nuchae, the spine of the seventh cervical vertebra, and the spines of the upper three or four thoracic vertebrae; *insertion*—the occipital bone inferior to the superior nuchal line and the mastoid process of the temporal bone; *innervation*—dorsal primary divisions of the middle cervical roots.

splenius cervicis: *Function*—brings the head and neck posteriorly and laterally with some rotation; *origin*—spines of the third to sixth thoracic vertebrae; *insertion*—posterior tubercles of the transverse processes of the upper two cervical vertebrae; *innervation*—dorsal primary divisions of the lower cervical roots.

stapedius: *Function*—pulls the head of the stapes posteriorly to increase tension of fluid in ear; *innervation*—the tympanic branch of the facial nerve.

sternocleidomastoid (sternomastoid): *Function*—rotates the head; *origin*—the upper part of the anterior surface of the manubrium sterni and the medial third of the clavicle; *insertion*—the mastoid process of the temporal bone; *innervation*—spinal part of the accessory nerve.

sternohyoid: *Function*—draws the hyoid bone inferiorly; *innervation*—branches of ansa cervicalis hypoglossi, including fibers from C1–C3.

sternomastoid: See *sternocleidomastoid.*

sternothyroid: *Function*—draws the larynx downward; *innervation*—branches of ansa cervicalis hypoglossi, including fibers from C1–C3.

styloglossus: *Function*—retracts and elevates the tongue; *innervation*—hypoglossal nerve.

stylohyoid: *Function*—elevates and retracts the hyoid bone; *innervation*—facial nerve.

stylopharyngeus: *Function*—elevates and dilates the pharynx; *innervation*—glossopharyngeal nerve.

subclavius: *Function*—depresses and pulls forward (anteriorly) the lateral end of the clavicle; *origin*—the junction of the first rib and its costal cartilage; *insertion*—the groove on the inferior surface of middle third of the clavicle; *innervation*—nerve to subclavius, C5–C6.

Continued on following page

subscapularis: *Function*—medially rotates the arm; *secondary function*—flexes, extends, abducts, and adducts the arm, depending on the arm position; *origin*—the medial two thirds of subscapular fossa; *insertion*—the lesser tubercle of the humerus; *innervation*—upper and lower subscapular nerves, C5–C6.

superior constrictor: *Function*—narrows the pharynx for swallowing; *innervation*—pharyngeal plexus.

superior gemellus: See *gemelli.*

superior oblique: See *obliquus superior.*

superior rectus: See *rectus superior.*

supinator: *Function*—supinates the forearm; *origin*—the lateral epicondyle of the humerus and the supinator crest of the ulna; *insertion*—the lateral surface of the proximal third of the radius; *innervation*—radial nerve, C6.

supraspinatus: *Function*—abducts the arm; *secondary function*—flexes and laterally rotates the arm; *origin*—the medial two thirds of the supraspinatus fossa; *insertion*—the superior facet of the greater tubercle of the humerus; *innervation*—suprascapular nerve, C5.

temporalis: *Function*—closes the jaw, and the posterior portion retracts the mandible; *origin*—the temporalis fossa; *insertion*—medial surface, apex, anterior, and posterior borders of the coronoid process and the anterior border of the ramus of the mandible; *innervation*—anterior and posterior deep temporal nerves of the mandibular division of the trigeminal nerve.

temporoparietalis: *Function*—draws the skin backward over temples and wrinkles the forehead; *innervation*—temporal branches of the facial nerve.

tensor fasciae latae: *Function*—flexes and abducts the thigh; *secondary function*—medially rotates the thigh; *origin*—the outer lip of the iliac crest and the lateral surface of the anterior superior iliac spine; *insertion*—iliotibial tract; *innervation*—superior gluteal nerve, L4–S1.

tensor tympani: *Function*—draws the tympanic membrane medially to increase tension on the membrane; *innervation*—mandibular division of the trigeminal nerve through the otic ganglion.

tensor veli palatini: *Function*—stretches the soft palate; *innervation*—trigeminal nerve.

teres major: *Function*—adducts and extends the arm; *secondary function*—medially rotates the arm; *origin*—the dorsal surface of the inferior angle of the scapula; *insertion*—the medial lip of the intertubercular sulcus of the humerus; *innervation*—lower subscapular nerve, C5–C6.

teres minor: *Function*—laterally rotates the arm; *secondary function*—adducts the arm; *origin*—the proximal two thirds of the lateral border of the scapula; *insertion*—inferior facet of the greater tubercle of the humerus; *innervation*—axillary nerve, C5.

thyroarytenoid (thyroarytenoideus): *Function*—relaxes the vocal cords; *innervation*—recurrent laryngeal nerve of the vagus nerve.

thyroepiglotticus: *Function*—depresses the epiglottis; *innervation*—recurrent laryngeal nerve of the vagus nerve.

thyrohyoid (thyroideus): *Function*—brings the hyoid bone inferiorly or raises the thyroid cartilage; *innervation*—fibers from C1.

tibialis anterior: *Function*—dorsiflexes, adducts, and inverts foot; *origin*—the lateral condyle and proximal half of the lateral surface of the tibial shaft; *insertion*—the medial cuneiform and the base of the first metatarsal bone; *innervation*—deep peroneal nerve, L4–S1.

tibialis posterior: *Function*—plantar flexes, adducts, and inverts the foot; *origin*—the posterior surface of the tibia and fibula; *insertion*—the tuberosity of the navicular, the three cuneiforms, the cuboid, and the bases of the second, third, and fourth metatarsals; *innervation*—tibial nerve, L5–S1.

transversus abdominis: *Function*—compresses the abdomen to assist in defecation, emesis, parturition, and forced expiration; *origin*—the lateral third of the inguinal ligament, the iliac crest, and the lower costal cartilages; *insertion*—primarily to the linear alba; *innervation*—branches of T7–T12, iliohypogastric and ilio-inguinal nerves.

transversus menti: *Function*—depresses the angle of the mouth; *innervation*—mandibular and buccal branches of the facial nerve.

transversus perinei profundus: *Function*—compresses the urethra; *innervation*—perineal branch of the pudendal nerve.

transversus perinei superficialis: *Function*—fixes the central tendinous part of the perineum; *innervation*—perineal branch of the pudendal nerve.

transversus thoracis: *Function*—brings the ventral ribs downward to decrease the size of the thoracic cavity; *origin*—the distal third of the posterior surfaces of the body of the sternum and the xiphoid process; *insertion*—lower borders of the costal cartilages of the second, third, fourth, fifth, and sixth ribs; *innervation*—intercostal nerves.

trapezius: *Function*—lower trapezius draws the scapula down, middle trapezius adducts the scapula, and upper trapezius draws the scapular upward; *origin*—the medial third of the superior nuchal line of the occipital bone, the external occipital protuberance, the ligamentum nuchae, the seventh cervical and all the thoracic vertebral spinous processes, and the corresponding supraspinous ligaments; *insertion*—the lateral third of the clavicle, the acromion process, and the spine of the scapula; *innervation*—spinal part of accessory nerve.

triceps brachii: *Function*—extends the forearm; *origin*—the long head arises from the infraglenoid tubercle of the scapula, the lateral head arises from the posterior surface of the shaft of the humerus along an oblique line above the radial groove, and the medial head arises from the posterior surface of the shaft of the humerus below the radial groove; *insertion*—the upper surface of the olecranon process of the ulna; *innervation*—radial nerve, C7–C8.

upper trapezius: See *trapezius*.

Continued on following page

vastus intermedius: *Function*—extends the leg; *origin*—anterior and lateral surfaces of the proximal two thirds of the femoral shaft; *insertion*—the patella, with some fibers passing over to blend with the ligamentum patellae; *innervation*—femoral nerve, L2–L4.

vastus lateralis: *Function*—extends the leg; *origin*—by a broad aponeurosis to the proximal part of the intertrochanteric line, anterior and inferior borders of the greater trochanter, the lateral lip of the gluteal tuberosity, and the proximal half of the lateral lip of the linea aspera; *insertion*—the lateral border of the patella; *innervation*—femoral nerve, L2–L4.

vastus medialis: *Function*—extends the leg; *origin*—the distal part of the intertrochanteric line, spiral line, the medial lip of the linea aspera, and the medial intermuscular septum; *insertion*—the medial border of the patella; *innervation*—femoral nerve, L2–L4.

vocalis: *Function*—closes the glottis; *innervation*—recurrent laryngeal branch of the vagus nerve.

zygomaticus major: *Function*—draws angle of mouth upward and backward; *origin*—the zygomatic bone in front of the zygomaticotemporal suture; *insertion*—the angle of the mouth; *innervation*—buccal branches of the facial nerve.

zygomaticus minor: *Function*—forms the nasolabial furrow; *origin*—the lateral surface of the zygomatic bone immediately behind the zygomaticomaxillary suture; *insertion*—the muscular substance of the upper lip; *innervation*—buccal branches of the facial nerve.

MUSCLES LISTED BY FUNCTION

For a more detailed description of muscle action, look under the muscle's name in the reference (alphabetized) list of muscles (starting on page 123). Here muscles are listed in the order of their relative importance in contributing to the movement listed. Nerves and innervating roots are in parentheses.

MUSCLES USED IN MOVEMENT OR STABILIZATION OF THE SCAPULA

Adduction	Abduction	Upward Rotation	Downward Rotation
Trapezius (spinal part of accessory nerve, sensory branches C3–C4)	Serratus anterior (long thoracic nerve, C5–C7)	Upper trapezius (spinal accessory nerve, sensory branches C3–C4)	Lower trapezius (spinal accessory nerve, sensory branches, C3–C4)
		Serratus anterior (long thoracic nerve, C5–C7)	Rhomboid major (dorsal scapular nerve, C5)
			Rhomboid minor (dorsal scapular nerve, C5)
			Levator scapulae (branches of C3 and C4, also frequently by the dorsal scapular nerve, C5)
			Pectoralis minor (medial pectoral nerve, C8–T1)

MUSCLES PRIMARILY ACTIVE AT THE GLENOHUMERAL JOINT			
Extension	*Flexion*	*Abduction*	*Adduction*
Latissimus dorsi (thoracodorsal nerve, C6–C8)	Pectoralis major (medial and lateral pectoral nerves, C5–T1)	Middle deltoid (axillary nerve, C5–C6)	Latissimus dorsi (thoracodorsal nerve, C6–C8)
Triceps brachii long head (radial nerve, C7–C8)	Anterior deltoid (axillary nerve, C5–C6)	Supraspinatus (suprascapular nerve, C5)	Pectoralis major (medial and lateral pectoral nerves, C5–T1)
Posterior deltoid (axillary nerve, C5–C6)	Supraspinatus (suprascapular nerve, C5)	Infraspinatus upper fibers C5 (suprascapular nerve, C5–C6)	Teres major (lower subscapular nerve, C5–C6)
Teres major (lower subscapular nerve, C5–C6)	Biceps brachii (musculocutaneous nerve, C5–C6)		Triceps brachii long head (radial nerve, C7–C8)
Subscapularis (upper and lower subscapular nerves, C5–C6)	Coracobrachialis (musculocutaneous nerve, C6–C7)		Teres minor (axillary nerve, C5)
	Subscapularis (upper and lower subscapular nerves, C5–C6)		Infraspinatus lower fibers (suprascapular nerve, C5–C6)

Medial Rotation	Lateral Rotation
Latissimus dorsi (thoracodorsal nerve, C6–C8)	Deltoid dorsal fibers (axillary nerve, C5–C6)
Pectoralis major (medial and lateral pectoral nerves, C5–T1)	Infraspinatus (suprascapular nerve, C5–C6)
Subscapularis (upper and lower subscapular nerves, C5–C6)	Supraspinatus (suprascapular nerve, C5)
Teres major (lower subscapular nerve, C5–C6)	Teres minor (axillary nerve, C5)
Deltoid ventral fibers (axillary nerve, C5–C6)	

MUSCLES OF THE ELBOW AND RADIOULNAR JOINTS

Extension	Flexion	Supination	Pronation
Triceps brachii long head (radial nerve, C7–C8)	Biceps brachii (musculocutaneous nerve, C5–C6)	Biceps brachii (musculocutaneous nerve, C5–C6)	Pronator teres (median nerve, C6–C7)
Anconeus (radial nerve, C7–C8)	Brachialis (musculocutaneous nerve, C5–C6, and radial nerve for sensory)	Supinator (radial nerve, C6)	Pronator quadratus (median nerve, C8–T1)
	Brachioradialis (radial nerve, C5–C6)		

MUSCLES OF THE WRIST

Extension	Flexion	Abduction	Adduction
Extensor carpi radialis longus (radial nerve, C6–C8)	Flexor carpi radialis (median nerve, C6–C7)	Flexor carpi radialis (median nerve, C6–C7)	Flexor carpi ulnaris (ulnar nerve, C8–T1)
Extensor carpi radialis brevis (radial nerve, C6–C7)	Flexor carpi ulnaris (ulnar nerve, C8–T1)	Extensor carpi radialis longus (radial nerve, C6–C8)	Extensor carpi ulnaris (radial nerve, C6–C8)
Extensor carpi ulnaris (radial nerve, C6–C8)	Palmaris longus (median nerve, C6–C7)	Extensor carpi radialis brevis (radial nerve, C6–C7)	
Extensor digitorum (radial nerve, C6–C8)	Flexor digitorum superficialis (median nerve, C7–C8)	Abductor pollicis longus (radial nerve, C6–C7)	
	Flexor digitorum profundus (median and ulnar nerves, C8–T1)	Extensor pollicis longus (radial nerve, C6–C8)	
		Extensor pollicis brevis (radial nerve, C6–C7)	

2

MUSCLES USED IN MOVEMENT OF THE FINGERS

Extension	Flexion	Abduction	Adduction
Extensor digitorum (radial nerve, C6–C8)	Flexor digitorum superficialis (median nerve, C7–C8)	Dorsal interossei (ulnar nerve, C8–T1)	Palmar interossei (ulnar nerve, C8–T1)
Extensor indicis (proprius) (radial nerve, C6–C8)	Flexor digitorum profundus (median and ulnar nerves, C8–T1)	Abductor digiti minimi (ulnar nerve, C8–T1)	
Extensor digiti minimi (radial nerve, C6–C8)	Flexor digiti minimi (ulnar nerve, C8–T1)	Opponens digiti minimi (ulnar nerve, T1)	
Lumbricals (1 and 2 by median nerve, C8–T1; 3 and 4 by ulnar nerve, C8–T1)	Opponens digiti minimi (ulnar nerve, T1)	Extensor indicis (radial nerve, C6–C8)	
Interossei (dorsal and palmar, IP extension) (ulnar nerve, C8–T1)	Lumbricals (1 and 2 by median nerve, C8–T1; 3 and 4 by ulnar nerve, C8–T1)		
	Interossei (dorsal and palmar, MTP flexion) (ulnar nerve, C8–T1)		

IP = interphalangeal, MTP = metatarsophalangeal.

MUSCLES USED IN MOVEMENT OF THE THUMB

Extension	Flexion	Abduction	Adduction
Extensor pollicis longus (radial nerve, C6–C8)	Flexor pollicis longus (median nerve, C8–T1)	Abductor pollicis longus (radial nerve, C6–C7)	Adductor pollicis (ulnar nerve, C8–T1)
Extensor pollicis brevis (radial nerve, C6–C7)	Flexor pollicis brevis (median nerve to superficial head, C8–T1; ulnar nerve to deep head, C8–T1)	Abductor pollicis brevis (median nerve, C8–T1)	Opponens pollicis (median nerve and sometimes by a branch of the ulnar, C8–T1)
	Opponens pollicis (median nerve and sometimes by a branch of the ulnar, C8–T1)		Flexor pollicis longus (median nerve, C8–T1)
			Flexor pollicis brevis (median nerve to superficial head, C8–T1; ulnar nerve to deep head, C8–T1)

2

MUSCLES USED IN MOVEMENT OF THE HIP

Flexion	Extension	Abduction	Adduction	Medial Rotation	Lateral Rotation
Psoas major (lumbar plexus, L2–L3)	Gluteus maximus (inferior gluteal nerve, L5–S2)	Gluteus medius (superior gluteal nerve, L4–S1)	Adductor magnus (obturator nerve, L2–L4; tibial portion of sciatic nerve, L2–L4)	Gluteus medius (superior gluteal nerve, L4–S1)	Gluteus maximus (inferior gluteal nerve, L5–S2)
Psoas minor (lumbar plexus, L1)	Gluteus medius (posterior portion) (superior gluteal nerve, L4–S1)	Gluteus minimus (superior gluteal nerve, L4–S1)	Gracilis (obturator nerve, L2–L3)	Gluteus minimus (superior gluteal nerve, L4–S1)	Sartorius (femoral nerve, L2–L3)
Iliacus (femoral nerve, L2–L3)	Biceps femoris (long head) (tibial portion of sciatic nerve, S1–S3)	Piriformis (sacral plexus, S1)	Adductor longus (obturator nerve, L2–L4)	Tensor fasciae latae (superior gluteal nerve, L4–S1)	Piriformis (sacral plexus, S1)
Sartorius (femoral nerve, L2–L3)	Semimembranosus (tibial portion of sciatic nerve, L5–S2)	Obturator internus (nerve to obturator internus, L5–S2)	Adductor brevis (obturator nerve, L2–L4)	Adductor longus (obturator nerve, L2–L4)	Obturator internus (nerve to obturator internus, L5–S2)
Rectus femoris (femoral nerve, L2–L4)	Semitendinosus		Pectineus (femoral, obturator, or	Pectineus (femoral, obturator, or	Gemellus superior (nerve to obturator internus, L5–S2)
Pectineus (femoral, obturator, or accessory obturator nerves, L2–L4)					

Gluteus medius (anterior portion) (superior gluteal nerve, L4–S1)
Gluteus minimus (superior gluteal nerve, L4–S1)
Adductor longus (obturator nerve, L2–L4)
Adductor brevis (obturator nerve, L2–L4)
Adductor magnus (upper portion) (obturator nerve, L2–L4; tibial portion of sciatic nerve, L2–L4)

(tibial portion of sciatic nerve, L5–S2)
Adductor magnus (lower portion) (obturator nerve, L2–L4; tibial portion of sciatic nerve, L2–L4)
Piriformis (sacral plexus, S1)
Obturator internus (nerve to obturator internus, L5–S2)

accessory obturator nerves, L2–L4

accessory obturator nerves, L2–L4
Adductor brevis (obturator nerve, L2–L4)
Adductor magnus (upper portion) (obturator nerve, L2–L4; tibial portion of sciatic nerve, L2–L4)

Adductor magnus (lower portion) (obturator nerve, L2–L4; tibial portion of sciatic nerve, L2–L4)
Gemellus inferior (nerve to quadratus femoris, L4–S1)
Obturator externus (obturator nerve, L3–L4)

2

MUSCLES USED IN MOVEMENT OF THE KNEE

Flexion	Extension	Medial Rotation of the Tibia	Lateral Rotation of the Tibia
Biceps femoris (long head: tibial portion of sciatic nerve, S1–S3; and short head: peroneal portion of sciatic nerve, L5–S2)	Rectus femoris (femoral nerve, L2–L4)	Sartorius (femoral nerve, L2–L3)	Biceps femoris (long head: tibial portion of sciatic nerve, S1–S3; and short head: peroneal portion of sciatic nerve, L5–S2)
Semitendinosus (tibial portion of sciatic nerve, L5–S2)	Vastus medialis (femoral nerve, L2–L4)	Gracilis (obturator nerve, L2–L3)	
Semimembranosus (tibial portion of sciatic nerve, L5–S2)	Vastus intermedius, (femoral nerve, L2–L4)	Semitendinosus (tibial portion of sciatic nerve, L5–S2)	
Gastrocnemius (tibial nerve, S1–S2)	Vastus lateralis (femoral nerve, L2–L4)	Semimembranosus (tibial portion of sciatic nerve, L5–S2)	
Plantaris (tibial nerve, L4–S1)	Articularis genus (femoral nerve, L3–L4)		
Sartorius (femoral nerve, L2–L3)			

MUSCLES USED IN MOVEMENT OF THE ANKLE AND SUBTALAR JOINTS					
Dorsiflexion	**Plantar Flexion**	**Inversion**	**Eversion**	**Adduction**	**Abduction**
Tibialis anterior (deep peroneal nerve, L4–S1)	Gastrocnemius (tibial nerve, S1–S2)	Tibialis posterior (tibial nerve, L5–S1)	Peroneus longus (superficial peroneal nerve, L4–S1)	Tibialis anterior (deep peroneal nerve, L4–S1)	Extensor digitorum longus (deep peroneal nerve, L4–S1)
Extensor hallucis longus (deep peroneal nerve, L4–S1)	Soleus (tibial nerve, S1–S2)	Flexor digitorum longus (tibial nerve, L5–S1)	Peroneus brevis (superficial peroneal nerve, L4–S1)	Tibialis posterior (tibial nerve, L5–S1)	Peroneus longus (superficial peroneal nerve, L4–S1)
Extensor digitorum longus (deep peroneal nerve, L4–S1)	Flexor hallucis longus (tibial nerve, L5–S2)	Flexor hallucis longus (tibial nerve, L5–S2)	Peroneus tertius (deep peroneal nerve, L5–S1)	Flexor hallucis longus (tibial nerve, L5–S2)	Peroneus brevis (superficial peroneal nerve, L4–S1)
	Flexor digitorum longus (tibial nerve, L5–S1)	Tibialis anterior (deep peroneal nerve, L4–S1)		Flexor digitorum longus (tibial nerve, L5–S2)	

Continued on following page

155

MUSCLES USED IN MOVEMENT OF THE ANKLE AND SUBTALAR JOINTS (Continued)

Dorsiflexion	Plantar Flexion	Inversion	Eversion	Adduction	Abduction
Peroneus tertius (deep peroneal nerve, L5–S1)	Tibialis posterior (tibial nerve, L5–S1)	Extensor hallucis longus (deep peroneal nerve, L4–S1)	Extensor digitorum longus (deep peroneal nerve, L4–S1)	Extensor hallucis longus (deep peroneal nerve, L5–S1)	Peroneus tertius (deep peroneal nerve, L5–S1)
	Plantaris (tibial nerve, L4–S1)		Extensor digitorum brevis (deep peroneal nerve, L5–S1)		
	Peroneus longus (superficial peroneal nerve, L4–S1)				
	Peroneus brevis (superficial peroneal nerve, L4–S1)				

MUSCLES USED IN MOVEMENT OF THE TOES

Extension	Flexion	Abduction	Adduction
Extensor digitorum longus (deep peroneal nerve, L4–S1)	Flexor digitorum longus (tibial nerve, L5–S1)	Abductor hallucis (medial plantar nerve, L5–S1)	Adductor hallucis (lateral plantar nerve, S2–S3)
Extensor hallucis longus (deep peroneal nerve, L4–S1)	Flexor hallucis longus (tibial nerve, L5–S2)	Abductor digiti minimi (lateral plantar nerve, S2–S3)	Plantar interossei (lateral plantar nerve, S2–S3)
Extensor digitorum brevis (deep peroneal nerve, L5–S1)	Flexor digitorum brevis (medial plantar nerve, L5–S1)	Dorsal interossei (lateral plantar nerve, S2–S3)	
Lumbricals (distal IP extension) (first lumbrical by medial plantar nerve, L5–S1; and second through fourth lumbricals by the lateral plantar nerve S2–S3)	Flexor hallucis brevis (medial plantar nerve, L5–S1)		
Interossei, dorsal and plantar (IP extension) (lateral plantar nerve, S2-S3)	Lumbricals (MTP flexion) (first lumbrical by medial plantar nerve, L5–S1; and second through fourth lumbricales by the lateral plantar nerve, S2–S3)		
	Interossei (MTP flexion) (lateral plantar nerve, S2–S3)		

Continued on following page

MUSCLES USED IN MOVEMENT OF THE TOES (Continued)			
Extension	**Flexion**	**Abduction**	**Adduction**
	Flexor digiti minimi (lateral plantar nerve, S2–S3)		
	Quadratus plantae (lateral plantar nerve, S2–S3)		

IP = interphalangeal, MTP = metatarsophalangeal.

MUSCLES LISTED BY REGION

Muscles are listed by body region. See the alphabetized reference list of muscles (starting on page 123) for descriptions that include function, innervation, origin, and insertion.

Muscles of the External Ear
Auricularis anterior
Auricularis posterior
Auricularis superior

Muscles of Facial Expression
Buccinator
Corrugator supercilii
Depressor anguli oris
Depressor labii inferioris
Depressor septi
Levator anguli oris
Levator labii superioris
Levator labii superioris alaeque nasi
Levator palpebrae superioris
Mentalis
Nasalis
Occipitofrontalis
Orbicularis oculi
Orbicularis oris
Platysma
Procerus
Risorius
Temporoparietalis
Transversus menti

Zygomaticus major
Zygomaticus minor

Muscles of Mastication
Buccinator
Lateral pterygoid
Masseter
Medial pterygoid
Temporalis

Muscles of the Eye
Ciliaris
Dilator pupillae
Levator palpebrae superioris
Obliquus inferior (inferior oblique)
Obliquus superior (superior oblique)
Rectus inferior (inferior rectus)
Rectus lateralis (lateral rectus)
Rectus medialis (medial rectus)
Rectus superior (superior rectus)
Sphincter pupillae

Muscles of the Internal Ear
Stapedius
Tensor tympani

Muscles of the Tongue
Chondroglossus
Genioglossus
Hyoglossus
Palatoglossus
Styloglossus

Muscles of the Palate
Levator veli palatini
Musculus uvulae
Palatoglossus
Palatopharyngeus
Tensor veli palatini

Muscles of the Pharynx
Inferior constrictor (constrictor inferior)
Middle constrictor (constrictor medius)
Palatopharyngeus
Salpingopharyngeus
Stylopharyngeus
Superior constrictor (constrictor superior)

Muscles of the Larynx
Aryepiglotticus
Arytenoid (arytenoideus)
Cricothyroid (cricothyroideus)
Lateral cricoarytenoid (cricoarytenoideus lateralis)
Posterior cricoarytenoid (cricoarytenoideus posterior)
Thyroarytenoid (thyroarytenoideus)
Thyroepiglotticus
Vocalis

Muscles of the Neck
Digastricus (anterior and posterior bellies)
Geniohyoid
Longus capitis
Longus colli
Mylohyoid
Omohyoid
Rectus capitis anterior
Rectus capitis lateralis
Scalenus anterior
Scalenus medius
Scalenus posterior
Sternohyoid
Sternothyroid
Stylohyoid
Thyrohyoid

Muscles Behind the Cranium
Obliquus capitis inferior
Obliquus capitis superior
Rectus capitis posterior major
Rectus capitis posterior minor

Muscles of the Back
Iliocostalis cervicis
Iliocostalis lumborum
Iliocostalis thoracis
Intertransversarii
Longissimus capitis
Longissimus cervicis
Longissimus thoracis
Multifidus
Rotatores
Semispinalis capitis
Semispinalis cervicis
Semispinalis thoracis
Spinalis capitis
Spinalis cervicis
Spinalis thoracis
Splenius capitis
Splenius cervicis

Muscles of the Thorax
Diaphragm
Innermost intercostals
Intercostales externi (external intercostals)
Intercostales interni (internal intercostals)
Levatores costarum
Serratus anterior
Serratus posterior inferior
Serratus posterior superior
Transversus thoracis

Muscles of the Abdominal Region
Cremaster
Obliquus externus abdominis (external oblique)
Obliquus internus abdominis (internal oblique)
Rectus abdominis
Transversus abdominis

Muscles of the Pelvis
Coccygeus
Levator ani iliococcygeus
Levator ani pubococcygeus

Muscles of the Perineum
Anal sphincter (external)
Anal sphincter (internal)
Bulbospongiosus (bulbocavernosus)
Continued on following page

Ischiocavernosus
Sphincter urethrae
Transversus perinei profundus
Transversus perinei superficialis

Muscles Connecting the Trunk or the Head to the Scapula
Levator scapulae
Lower trapezius
Pectoralis minor
Rhomboid major
Rhomboid minor
Serratus anterior
Sternocleidomastoid
   (sternomastoid)
Upper trapezius

Muscles of the Shoulder
Deltoid (anterior, middle,
   posterior)
Infraspinatus
Latissimus dorsi
Pectoralis major
Subscapularis
Supraspinatus
Teres major
Teres minor

Muscles of the Arm
Anconeus
Biceps brachii
Brachialis
Coracobrachialis
Triceps brachii

Muscles of the Forearm
Abductor pollicis longus
Brachioradialis
Extensor carpi radialis brevis
Extensor carpi radialis longus
Extensor carpi ulnaris
Extensor digiti minimi
Extensor digitorum
Extensor indicis
Extensor pollicis brevis
Extensor pollicis longus
Flexor carpi radialis
Flexor carpi ulnaris
Flexor digitorum profundus
Flexor digitorum superficialis
Flexor pollicis longus
Palmaris longus
Pronator quadratus
Pronator teres
Supinator

Muscles of the Hand
Abductor digiti minimi
Abductor pollicis brevis
Adductor pollicis
Flexor digiti minimi
Flexor pollicis brevis
Interossei (dorsal and palmar)
Lumbricales
Opponens digiti minimi
Opponens pollicis
Palmaris brevis

Muscles of the Iliac Region
Iliacus
Psoas major
Psoas minor
Quadratus lumborum

Muscles of the Thigh
Adductor brevis
Adductor longus
Adductor magnus
Articularis genus
Biceps femoris
Gemelli (superior and inferior)
Gluteus maximus
Gluteus medius
Gluteus minimus
Gracilis
Obturator externus
Obturator internus
Pectineus
Piriformis
Rectus femoris
Sartorius
Semimembranosus
Semitendinosus
Tensor fasciae latae
Vastus intermedius
Vastus lateralis
Vastus medialis

Muscles of the Leg
Extensor digitorum longus
Extensor hallucis longus
Flexor digitorum longus
Flexor hallucis longus
Gastrocnemius
Peroneus brevis
Peroneus longus
Peroneus tertius
Plantaris
Popliteus
Soleus
Tibialis anterior
Tibialis posterior

Muscles of the Foot
Abductor digiti minimi
Abductor hallucis
Adductor hallucis
Extensor digitorum brevis
Flexor digiti minimi brevis

Flexor digitorum brevis
Flexor hallucis brevis
Interossei (dorsal and plantar)
Lumbricales
Quadratus plantae (flexor
   digitorum accessorius)

MANUAL MUSCLE TESTING POSITIONS

There are two major texts on muscle testing: Kendall, FP, Mc-Creary, EK, and Provance, PG: Muscles: Testing and Function, ed 4. Williams & Wilkins, Baltimore, 1993; and Hislop, HJ and Montgomery, J: Daniels and Worthingham's Muscle Testing: Techniques of Manual Examination, ed 6. WB Saunders, Philadelphia, 1995. Each suggests different positions for testing. See manual muscle testing grading scales (on page 165) for differences in how they grade muscles. To facilitate testing patients once they have been positioned, the following table lists the positions suggested by the two texts.

SUPINE POSITION	
Daniels and Worthingham	*Kendall, McCreary, & Provance*
Cervical flexion—all tests	Toe extensors
Cervical rotation—normal, good, and fair	Toe flexors
Trunk flexion—all tests	Tibialis anterior
Trunk rotation—all tests	Tibialis posterior
Elevation of pelvis—all tests	Peroneals
Hip flexion—trace and zero	Tensor fasciae latae
Hip flexion with abduction and external rotation—poor, trace, and zero	Sartorius
	Iliopsoas
	Abdominals
Hip abduction—poor, trace, and zero	Neck flexors
	Finger flexors
Hip adduction—poor, trace, and zero	Finger extensors
	Thumb muscles
Hip external rotation—poor, trace, and zero	Wrist extensors
	Wrist flexors
Hip internal rotation—poor, trace, and zero	Supinators
	Pronators
Knee extension—trace and zero	Biceps brachii
	Brachioradialis
Shoulder horizontal adduction—normal, good, and fair	Triceps brachii—supine test

Continued on following page

SUPINE POSITION (Continued)	
Daniels and Worthingham	*Kendall, McCreary, & Provance*
Elbow flexion—trace and zero	Pectoralis major—upper part
	Pectoralis major—lower part
	Pectoralis minor
	Shoulder medial rotators—supine test
	Shoulder lateral rotators—supine test
	Serratus anterior
	Anterior deltoid—supine test

PRONE POSITION	
Daniels and Worthingham	*Kendall, McCreary, & Provance*
Cervical extension—all tests	Soleus
Trunk extension—all tests	Hamstrings—medial and lateral
Hip extension—all tests except poor	Gluteus maximus
Knee flexion—all tests except poor	Neck extensors
	Posterolateral neck extensors
Ankle plantar flexion—poor, trace, and zero	Back extensors
Scapular adduction—all tests	Quadratus lumborum
	Latissimus dorsi
Scapular adduction with downward rotation—normal, good, and fair	Lower trapezius
	Middle trapezius
Scapular elevation—poor, trace, and zero	Rhomboids and levator scapulae
Scapular depression with adduction—all tests	Posterior deltoid—prone test
	Triceps brachii—prone test
Shoulder extension—all tests	Teres major
Shoulder horizontal abduction—normal, good, and fair	Shoulder medial rotators—prone test
Shoulder external rotation—all tests	Shoulder lateral rotators—prone test
Shoulder internal rotation—all tests	
Elbow extension—normal, good, and fair	

Daniels and Worthingham	Kendall, McCreary, & Provance
Hip flexion—poor	Gluteus medius
Hip extension—poor	Gluteus minimus
Hip abduction—normal, good, and fair	Hip adductors
	Trunk lateral flexors
Hip abduction from the flexed position—normal, good, and fair	
Hip adduction—normal, good, and fair	
Knee flexion—poor	
Knee extension—poor	

Daniels and Worthingham	Kendall, McCreary, & Provance
Cervical rotation—poor, trace, and zero	Quadriceps femoris
Hip flexion—normal, good, and fair	Hip medial rotators
	Hip lateral rotators
Hip flexion with abduction and hip rotation—normal, good, and fair	Hip flexors—group test
	Popliteus
Hip abduction from the flexed position—poor, trace, and zero	Deltoid—all parts
	Coracobrachialis
Hip external rotation—normal, good, and fair	Upper trapezius
Hip internal rotation—normal, good, and fair	Serratus anterior—preferred test
Knee extension—normal, good, and fair	
Foot dorsiflexion with inversion—all tests	
Foot inversion—all tests	
Foot eversion—all tests	
Toe motions—all tests	
Hallux motions—all tests	

Continued on following page

SITTING POSITION (Continued)

Daniels and Worthingham	Kendall, McCreary, & Provance
Scapular abduction with upward rotation—all tests	
Scapular adduction with downward rotation—poor, trace, and zero	
Scapular elevation—normal, good, and fair	
Shoulder flexion—all tests	
Shoulder abduction—all tests	
Shoulder horizontal abduction—poor, trace, and zero	
Shoulder horizontal adduction—poor, trace, and zero	
Elbow flexion—normal, good, fair, and poor	
Elbow extension—poor, trace, and zero	
Forearm motions—all tests	
Wrist motions—all tests	
Finger motions—all tests	
Thumb motions—all tests	

STANDING POSITION

Daniels and Worthingham	Kendall, McCreary, & Provance
Ankle plantar flexion—normal, good, and fair	Serratus anterior
	Ankle plantar flexors

GRADING SYSTEMS FOR MANUAL MUSCLE TESTING

Manual muscle testing has been used to describe the performance of muscles and muscle groups. Three systems are in common use for testing and grading. The tests and the grading scales are described here without modification.

GRADING SYSTEM OF KENDALL, McCREARY, AND PROVANCE

Kendall and coauthors until recently utilized a percentage-based system for "muscle grading." In the 1993 edition of their text, the percentage-based system was dropped. A 0–10 numeric grading scale was introduced and attempts were made to standardize this system with other muscle grading systems.

Grade		Definition
10	Normal	In antigravity position holds test position against strong pressure.
9	Good+	In antigravity position holds test position against moderate to strong pressure.
8	Good	In antigravity position holds test position against moderate pressure.
7	Good−	In antigravity position holds test position against slight to moderate pressure.
6	Fair+	In antigravity position holds test position against slight pressure.
5	Fair	In antigravity position holds position (no added pressure).
4	Fair−	In antigravity position a gradual release from test position.
3	Poor+	In horizontal plane: Moves to completion of range against resistance or moves to completion of range and hold against pressure. In antigravity position: Moves through partial range of motion.
2	Poor	Moves through complete range of motion in horizontal plane.
1	Poor−	Moves through partial range of motion in horizontal plane.
T	Trace	Tendon becomes prominent or feeble contraction felt in the muscle, but no visible movement of the part.
0	Zero	No contraction felt in the muscle.

From Kendall, FP, McCreary, EK, and Provance, PG: Muscles: Testing and Function, ed 4. Williams & Wilkins, Baltimore, 1993, p 189, with permission.

GRADING SYSTEM OF HISLOP AND MONTGOMERY

Grade	Definition
5 (Normal)	Completes full range of motion against gravity; maintains end-range position against maximal resistance
4 (Good)	Completes full range of motion against gravity; maintains end-range position against strong resistance
3+ (Fair+)	Completes full range of motion against gravity; maintains end-range position against mild resistance
3 (Fair)	Completes full range of motion against gravity; unable to maintain end-range position against any resistance
2 (Poor)	Completes full range of motion in a gravity-eliminated position
2− (Poor−)	Completes partial range of motion in a gravity-eliminated position
1 (Trace)	The examiner observes or palpates contractile activity in the muscle; no movement
0 (Zero)	No activity detected in the muscle

Based on Hislop, HJ and Montgomery, J: Daniels and Worthingham's Muscle Testing: Techniques of Manual Examination, ed 6. WB Saunders, Philadelphia, 1995, pp 2–6.

MEDICAL RESEARCH COUNCIL'S GRADING SYSTEM

Grade	Definition
5	Normal power
4+	Active movement against gravity and strong resistance
4	Active movement against gravity and moderate resistance
4−	Active movement against gravity and slight resistance
3	Active movement against gravity
2	Active movement, with gravity eliminated
1	Flicker or trace of contraction
0	No contraction

From Medical Research Council: Aids to the Examination of the Peripheral Nervous System: Memorandum No. 45. Her Majesty's Stationary Office, London, 1976, p1, with permission.

ORTHOPEDIC TESTS

The following table lists orthopedic tests by body region and the pathology to be tested. Regions are listed from cephalad to caudal. For details on each test, consult the list of orthopedic tests (see page 172).

ORTHOPEDIC TESTS BY BODY REGION	
Body Region and Pathology	*Test*
Cervical Region	
Dural irritation	L'hermitte's sign
Nerve root lesions	Brachial plexus tension test
	Distraction test
	Foraminal compression test
	Shoulder abduction test
	Shoulder depression test
	Valsalva test
Subluxation of the axis	Sharp-Purser test
Vascular compression	Vertebral artery test
Shoulder	
Anterior shoulder dislocation	Apprehension test
Biceps tendon instability	Ludington's test (for ruptured biceps tendon)
	Speed's test (biceps test) (for bicipital tendinitis)
	Transverse humeral ligament test
	Yergason's test (for bicipital tendonitis)
Glenoid labrum tear	Clunk test
Inferior shoulder instability	Sulcus sign
Neurovascular compression syndromes	Adson's maneuver (for thoracic outlet syndrome)
	Allen maneuver (for thoracic outlet syndrome)
	Halstead maneuver (for thoracic outlet syndrome)
	Costoclavicular syndrome test (for thoracic outlet syndrome)
	Hyperabduction syndrome test
	Suprascapular nerve entrapment test

Continued on following page

Body Region and Pathology	Test
Posterior shoulder dislocation	Apprehension test
Rotator cuff tendinitis	Drop-arm test
	Hawkins-Kennedy impingement test
	Impingement sign
	Supraspinatus test
Elbow	
Ligamentous instability	Ligamentous instability tests (for medial and lateral collateral ligaments)
Neurovascular compression	Elbow flexion test (for cubital tunnel syndrome)
Tendinitis	Golfer's elbow test
	Tennis elbow tests
Wrist and Hand	
Contractures	Bunnel-Littler test (for limitations at the PIP joints)
	Tight retinacular ligament test (PIP, DIP joint, or collateral ligaments)
Neurovascular compression	Allen test (for vascular insufficiency to the hand)
	Froment's sign (for ulnar nerve damage)
	Jeanne's sign (for ulnar nerve damage)
	Phalen's test (wrist flexion test) (for carpal tunnel syndrome)
	Tinel's sign (for carpal tunnel syndrome)
Rheumatoid arthritis	Intrinsic-plus test (for limitations of the intrinsic hand muscles)
Tendinitis	Finkelstein's test (for de Quervain's disease)
Low Back	
Malingering	Hoover's test (for differentiating lower limb weakness from malingering)

Body Region and Pathology	*Test*
Nerve compression	Bowstring test (cram test or popliteal pressure sign) (for the sciatic nerve)
	Brudzinski's sign (for root, meningeal, or dural irritations)
	Femoral nerve traction test (for roots L2 to L4)
	Kernig's sign (Brudzinski's sign) (for root, meningeal, or dural irritations)
	Naffziger's test (for nerve root inflammation)
	Prone knee flexion test (reverse Lasègue test) (for roots L2, L3)
	Sitting root test (slump test) (for the sciatic nerve)
	Straight leg raising test (Lasègue's test) (for the sciatic nerve)
Sacroiliac Joint	Palpation of anterior superior iliac spines (patient sitting)
	Palpation of anterior superior iliac spines (patient standing)
	Palpation of iliac crests (patient sitting)
	Palpation of iliac crests (patient standing)
	Palpation of posterior superior iliac spines (patient sitting)
	Palpation of posterior superior iliac spines (patient standing)
	Prone knee flexion test
	Side-lying iliac compression test
	Sitting flexion test
	Standing flexion test
	Standing Gillet test
	Supine iliac gapping test
	Supine to long sitting test

Continued on following page

Body Region and Pathology	Test
Hip	
Arthritis	Patrick's test (fabere test, faber test, or figure-of-four test)
Contractures	Ober's test (for a tight iliotibial band)
	Thomas test (for tight hip flexor muscles)
Dislocation	Ortolani's test
	Galeazzi's test
	Barlow's provocative test
	Trendelenburg's test (for detecting dislocation, weakness of the gluteus medius muscle, or extreme coxa vara)
Knee	
Anterior instability	Anterior drawer test (for anterior instability)
	Crossover test (for anterolateral instability)
	Hughston test (jerk sign) (for anterolateral instability; it is a modification of the MacIntosh test)
	Lachman's test (for anterior instability)
	Losee test (for anterolateral rotary instability)
	MacIntosh test (lateral pivot shift, or anterolateral rotary instability)
	Slocum ALRI test (for anterolateral rotary instability)
	Slocum's test (for anterolateral rotary instability; it is a modification of the MacIntosh test)
Effusion	Brush (stroke or wipe) test (for slight effusions)
	Patellar tap test
	Fluctuation test (for significant effusions)

Body Region and Pathology	Test
Lateral instability	Adduction (varus) stress test
Medial instability	Abduction (valgus) stress test
Meniscus and tibiofemoral joint lesions	Apley grinding test (for meniscal or ligamentous lesions)
	Bounce home test (for meniscal lesions)
	Helfet test (for meniscal lesions)
	Hughston plica test (for abnormal suprapatellar plica, which can mimic a torn meniscus)
	McMurray test (for meniscal lesions)
	O'Donoghue's test (for meniscal lesions or capsular irritation)
	Wilson test (for osteochondritis dissecans)
Patellar lesions	Apprehension test (for a dislocating patella)
	Clarke's sign (for chondromalacia of the patella)
	Perkin's test (for patellar tenderness)
	Waldron test (for chondromalacia of the patella)
Posterior instability	External rotation recurvatum test (for posterolateral rotary instability)
	Hughston posterolateral drawer test (for posterolateral rotary instability)
	Hughston posteromedial drawer test (for posteromedial rotary instability)
	Jakob test (for posterolateral rotary instability)
	Posterior drawer test (for posterior instability)
	Posterior sag sign (gravity drawer test) (for posterior instability)

Continued on following page

Body Region and Pathology	Test
Foot and Ankle	
Achilles tendon	Thompson's test (for Achilles tendon rupture)
Deep vein thrombosis	Homans' sign (for deep vein thrombosis of the leg)
Ligamentous instability	Anterior drawer test (for anterior ankle instability)
	Kleiger test (for medial instability)
	Talar tilt (for the calcaneofibular ligament)

FOR MORE INFORMATION

Blauvelt, CT and Nelson, FRT: A Manual of Orthopaedic Terminology, ed 5. Mosby-Year Book, St. Louis, 1994.

D'Ambrosia, RD: Musculoskeletal Disorders: Regional Examination and Differential Diagnosis, ed 2. JB Lippincott, Philadelphia, 1986.

Magee, DJ: Orthopedic Physical Assessment, ed 2. WB Saunders, Philadelphia, 1992.

Orthopedic Tests Listed by Region

Common orthopedic tests described here are listed by body region, with the most cephalad regions listed first. Within body regions, the tests are listed in alphabetical order.

Cervical Spine

brachial plexus tension test: A test designed to detect nerve root compression. The patient lies supine and slowly abducts and externally rotates the arm just to the point of pain. The forearm is then supinated and flexed, with the examiner supporting the shoulder and forearm. The test result is positive if the patient's symptoms are reproduced or increased.

distraction test: A test designed to identify nerve root compression. The examiner places one hand under the patient's chin and the other under the occiput. The head is slowly lifted (distraction), and the test is considered positive if the radiating pain is decreased.

foraminal compression test (Spurling's test): A test designed to identify nerve root compression. The patient laterally flexes the head. The examiner carefully presses down (compression) on the head. The test result is positive if pain radiates into the arm toward the flexed side.

L'hermitte's sign: A test designed to identify dural irritation. The patient is in the long leg sitting position. While keeping the patient's knees extended, the examiner flexes the patient's head and hips simultaneously. The test result is positive if there is a sharp pain down the spine and into the upper or lower extremities.

Sharp-Purser test: A test designed to determine subluxation of the atlas on the axis. The examiner places one hand on the patient's forehead while the thumb of the other hand is placed over the spinous process of the axis to stabilize it. The patient is asked to slowly flex the head; at the same time the examiner presses backwards with the palm. A positive test is indicated if the examiner feels the head slide backwards during the movement.

shoulder abduction test: A test designed to identify extradural compression, such as a herniated disk, epidural vein compression, or nerve root compression most commonly at C5 or C6. The patient is in a sitting or lying position. The patient's arm is abducted actively or passively so that the hand or forearm of the patient rests on the patient's head. The test result is positive if there is a decrease in symptoms.

shoulder depression test: A test designed to detect nerve root compression or dural adhesions to the nerve or joint capsule. The examiner flexes the patient's head to one side while applying downward pressure on the opposite shoulder. The test result is positive if pain is increased.

Spurling's test: See *foraminal compression test.*

Valsalva test: A test designed to detect a space-occupying lesion in the cervical spine, such as a herniated disk or an osteophyte. The examiner instructs the patient to take a deep breath and hold the breath, as if the patient is having a bowel movement. The test result is positive if symptoms are reproduced or increased.

vertebral artery test: A test designed to detect compression of the vertebral artery. The patient is in a supine position. The examiner places the patient's head into a position of extension, lateral flexion, and rotation and holds that position for 30 s. Each side is tested separately. The test is positive if the patient reports having a feeling of dizziness or nausea, or if nystagmus is observed.

Shoulder

Adson's maneuver: A test designed to determine the presence of thoracic outlet syndrome. The patient turns the head toward the shoulder on the side being tested. The examiner externally rotates and extends the shoulder while the patient extends the head. The test result is positive if the radial pulse disappears while the patient holds a deep breath.

Allen maneuver: A test designed to identify the presence of thoracic outlet syndrome. With the patient seated, the examiner flexes the patient's elbow to 90° while the patient's shoulder is abducted 90° and externally rotated. The examiner then palpates the radial pulse while the patient rotates the head away from the test side. The test result is positive if the pulse disappears.

Continued on following page

apprehension test for anterior shoulder dislocation: A test designed to determine whether a patient has a history of anterior dislocations. With the patient supine, the examiner slowly abducts and externally rotates the patient's arm. The test is positive if the patient becomes apprehensive and resists further motion.

apprehension test for posterior shoulder dislocation: A test designed to determine whether a patient has a history of posterior dislocations. With the patient supine, the examiner slowly flexes the patient's arm to 90° and the patient's elbow to 90°. The examiner then internally rotates the patient's arm. A posterior force is then applied to the patient's elbow. The test result is positive if the patient becomes apprehensive and resists further motion.

biceps test: See *Speed's test.*

clunk test: A test designed to determine the presence of a tear of the glenoid labrum. With the patient supine, the examiner places one hand on the posterior aspect of the shoulder over the humeral head. The examiner fully abducts the arm over the patient's head and then pushes anteriorly with the hand over the humeral head. The test is positive if a "clunk" or grinding is palpated. The test may also cause apprehension if anterior instability is present.

costoclavicular syndrome test: A test designed to determine the presence of thoracic outlet syndrome. The patient is asked to adduct the scapula while the examiner extends the patient's shoulder. For a positive test, symptoms should be reproduced with a decreased radial pulse to confirm the diagnosis.

drop-arm test: A test designed to determine the presence of a torn rotator cuff. With the patient seated, the examiner abducts the patient's shoulder to 90°. The test result is positive if the patient is unable to lower the arm slowly to the side in the same arc of movement or has severe pain when attempting to do so.

Halstead maneuver: A test designed to determine the presence of thoracic outlet syndrome. With the patient seated, the examiner palpates the radial pulse and applies a downward force on the arm. The patient extends the neck and rotates the head toward the opposite side of the limb being tested. The test result is positive if the pulse disappears following this maneuver.

Hawkins-Kennedy impingement test: A test designed to identify supraspinatus tendinitis. The patient stands while the examiner flexes the arm to 90° and then forcibly internally rotates the shoulder. The test result is positive if pain is present during the maneuver.

hyperabduction syndrome test: A test designed to determine the presence of thoracic outlet syndrome. The patient abducts the arm above the head. Compression of the neurovascular bundle under the coracoid process and under the pectoralis minor muscle reproduces symptoms and results in a diminished radial pulse.

impingement sign: A test designed to identify inflammation of tissues within the subacromial space. The patient's upper extremity is forcibly flexed forward by the examiner. The maneuver is thought to decrease the space between the head of the humerus and acromion process. The test result is positive if the patient reports pain.

Ludington's test: A test designed for determining whether there has been a rupture of the long head of the biceps tendon. The patient is seated and clasps both hands on top of the head, supporting the weight of the upper limbs. The patient then alternately contracts and relaxes the biceps muscles. The test result is positive if the examiner cannot palpate the long head of the biceps tendon of the affected arm during the contractions.

Speed's test (biceps test): A test designed to determine whether bicipital tendonitis is present. With the forearm supinated and elbow fully extended, the patient tries to flex the arm against resistance applied by the examiner. The test result is positive if the patient reports increased pain in the area of the bicipital groove.

sulcus sign: A test designed to determine the presence of inferior instability. The patient stands with the arm by the side and the shoulder muscles relaxed. The examiner grasps the patient's forearm and pulls distally. The test result is positive if a space larger than one thumb width appears between the acromion and the humeral head.

suprascapular nerve entrapment test: A test designed to identify entrapment of the suprascapular nerve in the suprascapular notch. Patients report pain when horizontally adducting their arm across their chest. The pain is poorly localized to the posterior aspect of the shoulder.

supraspinatus test: A test designed to identify a tear in the supraspinatus tendon. The seated patient's upper limbs are positioned horizontally at 30° anterior to the frontal plane and internally rotated. The examiner applies a downward force on the patient's limbs. The test result is positive if pain and weakness are present on the involved side.

transverse humeral ligament test: A test designed to identify a torn transverse humeral ligament. The examiner abducts and internally rotates the patient's shoulder. The examiner then palpates the bicipital groove while externally rotating the patient's shoulder. The test result is positive if the biceps tendon can be felt to "snap" in and out of the groove with shoulder external rotation.

Yergason's test: A test designed to identify tendonitis of the long head of the biceps. The seated patient's arm is positioned at the side with the elbow flexed to 90°. Supination of the forearm against resistance produces pain in the biceps tendon in the area of the bicipital groove.

Elbow

elbow flexion test: A test designed to identify cubital tunnel syndrome. The patient is asked to hold his or her elbow fully flexed for 5 min. The test result is positive if tingling or paresthesias are felt in the ulnar nerve distribution of the forearm and hand.

golfer's elbow test: A test designed to identify the presence of inflammation in the area of the medial epicondyle. The patient flexes the elbow and wrist, supinates the forearm, and then extends the elbow. The test result is positive if the patient complains of pain over the medial epicondyle.

Continued on following page

ligamentous instability tests: Tests designed to assess the integrity of the lateral and medial collateral ligaments of the elbow. The patient's arm is held by the examiner so that the examiner is supporting the elbow and wrist. The examiner tests the lateral collateral ligament by applying an adduction or varus force to the distal forearm with the patient's elbow held in 20° to 30° of flexion. The medial collateral ligament is similarly tested by the application of an abduction or valgus force at the distal forearm. The test result is positive if pain or altered mobility is present.

tennis elbow tests: The following tests are designed to determine the presence of inflammation in the area of the lateral epicondyle:

- The patient flexes the elbow to approximately 45° and fully supinates the forearm while making a fist. The patient is then asked to pronate the forearm and radially deviate and extend the wrist while the examiner resists these motions. For a positive test result, pain is elicited in the area of the lateral epicondyle.
- The examiner pronates the patient's forearm, fully extends the elbow, and fully flexes the wrist. For a positive test result, pain is elicited in the area of the lateral epicondyle.
- The examiner resists extension of the third digit of the hand distal to the proximal interphalangeal (PIP) joint. A positive test is indicated by pain in the area of the lateral epicondyle of the humerus.

Wrist and Hand

Allen test: A test designed to determine the patency of the vascular communication in the hand. The examiner first palpates and occludes the radial and ulnar arteries. The patient is then asked to open and close the fingers rapidly from three to five times to cause the palmar skin to blanch. Pressure is then released from either the radial or ulnar artery, and the rapidity with which the hand regains color is noted. The test is repeated with release of the other artery. A positive Allen test result indicates that there is a diminished or absent communication between the superficial ulnar arch and the deep radial arch.

Bunnel-Littler test: A test designed to identify intrinsic muscle or joint contractures at the PIP joints. The examiner flexes the PIP joint maximally while maintaining the metacarpophalangeal (MCP) joint in slight extension. The test result is positive for a joint capsule contracture if the PIP joint cannot be flexed. The test is positive for intrinsic muscle contracture if the MCP is slightly flexed and the PIP flexes fully.

Finkelstein's test: A test designed to determine the presence of tenosynovitis of the abductor pollicis longus and extensor pollicis brevis tendons. The test is commonly used to determine the presence of de Quervain's disease. The patient makes a fist while holding the thumb inside the fingers. The patient then attempts to deviate ulnarly the first metacarpal and extend the proximal joint of the thumb. If the patient experiences pain, this is recorded as a positive test result.

Froment's sign: A test designed for determining the presence of adductor pollicis weakness from ulnar nerve paralysis. The patient attempts to grasp a piece of paper between the tips of the thumb and the radial side of the index finger. The test result is positive if the terminal phalanx of the patient's thumb flexes or if the MCP joint of the thumb hyperextends (Jeanne's sign) as the examiner attempts to pull the paper from the patient's grasp.

intrinsic-plus test: A test designed to identify shortening of the intrinsic muscles of the hand. This test is useful and specific when examining the hand of the patient with rheumatoid arthritis, particularly in the early stages prior to any destruction or deformity of the hand. In this test, the MCP joint of the finger being tested is hyperextended. The middle and distal joints flex slightly owing to passive action of tissues. The examiner then further attempts to flex passively the PIP joint of the finger. Any severe restriction to this movement is considered a positive sign.

Jeanne's sign: See *Froment's sign.*

Phalen's (wrist flexion) test: A test designed to determine the presence of carpal tunnel syndrome. The patient's wrists are maximally flexed by the examiner, who maintains this position by holding the patient's wrists together for 1 min. The test result is positive if paresthesias are present in the thumb, index finger, and the middle and lateral half of the ring finger.

tight retinacular ligament test: A test designed to determine the presence of shortened retinacular ligaments or a tight distal interphalangeal (DIP) joint capsule. The examiner holds the patient's PIP joint in a fully extended position while attempting to flex the DIP joint. If the DIP joint does not flex, the test is positive for either a contracted collateral ligament or joint capsule. The test is positive for tight retinacular (collateral) ligaments and a normal joint capsule if, when the PIP joint is flexed, the DIP joint flexes easily.

Tinel's sign: A test designed to detect carpal tunnel syndrome. The examiner taps over the carpal tunnel of the wrist. The test result is positive if the patient reports paresthesia distal to the wrist.

wrist flexion test: See *Phalen's test.*

Low Back (also see Sacroiliac Joint)

bowstring test (cram test or popliteal pressure sign): A test designed to identify the presence of sciatic nerve compression. A straight leg raising test is first carried out by the examiner. The leg is raised to the point where the patient reports pain. The knee is slightly flexed to reduce the symptoms. Digital pressure is then applied to the popliteal fossa. The test result is positive if pain is increased.

Brudzinski's sign: See *Kernig's sign.*

cram test: See *bowstring test.*

femoral nerve traction test: A test designed to identify nerve root compression of the midlumbar area (L2, L3, and L4). The patient lies on the unaffected side with the unaffected limb flexed slightly for support. The examiner grasps the affected limb and extends the knee while gently extending the hip approximately 15°, being sure not to extend the back. The patient's knee is then flexed, further

Continued on following page

stretching the femoral nerve. The test result is positive if pain radiates down the anterior thigh.

Hoover's test: A test designed to discriminate lower limb weakness from possible malingering. The patient relaxes in a supine position while the examiner places one hand under each heel. The patient is then asked to do a straight leg raise (knee extended). The test result is positive if the patient is unable to lift the leg and there is no downward pressure from the opposite leg.

Kernig's sign: A test designed to identify meningeal irritation, nerve root involvement, or dural irritation. The patient lies in the supine position with hands cupped behind the head. The patient flexes the head onto the chest (Brudzinski's sign) and raises the lower extremity with knee extended (Kernig's sign). The test result is positive if radiating pain is elicited.

Lasègue's test: See *straight leg raising test.*

Naffziger's test: A test designed to detect a space-occupying lesion in the spine. The patient lies supine while the examiner gently compresses the jugular veins for approximately 10 s. The patient is then asked to cough. The test result is positive if coughing produces pain in the lower back.

popliteal pressure sign: See *bowstring test.*

prone knee flexion test (reverse Lasègue test): A test designed to identify L2 or L3 nerve root lesions. The patient lies prone while the examiner passively flexes the knee so that the patient's heel touches the patient's buttocks. The test result is positive if unilateral symptoms are elicited or increased in the lumbar area or anterior thigh. Pain in the anterior thigh may indicate a tight quadriceps muscle.

reverse Lasègue test: See *prone knee flexion test.*

sitting root test (slump test): A test designed to identify compression of the sciatic nerve. The patient is seated with neck flexed. The knee is actively extended while the hip remains flexed. The test result is positive if pain increases.

slump test: See *sitting root test.*

straight leg raising test (Lasègue test): A test designed to identify sciatic nerve root compression. With the patient supine, the examiner raises the patient's extended leg while watching the patient's reaction. The examiner stops when the patient complains of back or leg pain (and not hamstring tightness). The examiner may also dorsiflex the ankle to further increase the traction on the sciatic nerve. Back pain suggests a central herniation, and leg pain suggests a lateral disk protrusion. The test is repeated for both sides.

Sacroiliac Joint

palpation of anterior superior iliac spines (patient sitting): A test designed to identify the presence of asymmetry of the sacroiliac joints that may be associated with subluxation or other pain-producing causes. The patient sits erect on a flat surface. The examiner, who is standing or squatting in front of the patient, places his or her thumbs on the inferior margins of the anterior superior iliac spines (ASISs). The examiner then moves the thumbs upward so that they are stopped by the bony prominence of the ASISs. The test result is positive if one ASIS is higher than the other.

palpation of anterior superior iliac spines (patient standing): A test designed to identify the presence of asymmetry of the sacroiliac joints that may be associated with subluxation or other pain-producing causes. The patient stands with feet 12 in apart. The examiner, standing or squatting in front of the patient, places her or his thumbs on the inferior margins of the ASISs. The examiner then moves the thumbs upward so that they are stopped by the bony prominence of the ASISs. The test result is positive if one ASIS is higher than the other.

palpation of iliac crests (patient sitting): A test designed to identify the presence of asymmetry of the sacroiliac joints that may be associated with subluxation or other pain-producing causes. The patient sits erect on a flat surface. The examiner, who is standing or squatting behind the patient, places the radial borders of his or her hands on the patient's waist. The hands are then moved gently downward to move aside soft tissues before the examiner's movement is stopped by the iliac crests. The test result is positive if one crest is higher than the other.

palpation of iliac crests (patient standing): A test designed to identify the presence of asymmetry of the sacroiliac joints that may be associated with subluxation or other pain-producing causes. The patient stands with feet 12 in apart. The examiner, who is standing or squatting behind the patient, places the radial borders of her or his hands on the patient's waist. The hands are then moved gently downward to move aside soft tissues before the examiner's movement is stopped by the iliac crests. The test result is positive if one crest is higher than the other.

palpation of posterior superior iliac spines (patient sitting): A test designed to identify the presence of asymmetry of the sacroiliac joints that may be associated with subluxation or other pain-producing causes. The patient sits erect on a flat surface. The examiner, who is standing or squatting behind the patient, places his or her thumbs on the inferior margin of the posterior superior iliac spines (PSISs). The examiner then moves her or his thumbs upward so that they are stopped by the bony prominence of the PSISs. The test result is positive if one PSIS is higher than the other.

palpation of posterior superior iliac spines (patient standing): A test designed to identify the presence of asymmetry of the sacroiliac joints that may be associated with subluxation or other pain-producing causes. The patient stands with feet 12 in apart. The examiner, who is standing or squatting behind the patient, places his or her thumbs on the inferior margin of the PSIS. The examiner then moves his or her thumbs upward so that they are stopped by the bony prominence of the PSIS. The test result is positive if one PSIS is higher than the other.

prone knee flexion test: A test designed to identify the presence of rotation of the innominate bones relative to the sacroiliac joint. The patient, who should be wearing shoes, lies prone with arms at sides and the cervical spine in a neutral position. The examiner stands at
Continued on following page

the patient's feet and grasps the heels of the patient's shoes. The examiner places his or her index fingers just posterior to the lateral malleoli and holds the feet in a neutral position relative to pronation and supination. The examiner then flexes the patient's knees to 90° of flexion. A change in the relative position of the patient's heels is said to indicate innominate rotation. An apparent increase in leg length is said to indicate a posterior innominate rotation on the same side. An apparent decrease in leg length is said to indicate an anterior innominate rotation on the same side.

side-lying iliac gapping test: A test designed to identify the presence of sacroiliac joint dysfunction. The patient lies on the side. The examiner stands above the patient and, with elbows fully extended, interlocks palms and places them over the most cephalad margin of the iliac crest. The examiner then exerts a downward and cephalad directed force on the crest. The test result is positive if the patient's painful symptoms in the sacroiliac, gluteal, or crural regions are reproduced.

sitting flexion test: A test designed to identify the presence of sacroiliac joint dysfunction. The patient sits erect on a flat surface, with feet flat on the floor and knees flexed to 90°. The hips are sufficiently abducted that the patient can bend forward between them. The examiner, who is kneeling or squatting behind the patient, places his or her thumbs on the inferior margin of the PSISs. The patient bends forward as far as possible, reaching the hands toward the floor. A positive test results occurs when one PSIS moves more in a cranial direction than does the other. The side with the greater movement is said to have articular restriction.

standing flexion test: A test designed to identify the presence of sacroiliac joint dysfunction. The patient stands with feet 12 in apart. The examiner, who is standing or squatting behind the patient, places his or her thumbs on the inferior margin of the PSISs. The patient then bends forward while keeping the knees straight. A positive test result occurs when one PSIS moves more in a cranial direction than does the other. The side with the greater movement is said to have articular restriction. Because hamstring tightness may also cause these findings, the test is not considered positive until hamstring tightness has been ruled out.

standing Gillet test: A test designed to identify the presence of sacroiliac joint dysfunction. The patient stands with feet 12 in apart. The examiner, who is standing behind the patient, places one thumb directly under one PSIS and the other thumb on the ipsilateral tubercle of S2 (which is on the sacrum at the level of the PSIS). The patient flexes the hip and knee on the side being palpated so that she or he is standing on one leg. A positive test result is one in which the PSIS does not dip downward as the extreme of hip flexion is reached. The test is repeated on the contralateral side.

supine iliac compression test: A test designed to identify sacroiliac joint dysfunction. The patient lies supine. The examiner crosses his or her arms, placing the palms of her or his hands on the patient's ASISs. The examiner then presses down and laterally to strain the sacroiliac ligaments. A positive test result occurs when the patient reports pain in the gluteal or posterior crural areas. If pain is felt in the lumbar region, the test is repeated after using more support for the lumbar spine.

supine to long sitting test: A test designed to identify the presence of rotation of the innominate bones relative to the sacroiliac joint. The patient lies supine while the examiner places her or his thumbs on the inferior borders of the medial malleoli. The patient then sits up, being careful to do so in a symmetrical, nontwisting fashion. Changes in the relative positions of the medial malleoli are noted. If one leg appears to lengthen when the patient sits up, that is interpreted as indicating a posterior innominate rotation on that side. If one leg appears to shorten when the patient sits up, that is interpreted as indicating an anterior innominate rotation on that side.

Hip

Barlow's provocative test: See also *Ortolani's test.* A test designed to identify hip instability in infants. The test is performed after the Ortolani test has been conducted. With the infant in the same position used for Ortolani's test, the examiner stabilizes the pelvis between the symphysis and sacrum with one hand. With the thumb of the other hand, the examiner attempts to dislocate the hip by gentle but firm posterior pressure.

faber test: See *Patrick's test.*

fabere test: See *Patrick's test.*

figure-of-four test: See *Patrick's test.*

Galeazzi's test: A test designed to detect unilateral congenital dislocations of the hip in children. The child is positioned supine with the hips flexed to 90° and the knees fully flexed. The test result is positive if one knee is positioned higher than the other.

Ober test: A test designed to determine the presence of a shortened (tight) iliotibial band. With the patient lying on one side, the lower limb closest to the table is flexed. The other lower limb, which is being tested, is abducted and extended. The knee of the limb is flexed to 90° and is then allowed to drop to the table. If the limb does not, this indicates that the iliotibial band is shortened (tight).

Ortolani's test: A test designed to identify a congenital hip dislocation in infants. The infant is positioned supine with the hips flexed 90° and the knees fully flexed. The examiner grasps the legs so that the examiner's thumbs are placed on the infant's medial thighs and the examiner's fingers are placed on the infant's lateral thighs. The thighs are gently abducted, and the examiner applies a gentle force to the greater trochanters with the fingers of each hand. Resistance will be felt at about 30° of abduction and, if there is a dislocation, a click will be felt as the dislocation is reduced (see the related *Barlow's provocative test*).

Patrick's test (fabere test, faber test, or figure-of-four test): A test designed to identify arthritis of the hip. With the patient lying supine, the knee is flexed and the hip is flexed, abducted, and externally rotated until the lateral malleolus rests on the opposite knee just above the patella. In this position the knee on the side being tested is gently forced downward; if pain is produced, the test result is positive for the presence of osteoarthritis of the hip.

Continued on following page

Thomas test: A test designed to test for contracture of the hip flexor muscles. In supine position, the patient holds one flexed hip against the chest. The test is positive if the other thigh does not remain against the surface.

Trendelenburg's test: A test designed to identify the presence of an unstable hip. The patient stands on the leg to be tested. The test is positive if the non-weight-bearing side does not rise as the patient stands on one lower extremity. A positive test result may be caused by a hip dislocation, weakness of the hip abductors, or coxa vara.

Knee

abduction (valgus stress) test: A test designed to identify medial instability of the knee. The examiner applies a valgus stress to the patient's knee while the patient's ankle is stabilized in slight lateral rotation. The test is first conducted with the knee fully extended and then repeated with the knee at 20° of flexion. Excessive movement of the tibia away from the femur indicates a positive test result. Positive findings with the knee fully extended indicate a major disruption of the knee ligaments. A positive test result with the knee flexed is indicative of damage to the medial collateral ligament.

adduction (varus stress) test: A test designed to identify lateral instability of the knee. The examiner applies a varus stress to the patient's knee while the ankle is stabilized. The test is done with the patient's knee in full extension and then with the knee in 20°–30° of flexion. A positive test result with the knee extended suggests a major disruption of the knee ligaments, whereas a positive test result with the knee flexed is indicative of damage to the lateral collateral ligament.

ALRI test: See *Slocum ALRI test.*

anterior drawer (sign) test: A test designed to detect anterior instability of the knee. The patient lies supine with the knee flexed 90°. The examiner sits across the forefoot of the patient's flexed lower limb. With the patient's foot in neutral rotation, the examiner pulls forward on the proximal part of the calf. Both lower limbs are tested. The test result is positive if there is excessive anterior movement of the tibia with respect to the femur.

Apley grinding test: A test designed to detect meniscal lesions. The patient lies prone with the knees flexed 90°. The examiner applies a compressive force through the foot and rotates the tibia back and forth while palpating the joint line with the other hand feeling for crepitation. The test result is positive if the patient reports pain or the examiner feels crepitation. This test is then repeated by applying a distractive force to the leg, and if pain is elicited it is indicative of a ligamentous injury rather than a meniscal injury.

apprehension test: A test designed to identify dislocation of the patella. The patient lies supine with the knee resting at 30° flexion. The examiner carefully and slowly displaces the patella laterally. If the patient looks apprehensive and tries to contract the quadriceps muscle to bring the patella back to neutral, the test result is positive.

bounce home test: A test designed to identify meniscal lesions. The patient lies supine, and the heel of the patient's foot is cupped by the examiner. The patient's knee is completely flexed and then allowed to extend passively. If extension is not complete or has a rubbery end-feel ("springy block"), the test result is positive.

brush (stroke or wipe) test: A test designed to identify a mild effusion in the knee. Starting below the joint line on the medial side of the patella, the examiner strokes proximally with the palm and fingers as far as the suprapatellar pouch. With the opposite hand, the examiner strokes down the lateral side of the patella. The test result is positive if a wave of fluid appears as a slight bulge at the medial distal border of the patella.

Clarke's sign: A test designed to identify the presence of chondromalacia of the patella. The patient lies relaxed with knees extended as the examiner presses down slightly proximal to the base of the patella with the web of the hand. The patient is then asked to contract the quadriceps muscle as the examiner applies more force. The test result is positive if the patient cannot complete the contraction without pain.

crossover test: A test designed to identify anterolateral instability of the knee. With the patient standing and the uninvolved leg crossed in front of the test leg, the examiner secures the foot of the test leg by carefully stepping on it. The patient rotates the upper torso away from the injured leg approximately 90°. In this position the patient is asked to contract the quadriceps muscles. If this action produces a feeling of "giving way" in the knee, the test result is positive.

drawer sign test: See *anterior drawer test* and *posterior drawer test*.

external rotation recurvatum test: A test designed to identify posterolateral rotary instability of the knee. There are two methods for this test. Both are conducted with the patient in supine position:

- The examiner elevates the patient's legs by grasping the patient's great toes. The test result is positive if the tibial tubercle is observed to rotate laterally while the knee goes into recurvatum.
- The examiner flexes the knee to 30° or 40°. The knee is then slowly extended while the examiner's other hand holds the posterolateral aspect of the knee to palpate for movement. The test result is positive if hyperextension and excessive lateral rotation occur in the injured limb.

fluctuation test: A test designed to identify significant knee effusion. The knee is placed in a position of 15° flexion. The examiner then places the palm of one hand over the suprapatellar pouch and the other hand anterior to the joint, with the thumb and index finger adjacent to the patellar margins. The examiner tries to feel and assess the shifting or fluctuation of synovial fluid while alternately pressing down with one hand and then the other.

gravity drawer test: See *posterior sag sign*.

Helfet test: A test designed to identify meniscal lesions. The "screw home" mechanism is observed during full extension. With a torn meniscus blocking the joint, the tibial tubercle remains slightly medial in relation to the midline of the patella, and the final limit of external rotation is prevented.

Continued on following page

Hughston plica test: A test designed to identify an abnormal supra-patellar plica. The patient lies supine, and the examiner flexes the knee and medially rotates the tibia with one arm and hand while with the other hand the patella is displaced slightly medially with the fingers over the course of the plica. The test result is positive if a "pop" is elicited at the plica while the knee is flexed and extended by the examiner.

Hughston posterolateral drawer test: A test designed to identify the presence of posterolateral rotary knee instability. The procedure is similar to the Hughston posteromedial test except the patient's foot is slightly laterally rotated. The test result is positive if the tibia rotates posteriorly on the lateral side an excessive amount when the examiner pushes the tibia posteriorly.

Hughston posteromedial drawer test: A test designed to identify posteromedial rotary instability of the knee. The patient lies in a supine position with the knee flexed to 90°. The examiner fixes the foot in slight medial rotation by sitting on the foot. The examiner pushes the tibia posteriorly. The test result is positive if the tibia moves or rotates posteriorly on the medial aspect an excessive amount.

Hughston test (jerk sign): A test designed to identify the presence of anterolateral rotary instability of the knee. The test is a modification of the MacIntosh test for anterolateral instability. The patient lies supine with the knee flexed to 90°. The extremity is grasped at the foot with one hand while the examiner's other hand rests over the proximal, lateral aspect of the leg just distal to the knee. A valgus stress is applied to the knee and the tibia is internally rotated while the knee is slowly moved into extension. The test result is positive if, when the knee is gradually extended, at 30°–40° of flexion the lateral tibial plateau suddenly subluxes forward and does so with a jerking sensation. The knee will spontaneously reduce if the leg is further extended.

Jakob test (reverse pivot shift): A test designed to identify postero-lateral rotary instability of the knee. This test can be performed with the patient either standing or supine:

- In the standing position, the patient leans against a wall with the involved extremity toward the examiner. The examiner's hands are placed above and below the test knee, and a valgus stress is applied while the patient flexes the knee. The test result is positive if there is a jerk in the knee or the tibia shifts posteriorly and the knee gives way.
- The patient lies supine. The examiner supports the patient's knee posteriorly with one hand and the heel with the other hand. The patient's foot is then laterally rotated.

jerk sign: See *Hughston test.*

Lachman's test: A test designed to identify injury to the anterior cruciate ligament. The patient lies supine with the examiner stabilizing the distal femur with one hand and grasping the proximal tibia with the other hand. With the knee held in slight flexion, the tibia is moved forward on the femur. A positive test result is indicated by a soft end-feel and excessive observable movement of the tibia.

lateral pivot shift: See *MacIntosh test*.

Losee test: A test designed to identify anterolateral rotary instability (ALRI) of the knee. With the patient supine and relaxed, the examiner cradles the patient's foot so that the knee is flexed to 30° and the leg is externally rotated and braced against the examiner's abdomen. With the patient's hamstrings relaxed, the examiner extends the knee while the examiner's thumb pushes the fibula anteriorly and a valgus stress is applied to the knee. The knee is allowed to rotate internally during extension. The test result is positive if the lateral tibial plateau subluxes anteriorly just before full extension.

MacIntosh test (lateral pivot shift): A test designed to identify ALRI. The examiner grasps the leg with one hand and places the other hand over the lateral, proximal aspect of the leg. With the knee in extension, a valgus stress is applied and the leg internally rotated as the knee is flexed. At about 30°–40° of flexion, a sudden jump is noted as the lateral tibial plateau, which has subluxed anteriorly in relation to the femoral condyle, suddenly reduces.

McMurray test: A test designed to identify meniscal lesions. The patient lies supine while the examiner grasps the foot with one hand and palpates the joint line with the other. The knee is fully flexed and the tibia rotated back and forth and then held alternately in internal and external rotation as the knee is extended. A click or crepitation may be felt over the joint line with a posterior meniscal lesion, as the knee is extended.

O'Donoghue's test: A test designed to detect meniscal injuries or capsular irritation. The patient lies supine, and the examiner flexes the knee to 90°, rotates it medially and laterally twice, and then fully flexes and rotates it again. The test result is positive if pain increases on rotation.

patellar tap test: A test designed to identify significant joint effusion. The knee is flexed or extended to discomfort, and the examiner taps the surface of the patella. The test result is positive if a floating of the patella is felt.

Perkin's test: A test for patellar tenderness. With the knee supported in full extension, the borders of the medial and lateral facets are palpated while the patella is displaced medially and laterally. With chondromalacia, this maneuver reveals varying degrees of tenderness.

plica test: See *Hughston plica test*.

posterior drawer test: A test designed to identify posterior instability of the knee. The patient lies supine with the knee flexed to 90° as the foot is held in a neutral position by the examiner sitting on it. The examiner's hands grasp the leg around the proximal tibia and attempt to move the tibia backward on the femur. The test result is positive if there is excessive posterior movement of the tibia on the femur.

posterior sag sign (gravity drawer test): A test designed to identify posterior instability of the knee. The patient lies supine with the knees flexed to 90° and the feet supported. The test result is positive if the tibia sags back on the femur.

Continued on following page

posterolateral drawer sign: See *Hughston posterolateral drawer test.*

posteromedial drawer sign: See *Hughston posteromedial drawer test.*

reverse pivot shift: See *Jakob test.*

Slocum ALRI test: A test designed to identify anterolateral rotary instability. The patient is lying on the side of the uninvolved leg, which is positioned with the hips and knees flexed 45°. The foot of the test leg rests on the table in medial rotation with the knee in extension. The examiner applies a valgus stress to the knee while flexing the knee. The test result is positive if the subluxation of the knee is reduced between 25° and 45°.

Slocum's test: A test designed to identify anterolateral instability of the knee. The patient is positioned supine with the knee flexed to 90° and the hip flexed to 45°. The examiner sits on the patient's forefoot, which is internally rotated 30°. The examiner grasps the tibia and applies an anteriorly directed force to the tibia. The test result is positive if tibial movement occurs primarily on the lateral side. The test can also be used to identify anteromedial rotary instability. This version of the test is performed with the foot laterally rotated 15°; it is positive if tibial movement primarily occurs on the medial side.

stroke test: See *brush test.*

valgus stress test: See *abduction test.*

varus stress test: See *adduction test.*

Waldron test: A test designed to identify chondromalacia of the patella. The patient does several slow deep knee bends while the examiner palpates the patella. The test result is positive if pain and crepitus are present during the range of movement.

Wilson test: A test designed to identify osteochondritis dissecans. The patient is seated with the leg in the dependent position. The patient extends the knee with the tibia medially rotated until the pain increases. The test is repeated with the tibia laterally rotated during extension. The test result is positive if the pain does not occur when the tibia is laterally rotated.

wipe test: See *brush test.*

Foot and Ankle

Achilles tendon test: See *Thompson's test.*

anterior drawer sign: A test designed to identify anterior ankle instability. The patient lies supine, and the examiner stabilizes the distal tibia and fibula with one hand while the examiner's other hand holds the foot in 20° of plantar flexion. The test result is positive if, while drawing the talus forward in the ankle mortise, there is straight anterior translation that exceeds that of the uninvolved side.

Homans' sign: A test designed to detect deep vein thrombosis in the lower part of the leg. The ankle is passively dorsiflexed, and any sudden increase of pain in the calf or popliteal space is noted.

Kleiger test: A test for detecting lesions of the deltoid ligament. The patient is seated with the knees flexed to 90°. The examiner holds the foot and attempts to abduct the forefoot. The test result is positive if the patient complains of pain medially and laterally. The talus may be felt to displace slightly from the medial malleolus.

Talar tilt: A test designed to identify lesions of the calcaneofibular ligament. The patient is supine or lying on one side with the knee flexed to 90°. With the foot in a neutral position, the talus is tilted medially. The test result is positive if the amount of adduction on the involved side is excessive.

Thompson's test: A test designed to detect ruptures of the Achilles tendon. The patient is placed in a prone position or on the knees with the feet extended over the edge of the bed. The middle third of the calf muscle is squeezed by the examiner. If a normal plantar flexion response is not elicited, an Achilles tendon rupture is suspected.

FOR MORE INFORMATION

Blauvelt, CT and Nelson, FRT: A Manual of Orthopaedic Terminology, ed 5. Mosby-Year Book, St. Louis, 1994.

D'Ambrosia, RD: Musculoskeletal Disorders: Regional Examination and Differential Diagnosis, ed 2. JB Lippincott, Philadelphia, 1986.

Magee, DJ: Orthopedic Physical Assessment, ed 2. WB Saunders, Philadelphia, 1992.

McCONNELL'S CLASSIFICATION OF PATELLAR ALIGNMENT

medial and lateral displacement: Lateral displacement is determined by the examiner palpating the medial and lateral femoral epicondyles with the index fingers and simultaneously palpating the midpatella with the thumbs. The distance between the index fingers and the thumbs should be approximately the same. If a displacement is present, the distance from the index finger to the thumbs will be less on the side of the displacement.

medial and lateral tilt: The degree of medial or lateral tilting is determined by comparing the height of the medial patella border with the lateral patellar border. The examiner places the thumb and index finger on the medial and lateral borders of the patella. Both digits should be of equal height. If one digit is higher than the other digit, the patella is tilted in the direction of the lower digit.

Continued on following page

anterior tilt: Anterior tilt is determined by the examiner palpating the inferior pole of the patella. If no anterior tilt exists, the inferior pole should be easily palpated. An anterior tilt is present if the examiner must place a downward pressure on the superior pole of the patella so that the inferior pole becomes superficial enough to palpate.

patellar rotation: Patellar rotation is determined by examining the relationship between the longitudinal axis of the patella and the longitudinal axis of the femur. The longitudinal axis of the patella should normally be in line with the anterior superior iliac spine. If the distal end of the patella is angled medially or laterally from the anterior superior iliac spine, the patella is considered to be rotated medially or laterally respectively.

FOR MORE INFORMATION

Fitzgerald, GK and McClure, PW: Reliability of measurements obtained with four tests for patellofemoral alignment. Phys Ther 75:84, 1995.

McConnell, J: The management of chondromalacia patellae: A long term solution. Australian Journal of Physiotherapy 32:215, 1986.

CYRIAX TERMS

End-feels According to Cyriax

end-feel: The type of resistance felt by an examiner at the end-range of a passive range-of-motion test.

> **bone to bone:** The abrupt halt to the movement that is felt when two hard surfaces meet, for example, at the extreme of passive extension of the normal elbow.

> **capsular:** The feeling of immediate stoppage of movement with some give. The type of end-feel felt at the end of the range of normal shoulder extension or hip extension.

> **empty:** The end-feel felt when the patient complains of considerable pain during passive movement but the examiner perceives no increase in resistance to joint movement.

> **spasm:** The feeling of muscle "spasm" coming actively into play. It is said to indicate the presence of acute or subacute arthritis.

> **springy block:** A rebound is seen and felt at the end of the range. It is said to occur with displacement of an intra-articular structure, for example, when a torn meniscus in the knee engages between the tibia and femur and prevents the last few degrees of extension.

> **tissue approximation:** The end-feel felt when a limb segment cannot be moved further because the soft tissues surrounding the joint cannot be compressed any further. It is the sensation felt at the end-range of elbow or knee flexion.

Cyriax's Selective Tissue Tension Tests

The following terms, developed by Cyriax, relate to a method that can be used to identify the source of the patient's pain complaints. In his system the diagnosis depends on asking the patient to move or on applying forces. In either case, patients report what they feel. Equal importance is placed on determining which movements are painful and/or limited and which movements are full range and/or pain-free.

active range of movements: These assess the patient's ability and willingness to perform the movements requested, the range of active movements available, and the patient's ability to produce the muscle forces required for active movement. These movements are also used to determine the region of the body from which the symptoms are originating and to determine which movements and muscles to examine in detail.

painful arc: The excursion (arc) near the mid-range in which pain is felt during an active movement test. The pain disappears as this position is passed in either direction. The pain may reappear at the end-range. According to Cyriax, a painful arc implies that a structure is pinched between two bony surfaces.

passive range of movements: These assess the ability of the "inert" (noncontractile, according to Cyriax) tissues to allow motion at a joint. The patient states whether pain is provoked. Each motion possible for the joint being tested must be examined to distinguish between capsular and noncapsular patterns of movement restrictions. Any discrepancy between the range of movement obtained actively and passively is noted.

resisted movements: These are resisted isometric contractions with the limb segment near the mid-range. These movements assess the tension-producing capabilities of specific muscle groups and whether the patient's pain is originating from these muscle groups.

BASED ON

Cyriax, J: Textbook of Orthopaedic Medicine, ed 11. Bailliere Tindall, London, 1984.

SIGNIFICANCE OF DIAGNOSTIC MOVEMENTS IN SELECTIVE TISSUE TENSION TESTS OF CYRIAX		
Tests	Results of Tests	Conclusion According to Cyriax
Active and passive movements	Pain is felt in one direction during the passive movement and in the opposite direction during the active movement.	A contractile structure is at fault.
Passive movements	Excessive range of motion is found.	Capsular or ligamentous laxity is evident.
Active and passive movements, resisted movements	Pain is felt at the end-range of active and passive movements; resisted movements are pain-free.	An "inert" noncontractile structure is at fault.
Resisted movements	Pain is not felt; strength is normal.	No lesion is present.
Resisted movements	Pain is felt; strength is normal.	A minor lesion of muscle or tendon may be present.
Resisted movements	Pain is felt; strength is decreased.	A serious lesion of the muscle or tendon may be present.
Resisted movements	Pain is not felt; strength is decreased.	A complete rupture of the muscle or tendon may be present.
Resisted movements	Pain is felt after a number of repetitions.	Intermittent claudication may be present.
Resisted movements	Pain is felt with all resisted movements.	There is evidence of emotional hypersensitivity or an organic cause of pain.

Based on Cyriax, J: Textbook of Orthopaedic Medicine, ed 11. Bailliere Tindall, London, 1984.

Capsular Patterns of the Joints According to Cyriax

capsular pattern: A limitation of movement or a pattern of pain at a joint that occurs in a predictable pattern. According to Cyriax, these patterns are due to lesions in either the joint capsule or the synovial membrane. Limitations of motion at a joint that do not fall into these predictable patterns are said to exhibit noncapsular patterns. Causes of noncapsular patterns are said to be ligamentous adhesions, internal derangements, and extra-articular lesions.

acromioclavicular joint: Pain only at the extremes of range.

ankle joint: If the calf muscles are of adequate length, there will be a greater limitation of plantar flexion than of dorsiflexion.

cervical spine (facet joints): Lateral flexion and rotation are equally limited, flexion is full range and painful, and extension is limited.

elbow: Greater limitation in flexion than in extension.

facet joints: See specific body region—*cervical spine, lumbar spine,* or *thoracic spine.*

finger joints: Greater limitation in flexion than in extension.

glenohumeral joint: Greatest limitation in external rotation, followed by abduction, with less limitation in internal rotation.

hip joint: Equal limitations in flexion, abduction, and medial rotation, with a slight loss in extension. There is little or no loss in lateral rotation.

knee joint: Greater limitation in flexion than in extension.

lumbar spine (facet joints): The capsular pattern for the joints of the lumbar spine cannot be determined because of the difficulty of assessing the amount of motion in these joints.

metatarsophalangeal joint (first): Greater limitation in extension than in flexion.

metatarsophalangeal joints (second through fifth): Variable.

midtarsal joint: Equal limitations in dorsiflexion, plantar flexion, adduction, and medial rotation.

radioulnar joint (distal): Full range of motion with pain at both extremes of rotation.

sacrococcygeal joints: Pain produced when forces are applied to these joints.

sacroiliac joint: Pain produced when forces are applied to these joints.

sternoclavicular joint: Pain only at the extremes of range.

symphysis pubis: Pain produced when forces are applied to this joint.

talocalcaneal joint: Limitation in varus.

thoracic spine (facet joints): The capsular pattern for the joints of the thoracic spine cannot be determined because of the difficulty of assessing the amount of motion in these joints.

Continued on following page

Cyriax Terms **191**

thumb joints: Greater limitation in flexion than in extension.

trapeziometacarpal joint: Limitations in abduction and in extension with full flexion.

wrist: Equal limitation in flexion and extension.

BASED ON

Cyriax J: Textbook of Orthopaedic Medicine, ed 11. Bailliere Tindall, London, 1984.

KALTENBORN TERMS
Grading System for Classifying Joint Motion

Hypomobility	0 =	No movement (ankylosis)
	1 =	Considerable decrease in movement
	2 =	Slight decrease in movement
Normal	3 =	Normal
Hypermobility	4 =	Slight increase in movement
	5 =	Considerable increase in movement
	6 =	Complete instability

convex-concave rule: The rule is used to guide therapists as to which direction they should move limb segments when examining joints with limitations in range of motion. When a therapist moves a convex joint surface on a concave joint surface, the convex joint surface is moved in a direction opposite the range-of-motion limitation. Conversely, when a therapist moves a concave joint surface on a convex joint surface, the concave joint surface is moved in the same direction as the range-of-motion limitation.

Grades of Movement According to Kaltenborn

Grade I traction: Movements are of small amplitude, and there is no appreciable joint separation. Traction force to nullify the compressive forces acting on the joint is applied.

Grade II traction and gliding: The slack of tissues surrounding the joint is taken up, and the tissues surrounding the joint are tightened.

Grade III traction and gliding: After the slack has been taken up, more force is applied, and the tissues crossing the joint are stretched.

End-feels According to Kaltenborn

end-feel: The type of resistance felt by an examiner at the end-range of a passive range-of-motion test.

firm end-feel: Results from capsular or ligamentous stretching. An example is the resistance felt by the examiner at the end-range of external rotation of the glenohumeral joint.

hard end-feel: Occurs when bone meets bone. An example is the resistance felt by the examiner at the end-range of extension of the elbow.

soft end-feel: Is due to soft tissue approximation or soft tissue stretching. An example is the resistance felt by the examiner at the end-range of knee flexion.

BASED ON

Kaltenborn, FM: Manual Mobilization of the Extremity Joints: Basic Examination and Treatment Techniques, ed 4. Olaf Norlis Bokhandel, Oslo, 1989.

MACCONNAILL TERMS

arthrokinematics: The study of movements within joints.

osteokinematics: The study of the movement of bony segments around a joint axis.

roll: The movement that occurs when equidistant points on a convex surface come into contact with equidistant points on the concave surface. Roll also occurs when equidistant points on a concave surface come into contact with equidistant points on the convex surface.

slide: The movement that occurs when the same point on the convex surface comes into contact with new points on the concave surface. Slide also occurs when the same point on the concave surface comes into contact with new points on the convex surface.

spin: Rotation of a convex joint surface about a longitudinal axis on a concave joint surface. Spin also occurs when a concave surface rotates about a longitudinal axis on the convex surface.

FOR MORE INFORMATION

Warwick, R and Williams, PL: Gray's Anatomy, ed 36. WB Saunders, Philadelphia, 1980.

MAITLAND TERMS

comparable sign: Any form of joint movement testing that causes the patient to report symptoms comparable to those associated with the patient's chief complaint.

mobilization: Passive movement test performed by an examiner in such a way that the patient can prevent the movement if he or she so chooses. Two main types of movement are:
- Passive oscillatory movements that are done at a rate of two or three per second. They are of small or large amplitude and are applied anywhere in a range of movement.
- Sustained stretching that is performed with small-amplitude oscillations at the end of the range of motion.

manipulation: Manipulation is a sudden movement or thrust, of small amplitude, performed at a speed that makes the patient unable to prevent the motion. Manipulation under anesthesia is a procedure performed with the patient under anesthesia that is used to stretch a joint to restore a full range of movement by breaking adhesions. The procedure does not consist of a sudden, forceful thrust that is per-
Continued on following page

formed when the patient is awake but is done as a steady and controlled stretch.

Grades of Movement According to Maitland

Grade I: Small-amplitude movements performed at the beginning of the range.

Grade II: Large-amplitude movements that do not reach the limit of the range. If the movement is performed near the beginning of the range, it is a II −; if taken deeply into the range, yet still not reaching the limit, it is a II +.

Grade III: Large-amplitude movements performed up to the limit of the range. If the movement is applied forcefully at the limit of the range, it is a III +; if applied gently at the limit of the range, it is a III −.

Grade IV: Small-amplitude movements performed at the limit of the range. Depending on the vigor of the motion, the grades can be a IV − or IV +.

BASED ON

Maitland, GD: Peripheral Manipulation, ed 3. Butterworths, Boston, 1991.

CRITERIA FOR CLASSIFICATION INTO THE LUMBAR SYNDROMES ACCORDING TO McKENZIE

The following describes the common findings associated with each syndrome. Information usually obtained during the history is listed first, followed by the information obtained during the physical examination (which consists of the examination, tests for movement loss, and the use of test movements).

Postural Syndrome

History

- Patients are usually 30 years of age or younger.
- Patients frequently have sedentary occupations.
- Pain is always intermittent and produced when the patient stays in one position (especially sitting and forward bending) for a prolonged period of time.
- Pain ceases with movement and activity.

Physical Examination

- Deformity of the lumbar spine is not present (i.e., there is no lateral shift or reduced or accentuated lumbar lordosis during standing).
- All test movements are pain-free.
- No loss of motion is noted during the test movements.
- Poor sitting and standing posture is often the only positive finding.

- Pain cannot be reproduced by test movements. The patient must assume and maintain a position that is stated to cause pain.

Dysfunction Syndrome

History

- Patients are likely to be older than 30 years of age.
- Pain is felt at the end-range of some movements and may interfere with the performance of certain simple tasks.
- Rapid changes in symptoms do not occur.
- Patients complain in the early stages of low back stiffness that occurs in the morning and that decreases as the day progresses.
- Patients with a longstanding history of a dysfunction syndrome are likely to have reduced flexion and extension and are likely to have stiffness that persists throughout the day.
- Patients often feel better when active and moving about than when they are at rest.
- Pain is intermittent and occurs only when the patient's back is placed in a position near the patient's limitation of motion.
- Pain is sometimes triggered by activity that the patient is not used to.

Physical Examination

- The posture is poor.
- Deformities (i.e., a lateral shift, reduced or accentuated lumbar lordosis during standing) are not typically seen except in elderly patients.
- A loss of movement is present.
- A loss of function may occur.
- Pain is easily reproduced with some test movements.
- Pain is elicited as soon as the end-range of limited movements is reached, but the pain subsides when the patient returns to his or her normal standing position.
- Patients who have an adherent nerve root may have peripheralization with flexion in standing, but flexion while lying supine does not cause peripheralization.
- Patients who have an adherent nerve root may laterally deviate during flexion toward the painful side.

Derangement Syndromes

History for All Derangement Syndromes

- Patients are likely to be between 20 and 35 years of age and are usually male.
- Derangements may arise from a single severe strain, a less severe strain applied more frequently, or a sustained flexion strain. A sustained flexion strain is the most common cause of derangement.
- Patients with derangement syndromes often have constant pain that varies in intensity, whereas patients with postural and dysfunction syndromes always have intermittent pain.

Continued on following page

- Pain is usually worse when the patient assumes certain positions. In general, if the derangement is small, patients feel better when they move and worse when they are at rest. If the derangement is large and causes significant deformity, patients usually feel better when they lie down.
- Pain is often increased when patients are in the sitting position.
- Patients often have difficulty finding a comfortable sleeping position.
- Patients have a loss of movement that is almost always asymmetrical.
- During the assessment of sagittal pain movements (flexion and extension), the patient's trunk often deviates to one side.
- Patients often have a history of recurring episodes of low back pain.
- Centralization of symptoms occurs only in derangement syndromes.
- Test movements can have a rapid effect on the condition. If a patient with derangement describes changes in the pain pattern after test movements, there should also be observable changes in range of motion and deformity.
- Symptoms are changed as a result of the test movements.
- Gross loss of movement may occur—severe cases have deformity.

History and Physical Examination for Derangement One

- Central or symmetrical low back pain is present (L4/L5 region).
- Buttock and thigh pain is only rarely present.
- Spinal extension is limited.
- The lumbar lordosis is normal, and there is no other lumbar postural deformity.

History and Physical Examination for Derangement Two

- Central or symmetrical low back pain is present (L4/L5 region).
- Buttock and/or thigh pain may be present.
- Extension is limited.
- The reduced lumbar lordosis deformity is present while the patient is standing.
- After painful extension of the lumbar spine, returning to a flexed position may result in relief from pain.

History and Physical Examination for Derangement Three

- Unilateral or asymmetrical low back pain is present (L4/L5 region).
- Buttock and/or thigh pain may be present.
- No deformity (i.e., a lateral shift, reduced or accentuated lumbar lordosis) is present.

History and Physical Examination for Derangement Four

- Unilateral or asymmetrical low back pain is present (L4/L5 region).

- Buttock and/or thigh pain may be present.
- A lateral shift deformity is present while the patient is standing.

History and Physical Examination for Derangement Five

- Unilateral or asymmetrical low back pain is present (L4/L5 region).
- Buttock and/or thigh pain may be present.
- Intermittent or constant pain extends below the knee.
- No deformity (i.e., a lateral shift, reduced or accentuated lumbar lordosis) is present.

History and Physical Examination for Derangement Six

- Unilateral or asymmetrical low back pain is present (L4/L5 region).
- Buttock and/or thigh pain may be present.
- Pain is usually constant and extends below the knee.
- A lateral shift and a reduced lumbar lordosis deformity is present.
- Neurologic deficit is often present.

History and Physical Examination for Derangement Seven

- Symmetrical or asymmetrical low back pain is present (L4/L5 region).
- Buttock and/or thigh pain may be present.
- An accentuated lumbar lordosis is present.
- The patient's lumbar spine remains lordotic even during flexion motions (e.g., during motion testing).
- Patients describe a sudden onset of pain and may say they were easily able to touch their toes the day before the onset of pain.

FOR MORE INFORMATION

McKenzie, RA: The Lumbar Spine: Mechanical Diagnosis and Therapy. Spinal Publications: Waikanae, New Zealand, 1981.

CRITERIA FOR CLASSIFICATION INTO THE CERVICAL SYNDROMES ACCORDING TO McKENZIE

The following describes the common findings associated with each syndrome. Information usually obtained during the history is listed first, followed by the information obtained during the physical examination (which consists of the examination, tests for movement loss, and the use of test movements).

Postural Syndrome

History

- Patients are usually 30 years of age or younger.
- Patients frequently have sedentary occupations.

Continued on following page

- Pain is always intermittent and produced when the patient stays in one position (especially sitting and lying) for a prolonged period of time.
- Pain ceases with movement and activity.

Physical Examination

- Deformity of the cervical spine is not present.
- All test movements are pain-free.
- No loss of motion will be noted during the test movements.
- Poor sitting and standing posture is often the only positive finding.
- Pain cannot be reproduced by test movements. The patient must assume and maintain a position that is stated to cause pain.
- Any change in position relieves the pain provided the structures are unloaded.

Dysfunction Syndrome

History

- Patients are likely to be older than 30 years of age.
- Pain is felt at the end-range of some movements and may interfere with the performance of certain simple tasks.
- Rapid changes in symptoms do not occur.
- Patients complain in the early stages of neck stiffness that occurs in the morning and that decreases as the day progresses.
- Patients with a longstanding history of a dysfunction syndrome are likely to have reduced flexion and extension and are likely to have stiffness that persists throughout the day.
- Patients often feel better when they are active and moving about than when they are at rest.
- Pain is intermittent and occurs only when the patient's neck is placed in a position near the patient's limitation of motion.
- Pain is sometimes triggered by activity that the patient is not used to.

Physical Examination

- The posture is poor.
- Deformities (e.g., Dowager's hump) are not typically seen except in elderly patients.
- A loss of movement is present.
- A loss of function may occur.
- Pain is easily reproduced with some test movements.
- Pain is elicited as soon as the end-range of limited movements is reached, but the pain subsides when the patient returns to his or her normal standing position.
- Pain is localized in the neck adjacent to the spine, bilateral or unilateral.
- Pain may radiate locally to midscapular region and upper trapezius, especially after prolonged end-range positioning.

Derangement Syndromes

History for All Derangement Syndromes

- Patients are likely to be between 12 and 55 years of age.
- Derangements may arise from a single severe strain, a less severe

strain applied more frequently, or a sustained flexion strain. A sustained flexion strain is the most common cause of derangement.

- Patients with derangement syndromes often have constant pain that varies in intensity, whereas patients with postural and dysfunction syndromes always have intermittent pain.
- Pain is usually worse when the patient assumes certain positions.
- Pain is often increased when patients are in the sitting position.
- Patients often have difficulty finding a comfortable sleeping position.
- Patients have a loss of movement that is almost always asymmetrical.
- During the assessment of sagittal pain movements (flexion and extension), the patient's neck often deviates to one side.
- Patients often have a history of recurring episodes of neck pain.
- The posture may be poor.
- Pain may be felt adjacent to the midline of the spine and may radiate and be referred distally in the form of pain, paraesthesia, or numbness.

History and Physical Examination for Derangement One

- Central or symmetrical pain about C5 to C7 is present.
- Scapular or shoulder pain is only rarely present.
- Cervical extension is limited.
- The cervical lordosis is normal, and there is no other cervical postural deformity.
- This form of derangement is rapidly reversible.

History and Physical Examination for Derangement Two

- Central or symmetrical pain about C5 to C7 is present.
- Scapular, shoulder, or upper arm pain may be present.
- Cervical extension is limited.
- Reduced cervical lordosis deformity is present.
- This form of derangement is rarely rapidly reversible.

History and Physical Examination for Derangement Three

- Unilateral or asymmetrical pain about C3 to C7 is present.
- Scapular, shoulder, or upper arm pain may be present.
- No deformity is present.
- Cervical extension, rotation, and lateral flexion may be individually or collectively obstructed.
- This form of derangement is rapidly reversible.

History and Physical Examination for Derangement Four

- Unilateral or asymmetrical pain about C5 to C7 is present.
- Scapular, shoulder, or upper arm pain may be present.
- Acute wry neck or torticollis deformity is present.
- Cervical extension, rotation, and lateral flexion are obstructed.
- This form of derangement is rapidly reversible.

Continued on following page

History and Physical Examination for Derangement Five

- Unilateral or asymmetrical pain about C5 to C7 is present.
- Scapular, shoulder, or upper arm pain may be present.
- No deformity is present.
- Cervical extension and lateral flexion toward the side of pain are obstructed.
- This form of derangement is often rapidly reversible.
- A small percentage of patients fail to respond to mechanical therapy.

History and Physical Examination for Derangement Six

- Unilateral or asymmetrical pain about C5 to C7 is present.
- Arm symptoms distal to the elbow may be present.
- Pain is usually constant and extends below the elbow.
- A cervical kyphosis, acute wry neck, or torticollitis deformity is present.
- Neurologic motor deficit is often present.
- This form of derangement is not rapidly reversible.

History and Physical Examination for Derangement Seven

- Symmetrical or asymmetrical pain about C4 to C6 is present.
- Anterior and anterolateral neck pain may be present.
- No deformity is present.
- Dysphagia is common.
- Cervical flexion is obstructed.
- This form of derangement is rapidly reversible.

FOR MORE INFORMATION

McKenzie, RA: The Cervical and Thoracic Spine: Mechanical Diagnosis and Therapy. Spinal Publications, Waikanae, New Zealand, 1990.

WADDELL'S NONORGANIC PHYSICAL SIGNS IN LOW BACK PAIN

tenderness: Tenderness not related to a particular skeletal or neuromuscular structure, may be either superficial or nonanatomic.

> **superficial:** The skin is tender to light pinch over a wide area of lumbar skin not in a distribution associated with a posterior primary ramus.

> **nonanatomic:** Deep tenderness, which is not localized to one structure, is felt over a wide area and often extends to the thoracic spine, sacrum, or pelvis.

simulation tests: These tests give the patient the impression that a particular examination is being carried out when in fact it is not.

> **axial loading:** Low back pain is reported when the examiner presses down on the top of the patient's head. Neck pain is common and should not be considered indicative of a nonorganic sign.

> **rotation:** Back pain is reported when the shoulders and pelvis are passively rotated in the same plane as the patient stands relaxed with the feet together. In the presence of root irritation, leg pain may be produced and should not be considered indicative of a nonorganic sign.

distraction tests: A positive physical finding is demonstrated in the routine manner; this finding is then checked while the patient's attention is distracted. A nonorganic component may be present if the finding disappears when the patient is distracted.

> **straight leg raising:** The examiner lifts the patient's foot as when testing the plantar reflex in the sitting position. A nonorganic component may be present if the leg is lifted higher than when tested in the supine position.

regional disturbances: Dysfunction (e.g., sensory or motor) involving a widespread region of body parts in a manner that cannot be explained based on anatomy. Care must be taken to distinguish from multiple nerve root involvement.

> **weakness:** Demonstrated on testing by a partial cogwheel "giving way" of many muscle groups that cannot be explained on a localized neurologic basis.

> **sensory:** Include diminished sensation to light touch, pinprick or other neurologic tests fitting a "stocking" rather than a dermatomal pattern.

overreaction: May take the form of disproportionate verbalization, facial expression, muscle tension and tremor, collapsing or sweating. Judgments should be made with caution minimizing the examiner's own emotional reaction.

> SCORING. Any individual sign counts as a positive sign for that type; a finding of three or more of the five types is clinically significant.

BASED ON

Waddell, G, et al: Nonorganic physical signs in low-back pain. Spine 5:117, 1980, with permission.

QUEBEC TASK FORCE CLASSIFICATION OF ACTIVITY-RELATED SPINAL DISORDERS

Classification	Symptoms	Duration of Symptoms from Onset	Working Status at Time of Evaluation
1	Pain without radiation	a (<7 d)	W (working)
2	Pain + radiation to extremity, proximally	b (7 d–7 wk)	I (idle)
3	Pain + radiation to extremity, distally*	c (>7 wk)	
4	Pain + radiation to upper/lower limb neurologic signs		
5	Presumptive compression of a spinal nerve root on a simple roentgenogram (i.e., spinal instability or fracture)		
6	Compression of a spinal nerve root confirmed by Specific imaging techniques (i.e., computerized axial tomography, myelography, or magnetic resonance imaging) Other diagnostic techniques (e.g., electromyography, venography)		
7	Spinal stenosis		
8	Postsurgical status, 1–6 mo after intervention		
9	Postsurgical status, > 6 mo after intervention 9.1 Asymptomatic 9.2 Symptomatic		
10	Chronic pain syndrome		W (working)
11	Other diagnoses		I (idle)

*Not applicable to the thoracic segment.
From Quebec Task Force on Spinal Disorders: Scientific approach to the assessment and management of activity-related spinal disorders: A monograph for clinicians. Report of the Quebec Task Force on Spinal Disorders. Spine 12:S17, 1987, with permission.

WARNING SIGNS ("RED-FLAGS")
IN ASSESSMENT OF ACUTE LO\
PROBLEMS IN ADULTS
According to Clinical Practice Gui\
No. 14 of the Agency for Health Care
and Research

Red flags are indicators of potentially serious pat\
identification of red flags indicates the need for additional n., , or
investigations.

ASSESSMENT OF ACUTE LOW BACK PAIN	
Red Flag	*Reason Why Information Is Important*
Past history of: Cancer Unexplained weight loss Immunosuppression Intravenous drug use Urinary infection Pain increasing with rest	Indications of possible cancer or infections
Presence of fever	Indications of possible cancer or infections
Presence of bladder dysfunction	Indication of cauda equina syndrome
Presence of saddle anaesthesia	Indication of cauda equina syndrome
Presence of major weakness in the limb of the lower extremity	Indication of cauda equina syndrome
Trauma that could have caused a fracture, taking into account consideration of the patient's age and likelihood of having osteoporosis	Avoidance of delays in diagnosing possible fracture

FOR MORE INFORMATION

Bigos, SJ, et al: Acute Low Back Problems in Adults: Clinical Practice
Guideline No. 14. AHCPR Publication No. 95-0642. Agency for
Health Care Policy and Research, Rockville, MD, 1994.

LOW BACK DISABILITY QUESTIONNAIRES

Roland and Morris Disability Questionnaire: Description

Roland and Morris derived a "disability index" from 24 items on the Sickness Impact Profile (SIP). By adding the phrase "because of my back" to each statement from the SIP, their index was disease specific for low back. The Roland and Morris Disability Index also ignores the established scoring scale of the SIP and instead each answer is scaled as 0 or 1, resulting in a range of scores 0 to 24.

Roland and Morris Disability Questionnaire: Instrument

When your back hurts, you may find it difficult to do some of the things you normally do.

This list contains some sentences that people have used to describe themselves when they have back pain. When you read them, you may find that some stand out because they describe you *today*. As you read the list, think of yourself *today*. When you read a sentence that describes you today, put a check beside the number of the sentence. If the sentence does not describe you, then leave the space blank and go on to the next one. Remember, only check the sentence if you are sure that it describes you *today*.

_____ 1. I stay at home most of the time because of my back.
_____ 2. I change position frequently to try and get my back comfortable.
_____ 3. I walk more slowly than usual because of my back.
_____ 4. Because of my back, I am not doing any of the jobs that I usually do around the house.
_____ 5. Because of my back, I use a handrail to get upstairs.
_____ 6. Because of my back, I lie down to rest more often.
_____ 7. Because of my back, I have to hold onto something to get out of an easy chair.
_____ 8. Because of my back, I try to get other people to do things for me.
_____ 9. I get dressed more slowly than usual because of my back.
_____ 10. I only stand up for short periods of time because of my back.
_____ 11. Because of my back, I try not to bend or kneel down.
_____ 12. I find it difficult to get out of a chair because of my back.
_____ 13. My back is painful almost all the time.
_____ 14. I find it difficult to turn over in bed because of my back.
_____ 15. My appetite is not very good because of my back pain.
_____ 16. I have trouble putting on my socks (or stockings) because of the pain in my back.
_____ 17. I only walk short distances because of my back pain.
_____ 18. I sleep less well because of my back.
_____ 19. Because of my back pain, I get dressed with help from someone else.
_____ 20. I sit down for most of the day because of my back.
_____ 21. I avoid heavy jobs around the house because of my back.

_____22. Because of my back pain, I am more irritable and bad tempered with people than usual.
_____23. Because of my back, I go upstairs more slowly than usual.
_____24. I stay in bed most of the time because of my back.

From Roland, M and Morris, R: A study of the natural history of back pain, part I: The development of a reliable and sensitive measure of disability in low back pain. Spine 8:141, 1983.

Oswestry Low Back Pain Disability Questionnaire: Description

The Oswestry Low Back Pain Disability Questionnaire is an index described by Fairbanks et al. and later modified by Hudson-Cook et al. The questionnaire is an easily administered self-report that yields a patient's perceived disability based on 10 areas of limitation in performance. Each section is scored on a 6-point scale (0–5), with 0 representing no limitation and 5 representing maximal limitation. The subscales combined add up to a maximum of 50. The score is then doubled and presented as a percentage of the patient's perceived disability (the higher the score, the higher the disability). The Oswestry index has been used in treatment efficacy studies involving manipulation and exercise as well as correlational studies of physical impairments and functional limitations.

Oswestry Low Back Pain Disability Questionnaire: Instrument

Please read:
This questionnaire has been designed to give the doctor information as to how your back pain has affected your ability to manage in everyday life. Please answer every section, and mark in each section only the one box which applies to you. We realize you may consider that two of the statements in any one section relate to you, but please just mark the box which most closely describes your problem.

Section 1—Pain Intensity
☐ I can tolerate the pain I have without having to use pain killers.
☐ The pain is bad but I manage without taking pain killers.
☐ Pain killers give complete relief from pain.
☐ Pain killers give moderate relief from pain.
☐ Pain killers give very little relief from pain.
☐ Pain killers have no effect on the pain and I do not use them.

Section 2—Personal Care (Washing, Dressing, etc.)
☐ I can look after myself normally without causing extra pain.
☐ I can look after myself normally but it causes extra pain.
☐ It is painful to look after myself and I am slow and careful.
☐ I need some help but manage most of my personal care.
☐ I need help every day in most aspects of self care.
☐ I do not get dressed, wash with difficulty and stay in bed.

Continued on following page

Section 3—Lifting
- ☐ I can lift heavy weights without extra pain.
- ☐ I can lift heavy weights but it gives extra pain.
- ☐ Pain prevents me from lifting heavy weights off the floor, but I can manage if they are conveniently positioned, eg, on a table.
- ☐ Pain prevents me from lifting heavy weights but I can manage light to medium weights if they are conveniently positioned.
- ☐ I can lift only very light weights.
- ☐ I cannot lift or carry anything at all.

Section 4—Walking
- ☐ Pain does not prevent me walking any distance.
- ☐ Pain prevents me walking more than 1 mile.
- ☐ Pain prevents me from walking more than $\frac{1}{2}$ mile.
- ☐ Pain prevents me from walking more than $\frac{1}{4}$ mile.
- ☐ I can only walk using a cane or crutches.
- ☐ I am in bed most of the time and have to crawl to the toilet.

Section 5—Sitting
- ☐ I can sit in any chair as long as I like.
- ☐ I can only sit in my favorite chair as long as I like.
- ☐ Pain prevents me sitting more than 1 hour.
- ☐ Pain prevents me from sitting more than $\frac{1}{2}$ hour.
- ☐ Pain prevents me from sitting more than 10 minutes.
- ☐ Pain prevents me from sitting at all.

Section 6—Standing
- ☐ I can stand as long as I want without extra pain.
- ☐ I can stand as long as I want but it gives me extra pain.
- ☐ Pain prevents me from standing for more than 1 hour.
- ☐ Pain prevents me from standing for more than 30 minutes.
- ☐ Pain prevents me from standing for more than 10 minutes.
- ☐ Pain prevents me from standing at all.

Section 7—Sleeping
- ☐ Pain does not prevent me from sleeping well.
- ☐ I can sleep well only by using tablets.
- ☐ Even when I take pills, I have less than six hours sleep.
- ☐ Even when I take pills, I have less than four hours sleep.
- ☐ Even when I take pills, I have less than two hours sleep.
- ☐ Pain prevents me from sleeping at all.

Section 8—Sex Life
- ☐ My sex life is normal and causes no extra pain.
- ☐ My sex life is normal but causes some extra pain.
- ☐ My sex life is nearly normal but is very painful.
- ☐ My sex life is severely restricted by pain.
- ☐ My sex life is nearly absent because of pain.
- ☐ Pain prevents any sex life at all.

Section 9—Social Life
☐ My social life is normal and gives me no extra pain.
☐ My social life is normal but increases the degree of pain.
☐ Pain has no significant effect on my social life apart from limiting my more energetic interests, eg, dancing, etc.
☐ Pain has restricted my social life and I do not go out as often.
☐ Pain has restricted my social life to my home.
☐ I have no social life because of pain.

Section 10—Traveling
☐ I can travel anywhere without extra pain.
☐ I can travel anywhere but it gives me extra pain.
☐ Pain is bad but I manage journeys over two hours.
☐ Pain restricts me to journeys of less than one hour.
☐ Pain restricts me to short necessary journeys under 30 minutes.
☐ Pain prevents me from traveling except to the doctor or hospital.

From Fairbank, JCT, et al: The Oswestry Low Back Disability Questionnaire. Physiotherapy 66:271, 1980, with permission.

FOR MORE INFORMATION

Hudson-Cook N et al. A revised Oswestry disability questionnaire. In Roland, MO and Jenner, JR (eds): Back Pain: New Approaches to Rehabilitation and Education. Manchester University Press, New York, 1989, pp 187–204.

SCOLIOSIS

Systems Used to Measure Curves

Cobb Method

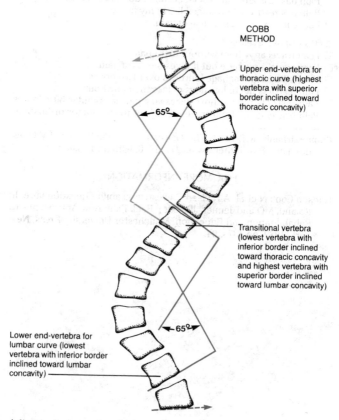

COBB
METHOD

Upper end-vertebra for thoracic curve (highest vertebra with superior border inclined toward thoracic concavity)

65°

Transitional vertebra (lowest vertebra with inferior border inclined toward thoracic concavity and highest vertebra with superior border inclined toward lumbar concavity)

Lower end-vertebra for lumbar curve (lowest vertebra with inferior border inclined toward lumbar concavity)

65°

A line is drawn perpendicular to the upper margin of the vertebra that inclines most toward the concavity. A line is also drawn on the inferior border of the lower vertebra with greatest angulation toward the concavity. The angle formed by these intersecting lines is the measure of curvature. The apical vertebra is also usually noted.

Risser-Ferguson Method

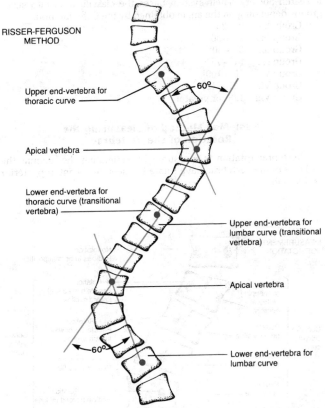

RISSER-FERGUSON
METHOD

Upper end-vertebra for thoracic curve

60°

Apical vertebra

Lower end-vertebra for thoracic curve (transitional vertebra)

Upper end-vertebra for lumbar curve (transitional vertebra)

Apical vertebra

60°

Lower end-vertebra for lumbar curve

The midpoints of the proximal, distal, and apical vertebrae of the curvature are identified. The proximal vertebra is the highest vertebra whose superior surface tilts to the concavity of the curve. The distal vertebra is the lowest vertebra whose inferior surface tilts to the concavity of the curve. The apical vertebra is between the proximal and distal vertebrae and is parallel to the horizontal or transverse plane of the body. The angle formed by the two lines that intersect the apex from the proximal and distal midpoints is the measure of the curvature. The method is still used but is no longer accepted internationally.

Continued on following page

Classification of Scoliotic Curves

Classifications of curves has been standardized by the Scoliosis Research Society. Their system bases the classification into seven groups depending on the angle obtained by the Cobb method.

Group I: 0°–20°
Group II: 21°–30°
Group III: 31°–50°
Group IV: 51°–75°
Group V: 76°–100°
Group VI: 101°–125°
Group VII: 126° or greater

Nash-Moe Method of Measuring the Rotation of the Vertebrae

Vertebral rotation is measured by estimating the amount the pedicles of the vertebrae have rotated as seen on an anteroposterior radiograph.

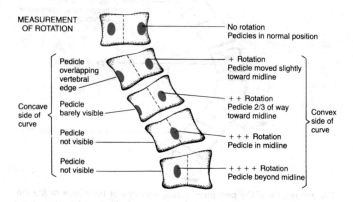

Glossary of Scoliosis Terms

adolescent scoliosis: Spinal curvature presenting at or about the onset of puberty and before maturity.

adult scoliosis: Spinal curvature existing after skeletal maturity.

angle of thoracic inclination: With the trunk flexed 90 degrees at the hips, this is the angle between the horizontal plane and a plane across the posterior rib cage at the greatest prominence of a rib hump.

apical vertebra: The most rotated vertebra in a curve; the most deviated vertebra from the vertical axis of the patient.

body alignment, balance, compensation: 1) The alignment of the midpoint of the occiput over the sacrum in the same vertical plane as the shoulders over the hips. 2) In roentgenology, when the sum of the angular deviations of the spine in one direction is equal to that in the opposite direction.

café au lait spots: Light brown, irregular areas of skin pigmentation. If they are sufficient in number and have smooth margins, they suggest neurofibromatosis.

compensatory curve: A curve, which can be structural, above or below a major curve that tends to maintain normal body alignment.

congenital scoliosis: Scoliosis due to congenitally anomalous vertebral development.

curve measurement: Cobb method: Select the upper and lower end vertebrae. Erect lines perpendicular to their transverse axes. They intersect to form the angle of the curve. If the vertebral end plates are poorly visualized, a line through the bottom or top of the pedicles may be used.

double major scoliosis: Scoliosis with two structural curves.

double thoracic curves (scoliosis): Two structural curves within the thoracic spine.

end vertebra: 1) The most cephalad vertebra of a curve, whose superior surface tilts maximally toward the concavity of the curve. 2) The most caudad vertebra whose inferior surface tilts maximally toward the concavity of the curve.

fractional curve: A compensatory curve that is incomplete because it returns to the erect [position]. Its only horizontal vertebra is its caudad or cephalad one.

full curve: A curve in which the only horizontal vertebra is at the apex.

gibbus: A sharply angular kyphos.

hyperkyphosis: A sagittal alignment of the thoracic spine in which there is more than the normal amount of kyphosis (a kyphos).

hypokyphosis: A sagittal alignment of the thoracic spine in which there is less than the normal amount of kyphosis, but it is not so severe as to be truly lordotic.

hysterical scoliosis: A nonstructural deformity of the spine that develops as a manifestation of a conversion reaction.

idiopathic scoliosis: A structural spinal curvature for which no cause is established.

iliac epiphysis, iliac apophysis: The epiphysis along the wing of an ilium.

inclinometer: An instrument used to measure the angle of thoracic inclination or rib hump.

infantile scoliosis: Spinal curvature developing during the first 3 years of life.

juvenile scoliosis: Spinal curvature developing between the skeletal age of 3 years and the onset of puberty.

Continued on following page

kyphos: A change in alignment of a segment of the spine in the sagittal plane that increases the posterior convex angulation; an abnormally increased kyphosis.

kyphoscoliosis: A spine with scoliosis and a true hyperkyphosis. A rotatory deformity with only *apparent* kyphosis should not be described by this term.

kyphosing scoliosis: A scoliosis with marked rotation such that lateral bending of the rotated spine mimics kyphosis.

lordoscoliosis: A scoliosis associated with an abnormal anterior angulation in the sagittal plane.

major curve: Term used to designate the largest structural curve.

minor curve: Term used to refer to the smallest curve, which is always more flexible than the major curve.

nonstructural curve: A curve that has no structural component and that corrects or overcorrects on recumbent side-bending roentgenograms.

pelvic obliquity: Deviation of the pelvis from the horizontal in the frontal plane. Fixed pelvic obliquities can be attributable to contractures either above or below the pelvis.

primary curve: The first or earliest of several curves to appear, if identifiable.

rotational prominence: In the forward-bending position, the thoracic prominence on one side is usually due to vertebral rotation, causing rib prominence. In the lumbar spine, the prominence is usually due to rotation of the lumbar vertebrae.

skeletal age, bone age: The age obtained by comparing an anteroposterior roentgenogram of the left hand and wrist with the standards of the Gruelich and Pyle Atlas.

structural curve: A segment of the spine with a lateral curvature that lacks normal flexibility. Radiographically, it is identified by the complete lack of a curve on a supine film or by the failure to demonstrate complete segmental mobility on supine side-bending films.

vertebral end plates: The superior and inferior plates of cortical bone of the vertebral body adjacent to the intervertebral disc.

vertebral growth plate: The cartilaginous surface covering the top and bottom of a vertebral body, which is responsible for the linear growth of the vertebra.

vertebral ring apophyses: The most reliable index of vertebral immaturity, seen best in lateral roentgenograms or in the lumbar region in side-bending anteroposterior views.

FROM

Winter, RB: Classification and terminology. In Lonstein, JE, et al: Moe's Textbook of Scoliosis and Other Spinal Deformities, ed 3. WB Saunders, Philadelphia, 1995, pp 41–42, with permission.

SALTER-HARRIS CLASSIFICATION OF EPIPHYSEAL PLATE INJURIES

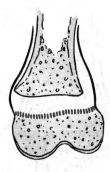

2

Type of Injury
Type I

Description and Prognosis
Complete separation of the epiphysis from the metaphysis without fracture of the bone. Type I injuries are usually caused by shear forces and are most common in newborns (birth injuries) and young children. Closed reduction is not difficult, and the prognosis is excellent, provided the blood supply to the epiphysis is intact.

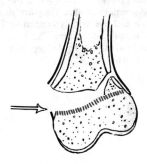

Type of Injury
Type II

Description and Prognosis
The line of separation extends a variable distance along the epiphyseal plate and then out through the metaphysis to produce a triangular fragment. Type II injuries are the most common type of epiphyseal fracture and occur as a result of shearing and bending forces. These injuries tend to occur in the older child. Closed reduction is relatively easy to maintain. The prognosis for growth is excellent, providing blood supply to plate is intact.

Continued on following page

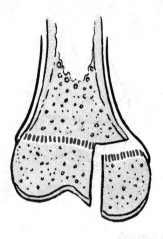

Type of Injury
Type III

Description and Prognosis
Intra-articular fracture extending from the joint surface to the deep zone of the epiphyseal plate and then along the plate to the periphery. Type III injuries are uncommon. They are caused by an intra-articular shearing force and are usually limited to the distal epiphysis. Open reduction is usually necessary. The prognosis for growth is good, provided the blood supply to the separated portion of the epiphysis has not been disrupted.

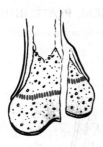
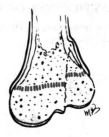

Type of Injury
Type IV

Description and Prognosis
An intra-articular fracture extending from the joint surface through the epiphysis, across the entire thickness of the plate, and through a portion of the metaphysis. Type IV injuries are commonly seen as fractures of the lateral condyle of the humerus. Except for undisplaced fractures, open reduction and internal skeletal fixation are necessary. Perfect reduction is necessary for a favorable prognosis of restored bone growth.

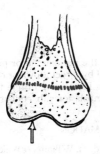
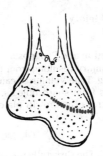

Type of Injury
Type V

Description and Prognosis
An uncommon injury that results from a severe crushing force applied through the epiphysis to one area of the plate. Type V injuries are most common in the ankle or the knee, resulting from a severe abduction or adduction injury to the joint. Weight bearing must be avoided for 3 weeks in the hope of preventing the almost inevitable premature cessation of growth. Prognosis for bone growth is usually poor.

Continued on following page

CLASSIFICATION OF EPIPHYSEAL PLATE INJURIES

Rang recognizes a sixth type of plate injury not described in the Salter-Harris system.

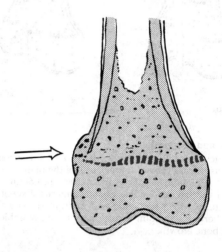

Type of Injury
Type VI

Description and Prognosis
A rare injury resulting from damage to the periosteum or perichondral ring. Type VI injuries can be caused by direct blows or deep lacerations from sharp objects. Because a local bony bridge tends to form across the growth plate, the prognosis for subsequent growth is poor.

FOR MORE INFORMATION

Rang, M: The Growth Plate and Its Disorders. Williams & Wilkins, Baltimore, 1969.

Salter, RB: Textbook of Disorders and Injuries of the Musculoskeletal System, ed 2. Williams & Wilkins, Baltimore, 1983.

Crenshaw, AH (ed): Campbell's Operative Orthopaedics, Vol 2, ed 8. Mosby-Year Book, St. Louis, 1992.

CONTRIBUTION OF THE EPIPHYSES TO BONE GROWTH

Bone	Proximal End (%)	Distal End (%)
Femur	30	70
Fibula	60	40
Humerus	80	20
Radius	25	75
Tibia	55	45
Ulna	20	80

From Rang, M: The Growth Plate and Its Disorders. Williams & Wilkins, Baltimore, 1969, with permission.

CRITERIA FOR THE CLASSIFICATION OF RHEUMATOID ARTHRITIS

THE 1987 REVISED CRITERIA FOR CLASSIFICATION OF RHEUMATOID ARTHRITIS TRADITIONAL FORMAT

Criterion	Definition
1. Morning stiffness	Morning stiffness in and around the joints lasting at least 1 h before maximal improvement.
2. Arthritis of three or more joint areas	At least three joint areas have simultaneously had soft-tissue swelling or fluid (not bony overgrowth alone) observed by a physician. The 14 possible joint areas are right or left PIP, MCP, wrist, elbow, knee, ankle, and MTP joints.
3. Arthritis of hand joints	At least one joint area swollen as above in a wrist, MCP, or PIP.
4. Symmetric arthritis	Simultaneous involvement of the same joint areas (as in 2) on both sides of the body (bilateral involvement of PIPs, MCPs, or MTPs is acceptable without absolute symmetry).
5. Rheumatoid nodules	Subcutaneous nodules, over bony prominences, or extensor surfaces, or in juxta-articular regions, observed by a physician.
6. Serum rheumatoid factor	Demonstration of abnormal amounts of serum "rheumatoid factor" by any method that has been positive in 5% of normal control subjects.

Continued on following page

Criterion	Definition
7. Radiologic changes	Radiologic changes typical of rheumatoid arthritis on PA hand and wrist roentgenograms, which must include erosions or unequivocal bony decalcification localized to or most marked adjacent to the involved joints (osteoarthritis changes alone do not qualify).

For classification purposes, a patient shall be said to have rheumatoid arthritis if he/she has satisfied at least four of the above seven criteria. Criteria 1–4 must have been present for at least 6 wk. Patients with two clinical diagnoses are not excluded. Designation as "classic," "definite," or "probable" rheumatoid arthritis is *not* to be made.

MCPs = metacarpophalangeal joints, MTP = metatarsophalangeal joints, PA = posteroanterior, PIPs = proximal interphalangeal joints.
From Arnett, FC, et al: The American Rheumatological Association 1987 revised criteria for the classification of rheumatoid arthritis. Arthritis & Rheum 31:315, 1988, with permission.

FOR MORE INFORMATION

Primer on the Rheumatic Diseases, ed 10. Arthritis Foundation, Atlanta, 1993.

THE 1958 DIAGNOSTIC CRITERIA FOR RHEUMATOID ARTHRITIS

1. Morning stiffness.
2. Pain on motion or tenderness in at least one joint (observed by a physician).
3. Swelling (soft-tissue thickening or fluid, not bony overgrowth alone) in at least one joint (observed by a physician).
4. Swelling of at least one other joint (observed by a physician).
5. Symmetrical joint swelling (observed by a physician) with simultaneous involvement of the same joint on both sides of the body (bilateral involvement of PIP, MCP, or MTP joints is acceptable without absolute symmetry). Terminal phalangeal joint involvement will not fulfill this criterion.
6. Subcutaneous nodules (observed by a physician) over bony prominences, on extensor surfaces, or in juxta-articular regions.

7. Roentgenographic changes typical of rheumatoid arthritis (which must include at least bony decalcification localized to or most marked adjacent to the involved joints and not just degenerative changes). Degenerative changes do not exclude patients from any group classified as having rheumatoid arthritis.

8. Positive agglutinin test—demonstration of the "rheumatoid factor" by any method that, in two laboratories, has been positive in not over 5% of normal control subjects, or positive streptococcal agglutinin test.

9. Poor mucin precipitate from synovial fluid (with shreds and cloudy solution). (An inflammatory synovial effusion with ≥ 2000 WBC/mm³, without crystals can be substituted for this criterion.)

10. Characteristic histologic changes in synovium with three or more of the following: marked villous hypertrophy; proliferation of superficial synovial cells often with palisading; marked infiltration of chronic inflammatory cells (lymphocytes or plasma cells predominating) with tendency to form "lymphoid follicles"; deposition of compact fibrin either on surface or interstitially; foci of necrosis.

11. Characteristic histologic changes in nodules showing granulomatous foci with central zones of cell necrosis, surrounded by a palisade of proliferated mononuclear cells and peripheral fibrosis and chronic inflammatory cell infiltration.

A. *Classic rheumatoid arthritis* requires seven of the above criteria. In criteria 1–5 the joint signs or symptoms must be continuous for at least 6 wk.

B. *Definite rheumatoid arthritis* requires five of the above criteria. In criteria 1–5 the joint signs or symptoms must be continuous for at least 6 wk.

C. *Probable rheumatoid arthritis* requires three of the above criteria. In criteria 1–5 the joint signs or symptoms must be continuous for at least 6 wk.

D. *Possible rheumatoid arthritis* (not used).

E. *Exclusions*

1. Typical rash of SLE

2. High concentrations of LE cells

3. Histologic evidence of periarteritis nodosa

4. Polymyositis and dermatomyositis

5. Scleroderma

6. Rheumatic fever

Continued on following page

7. Gouty arthritis
8. Tophi
9. Acute infectious arthritis
10. Tuberculous arthritis
11. Reiter's syndrome
12. Shoulder-hand syndrome
13. Hypertrophic pulmonary osteoarthropathy
14. Neuropathic arthropathy
15. Ochronosis
16. Sarcoidosis
17. Multiple myeloma
18. Erythema nodosum
19. Leukemia or lymphoma
20. Agammaglobulinemia

LE = lupus erythematosus; MCP = metacarpophalangeal; MTP = metatarsophalangeal; PIP = proximal interphalangeal; SLE = systemic lupus erythematosus.

From Ropes, MW, et al: 1958 Revision of diagnostic criteria for rheumatoid arthritis. Bull Rheum Dis 9: 175, 1958, with permission.

FOR MORE INFORMATION

Primer on the Rheumatic Diseases, ed 10. Arthritis Foundation, Atlanta, 1993.

RELATIVE PERFORMANCE OF OLD AND NEW CRITERIA SETS FOR RHEUMATOID ARTHRITIS

	Sensitivity	Specificity	Number Misclassified
Old ARA Criteria			
Mucin clot, synovial biopsy, and nodule biopsy excluded. At least five out of eight criteria must be present.	92%	85%	61

RELATIVE PERFORMANCE OF OLD AND NEW CRITERIA SETS FOR RHEUMATOID ARTHRITIS

	Sensitivity	Specificity	Number Misclassified
Old New York Criteria			
At least two out of four criteria must be present.	98%	76%	69
At least three out of four criteria must be present.	81%	94%	64
New RA Criteria			
At least four out of seven criteria must be present.	91.2%*	89.3%	51
New Classification Tree Criteria	93.5%†	89.3%	45

*Early disease onset (< 1 yr—sensitivity 80.9%, specificity 88.2%)
†Early disease onset (< 1 yr—sensitivity 85%, specificity 90%)
From the Bulletin on the Rheumatic Diseases, ed 10. Arthritis Foundation, Atlanta, 1993, with permission of the Arthritis Foundation.

FOR MORE INFORMATION

Arnett, FC: Revised criteria for classification of rheumatoid arthritis. Bull Rheum Dis 38:1, 1989.

CLASSIFICATION OF RHEUMATOID ARTHRITIS BY FUNCTIONAL CAPACITY

Class	Functional Capacity
Class I	Completely able to perform usual activities of daily living (self-care, vocational, and avocational)
Class II	Able to perform usual self-care and vocational activities, but limited in avocational activities
Class III	Able to perform usual self-care activities, but limited in vocational and avocational activities
Class IV	Limited in ability to perform usual self-care, vocational, and avocational activities

From Hochberg, MC, et al: The American College of Rheumatology 1991 revised criteria for the classification of global functional status in rheumatoid arthritis. Arthritis & Rheum 35:498, 1992, with permission.

CLASSIFICATION OF RHEUMATOID ARTHRITIS BY STAGES OF PROGRESSION

Stage I, Early

†1. No destructive changes on roentgenographic examination.

2. Roentgenologic evidence of osteoporosis may be present.

Stage II, Moderate

†1. Roentgenologic evidence of osteoporosis, with or without slight subchondral bone destruction; slight cartilage destruction may be present.

†2. No joint deformities, although limitation of joint mobility may be present.

3. Adjacent muscle atrophy.

4. Extra-articular soft-tissue lesions, such as nodules and tenosynovitis, may be present.

Stage III, Severe

†1. Roentgenologic evidence of cartilage and bone destruction, in addition to osteoporosis.

†2. Joint deformity, such as subluxation, ulnar deviation, or hyperextension, without fibrous or bony ankylosis.

3. Extensive muscle atrophy.

4. Extra-articular soft-tissue lesions, such as nodules and tenosynovitis, may be present.

Stage IV, Terminal

†1. Fibrous or bony ankylosis.

2. Criteria of stage III.

†The criteria prefaced by daggers are those that must be present to permit classification of a patient in any particular stage or grade.

From Primer on the Rheumatic Diseases, ed 10. Arthritis Foundation, Atlanta, 1993. Used by permission of the Arthritis Foundation.

CRITERIA FOR THE DIAGNOSIS OF JUVENILE RHEUMATOID ARTHRITIS

I. General

The JRA Criteria Subcommittee in 1982 again reviewed the 1977 Criteria (1) and recommended that *juvenile rheumatoid arthritis* be the name for the principal form of chronic arthritic disease in children and that this general class should be classified into three onset subtypes: systemic, polyarticular, and pauciarticular. The onset subtypes may be further subclassified into subsets as indicated below. The following classification enumerates the requirements for the diagnosis of JRA and the three clinical onset subtypes and lists subsets of each subtype that may be useful in further classification.

II. General criteria for the diagnosis of juvenile rheumatoid arthritis:

A. Persistent arthritis of at least six weeks duration in one or more joints.

B. Exclusion of other causes of arthritis (see list of exclusions)

III. JRA onset subtypes

The onset subtype is determined by manifestations during the first six months of disease and remains the principal classification, although manifestations more closely resembling another subtype may appear later.

A. Systemic onset JRA: This subtype is defined as JRA with persistent intermittent fever (daily intermittent temperatures to 103°F or more) with or without rheumatoid rash or other organ involvement. Typical fever and rash will be considered probable systemic onset JRA if not associated with arthritis. Before a definite diagnosis can be made, arthritis, as defined, must be present.

Continued on following page

1. JRA Criteria Subcommittee of the Diagnostic and Therapeutic Criteria Committee of the American Rheumatism Association: Current proposed revisions of the JRA criteria. Arthritis Rheum 20(suppl)195, 1977

B. Pauciarticular onset JRA: This subtype is defined as JRA with arthritis in four or fewer joints during the first six months of disease. Patients with systemic onset JRA are excluded from this onset subtype.

C. Polyarticular JRA: This subtype is defined as JRA with arthritis in five or more joints during the first six months of disease. Patients with systemic JRA onset are excluded from this subtype.

D. The onset subtypes may include the following subsets:
  1. Systemic onset (SO)
      a. Polyarthritis
      b. Oligoarthritis
  2. Oligoarthritis (OO) (Pauciarticular onset)
      a. Antinuclear antibody (ANA) positive-chronic uveitis
      b. Rheumatoid factor (RF) positive
      c. Seronegative, B27 positive
      d. Not otherwise classified
  3. Polyarthritis (PO)
      a. RF positivity
      b. Not otherwise classified

IV. Exclusions
  A. Other rheumatic diseases
      1. Rheumatic fever
      2. Systemic lupus erythematosus
      3. Ankylosing spondylitis
      4. Polymyositis and dermatomyositis
      5. Vasculitic syndromes
      6. Scleroderma
      7. Psoriatic arthritis
      8. Reiter's syndrome
      9. Sjögren's syndrome
      10. Mixed connective tissue disease
      11. Behçet's syndrome
  B. Infectious arthritis
  C. Inflammatory bowel disease
  D. Neoplastic diseases including leukemia
  E. Nonrheumatic conditions of bones and joints
  F. Hematologic diseases
  G. Psychogenic arthralgia
  H. Miscellaneous
      1. Sarcoidosis
      2. Hypertrophic osteoarthropathy
      3. Villonodular synovitis
      4. Chronic active hepatitis
      5. Familial Mediterranean fever

V. Other proposed terminology
  Juvenile chronic arthritis (JCA) and juvenile arthritis (JA) are new diagnostic terms currently in use in some places for the arthritides of childhood. The diagnoses of JCA and JA are not equivalent to each other, nor to the older diagnosis of juvenile rheumatoid arthritis or Still's disease. Hence reports of studies of JCA or JA cannot be directly compared with one another nor to reports of JRA or Still's disease. Juvenile chronic arthritis is

described in more detail in a report of the European Conference on the Rheumatic Diseases of Children (2) and juvenile arthritis in the report of the Ross Conference (3).

2. Ansell BW: Chronic arthritis in childhood. Ann Rheum Dis 37:107, 1978
3. Fink CW: Keynote address: Arthritis in childhood, Report of the 80th Ross Conference in Pediatric Research. Columbus, Ross Laboratories, 1979, pp 1–2

From the Primer on Rheumatic Diseases, ed 10. Arthritis Foundation, Atlanta, 1993, with permission.

DRUGS COMMONLY USED IN TREATMENT OF RHEUMATOID ARTHRITIS

CATEGORIES OF DRUGS USED IN RHEUMATOID ARTHRITIS

I. NONSTEROIDAL ANTI-INFLAMMATORY DRUGS

Aspirin (many trade names)	Ketoprofen (Orudis)
Diclofenac (Voltaren)	Meclofenamate (Meclofen, Meclomen)
Diflunisal (Dolobid)	Nabumetone (Relafen)
Etodolac (Lodine)	Naproxen (Anaprox, Naprosyn)
Fenoprofen (Nalfon)	Oxaprozin (Daypro)
Flurbiprofen (Ansaid)	Phenylbutazone (Butazolidin)
Ibuprofen (many trade names)	Piroxicam (Feldene)
Indomethacin (Indameth, Indocin)	Sulindac (Clinoril)
	Tolmetin (Tolectin)

II. CORTICOSTEROIDS

Betamethasone (Celestone)	Paramethasone (Haldrone)
Cortisone (Cortone acetate)	Prednisolone (Hydeltrasol, others)
Dexamethasone (Decadron)	Prednisone (Deltasone, others)
Hydrocortisone (Cortef, others)	Triamcinolone (Aristocort)
Methylprednisolone (Medrol, others)	

III. DISEASE-MODIFYING ANTIRHEUMATIC DRUGS

Auranofin (Ridaura)	Hydroxychloroquine (Plaquenil)
Aurothioglucose (Solganal)	Methotrexate (Rheumatrex)
Azathioprine (Imuran)	Penicillamine (Cuprimine, Depen)
Chloroquine (Aralen)	
Gold sodium thiomalate (Myochrysine)	

From Ciccone, CD: Pharmacology in Rehabilitation, ed 2. FA Davis, Philadelphia, 1996, p 215, with permission.

DISEASE-MODIFYING ANTIRHEUMATIC DRUGS

Drug	Trade Name	Usual Dosage	Special Considerations
Antimalarials			
Chloroquine	Aralen	Oral: Up to 4 mg/kg of lean body weight per day.	Periodic ophthalmic exams recommended to check for retinal toxicity.
Hydroxychloroquine	Plaquenil	Oral: Up to 6.5 mg/kg of lean body wieght per day.	Similar to chloroquine.
Azathioprine	Imuran	Oral: 1 mg/kg body weight per day; can be increased after 6–8 wk up to maximum dose of 2.5 mg/kg body weight.	Relatively high toxicity; should be used cautiously in debilitated patients or patients with renal body disease.
Gold compounds			
Auranofin	Ridaura	Oral: 6 mg one each day or 3 mg BID.	May have a long latency (6–9 mo) before onset of benefits.

Drug	Trade Name	Dosage	Special Considerations
Aurothioglucose	Solganal	Intramuscular: 10 mg the 1st wk, 25 mg the 2nd and 3rd wk, then 25–50 mg each wk until total dose of 1 g. Maintenance doses of 25–50 mg every 2–4 wk can follow.	Effects occur somewhat sooner than oral gold, but still has long delay (4 mo).
Gold sodium thiomalate	Myochrysine	Similar to aurothioglucose.	Similar to aurothioglucose.
Methotrexate	Rheumatrex	Oral: 2.5–5 mg every 12 h for total of 3 doses/wk or 10 mg once each week. Can be increased up to a maximum of 20–25 mg/wk.	Often effective in halting joint destruction, but long-term use limited by toxicity.
Penicillamine	Cuprimine, Depen	Oral: 125 or 250 mg one each day; can be increased to a maximum of 1.5 g/d.	Relatively high incidence of toxicity with long-term use.

From Ciccone, CD: Pharmacology in Rehabilitation, ed 2. FA Davis, Philadelphia, 1996, p 219, with permission.

COMMON NONSTEROIDAL ANTI-INFLAMMATORY DRUGS (NSAIDs)

Generic Name	Trade Name(s)	Specific Comments — Comparison to Other NSAIDs
Aspirin	Many trade names	Most widely used NSAID for analgesic and anti-inflammatory effects; also used frequently for antipyretic and anticoagulant effects.
Diclofenac	Voltaren	Substantially more potent than naproxen and several other NSAIDs; adverse side effects occur in 20% of patients.
Diflunisal	Dolobid	Has potency 3–4 times greater than aspirin in terms of analgesic and anti-inflammatory effects but lacks antipyretic activity.
Etodolac	Lodine	Effective as analgesic/anti-inflammatory agent with fewer side effects than most NSAIDs; may have gastric-sparing properties.
Fenoprofen	Nalfon	GI side effects fairly common but usually less intense than those occurring with similar doses of aspirin.
Flurbiprofen	Ansaid	Similar to aspirin's benefits and side effects; also available as topical ophthalmic preparation (Ocufen).
Ibuprofen	Motrin, Rufen, others	First nonaspirin NSAID also available in nonprescription form; fewer GI side effects than aspirin but GI effects still occur in 5%–15% of patients.
Indomethacin	Indameth, Indocin	Relative high incidence of dose-related side effects; problems occur in 25%–50% of patients.
Ketoprofen	Orudis	Similar to aspirin's benefits and side effects but has relatively short half-life (1–2 h).
Ketorolac	Toradol	Can be administered orally or by intramuscular injection; parenteral doses provide postoperative analgesia equivalent to opioids.

Meclofenamate	Meclofen, Meclomen	No apparent advantages or disadvantages compared to aspirin and other NSAIDs.
Mefenamic acid	Ponstel	No advantages; often less effective and more toxic than aspirin and other NSAIDs.
Nabumetone	Relafen	Effective as analgesic/anti-inflammatory agent with fewer side effects than most NSAIDs.
Naproxen	Anaprox, Naprosyn	Similar to ibuprofen in terms of benefits and adverse effects.
Oxaprozin	Daypro	Analgesic and anti-inflammatory effects similar to aspirin; may produce fewer side effects than other NSAIDs.
Phenylbutazone	Butazolidin, others	Potent anti-inflammatory effects but long-term use limited by high incidence of side effects (10%–45% of patients).
Piroxicam	Feldene	Long half-life (45 h) allows once-daily dosing; may be somewhat better tolerated than aspirin.
Sulindac	Clinoril	Relatively little effect on kidneys (renal-sparing), but may produce more GI side effects than aspirin.
Tolmetin	Tolectin	Similar to aspirin's benefits and side effects but must be given frequently (qid) because of short half-life (1 h).

From Ciccone, CD: Pharmacology in Rehabilitation, ed 2. FA Davis, Philadelphia, 1996, p 204, with permission.

COMMON NONSTEROIDAL ANTI-INFLAMMATORY DRUGS (NSAIDs)

Classes	Dosages (according to desired effect)	
	Analgesia	Anti-inflammation
Aspirin (many trade names)	325–650 mg every 4 h	3.6–5.4 g/d in divided doses
Diclofenac (Voltaren)	—	150–200 mg/d in 2–4 divided doses
Diflunisal (Dolobid)	1 g initially; 500 mg every 8–12 h as needed	250–500 mg bid
Fenoprofen (Nalfon)	200 mg every 4–6 h	300–600 mg tid or qid
Flurbiprofen (Ansaid)	—	200–300 mg/d in 2–4 divided doses
Ibuprofen (Advil, Amersol, Motrin, Nuprin, Rufen)	200–400 mg every 4–6 h as needed	1.2–3.2 g/d in 3–4 divided doses
Indomethacin (Indameth, Indocin)	—	25–50 mg 2–4 times each day initially; can be increased up to 200 mg/d as tolerated
Ketoprofen (Orudis)	50 mg every 6–8 h	150–300 mg/d in 3–4 divided doses

Drug		
Meclofenamate (Meclofen, Meclomen)	50 mg every 4–6 h	200–400 mg/d in 3–4 divided doses
Mefenamic acid (Ponstel)	500 mg initially; 250 mg every 6 h as needed	—
Naproxen (Naprosyn)	500 mg initially; 250 mg every 6–8 h	250, 375, or 500 mg bid
Naproxen sodium (Anaprox)	550 mg initially; 275 mg every 6–8 h	275 mg bid
Phenylbutazone (Butazolidin, Butazone)	—	300–600 mg/d in 3–4 divided doses initially; 100 mg 1–4 times each day for maintenance
Piroxicam (Feldene)	—	20 mg/d single dose; or 10 mg bid
Sulindac (Clinoril)	—	150 or 200 mg bid
Tolmetin (Tolectin)	—	400 mg tid initially; 600 mg–1.8 g/d in 3–4 divided doses

From Ciccone, CD: Pharmacology in Rehabilitation, ed 2. FA Davis, Philadelphia, 1996, p 204, with permission.

COMMON GASTROINTESTINAL SIDE EFFECTS ASSOCIATED WITH THE NONASPIRIN NSAIDS*

Drug	Mild to Moderate Stomach Cramps, Pain, or Discomfort	Bloated Feeling or Gas	Heartburn or Indigestion	Nausea	Vomiting	Diarrhea	Constipation
Diclofenac	M	L	M	M	R	M	M
Diflunisal	M	L	M	M	L	M	L
Fenoprofen	L	L	M	M	M	L	M
Flurbiprofen	M	L	M	M	L	M	L
Ibuprofen	M	L	M	M	L	L	L
Indomethacin	M	R	M	M	L	L	L
Ketoprofen	M	M	H	M	L	M	M
Meclofenamate	M	M	M	H	U	H	L
Mefenamic acid	M	L	M	M	U	M	L
Naproxen	M	U	M	M	R	L	M
Phenylbutazone	M	R	L	M	R	R	R
Piroxicam	M	L	M	M	R	L	L
Sulindac	H	L	M	M	L	M	M
Tometin	M	M	M	H	M	M	L

*Incidence of side effects: H = high incidence (10% or greater); M = more frequent (3%–9%); L = less frequent (1%–3%); R = rare (<1%); U = unknown.

Copied from *USP DI®, 14th Edition* Copyright 1994. The USP Convention, Inc. Permission granted. The USP is not responsible for any inaccuracy of quotation nor for any false or misleading implication that may arise due to the text used or due to the quotation of information subsequently changed in later editions.

SECTION 3

Neuroanatomy, Neurology, and Neurologic Therapy

3

THE BRAIN

Lateral Surface: Anatomic Features and Brodmann's Numbers

Anatomic Features

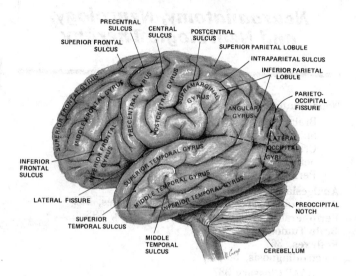

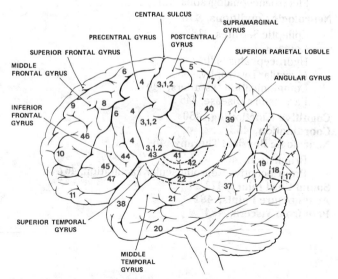

A lateral view of the surface of the brain, showing Brodmann's numbers.

Midsagittal View: Anatomic Features and Brodmann's Numbers

Anatomic Features

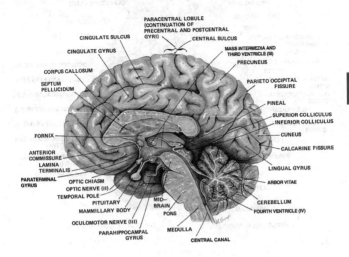

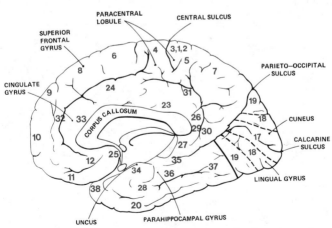

A medial view of the surface of the brain, showing Brodmann's numbers.
Continued on following page

View of the Inferior (Basilar) Surface of the Brain

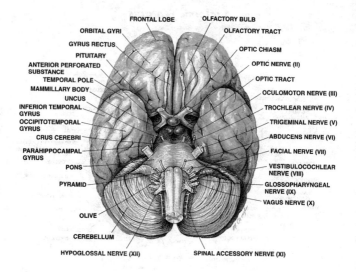

FRONTAL LOBE
OLFACTORY BULB
ORBITAL GYRI
OLFACTORY TRACT
GYRUS RECTUS
OPTIC CHIASM
PITUITARY
ANTERIOR PERFORATED SUBSTANCE
OPTIC NERVE (II)
TEMPORAL POLE
OPTIC TRACT
MAMMILLARY BODY
OCULOMOTOR NERVE (III)
UNCUS
INFERIOR TEMPORAL GYRUS
TROCHLEAR NERVE (IV)
OCCIPITOTEMPORAL GYRUS
TRIGEMINAL NERVE (V)
CRUS CEREBRI
ABDUCENS NERVE (VI)
PARAHIPPOCAMPAL GYRUS
FACIAL NERVE (VII)
PONS
VESTIBULOCOCHLEAR NERVE (VIII)
PYRAMID
GLOSSOPHARYNGEAL NERVE (IX)
VAGUS NERVE (X)
OLIVE
CEREBELLUM
HYPOGLOSSAL NERVE (XII)
SPINAL ACCESSORY NERVE (XI)

The Motor Cortex

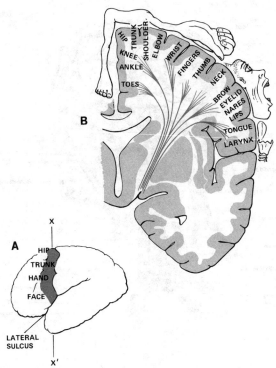

A *shows the somatotopical representation of the motor cortex. Illustrated is a left cortex.* B *shows the somatotopical organization of cortical neurons in a section taken along plane x-x' in* A.

BLOOD SUPPLY TO THE BRAIN

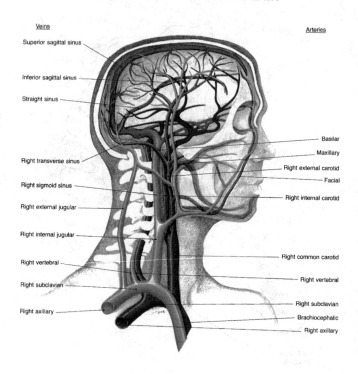

Circle of Willis

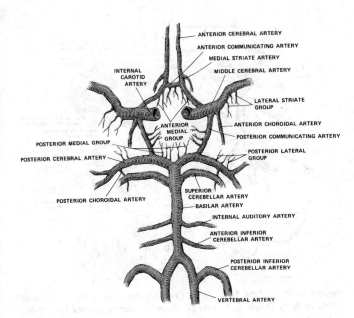

ANTERIOR CEREBRAL ARTERY

ANTERIOR COMMUNICATING ARTERY

MEDIAL STRIATE ARTERY

MIDDLE CEREBRAL ARTERY

INTERNAL CAROTID ARTERY

LATERAL STRIATE GROUP

ANTERIOR MEDIAL GROUP

ANTERIOR CHOROIDAL ARTERY

POSTERIOR COMMUNICATING ARTERY

POSTERIOR MEDIAL GROUP

POSTERIOR CEREBRAL ARTERY

POSTERIOR LATERAL GROUP

POSTERIOR CHOROIDAL ARTERY

SUPERIOR CEREBELLAR ARTERY

BASILAR ARTERY

INTERNAL AUDITORY ARTERY

ANTERIOR INFERIOR CEREBELLAR ARTERY

POSTERIOR INFERIOR CEREBELLAR ARTERY

VERTEBRAL ARTERY

3

Blood Supply to the Brain Stem

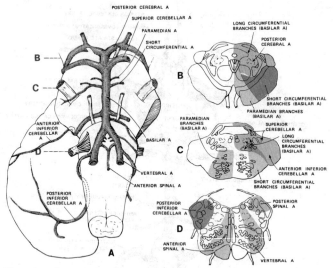

Ventral surface of the brain stem. Cross-sections are at the levels indicated in A by letters B, C, and D. Some territories served by arteries overlap.

Cerebral Circulation

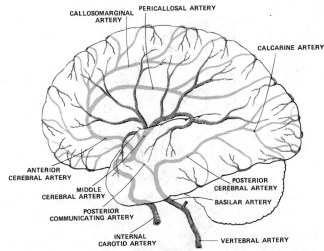

Lateral view of a left hemisphere. The anterior and posterior cerebral arteries are normally not visible from a lateral view. Here they are shown as they are positioned on the medial surface of the hemisphere.

Frontal Hemi-Section of the Cerebrum Showing Areas Supplied by Arteries

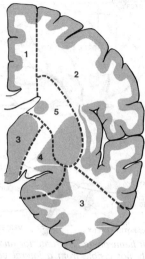

Section at the level of the central sulcus. The areas of distribution are (1) the anterior cerebral artery, including the callosomarginal and pericallosal arteries; (2) the middle cerebral artery; (3) the posterior cerebral artery to the diencephalon and occipital lobe; (4) the medial striate arteries to the internal capsule, globus pallidus, and amygdala; and (5) the lateral striate arteries to the caudate nucleus, putamen, and internal capsule.

THE BRAIN STEM AND DIENCEPHALON
Ventral Surface

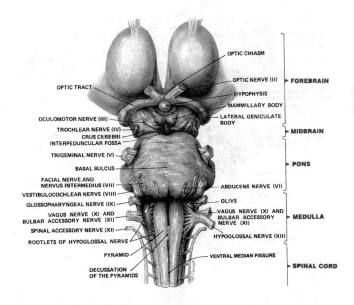

3

The Brain Stem and Diencephalon **243**

Dorsal Surface of the Brain Stem

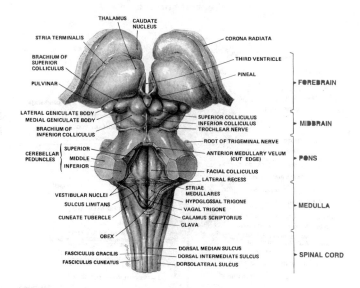

THALAMUS
CAUDATE NUCLEUS
STRIA TERMINALIS
CORONA RADIATA
BRACHIUM OF SUPERIOR COLLICULUS
THIRD VENTRICLE
PULVINAR
PINEAL
FOREBRAIN

LATERAL GENICULATE BODY
MEDIAL GENICULATE BODY
BRACHIUM OF INFERIOR COLLICULUS
SUPERIOR COLLICULUS
INFERIOR COLLICULUS
TROCHLEAR NERVE
MIDBRAIN

ROOT OF TRIGEMINAL NERVE
CEREBELLAR PEDUNCLES
SUPERIOR
MIDDLE
INFERIOR
ANTERIOR MEDULLARY VELUM (CUT EDGE)
FACIAL COLLICULUS
LATERAL RECESS
PONS

VESTIBULAR NUCLEI
SULCUS LIMITANS
CUNEATE TUBERCLE
STRIAE MEDULLARES
HYPOGLOSSAL TRIGONE
VAGAL TRIGONE
CALAMUS SCRIPTORIUS
CLAVA
MEDULLA

OBEX

FASCICULUS GRACILIS
FASCICULUS CUNEATUS
DORSAL MEDIAN SULCUS
DORSAL INTERMEDIATE SULCUS
DORSOLATERAL SULCUS
SPINAL CORD

Lateral Surface of the Brain Stem

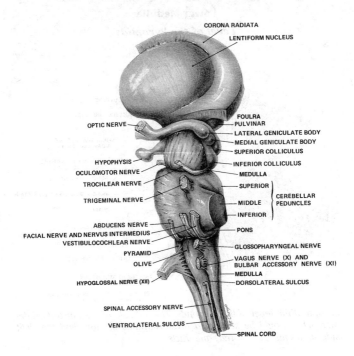

CORONA RADIATA
LENTIFORM NUCLEUS

OPTIC NERVE

FOULRA
PULVINAR
LATERAL GENICULATE BODY
MEDIAL GENICULATE BODY
SUPERIOR COLLICULUS

HYPOPHYSIS
OCULOMOTOR NERVE
TROCHLEAR NERVE
TRIGEMINAL NERVE

INFERIOR COLLICULUS
MEDULLA

SUPERIOR

MIDDLE   CEREBELLAR
                PEDUNCLES
INFERIOR

ABDUCENS NERVE
FACIAL NERVE AND NERVUS INTERMEDIUS
VESTIBULOCOCHLEAR NERVE
PYRAMID
OLIVE

PONS

GLOSSOPHARYNGEAL NERVE

VAGUS NERVE (X) AND
BULBAR ACCESSORY NERVE (XI)

HYPOGLOSSAL NERVE (XII)

MEDULLA
DORSOLATERAL SULCUS

SPINAL ACCESSORY NERVE

VENTROLATERAL SULCUS

SPINAL CORD

3

BRAIN STEM: CROSS-SECTIONAL VIEWS

Lower Medulla

Level of the Pyramids

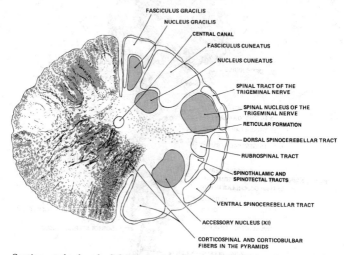

FASCICULUS GRACILIS

NUCLEUS GRACILIS

CENTRAL CANAL

FASCICULUS CUNEATUS

NUCLEUS CUNEATUS

SPINAL TRACT OF THE TRIGEMINAL NERVE

SPINAL NUCLEUS OF THE TRIGEMINAL NERVE

RETICULAR FORMATION

DORSAL SPINOCEREBELLAR TRACT

RUBROSPINAL TRACT

SPINOTHALAMIC AND SPINOTECTAL TRACTS

VENTRAL SPINOCEREBELLAR TRACT

ACCESSORY NUCLEUS (XI)

CORTICOSPINAL AND CORTICOBULBAR FIBERS IN THE PYRAMIDS

Section at the level of the pyramids. The left side of the illustration depicts what would be seen in a myelin-strained section, and the right side shows nuclei (colored) and tracts.

Level of Decussation of the Medial Lemniscus

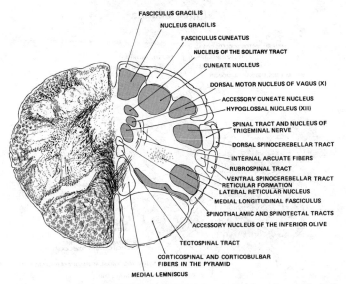

FASCICULUS GRACILIS
NUCLEUS GRACILIS
FASCICULUS CUNEATUS
NUCLEUS OF THE SOLITARY TRACT
CUNEATE NUCLEUS
DORSAL MOTOR NUCLEUS OF VAGUS (X)
ACCESSORY CUNEATE NUCLEUS
HYPOGLOSSAL NUCLEUS (XII)
SPINAL TRACT AND NUCLEUS OF TRIGEMINAL NERVE
DORSAL SPINOCEREBELLAR TRACT
INTERNAL ARCUATE FIBERS
RUBROSPINAL TRACT
VENTRAL SPINOCEREBELLAR TRACT
RETICULAR FORMATION
LATERAL RETICULAR NUCLEUS
MEDIAL LONGITUDINAL FASCICULUS
SPINOTHALAMIC AND SPINOTECTAL TRACTS
ACCESSORY NUCLEUS OF THE INFERIOR OLIVE
TECTOSPINAL TRACT
CORTICOSPINAL AND CORTICOBULBAR FIBERS IN THE PYRAMID
MEDIAL LEMNISCUS

Section at the level of the decussation of the medial lemniscus. The left side of the illustration depicts what would be seen in a myelin-stained section, and the right side shows nuclei (colored) and tracts. Brain stem cross-sectional views continued on pages 248–252.

BRAIN STEM: CROSS-SECTIONAL VIEWS
(Continued)
Upper Medulla

The left side of the illustration depicts what would be seen in a myelin-stained section, and the right side shows nuclei (colored) and tracts.

Pons

Abducens and Facial Nerves

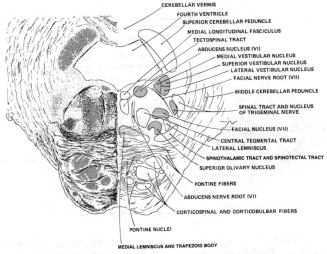

CEREBELLAR VERMIS
FOURTH VENTRICLE
SUPERIOR CEREBELLAR PEDUNCLE
MEDIAL LONGITUDINAL FASCICULUS
TECTOSPINAL TRACT
ABDUCENS NUCLEUS (VI)
MEDIAL VESTIBULAR NUCLEUS
SUPERIOR VESTIBULAR NUCLEUS
LATERAL VESTIBULAR NUCLEUS
FACIAL NERVE ROOT (VII)
MIDDLE CEREBELLAR PEDUNCLE
SPINAL TRACT AND NUCLEUS OF TRIGEMINAL NERVE
FACIAL NUCLEUS (VII)
CENTRAL TEGMENTAL TRACT
LATERAL LEMNISCUS
SPINOTHALAMIC TRACT AND SPINOTECTAL TRACT
SUPERIOR OLIVARY NUCLEUS
PONTINE FIBERS
ABDUCENS NERVE ROOT (VI)
CORTICOSPINAL AND CORTICOBULBAR FIBERS
PONTINE NUCLEI
MEDIAL LEMNISCUS AND TRAPEZOID BODY

Section at the level of the nuclei of the abducens and facial nerves. The left side of the illustration depicts what would be seen in a myelin-stained section, and the right side shows nuclei (colored) and tracts.

Trigeminal Nerve

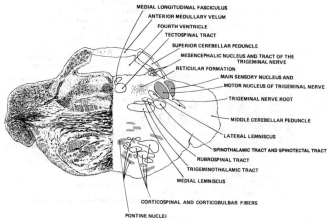

MEDIAL LONGITUDINAL FASCICULUS
ANTERIOR MEDULLARY VELUM
FOURTH VENTRICLE
TECTOSPINAL TRACT
SUPERIOR CEREBELLAR PEDUNCLE
MESENCEPHALIC NUCLEUS AND TRACT OF THE TRIGEMINAL NERVE
RETICULAR FORMATION
MAIN SENSORY NUCLEUS AND
MOTOR NUCLEUS OF TRIGEMINAL NERVE
TRIGEMINAL NERVE ROOT
MIDDLE CEREBELLAR PEDUNCLE
LATERAL LEMNISCUS
SPINOTHALAMIC TRACT AND SPINOTECTAL TRACT
RUBROSPINAL TRACT
TRIGEMINOTHALAMIC TRACT
MEDIAL LEMNISCUS
CORTICOSPINAL AND CORTICOBULBAR FIBERS
PONTINE NUCLEI

Section at the level of the main sensory and motor nuclei of the trigeminal nerve. The left side of the illustration depicts what would be seen in a myelin-stained section, and the right shows nuclei (colored) and tracts.

Lower Midbrain

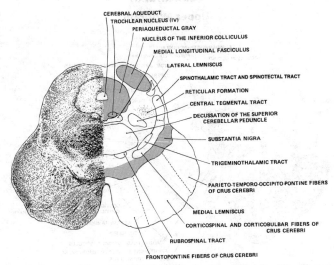

CEREBRAL AQUEDUCT
TROCHLEAR NUCLEUS (IV)
PERIAQUEDUCTAL GRAY
NUCLEUS OF THE INFERIOR COLLICULUS
MEDIAL LONGITUDINAL FASCICULUS
LATERAL LEMNISCUS
SPINOTHALAMIC TRACT AND SPINOTECTAL TRACT
RETICULAR FORMATION
CENTRAL TEGMENTAL TRACT
DECUSSATION OF THE SUPERIOR
CEREBELLAR PEDUNCLE
SUBSTANTIA NIGRA
TRIGEMINOTHALAMIC TRACT
PARIETO-TEMPORO-OCCIPITO-PONTINE FIBERS
OF CRUS CEREBRI
MEDIAL LEMNISCUS
CORTICOSPINAL AND CORTICOBULBAR FIBERS OF
CRUS CEREBRI
RUBROSPINAL TRACT
FRONTOPONTINE FIBERS OF CRUS CEREBRI

Section at the level of the inferior colliculus. The left side of the illustration depicts what would be seen in a myelin-stained section, and the right side shows nuclei (colored) and tracts.

BRAIN STEM: CROSS-SECTIONAL VIEWS
(Continued)

Upper Midbrain

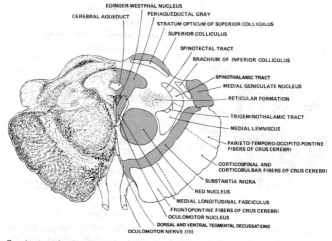

EDINGER-WESTPHAL NUCLEUS
CEREBRAL AQUEDUCT
PERIAQUEDUCTAL GRAY
STRATUM OPTICUM OF SUPERIOR COLLICULUS
SUPERIOR COLLICULUS
SPINOTECTAL TRACT
BRACHIUM OF INFERIOR COLLICULUS
SPINOTHALAMIC TRACT
MEDIAL GENICULATE NUCLEUS
RETICULAR FORMATION
TRIGEMINOTHALAMIC TRACT
MEDIAL LEMNISCUS
PARIETO-TEMPORO-OCCIPITO-PONTINE FIBERS OF CRUS CEREBRI
CORTICOSPINAL AND CORTICOBULBAR FIBERS OF CRUS CEREBRI
SUBSTANTIA NIGRA
RED NUCLEUS
MEDIAL LONGITUDINAL FASCICULUS
FRONTOPONTINE FIBERS OF CRUS CEREBRI
OCULOMOTOR NUCLEUS
DORSAL AND VENTRAL TEGMENTAL DECUSSATIONS
OCULOMOTOR NERVE (III)

Section at the level of the superior colliculus and the red nucleus. The left side of the illustration depicts what would be seen in a myelin-stained section, and the right side shows nuclei (colored) and tracts.

SPINAL CORD: CROSS-SECTIONAL VIEWS
Cervical, Thoracic, and Lumbar Sections

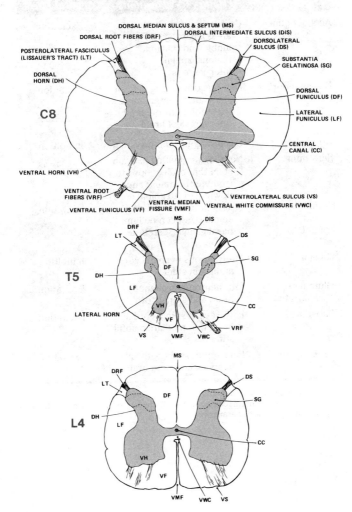

CENTRAL NEUROTRANSMITTERS

Transmitter	Primary CNS Locations	General Effect
Acetylcholine	Cerebral cortex (many areas), basal ganglia, limbic and thalamic regions, spinal interneurons	Excitation
Norepinephrine	Neurons originating in brain stem and hypothalamus that project throughout other areas of brain	Inhibition
Dopamine	Basal ganglia, limbic system	Inhibition
Serotonin	Neurons originating in brain stem that project upward (to hypothalamus) and downward (to spinal cord)	
γ-Aminobutyric acid (GABA)	Interneurons throughout spinal cord, cerebellum, basal ganglia, cerebral cortex	Inhibition
Glycine	Interneurons in spinal cord and brain stem	Inhibition
Glutamate, aspartate	Interneurons throughout brain and spinal cord	Excitation
Substance P	Pathways in spinal cord and brain that mediate painful stimuli	Excitation
Enkephalins	Pain suppression pathways in spinal cord and brain	Excitation

CNS = central nervous system.
From Ciccone, CD: Pharmacology in Rehabilitation, ed 2. FA Davis, Philadelphia, 1996, p 65, with permission.

SPINAL CORD: TRACTS AND LAMINA OF REXED

Cross-Section Approximately at C8–T1

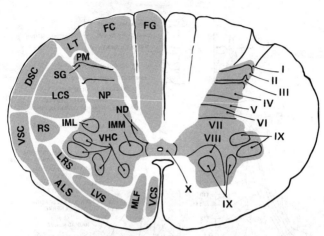

Tracts and nuclei of the cord are illustrated on the left; Rexed's laminar organization of the gray matter is illustrated on the right. DSC = dorsal spinocerebellar tract; FC = fasciculus cuneatus; FG = fasciculus gracilis; IC = intermediolateral cell column; LCS = lateral corticospinal tract; LRS = lateral reticulospinal tract; LST = lateral spinothalamic tract; LT = Lissauer's tract; MRS = medial reticulospinal tract; ND = nucleus dorsalis; NP = nucleus proprius; PM = posteromarginal nucleus; RS = rubrospinal tract; SG = substantia gelatinosa; TS = tectospinal tract; VCS = ventral corticospinal tract; VHC = ventral horn cell columns; VS = vestibulospinal tract; VSC = ventral spinocerebellar tract.

CUTANEOUS INNERVATION: DERMATOMES AND PERIPHERAL NERVE DISTRIBUTIONS

View of Ventral Surface

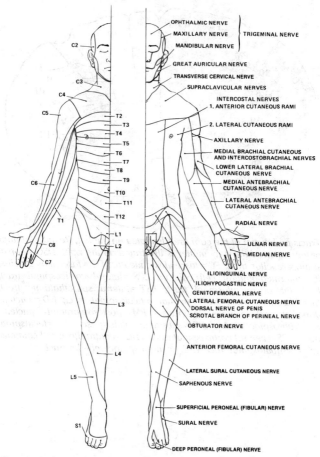

Cutaneous innervation of the front (ventral surface) of the body. Dermatomes are on the left, and peripheral nerves are on the right.

View of Dorsal Surface

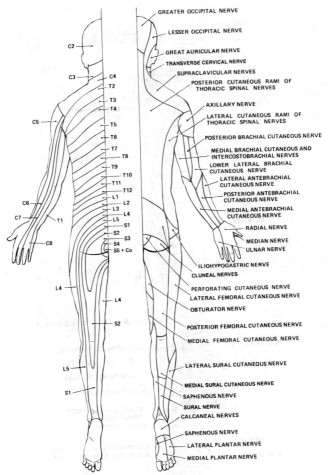

GREATER OCCIPITAL NERVE

LESSER OCCIPITAL NERVE

GREAT AURICULAR NERVE

TRANSVERSE CERVICAL NERVE

SUPRACLAVICULAR NERVES

POSTERIOR CUTANEOUS RAMI OF THORACIC SPINAL NERVES

AXILLARY NERVE

LATERAL CUTANEOUS RAMI OF THORACIC SPINAL NERVES

POSTERIOR BRACHIAL CUTANEOUS NERVE

MEDIAL BRACHIAL CUTANEOUS AND INTERCOSTOBRACHIAL NERVES

LOWER LATERAL BRACHIAL CUTANEOUS NERVE

LATERAL ANTEBRACHIAL CUTANEOUS NERVE

POSTERIOR ANTEBRACHIAL CUTANEOUS NERVE

MEDIAL ANTEBRACHIAL CUTANEOUS NERVE

RADIAL NERVE

MEDIAN NERVE

ULNAR NERVE

ILIOHYPOGASTRIC NERVE

CLUNEAL NERVES

PERFORATING CUTANEOUS NERVE

LATERAL FEMORAL CUTANEOUS NERVE

OBTURATOR NERVE

POSTERIOR FEMORAL CUTANEOUS NERVE

MEDIAL FEMORAL CUTANEOUS NERVE

LATERAL SURAL CUTANEOUS NERVE

MEDIAL SURAL CUTANEOUS NERVE

SAPHENOUS NERVE

SURAL NERVE

CALCANEAL NERVES

SAPHENOUS NERVE

LATERAL PLANTAR NERVE

MEDIAL PLANTAR NERVE

C2, C3, C4, C5, C6, C7, C8
T1, T2, T3, T4, T5, T6, T7, T8, T9, T10, T11, T12
L1, L2, L3, L4, L5
S1, S2, S3, S4, S5 + Co

3

Cutaneous innervation of the back (dorsal surface) of the body. Dermatomes are on the left, and peripheral nerves are on the right.

RELATIONSHIP BETWEEN SPINAL AND VERTEBRAL SEGMENTS

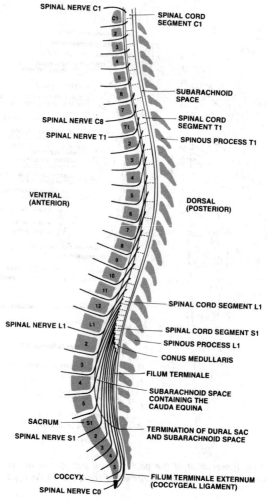

The figure shows the relationships between the spinal cord, spinal roots, vertebral segments, and dural sac. The dural sac, the filum terminale internus, and the filum terminale externus (coccygeal ligament) are shown in color.

AUTONOMIC NERVOUS SYSTEM

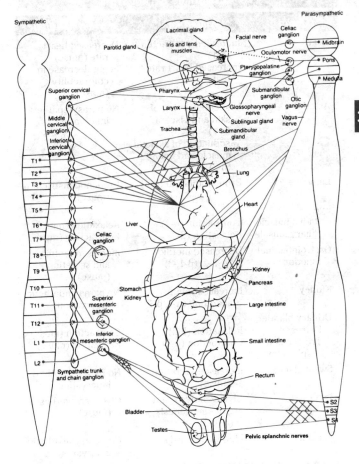

RESPONSE OF EFFECTOR ORGANS TO AUTONOMIC STIMULATION

Organ	Sympathetic*	Parasympathetic†
Heart	Increased contractility (β-1) Increased heart rate (β-1)	Decreased heart rate (musc) Slight decrease in contractility (musc)
Arterioles	Vasoconstriction of skin and viscera (α-1) Vasodilation of skeletal muscle and liver (β-2)	No parasympathetic innervation
Lung	Bronchodilation (β-2)	Bronchoconstriction (musc)
Eye		
Radial muscle	Contraction (α-1)	Relaxation (musc)
Ciliary muscle	Relaxation (β-2)	Contraction (musc)
Gastrointestinal function	Decreased motility (α-1,-2; (β-1,-2)	Increased motility and secretion (musc)
Kidney	Increased renin secretion (α-1, β-1)	No parasympathetic innervation
Urinary bladder		
Detrusor	Relaxation (β-2)	Contraction (musc)
Trigone and sphincter	Contraction (α-1)	Relaxation (musc)
Sweat glands	Increased secretion (musc‡)	No parasympathetic innervation
Liver	Glycogenolysis and gluconeogenesis (α, β-2)	Glycogen synthesis (musc)
Fat cells	Lipolysis (α, β-1)	No parasympathetic innervation

*The primary receptor subtypes that mediate each response are listed in parentheses (e.g., α-1, β-2). If no subtype is designated, it is because the particular α or β subtype has not been conclusively determined.
†All organ responses to parasympathetic stimulation are mediated via muscarinic (musc) receptors.
‡Response is due to sympathetic postganglionic cholinergic fibers.
From Ciccone, CD: Pharmacology in Rehabilitation, ed 2. FA Davis, Philadelphia, 1996, p 249, with permission.

AUTONOMIC RECEPTOR LOCATIONS AND RESPONSES

Receptor	Primary Location(s)	Response
CHOLINERGIC		
Nicotinic	Autonomic ganglia	Mediation of transmission to postganglionic neuron
Muscarinic	All parasympathetic effector cells:	
	Viscera and bronchiole smooth muscle	Contraction (generally)
	Cardiac muscle	Decreased heart rate
	Exocrine glands (salivary, intestinal, lacrimal)	Increased secretion
	Sweat glands	Increased secretion
ADRENERGIC		
α-1	Vascular smooth muscle	Contraction
	Intestinal smooth muscle	Relaxation
	Radial muscle iris	Contraction (mydriasis)
	Ureters	Increased motility
	Urinary sphincter	Contraction
	Spleen capsule	Contraction
α-2	CNS inhibitory synapses	Decreased sympathetic discharge from CNS
	Presynaptic terminal at peripheral adrenergic synapses	Decreased norepinephrine release
	Gastrointestinal tract	Decreased motility and secretion
	Pancreatic islet cells	Decreased insulin secretion
β-1	Cardiac muscle	Increased heart rate and contractility
	Kidney	Increased renin secretion
	Fat cells	Increased lipolysis

Continued on following page

AUTONOMIC RECEPTOR LOCATIONS AND RESPONSES
(Continued)

Receptor	Primary Location(s)	Response
β-2	Bronchiole smooth muscle	Relaxation (bronchodilation)
	Some arterioles (skeletal muscle, liver)	Vasodilation
	Gastrointestinal smooth muscle	Decreased motility
	Skeletal muscle and liver cells	Increased cellular metabolism
	Uterus	Relaxation
	Gallbladder	Relaxation

From Ciccone, CD: Pharmacology in Rehabilitation, ed 2. FA Davis, Philadelphia, 1996, p 255, with permission.

SUMMARY OF ADRENERGIC AGONIST/ANTAGONIST USE ACCORDING TO RECEPTOR SPECIFICITY

Primary Receptor Location: Response When Stimulated	Agonist Use(s)*	Antagonist Use(s)*
α-1 Receptor		
Vascular smooth muscle: vasoconstriction	Hypotension Nasal congestion Paroxysmal supraventricular tachycardia	Hypertension
α-2 Receptor		
CNS synapses (inhibitory): decreased sympathetic discharge from brain stem	Hypertension	No significant clinical use
β-1 Receptor		
Heart: increased heart rate and force of contraction	Cardiac decompensation	Hypertension Arrhythmia Angina pectoris Prevention of reinfarction

SUMMARY OF ADRENERGIC AGONIST/ANTAGONIST USE ACCORDING TO RECEPTOR SPECIFICITY

Primary Receptor Location: Response When Stimulated	Agonist Use(s)*	Antagonist Use(s)*
β-2 Receptor		
Bronchioles: bronchodilation	Prevent bronchospasm	No significant clinical use
Uterus: relaxation	Prevent premature labor	

*Primary clinical condition(s) that the agonists or antagonists are used to treat.
From Ciccone, CD: Pharmacology in Rehabilitation, ed 2. FA Davis, Philadelphia, 1996, p 272, with permission.

CIRCULATION OF THE CEREBROSPINAL FLUID

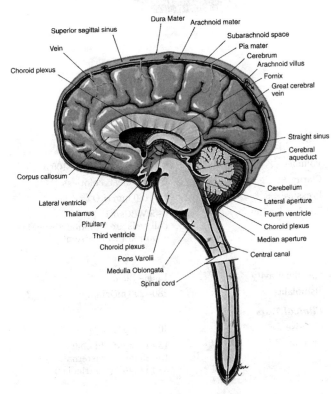

Circulation of the Cerebrospinal Fluid   **263**

Detail of Superior Sagittal Sinus Showing Arachnoid Granulation

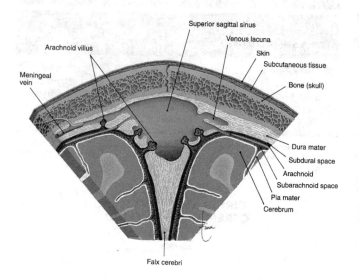

NORMAL CEREBROSPINAL FLUID VALUES IN ADULTS

Volume	90–150 ml; child: 60–100 ml
Clarity	Crystal clear, colorless
Pressure	50–180 mm H_2O
Total cell count	0–5 WBCs/μl (All cells are lymphocytes; PMNs and RBCs are absent.)
Specific gravity	1.006–1.008
Osmolality	280–290 mOsm/kg
Clinical Tests	
Glucose	40–70 mg/dl
Protein	15–45 mg/dl (lumbar) 15–25 mg/dl (cisternal) 5–15 mg/dl (ventricular)

Lactic acid	24 mg/dl
Glutamine	6–15 mg/dl
A/G ratio (albumin to globulin)	8:1
Chloride	118–132 mEq/L
Urea nitrogen	6–16 mg/dl
Creatinine	0.5–1.2 mg/dl
Cholesterol	0.2–0.6 mg/dl
Uric acid	0.5–4.5 mg/dl
Bilirubin	0 (none)
LDH	1/10 that of serum

Electrolytes and pH

pH	7.30–7.40
Chloride	118–132 mEq/L
Sodium	144–154 mEq/L
Potassium	2.0–3.5 mEq/L
CO_2 content	25–30 mEq/L (mmol)
P_{CO_2}	42–53 mm Hg
P_{O_2}	40–44 mm Hg
Calcium	2.1–2.7 mEq/L
Magnesium	2.4–3.1 mEq/L

Syphilis

VDRL	Negative

LDH = lactate dehydrogenase; PMNs = polymorphonuclear leukocytes; RBCs = red blood cells; WBC = white blood cells.

From Fischbach, FT: A Manual of Laboratory Diagnostic Tests, ed 4. JB Lippincott, Philadelphia, 1992, p 246, with permission.

ABNORMALITIES IN CEREBROSPINAL FLUID WITH VARIOUS CONDITIONS*

	Pressure	Cells/µl	Predominant Cell Type	Glucose	Protein
Normal	100–200 mm Hg	0–3	L	50–100 mg/dl	20–45 mg/dl
Acute bacterial meningitis	↑	500–5000	PMN	↓	About 100 mg/dl
Subacute meningitis (TB, *Cryptococcus*, sarcoid, leukemia, carcinoma)	N or ↑	100–700	L	↓	↑
Viral infections	N or ↑	100–2000	L	N	N or ↑
Brain abscess or tumor	N or ↑	0–1000	L	N	↑
Pseudotumor cerebri	↑	N	L	N	N or ↓
Lead encephalopathy	↑	0–500	L	N	↑
Acute syphilitic meningitis	N or ↑	25–2000	L	N	↑

Paretic neurosyphilis	N or ↑	15–2000	L	N	↑
Lyme disease of CNS	N or ↑	0–500	L	N	N or ↑
Guillain-Barré syndrome	N	0–100	L	N	>100 mg/dl
Cerebral hemorrhage	↑	Bloody	RBCs	N	↑
Cerebral thrombosis	N or ↑	0–100	L	N	N or ↑
Cord tumor	N	0–50	L	N	N or ↑

*Figures given for pressure, cell count, and protein are approximations; exceptions are frequent. Similarly, PMNs may predominate in conditions usually characterized by lymphocyte response, especially early in the course of viral infections or tuberculous meningitis. Alterations in glucose are less variable and more reliable.

Boldface indicates normal values.

N = normal; ↑ = increased; ↓ = decreased; L = lymphocyte.

From The Merck Manual, ed 16. Merck & Co, Rahway, NJ, 1992, p 1388, with permission.

CLASSIFICATION OF THE CRANIAL NERVES
Definitions
Afferent Components

general somatic afferents (GSA): Innervate receptors for touch, pain, or temperature sensibility of the skin; innervate sensory organs of muscle, joint, and tendon.

special somatic afferents (SSA): Innervate specialized receptors of ectodermal origin, specifically those for vision and vestibular and auditory sensibility.

general visceral afferents (GVA): Innervate touch, pain, or temperature receptors that are related to mucous or serous membranes, hollow organs, or glands; innervate chemoreceptors and baroreceptors.

special visceral afferents (SVA): Innervate specialized receptors found in the cranial region that are associated with visceral activity, specifically those for taste and smell.

Efferent Components

general somatic efferents (GSE): Motoneurons that innervate skeletal muscle that was not derived from the branchial arch mesoderm.

specialized visceral efferents (SVE): Motoneurons that innervate skeletal muscle that was derived from the embryonic branchial arch mesoderm, including muscles of the jaw, facial expression, pharynx, and larynx.

general visceral efferents (GVE): Motoneurons that are part of the autonomic nervous system and innervate smooth muscle, cardiac muscle, and glands.

FOR MORE INFORMATION

Gilman, S and Newman, SW: Manter and Gatz's Essentials of Clinical Neuroanatomy and Neurophysiology, ed 9. FA Davis, Philadelphia, 1996.

FUNCTIONAL COMPONENTS OF THE CRANIAL NERVES

Cranial Nerve Number	Name	Components
I	Olfactory	SVA
II	Optic	SSA
III	Oculomotor	GSE, GVE
IV	Trochlear	GSA, GSE
V	Trigeminal	GSA, SVE
VI	Abducens	GSA, GSE
VII	Facial	GSA, GVA, GVE, SVA, SVE

FUNCTIONAL COMPONENTS OF THE CRANIAL NERVES

Cranial Nerve		Components
Number	**Name**	
VIII	Vestibulocochlear	SSA
IX	Glossopharyngeal	GSA, GVA, GVE, SVA, SVE
X	Vagus	GSA, GVA, SVA, SVE, GVE
XI	Accessory	GSA, SVE
XII	Hypoglossal	GSA, GSE

OVERVIEW OF CRANIAL NERVE INNERVATIONS

SENSORY INNERVATION

Modality	*Number*	*Classification*
Olfaction	I	SVA
Vision	II	SSA
Taste	VII, IX, X	SVA
Hearing and vestibular organs	VIII	SSA
Skin overlying face and scalp to vertex	V	GSA
Majority of mucosal membranes	V	GSA
Remainder of mucosal membranes	VII, IX, X	GVA

MOTOR INNERVATION

Structure	*Number*	*Classification*
Muscles within orbit	III, IV, and VI	GSE
Muscles of the tongue	XII	GSE
Muscles of mastication, tensor tympani, tensor palati (tensor veli palatini), anterior belly of digastric, mylohyoid	V	Mandibular division, SVE
Muscles of facial expression and the stapedius, stylohyoid, posterior belly of digastric	VII	SVE

Continued on following page

MOTOR INNERVATION (Continued)		
Structure	*Number*	*Classification*
Mucosal and glandular secretions including lacrimal, mucous glands, nose, palate, oral cavity; submandibular and sublingual glands	VII	GVE
Parotid gland	IX	GVE

SYMPATHETIC AND PARASYMPATHETIC COMPONENTS OF THE CRANIAL NERVES

Sympathetic Components

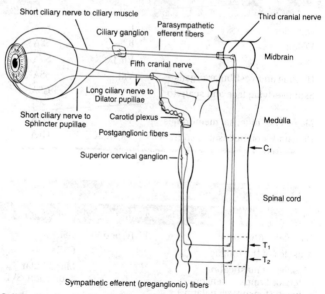

Cell bodies for the sympathetic nerve supply to the head are located in the superior cervical ganglion. Postganglionic fibers reach visceral targets such as the smooth muscle of blood vessels or the dilator pupillae by ascending with the internal carotid artery or any of its branches.

PARASYMPATHETIC DISTRIBUTION TO THE HEAD

Cranial Nerve	Ganglion	Innervates	Course
Oculomotor	Ciliary	Sphincter pupillae and the ciliary muscles	Short ciliary nerves to the sphincter pupillae (for pupillary constriction) and to the ciliary muscle (for increased lens convexity)
Facial	Pterygopalatine	Lacrimal gland and mucosa	Via lacrimal nerve and gland and glands of nose and palate
Facial	Submandibular	Submandibular and sublingual glands and mucosa	Via chorda tympani and submaxillary ganglion and on to the submandibular and sublingual salivary glands
Glossopharyngeal	Otic	Parotid gland	Lesser petrosal nerve through the otic ganglion to the parotid gland

3

DISTRIBUTION OF THE CRANIAL NERVES: MAJOR COMPONENTS

Cranial Nerve	Distribution	Function
Olfactory	Olfactory mucosa	Smell
Optic	Retina	Vision
Oculomotor	Superior division: rectus superior (superior rectus) and levator palpebra	Eye movements
	Inferior division: rectus inferior (inferior rectus) and rectus medialis (medial rectus) muscles; obliquus inferior (inferior oblique) muscle and parasympathetic accommodation fibers to the ciliary ganglion and on to the sphincter pupillae and ciliary muscles	Eye movements
Trochlear	Obliquus superior (superior oblique) muscle	Eye movements
Trigeminal	Ophthalmic nerve: eyeball and face	Sensation of the face, scalp, eyeball, and tongue (not for taste)
	Maxillary nerve: upper jaw and face	
	Mandibular nerve: muscles of mastication and to lower part of face and anterior two thirds of tongue	
Abducens	Rectus lateralis (lateral rectus) muscle	Eye movements
Facial	Muscles of face and scalp	Facial expression
	Anterior two thirds of the tongue	Taste

DISTRIBUTION OF THE CRANIAL NERVES: MAJOR COMPONENTS

Cranial Nerve	*Distribution*	*Function*
	Submandibular, sublingual, and lacrimal glands	Secretion (saliva and tears) lingual and lacrimal glands
	External auditory meatus	Pain and temperature of the external auditory meatus
Vestibulocochlear	Cochlear nerve	Hearing
	Vestibular nerve	To semicircular canals, utricle, and saccule
Glossopharyngeal	Tympanic	Sensory innervation to middle ear
	Lesser petrosal nerve	Innervation of parotid gland (via the otic ganglion)
	Carotid	Chemoreceptors and baroreceptors
	Pharyngeal	Mucosal membranes of the pharynx
	Muscular	Innervation of stylopharyngeus muscle
	Tonsillar	Sensation to the tonsils
	Lingual	General sensation and taste to the posterior one third of the tongue and papillae
Vagus	Meningeal	Dura mater and posterior fossa of the skull

Continued on following page

3

Cranial Nerve	Distribution	Function
Vagus (con't.)	Auricular	Sensation around the external acoustic meatus
	Pharyngeal	Motor nerves of the pharynx
	Superior laryngeal	Sensory innervation of the muscles and mucous membranes of the larynx
	Recurrent laryngeal (left and right)	Motor innervation to the muscles of the larynx, sensation to lower larynx, and branches to esophagus and trachea
	Cardiac	Joins cardiac plexus
	Pulmonary	Lung
	Esophageal	Esophagus and posterior pericardium
	Gastric	Stomach
	Celiac	Contributes to celiac plexus
	Hepatic	Liver
Accessory	Cranial with vagus and larynx	Muscles of pharynx and soft palate
	Spinal motor innervation to sternomastoid and trapezius	Neck movements
Hypoglossal	All muscles of the tongue except the palatoglossus	Movement of the tongue

CRANIAL NERVE TESTING
Nerve Examination and Types of Deficits

I. Olfactory — The patient is asked to identify familiar odors (tobacco, garlic, coffee) with eyes closed.

II. Optic — **field testing:** One eye is covered as patient looks at the examiner's nose. Starting at the peripheral extent of each quadrant, the examiner moves a finger in front of the patient toward the center of vision; patient states when she or he first sees the finger, thus revealing any gross deficits.

retinal lesion: Blind spot in affected eye.

optic nerve lesion: Partial or complete blindness.

Text continues on page 276.

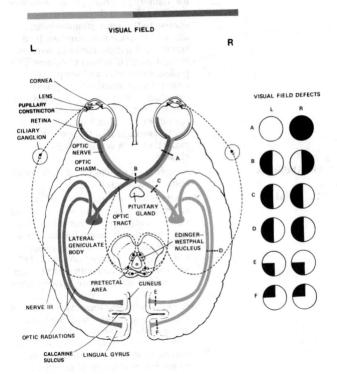

Lesions along the pathway from the eye to the visual cortex (lesions A through F) result in deficits in the visual fields, which are shown as black areas on the corresponding visual field diagrams. The pathway through the pretectum and cranial nerve III (oculomotor), which mediates reflex constriction of the pupil in response to light, is also shown.

complete lesion of optic tract or of one lateral geniculate body: Blindness in opposite halves of both visual fields.

temporal lobe abnormality: Blindness in upper quadrant of both visual fields on the side opposite lesion.

parietal lobe lesion: Contralateral blindness in lower quadrants of both eyes.

occipital lobe lesion: Contralateral blindness in corresponding half of each visual field.

III. Oculomotor

Examiner tests patient for an inability to elevate, depress, and adduct affected eye.

IV. Trochlear

Examiner tests patient for an inability to depress and adduct the affected eye.

V. Trigeminal

Examiner tests sensations in all areas of the patient's face bilaterally and looks for inability to sense specific stimuli or for differences in threshold in response to the same stimulus bilaterally. Corneal reflex is examined by determining if patient blinks in response to light touch of cotton to cornea. The patient's masseter and temporalis muscles are palpative in response to examiner's command to close jaw. Jaw reflex is tested by striking the middle of chin with a reflex hammer while patient's mouth is slightly open; normally there is a sudden, slight jaw closing.

VI. Abducens

Examiner tests patient for an inability to abduct the affected eye.

VII. Facial

Patient imitates examiner's facial expressions; patient maintains eye closure as examiner attempts to manually open eye. Sensation is tested by having patient identify taste of stimuli (sugar, salt, and so on) placed on one half of anterior tongue and with sips of water at a neutral temperature between stimuli.

facial muscle motor loss: Involvement of supranuclear fibers supplying facial nerve leads to a motor loss in lower half of face, whereas nuclear or peripheral nerve injury leads to loss of all motor function on the side of the lesion.

facial sensory loss: Sensory loss can be

caused by compromise of chorda tympani to anterior tongue.

VIII. Vestibulocochlear	**hearing:** For auditory portion, examiner moves ticking watch away from ear until sound is no longer heard; both ears are tested.

lateralization: Examiner places base of tuning fork atop patient's skull while inquiring whether the sound remains central or is referred to one side.

air and bone conduction: Examiner places tuning fork on mastoid process until patient no longer hears sound; then holds vibrating portion next to ear to determine air conduction (which is usually better than bone conduction). Deficits such as tinnitus, decreased hearing, or deafness may suggest involvement of cochlear nerve or cochlear nucleus at pontomedullary junction.

vestibular: Examiner tests for past-pointing by having the patient raise an arm and bring the index finger to the examiner's index finger; the test is performed with the patient's eyes opened and closed. With vestibular disorders the patient misses the examiner's finger by pointing to one side or the other. The patient may also have difficulty in performing the finger-to-nose test; nystagmus may also be present. Caloric testing (infiltrating one ear with cold water at 18°–20°C) should demonstrate vertigo, past-pointing, and nystagmus, whereas a patient with a defective vestibular system will not necessarily show such changes.

IX. Glossopharyngeal	See tests listed under the vagus nerve.
X. Vagus	Examiner touches side of patient's pharynx with applicator stick to elicit gag reflex and notes rise in uvula when its mucous membrane is stroked (the glossopharyngeal nerve supplies the sensory portion of this reflex). Patient's ability to swallow and to speak clearly without hoarseness as well as to demonstrate symmetrical vocal cord movements and soft palate movement suggest an intact vagus nerve to pharynx, larynx, and soft palate.

| XI. Accessory | Patient performs shoulder shrug against resistance (upper trapezius), resistance to lateral neck flexion with rotation (sternomastoid). |
| XII. Hypoglossal | Patient protrudes tongue while examiner checks for lateral deviation, atrophy, or tremor. |

FOR MORE INFORMATION

Waxman, SG and deGroot, J: Correlative Neuroanatomy, ed 22. Appleton & Lange, Norwalk, 1995.

MUSCLES THAT MOVE THE EYE

BY MOVEMENT

Adduction	*Abduction*
Rectus medialis (medial rectus)	Obliquus inferior (inferior oblique)
Rectus superioris (superior rectus)	Obliquus superior (superior oblique)
Rectus inferior (inferior rectus)	Rectus lateralis (lateral rectus)

Medial Rotation	*Lateral Rotation*
Obliquus superior (superior oblique)	Obliquus inferior (inferior oblique)
Rectus superior (superior rectus)	Rectus inferior (inferior rectus)

Depression	*Elevation*
Obliquus superior (superior oblique)	Rectus lateralis (lateral rectus)
Rectus inferior (inferior rectus)	Rectus superior (superior rectus)
	Obliquus inferior (inferior oblique)

BY MUSCLE

Muscle	*Innervation*	*Function*
Rectus superior (superior (rectus)	Oculomotor (III)	Elevation, adduction, medial rotation
Obliquus superior (superior oblique)	Trochlear (IV)	Depression, abduction, medial rotation
Rectus inferior (inferior rectus)	Oculomotor (III)	Depression, adduction, lateral rotation
Obliquus inferior (inferior oblique)	Oculomotor (III)	Elevation, abduction, lateral rotation
Rectus medialis (medial rectus)	Oculomotor (III)	Adduction
Rectus lateralis (lateral rectus)	Abducens (VI)	Abduction

3

CLINICAL TESTS FOR FUNCTION OF EXTRAOCULAR MUSCLES

Muscle	Movement of Eye Requested
Rectus lateralis (lateral rectus)	Outward (abduction)
Rectus medialis (medial rectus)	Inward (adduction)
Rectus superioris (superior rectus)	Elevation and adduction
Rectus inferioris (inferior rectus)	Depression and adduction
Obliquus superioris (superior oblique)	Depression and adduction
Obliquus inferioris (inferior oblique)	Elevation and adduction

THE EYE AND THE ORBIT

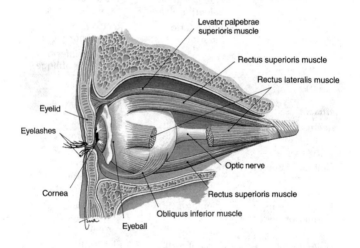

Levator palpebrae superioris muscle

Rectus superioris muscle

Rectus lateralis muscle

Eyelid

Eyelashes

Optic nerve

Cornea

Rectus superioris muscle

Obliquus inferior muscle

Eyeball

STRUCTURES OF THE EYE

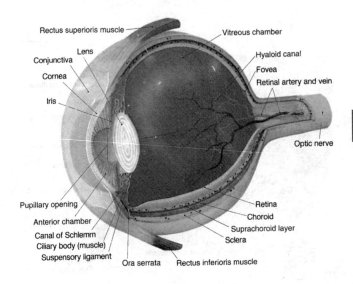

Rectus superioris muscle

Vitreous chamber

Lens

Conjunctiva

Hyaloid canal

Cornea

Fovea

Iris

Retinal artery and vein

Optic nerve

Pupillary opening

Retina

Anterior chamber

Choroid

Canal of Schlemm

Suprachoroid layer

Ciliary body (muscle)

Sclera

Suspensory ligament

Ora serrata

Rectus inferioris muscle

3

ANATOMY OF THE EAR

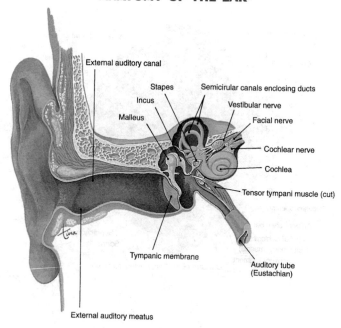

- External auditory canal
- Stapes
- Incus
- Malleus
- Semicirular canals enclosing ducts
- Vestibular nerve
- Facial nerve
- Cochlear nerve
- Cochlea
- Tensor tympani muscle (cut)
- Tympanic membrane
- Auditory tube (Eustachian)
- External auditory meatus

INNER EAR

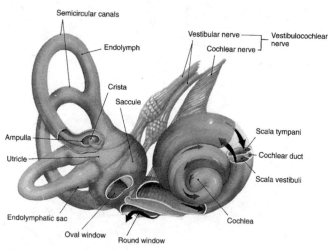

- Semicircular canals
- Endolymph
- Crista
- Saccule
- Ampulla
- Utricle
- Endolymphatic sac
- Oval window
- Round window
- Vestibular nerve
- Cochlear nerve
- Vestibulocochlear nerve
- Scala tympani
- Cochlear duct
- Scala vestibuli
- Cochlea

Shows direction of flow of endolymph in the cochlear duct and flow of the perilymph in the scala tympani and scale vestibuli.

CLASSIFICATION OF NERVE FIBERS

Sensory and Motor Fibers	Sensory Fibers	Largest Fiber Diameter (μm)	Fastest Conduction Velocity (m/s)	General Comments	
A-α	Ia	22	120	Motor:	The large α motoneurons of lamina IX, innervating extrafusal muscle fibers
				Sensory:	The primary afferents of muscle spindles
A-α	Ib	22	120	Sensory:	Golgi tendon organs, touch and pressure receptors
A-β	II	13	70	Motor:	The motoneurons innervating both extrafusal and intrafusal (muscle spindle) muscle fibers
				Sensory:	The secondary afferents of muscle spindles, touch and pressure receptors, and pacinian corpuscles (vibratory sensors)

Continued on following page

3

CLASSIFICATION OF NERVE FIBERS (Continued)

Sensory and Motor Fibers	Sensory Fibers	Largest Fiber Diameter (μm)	Fastest Conduction Velocity (m/s)	General Comments
A-γ		8	40	**Motor:** The small gamma motoneurons of lamina IX, innervating intrafusal fibers (muscle spindles)
A-δ	III	5	15	**Sensory:** Small, lightly myelinated fibers; touch, pressure, pain, and temperature
B		3	14	**Motor:** Small, lightly myelinated preganglionic autonomic fibers
C	IV	1	2	**Motor:** All postganglionic autonomic fibers (all are unmyelinated)
				Sensory: Unmyelinated pain and temperature fibers

From Gilman, S and Newman, SW: Manter and Gatz's Essentials of Clinical Neuroanatomy and Neurophysiology, ed 9. FA Davis, Philadelphia, 1996, p. 29, with permission.

RELATIVE SIZE AND SUSCEPTIBILITY TO BLOCK OF TYPES OF NERVE FIBERS					
Fiber Type*	Function	Diameter (μm)	Myelination	Conduction Velocity (m/s)	Sensitivity to Block
Type A					
α	Proprioception, motor	12–20	Heavy	70–120	+
β	Touch, pressure	5–12	Heavy	30–70	++
γ	Muscle spindles	3–6	Heavy	15–30	++
δ	Pain, temperature	2–5	Heavy	12–30	+++
Type B	Preganglionic autonomic	<3	Light	3–15	++++
Type C					
Dorsal root	Pain	0.4–1.2	None	0.5–2.3	++++
Sympathetic	Postganglionic	0.3–1.3	None	0.7–2.3	++++

*Fiber types are classified according to the system established by Gasser, HS and Erlanger, J: Role of fiber size in the establishment of nerve block by pressure or cocaine. Am J Physiol 88:581, 1929.

From Katzung, BG: Basic and Clinical Pharmacology, ed 5. Appleton & Lange, Stamford, 1992. As appearing in Ciccone, CD: Pharmacology in Rehabilitation, ed 2. FA Davis, Philadelphia, 1996, p 154, with permission.

ANALGESIA

OPIOID ANALGESICS

Drug	Route of Administration*	Onset of Action (min)	Time to Peak Effect (min)	Duration of Action (h)
	STRONG AGONISTS			
Fentanyl (Sublimaze)	IM	7–15	20–30	1–2
	IV	1–2	3–5	0.5–1
Hydromorphone (Dilaudid)	Oral	30	90–120	4
	IM	15	30–60	4
	IV	10–15	15–30	2–3
	Sub-Q	15	30–90	4
Levorphanol (Levo-Dromoran)	Oral	10–60	90–120	4–5
	IM	—	60	4–5
	IV	—	Within 20	4–5
	Sub-Q	—	60–90	4–5
Meperidine (Demerol)	Oral	15	60–90	2–4
	IM	10–15	30–50	2–4
	IV	1	5–7	2–4
	Sub-Q	10–15	30–50	2–4

Drug	Route			
Methadone (Dolophine)	Oral	30–60	90–120	4–6
	IM	10–20	60–120	4–5
	IV	—	15–30	3–4
Morphine (many trade names)	Oral	—	60–120	4–5
	IM	10–30	30–60	4–5
	IV	—	20	4–5
	Sub-Q	10–30	50–90	4–5
	Epidural	15–60	—	Up to 24
Oxymorphone (Numorphan)	IM	10–15	30–90	3–6
	IV	5–10	15–30	3–4
	Sub-Q	10–20	—	3–6
	Rectal	15–30	120	3–6
MILD-TO-MODERATE AGONISTS				
Codeine (many trade names)	Oral	30–40	60–120	4
	IM	10–30	30–60	4
	Sub-Q	10–30	—	4
Hydrocodone (Hycodan)	Oral	10–30	30–60	4–6
Oxycodone (Percodan)	Oral	—	60	3–4
Propoxyphene (Darvon, Dolene)	Oral	15–60	120	4–6

Continued on following page

3

ANALGESIA (Continued)

OPIOID ANALGESICS (Continued)

Drug	Route of Administration*	Onset of Action (min)	Time to Peak Effect (min)	Duration of Action (h)
MIXED AGONIST-ANTAGONIST				
Butorphanol (Stadol)	IM	10–30	30–60	3–4
	IV	2–3	30	2–4
Nalbuphine (Nubain)	IM	Within 15	60	3–6
	IV	2–3	30	3–4
	Sub-Q	Within 15	—	3–6
Pentazocine (Talwin)	Oral	15–30	60–90	3
	IM	15–20	30–60	2–3
	IV	2–3	15–30	2–3
	Sub-Q	15–20	30–60	2–3

*IM = intramuscular; IV = intravenous; sub-Q = subcutaneous.

From Ciccone, CD: Pharmacology in Rehabilitation, ed 2. FA Davis, Philadelphia, 1996, p 181, with permission.

OPIOID RECEPTORS

Receptor Subtype	Primary CNS Location	Primary Physiologic Response	Abuse Potential
μ	Supraspinal areas of pain modulation (periaqueductal gray, medial thalamic nuclei, hypothalamus, limbic system)	Supraspinal analgesia, euphoria, respiratory depression	High
κ	Dorsal horn of spinal gray matter (substantia gelatinosa); deep layers of cerebral cortex	Spinal analgesia, sedation, depressed flexor reflexes	Low
δ	Substantia nigra, globus pallidus, corpus striatum, other limbic structures	Euphoria, sedation	Low
σ	Hippocampus	Dysphoria, hallucinations, cardiovascular stimulation	Low

From Ciccone, CD: Pharmacology in Rehabilitation, ed 2. FA Davis, Philadelphia, 1996, p 179, with permission.

PATIENT-CONTROLLED ANALGESIA

Drug (Concentration)	Demand Dose	Lockout Interval (min)
Fentanyl (10 μg/ml)	10–20 μg	5–10
Hydromorphone (0.2 mg/ml)	0.05–0.25 mg	5–10
Meperidine (10 mg/ml)	5–30 mg	5–12
Methadone (1 mg/ml)	0.5–2.5 mg	8–20
Morphine (1 mg/ml)	0.5–3.0 mg	5–12
Nalbuphine (1 mg/ml)	1–5 mg	5–10
Oxymorphone (0.25 mg/ml)	0.2–0.4 mg	8–10

From Ferrante, FM: Patient-controlled analgesia. Anesthesiol Clin North Am 10:287, 1992, with permission.

ANALGESIA (Continued)

BASIC FEATURES OF SOME COMMON PATIENT-CONTROLLED ANALGESIA PUMPS			
Feature	Abbott PMP	Bard Ambulatory PCA Infuser	Pharmacia/Deltec Infuser
Size	$6.75 \times 4.0 \times 23$	$4.75 \times 3.4 \times 1.2$ (100-ml container) $4.75 \times 3.4 \times 2.75$ (250-ml container)	$1.1 \times 3.5 \times 4.7 \times 6.3$ (50-ml cassette) $1.1 \times 3.5 \times 7.8$ (100-ml cassette)
Power source	Wall plug in AC 2×9 alkaline battery; attachable battery pack	Lithium 3×3 V battery	Akaline 9 V
Drive mechanism	Rotary peristaltic	Linear peristaltic	Linear peristaltic
Bolus dose	0.1–25 ml (or mg/h)	0.1–20 ml (or mg/h)	0.1–6 ml (or mg/ml)
Reservoir	0.1–1000 ml (or mg or μg)	Maximum of 240 ml	50–100 ml
Lockout	5–99 min	3 min–10 h	5–999 min
Hourly limit	Maximum 25 ml	1–30 ml	0–6 ml

PCA = patient-controlled analgesia, PMP = pain management provider.
Based on Shaw, HL: Treatment of intractable cancer pain by electronically controlled parenteral infusion of analgesic drugs. Cancer 72(suppl):3416, 1993.

COMMON LOCAL ANESTHETICS

Generic Name	Trade Name	Relative Onset* of Action	Relative Duration* of Action	Principal Use(s)
Benzocaine	Americaine	—	—	Topical
Bupivicaine	Marcaine	Slow–medium	Long	Infiltration Peripheral nerve block Epidural Spinal Sympathetic block
Butamben	Butesin Picrate	—	—	Topical
Chloroprocaine	Nesacaine	Rapid	Short	Infiltration Peripheral nerve block Epidural
Dibucaine	Nupercainal	—	—	Topical
Etidocaine	Duranest	Rapid	Long	Infiltration Peripheral nerve block Epidural
Lidocaine	Xylocaine	Rapid	Intermediate	Infiltration Peripheral nerve block Epidural Spinal

Continued on following page

3

291

ANALGESIA (Continued)

COMMON LOCAL ANESTHETICS (Continued)

Generic Name	Trade Name	Relative Onset* of Action	Relative Duration* of Action	Principal Use(s)
Lidocaine (con't.)				Transdermal Topical Sympathetic block
Mepivacaine	Carbocaine	Medium–rapid	Intermediate	Infiltration Peripheral nerve block Epidural
Pramoxine	Tronothane	—	—	Topical
Prilocaine	Citanest	Rapid	Intermediate	Infiltration Peripheral nerve block
Procaine	Novacaine	Slow	Short	Infiltration Peripheral nerve block Spinal
Tetracaine	Pontocaine	Rapid	Intermediate–long	Topical Spinal

*Values for onset and duration refer to use during injection. Relative durations of action are as follows: short = 30–60 min; intermediate = 1–3 h; and long = 3–10 h of action.

From USP DI®, 14th Edition, copyright 1994. The USP Convention, Inc. Permission granted. The USP is not responsible for any inaccuracy of quotation nor for any false or misleading implication that may arise due to the text used or due to the quotation of information subsequently changed in later editions.

ANATOMICAL CLASSIFICATION OF PERIPHERAL NEUROPATHIES

SYMMETRICAL GENERALIZED NEUROPATHIES (POLYNEUROPATHIES)

DISTAL AXONOPATHIES

Toxic: drugs, industrial and environmental chemicals

Metabolic: uremia, diabetes, porphyria, endocrine

Deficiencies: thiamine, pyridoxine

Genetic: hereditary motor sensory neuropathy type II (HMSN II)

Malignancy associated: oat-cell carcinoma, multiple myeloma

MYELINOPATHIES

Toxic: diphtheria, buckthorn

Immunologic: acute inflammatory polyneuropathy (Guillain-Barré), chronic inflammatory polyneuropathy

Genetic: Refsum's disease, metachromatic leukodystrophy

NEURONOPATHIES

Somatic Motor

Undetermined: amyotrophic lateral sclerosis

Genetic: hereditary motor neuropathies

Somatic Sensory

Infectious: herpes zoster neuronitis

Malignancy associated: sensory neuropathy syndrome

Toxic: pyridoxine sensory neuropathy

Undetermined: subacute sensory neuropathy syndrome

Autonomic

Genetic: hereditary dysautonomia (hereditary sensory neuropathy type IV [HSN IV])

Classification of Neuropathies continued on page 294.

FOCAL (MONONEUROPATHY) AND MULTIFOCAL (MULTIPLE MONONEUROPATHY) NEUROPATHIES

Ischemia: polyarteritis, diabetes, rheumatoid arthritis

Infiltration: leukemia, lymphoma, granuloma, schwannoma, amyloid

Physical injuries: severance, focal crush, compression, stretch and traction, entrapment

Immunologic: brachial and lumbar plexopathy

FOR MORE INFORMATION

Schaumburg, HH, et al: Disorders of Peripheral Nerves, ed 2. FA Davis, Philadelphia, 1992.

ANATOMICAL CLASSIFICATIONS OF ACUTE NERVE INJURIES

TERMS USED TO DESCRIBE ACUTE NERVE INJURIES: LESIONS AND CLINICAL FEATURES
(see figures for illustrations of each lesion type)

Suggested Nomenclature	Previous Nomenclature	Anatomic Lesion	Common Clinical Features
Class 1	Neuropraxia Transient Delayed reversible	Conduction block Ischemia Demyelination	A rapidly reversible loss of nerve function occurs Dysfunction of the nerve persists for a few weeks
Class 2	Axonotmesis	Axonal interruption	Total loss of function occurs in the nerve until there is regeneration of the damaged axon; wallerian degeneration occurs distal to the site of the lesion; regenerating axons are guided back to their terminations via the intact Schwann cell tubes and other endoneural connective tissue
Class 3	Neurotmesis Partial	Nerve fiber interruption Damage to Schwann cell tube and endoneural connective tissue	Reinnervation may be incomplete because of a failure of the regenerating axon to find its proper terminus
	Complete	Total nerve severance	Reinnervation will not occur unless the nerve is surgically repaired; neuroma formation and aberrant regeneration are common

3

Based on Schaumburg, HH, et al: Disorders of Peripheral Nerves, ed 2. FA Davis, Philadelphia, 1992, p 209.

Class 1 (Neurapraxia) Nerve Injury

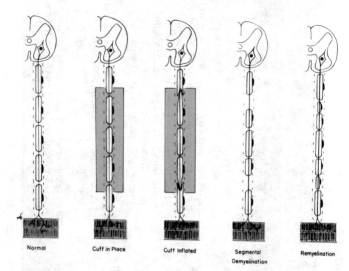

Normal   Cuff in Place   Cuff Inflated   Segmental Demyelination   Remyelination

CLASS I — ACUTE NERVE INJURY
(e.g. Compression)

Class 1 (neurapraxia) nerve injury associated with compression by a cuff. Axon movement at both edges of the cuff causes intussusception of the attached myelin across the node of Ranvier into the adjacent paranode. Affected paranodes demyelinate. Remyelination begins following cuff removal, and conduction eventually resumes. Conduction is normal in the nerve above and below the cuff since the axon has not been damaged.

Class 2 (Axonotmesis) Nerve Injury

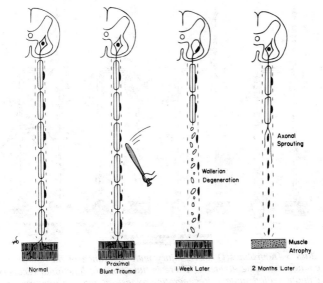

CLASS 2 NERVE INJURY

Class 2 (axonotmesis) nerve injury from a crush injury to a limb. Axonal disruption occurs at the site of injury. Wallerian degeneration takes place throughout the axon distal to the injury with loss of axon, myelin, and nerve conduction. Preservation of Schwann cell tubes and other endoneurial connective tissue ensures that regenerating axons have the opportunity to reach their previous terminals and, hopefully, re-establish functional connections.

Class 3 (Neurotmesis) Nerve Injury

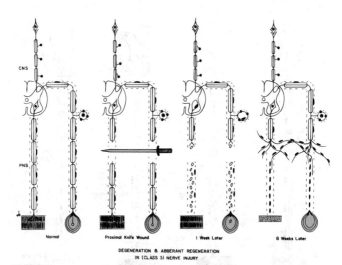

DEGENERATION & ABBERANT REGENERATION
IN (CLASS 3) NERVE INJURY

Class 3 (neurotmesis) nerve injury with severance of all neural and connective tissue elements. There is little hope of functional recovery without skilled surgery. Regenerating axons are entering inappropriate Schwann cell tubes (aberrant regeneration).

PERIPHERAL NERVE ENTRAPMENT SYNDROMES

The conditions presented in this section are listed alphabetically under upper and lower extremity syndromes:

Upper Extremity Syndromes

anterior interosseous nerve syndrome: The anterior interosseus nerve is compromised at or near its site of origin from the median nerve. Entrapment may occur as a result of thrombosis of the vessels that accompany the nerve, an accessory head of the flexor pollicis longus, an enlarged bicipital bursa, a tendinous origin of the deep head of the pronator muscle, or from either forearm fracture undergoing open reduction or supracondylar fractures in children. This syndrome is characterized by pain or discomfort in the volar aspect of the proximal forearm area with eventual weakness or paralysis of the pronator quadratus and flexor pollicis longus, and the flexor digitorum profundus slips to the index and middle finger.

carpal tunnel syndrome: The median nerve is compressed as it passes through the tunnel formed by the concavity in the two rows of carpal bones and the flexor retinaculum. The causes may be inflammatory, as in tenosynovitis of the flexor tendons or rheumatoid arthritis, hormonal dysfunction, or bony deformity secondary to fracture, acromegaly, or congenital stenosis. The syndrome presents as pain and paresthesias, usually worse at night, involving the digits supplied by the median nerve. There may be weakness and atrophy of the abductor pollicis brevis, the opponens pollicis, and the first and second lumbricales.

cubital tunnel syndrome: The ulnar nerve becomes entrapped at the cubital tunnel, which is formed by the ulnar groove between the medial epicondyle of the humerus and the olecranon. This syndrome can be caused by ganglion formation, arthritis, an old fracture of the lateral humeral epicondyle, and dislocation of the ulnar nerve when the elbow is flexed. Sensory involvement is localized over the ulnar aspect of the hand on both the palmar and dorsal aspects. The motor weakness is manifested in the forearm by the flexor carpi ulnaris and in the hand by the adductor pollicis, and the flexor digitorum profundus, lumbricales, and interosseus muscles (fourth and fifth digits). These weaknesses result in a radial deviation on wrist flexion and a mild clawing of the fourth and fifth fingers.

flexor carpi ulnaris syndrome: The ulnar nerve becomes entrapped as it passes under the arcuate ligament between the two heads of the flexor carpi ulnaris muscle. The symptoms are similar to those described for cubital tunnel syndrome.

posterior interosseous nerve entrapment: The posterior interosseous nerve, a branch of the radial nerve, may be entrapped as it passes through the two heads of the supinator muscle via an aponeurotic arch (arcade of Frohse). Most cases of this syndrome are found to be secondary to either thickening or narrowing of the arcade of Frohse. Predisposing factors are diabetes mellitus, leprosy, periarteritis nodosa, and heavy metal poisoning. The complete syndrome presents as pain or discomfort over the proximal or lateral aspect of the forearm. The patient radially deviates on dorsiflexion of the wrist and the fingers and thumb cannot be extended at the metacarpophalangeal (MCP) joints.

pronator teres syndrome: This syndrome occurs when the median nerve is entrapped as it passes between the two heads of the pronator teres. Symptoms are pain or discomfort over the volar proximal third of the forearm, which is aggravated when the forearm is overly pronated and the wrist flexed. Paresthesias may be present in the radial three half digits. Muscle weakness is highly variable. The flexor carpi radialis, the flexor digitorum superficialis, and the median lumbricales are often weak. The most common causes of this syndrome are:
1. Narrowing of the space between the two heads of the pronator
2. Direct trauma of the volar upper third of the forearm
3. Repetitive motion of the limb (forearm pronation with finger flexion)
4. An anatomic variation
5. Chronic external compression of the upper forearm

spiral groove syndrome: This syndrome results from entrapment or direct trauma to the radial nerve at the spiral groove of the humerus between the medial and lateral heads of the triceps. It usually occurs

Continued on following page

as a complication of humeral fractures or direct pressure on the nerve (Saturday night palsy). Fully manifested, its symptoms are a drop wrist with a flexed MCP joint and an adducted thumb. All muscles innervated by the radial nerve may be paralyzed, except for the triceps.

supracondylar process syndrome: The median nerve, accompanied by the brachial or ulnar artery, may become entrapped beneath the ligament of Struthers. This ligament originates from a bony process above the medial condyle and runs to the medial epicondyle of the elbow (it is present in about 1% of limbs). The patient presents with pronator teres weakness, and the radial or ulnar pulse may decrease or vanish when the arm is fully extended and supinated.

ulnar (Guyon's) tunnel syndrome: The ulnar nerve becomes entrapped as it travels through the ulnar tunnel from the forearm into the hand. This tunnel is formed by the pisohamate ligament at the wrist. Entrapment occurs usually as a result of a space-occupying lesion within the tunnel such as with rheumatoid arthritis or from the formation of ganglions. The symptoms are pain over the palmar aspect of the ulnar side of the hand and the fifth digit and the ulnar aspect of the fourth digit. Motor function shows the typical "preacher" or "benediction" hand. Atrophy of the hypothenar and interosseus muscles (especially the first dorsal interossei) may become very noticeable.

Lower Extremity Syndromes

anterior compartment syndrome: The anterior tibial artery and veins and the deep branch of the peroneal nerve are compressed as a result of increased pressure within the confines of the anterior compartment. Blood supply to the muscles within this osteofascial compartment is compromised. This syndrome may result from anterior tibial tendonitis associated with running long distances, a direct blow to the anterior aspect of the leg, or an overly tight cast to the leg. Early symptoms are intense pain in the anterior aspect of the leg with signs of vascular depletion in the foot. Muscular loss appears as an inability to dorsiflex the ankle, the toes, and the big toe. There is hypesthesia or anesthesia in the dorsal aspect of the first web space.

common peroneal nerve syndrome: The common peroneal nerve at the fibular head and neck is injured or entrapped as it winds around the fibula head. Some of the most common causes of this syndrome are excessive pressure from poorly applied casts or bandages, excessive pressure in bedridden patients allowed to remain in external rotation, fracture of the neck of the fibula, severe acute genu varum, and direct trauma to the nerve. In patients with a fully developed syndrome, the patient's foot appears in full plantar flexion and slight inversion as a result of weakness or paralysis in all the muscles of the anterior and lateral compartment of the leg. The patient has a steppage gait.

meralgia paresthetica: The lateral femoral cutaneous nerve is compressed as it passes into the thigh under the inguinal ligament just medial to the anterior superior iliac spine. It is brought on by trauma, postural abnormalities, occupations requiring long periods of hip flexion, obesity, and wearing of a tight belt or truss. The patient usually complains of discomfort or pain in the lateral aspect of the thigh.

piriformis syndrome: The sciatic nerve becomes entrapped as it emerges from the pelvis through the greater sciatic foramen, passing between the piriformis muscle above and the obturator internus below. The common causes of this syndrome are sustained piriformis muscle contraction and fibrotic muscle changes secondary to direct trauma, as in posterior dislocation of the hip joint. The patient has motor and sensory changes involving the posterior aspect of the thigh and the entire leg and foot. Muscle weakness of the hamstrings, gluteus maximus, ankle dorsiflexors, plantar flexors, and the intrinsics of the foot can result in a gluteus maximus lurch as well as difficulty in walking on toes or heels.

popliteal fossa entrapment: The tibial nerve is compressed as it passes through the popliteal fossa. It is usually caused by a Baker's cyst. Enlarged cysts may also compress the common peroneal and sural nerves. Other causes are proliferation of the synovial tissue in patients with rheumatoid arthritis. The patient presents with incomplete flexion of the knee joint and pain behind the knee or in the calf muscles when the foot is dorsiflexed. The gastrocnemius, tibialis posterior, flexor hallucis longus, flexor digitorum longus, and the intrinsic muscles of the foot (except for extensor digitorum brevis) are weak or paralyzed. The entire plantar surface of the foot is hypesthetic or anesthetic.

tarsal tunnel syndrome: The posterior tibial nerve or its branches are compressed as it passes under the flexor retinaculum behind the medial malleolus of the ankle joint. The most common causes of this syndrome are tenosynovitis of the flexor hallucis longus, flexor digitorum longus, or tibialis posterior caused by local trauma or systemic connective tissue diseases; venous distension or engorgement within the tunnel from chronic venous insufficiency or distortion of the canal from either developmental (pes planus, pes valgus); or traumatic deformities (fracture of the medial malleolus or fracture or dislocation of the calcaneus or talus). There is severe weakness of plantar flexion and edema in the back of the leg.

BASED ON

Perotto, A and Delagi, E: Peripheral nerve entrapment syndromes. In Ruskin, A (ed): Current Therapy in Physiatry, Physical Medicine and Rehabilitation. WB Saunders, Philadelphia, 1984.

CERVICAL PLEXUS
Anatomy

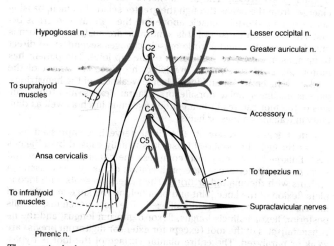

Hypoglossal n. ———

C1

C2 ——— Lesser occipital n.
——— Greater auricular n.

To suprahyoid
muscles

C3

C4 ——— Accessory n.

C5

Ansa cervicalis

——— To trapezius m.

To infrahyoid
muscles

——— Supraclavicular nerves

Phrenic n.

The cervical plexus is formed by anterior primary rami of C1, C2, C3, and C4. The plexus lies almost entirely beneath the sternomastoid muscle.

BRACHIAL PLEXUS

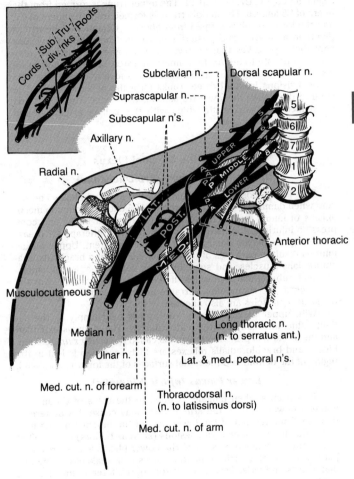

Note that extensor muscles are innervated by posterior divisions, and anterior divisions innervate flexors. Each of the three trunks (upper, middle, and lower) has an anterior and posterior division. The posterior divisions form the posterior cord, and the anterior divisions form the lateral and medial cords.

Continued on following page

Anatomy

The brachial plexus is formed by anterior primary rami of spinal segments C5, C6, C7, C8, and T1. The upper trunk is formed from the fibers of C5 and C6. The middle trunk is formed from the fibers of C7, and the lower trunk is formed from fibers of C8 and T1. The trunks divide into anterior and posterior divisions. The anterior divisions contribute to nerves that innervate flexors, and the posterior divisions contribute to nerves that innervate extensors. The anterior divisions of the middle and upper trunk form the lateral cord. The posterior divisions from all three trunks form the posterior cord. The anterior division of the lower trunk forms the medial cord. The cords are named for their relationships with the axillary artery, around which the plexus wraps.

Injuries to the Brachial Plexus

Upper Plexus Injury (Erb-Duchenne)

This is the most common injury to the brachial plexus and occurs when damage is done to the roots of C5 and C6. Common mechanisms of injury are traction injuries (as occur at birth) and compression injuries. Months or years after radiation therapy for breast cancer, upper plexus damage may become apparent. Upper plexus injuries result in paralysis of the deltoid, biceps, and brachialis, brachioradialis muscles, and sometimes the supraspinatus, infraspinatus, and subscapularis muscles. If the roots are avulsed from the spinal cord, the rhomboids, serratus anterior, levator scapula, and the scalene muscles are also affected.

With upper plexus injuries, the arm is held limply at the patient's side, internally rotated and adducted. The elbow is extended and the forearm is pronated in what is called the *waiter's tip* position. Biceps and brachioradialis reflexes are lost. Sensation is lost in the region of the deltoid and the radial surfaces of the forearm and hand.

Lower Plexus Injury (Klumpke)

This occurs when damage is done to the roots of C8 and T1. Forceful upward pull of the arm at birth may cause this pattern of damage. Compression of the lower part of the brachial plexus may occur due to space-occupying lesions (such as tumors) and is often due to the presence of a cervical rib. Lower plexus injuries result in paralysis of all the intrinsic hand muscles and weakness of the medial fingers and wrist flexors. Extensors of the forearm may also be weak.

A clawhand deformity is seen with lower plexus injuries; that is, the fourth and fifth digits are hyperextended at the MCP joints and flexed at the interphalangeal (IP) joints, the first phalanx is hyperextended, and the fifth finger remains abducted. Guttering of the hand may be seen due to atrophy of the intrinsic muscles. Sensation is lost in the region of the ulnar side of the arm, forearm, and hand. Lower plexus lesions are often accompanied by disturbances in the sympathetic nervous system (e.g., Horner's syndrome). Trophic changes in the arm may occur that can include edema and changes in the appearance of the skin and nails.

BRACHIAL PLEXUS LATENCY DETERMINATIONS FROM SPECIFIC NERVE ROOT STIMULATION

Plexus	Site of Stimulation	Recording Site	Latency Across Plexus (ms) Range	Latency Across Plexus (ms) Mean ± SD
Brachial (upper trunk and lateral cord)	C5 and C6	Biceps	4.8–6.2	5.3 ± 0.4
Brachial (posterior cord)	C6, C7, C8	Triceps	4.4–6.1	5.4 ± 0.4
Brachial (lower trunk and medial cord)	C8, T1, ulnar nerve	Abductor digiti minimi	3.7–5.5	4.7 ± 0.5

Based on MacLean, IC: Nerve root stimulation to evaluate conduction across the brachial and lumbosacral plexuses. Third Annual Continuing Education Course, American Association of Electromyography and Electrodiagnosis, September 25, 1980, Philadelphia.

NERVE CONDUCTION TIMES FROM ERB'S POINT TO MUSCLE			
Muscle	n*	Distance (cm)	Latency (ms)†
Biceps	19	20	4.6 ± 0.6
	15	24	4.7 ± 0.6
	14	28	5.0 ± 0.5
Deltoid	20	15.5	4.3 ± 0.5
	17	18.5	4.4 ± 0.4
Triceps	16	21.5	4.5 ± 0.4
	23	26.5	4.9 ± 0.5
	16	31.5	5.3 ± 0.5
Supraspinatus	19	8.5	2.6 ± 0.3
	16	10.5	2.7 ± 0.3
Infraspinatus	20	14	3.4 ± 0.4
	15	17	3.4 ± 0.5

*Number of subjects tested to obtain values.
†Mean ± SD.
From Kimura, J: Electrodiagnosis in Diseases of Nerve and Muscle: Principles and Practice, ed 2. FA Davis, Philadelphia, 1989, p 119, with permission.

LONG THORACIC NERVE, ANTERIOR THORACIC NERVE, LATERAL PECTORAL NERVE, AND THE MEDIAL PECTORAL NERVE

Course and Distribution

Muscles innervated by nerves are listed in italics.

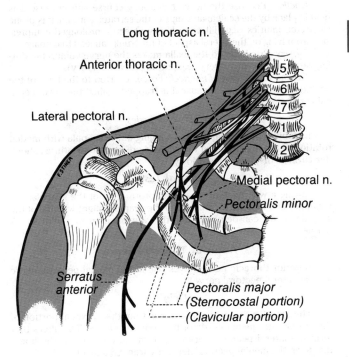

LONG THORACIC NERVE AND ANTERIOR THORACIC NERVES

Long Thoracic Nerve

Long thoracic nerve, also called the external respiratory nerve of Bell, nerve to serratus anterior, or posterior thoracic nerve (a term that also includes the dorsal scapular nerve).

Origin

The long thoracic nerve arises from anterior primary rami of C5, C6, and C7.

Continued on following page

Innervation

Motor

The long thoracic nerve innervates the serratus anterior muscle.

Cutaneous and Joint

None.

Common Injuries

Traction: Because the nerve has a long course and because it is held in place by the scaleni and slips of the serratus anterior, it is prone to stretch injuries (e.g., lifting of heavy objects); prolonged compression from lying on the lateral aspect of the trunk can lead to damage.

Surgery: Proximity to the axilla makes the nerve vulnerable during various forms of surgery (e.g., during breast surgery).

Trauma to the base of the neck: Forces exerted to the base of the neck damage the nerve because it is trapped against the lower cervical vertebrae.

Effects of Injuries

Instability of the scapula and winging of the scapula with medial rotation of the lower part of the scapula are common features; shoulder girdle is displaced posteriorly.

Special Tests

During a wall push-up or during protraction of the scapula, the examiner should look for winging of the scapula; slight winging of the scapula at rest can be noted, and this winging increases with shoulder flexion.

Anterior Thoracic Nerve

Anterior thoracic nerve (gives rise to the medial pectoral nerve and the lateral pectoral nerve).

Origin

The anterior thoracic nerve arises from the proximal portion of the lateral and medial cords of the brachial plexus. The fibers that form the lateral pectoral nerve are from C5, C6, and C7; the fibers that form the medial pectoral nerve are from C8 and T1.

Innervation

Motor

The lateral pectoral nerve innervates the superior and clavicular portions of the pectoralis major muscle. The medial pectoral nerve innervates pectoralis minor muscle and the inferior part of the sternocostal portion of the pectoralis major muscle.

Cutaneous and Joint

None.

Common Injuries

Isolated injuries to these nerves are rare. Fibers that form the nerves may be damaged when there is a nerve root or brachial plexus injury.

Depending on the extent of injury, weakness or paralysis of the pectoral muscles may result; the shoulder is held slightly posterior and may be elevated or depressed.

Special Tests

When the examiner elevates the patient's shoulders by placing his hands in the axillae, the shoulder of the affected side rises higher than that of the normal side; when the patient flexes both arms to approximately 90°, the affected arm deviates laterally.

DORSAL SCAPULAR NERVE, NERVE TO SUBCLAVIUS, AND SUPRASCAPULAR NERVE

Course and Distribution: Posterior View

Muscles innervated by nerves are listed in italics.

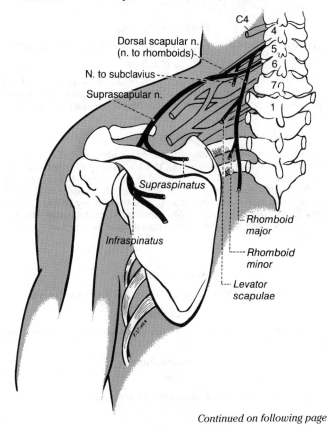

Continued on following page

Dorsal Scapular Nerve

The dorsal scapular nerve is also called the posterior scapular nerve or the nerve to the rhomboids.

Origin

The dorsal scapular nerve arises from anterior primary rami of C5.

Innervation

Motor

The dorsal scapular nerve innervates the rhomboid minor and rhomboid major muscles and contributes innervation to the levator scapulae muscle, which also receives innervation from C3 and C4.

Cutaneous and Joint

None.

Common Injuries

Injury to the C5 root is more common than injury to the nerve.

Effects of Injuries

Depending on the extent of injury, weakness or paralysis of the rhomboid muscles and paresis of the levator scapulae may result; the inferior portion of the vertebral border of the scapula wings posteriorly.

Special Tests

When the patient is asked to brace the shoulders (i.e., stand at attention with shoulders square), the scapula of the affected shoulder is obliquely positioned with the upper vertebral border lying medially and the inferior portion lying laterally; damage to the dorsal scapular nerve can be differentiated from injury to the C5 root only by electromyographic (EMG) testing, which indicates that the lesion is isolated to the rhomboid muscles and the levator scapulae muscle.

Nerve to Subclavius

The nerve to subclavius is also called the subclavian nerve.

Origin

The subclavian nerve arises from the upper trunk of the brachial plexus from fibers originating at C5 and C6.

Innervation

Motor

The subclavian nerve innervates the subclavius muscle.

Cutaneous and Joint

None.

Common Injuries

Isolated injury to the nerve is uncommon.

Effects of Injuries

Depending on the extent of injury, weakness or paralysis of the subclavius muscle results in slight forward displacement of the lateral end of the clavicle.

Special Tests

None.

Suprascapular Nerve

Origin

The suprascapular nerve arises from the upper trunk of the brachial plexus from fibers originating at C5 and C6.

Innervation

Motor

The suprascapular nerve innervates the supraspinatus muscle and the infraspinatus muscle.

Cutaneous and Joint

There is no cutaneous distribution; the nerve supplies posterior capsule of the glenohumeral joint.

Common Injuries

Traction and pressure: Downward displacement on the shoulder stretches the nerve and can cause injury (e.g., as occurs with Erb's palsy or due to gymnastics).

Trauma: Wounds above the scapula will frequently affect the nerve.

Effects of Injuries

Atrophy of the supraspinatus muscle and the infraspinatus muscle are common features. There is difficulty initiating abduction and external rotation at the glenohumeral joint. When at rest, the arm may be kept slightly medially rotated.

Special Tests

To test for loss of function of the infraspinatus muscle, the examiner tests for lateral rotation; EMG testing reveals only denervation of supraspinatus and infraspinatus muscles without any denervation to other muscles innervated by C5 and C6.

THORACODORSAL NERVE AND SUBSCAPULAR NERVES

Course and Distribution

Muscles innervated by nerves are listed in italics.

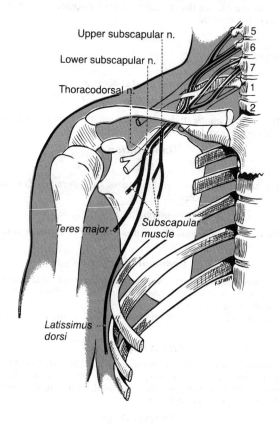

Thoracodorsal Nerve

Origin

The thoracodorsal nerve arises from the posterior cord of the brachial plexus from fibers originating at C6, C7, and C8.

Innervation

Motor

The thoracodorsal nerve innervates the latissimus dorsi muscle.

Cutaneous and Joint

None.

Common Injuries

Isolated injuries to the nerve are rare; damage is associated with injuries to the posterior cord of the brachial plexus.

Effects of Injuries

Paralysis of the latissimus dorsi muscle may result in winging of the inferior angle of the scapula and an inability to extend the arm powerfully.

Special Tests

The examiner resists shoulder extension; if the latissimus dorsi muscle is denervated, there is weakness.

Subscapular Nerves

Origin

The upper (superior) subscapular nerve and the lower (inferior) subscapular nerve arise from the posterior cord of the brachial plexus from fibers originating at C5 and C6 (the upper subscapular nerve is also called the short subscapular nerve).

Innervation

Motor

The upper subscapular nerve innervates the subscapularis muscle; the lower subscapular nerve innervates the subscapularis muscle and the teres major muscle.

Cutaneous and Joint

None.

Common Injuries

Isolated injuries to the nerves are rare; damage is associated with injuries to the posterior cord of the brachial plexus.

Effects of Injuries

Paralysis of the subscapularis muscle results in weakness of medial rotation. Paralysis of the teres major muscle does not significantly affect function.

Special Tests

The examiner resists medial rotation; there is weakness rather than loss of motion if the nerve is damaged because other medial rotators are still innervated.

AXILLARY NERVE

Course and Distribution: Posterior View

Muscles innervated by nerves are listed in italics.

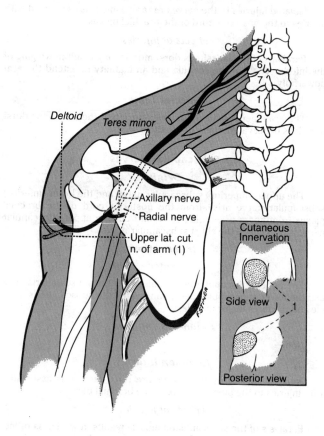

The axillary nerve is also called the circumflex nerve.

Origin

The axillary nerve arises from the posterior cord of the brachial plexus from fibers originating at C5 and C6.

Innervation

Motor

The axillary nerve innervates the deltoid muscle (all three parts) and the teres minor muscle.

Cutaneous and Joint

Cutaneous in the area of the deltoid muscle.

Common Injuries

Fractures: Because the axillary nerve wraps around the proximal humerus, any fracture in the region of the surgical neck of the humerus may be accompanied by an axillary nerve lesion.

Dislocations: Movement of the humerus after a dislocation at the glenohumeral joint may result in an axillary nerve lesion.

Forceful hyperextension of the shoulder: With hyperextension of the shoulder (as might occur during a wrestling match), the axillary nerve may be compromised.

Inappropriate use of crutches: Pressure on the axillary region due to leaning on crutches can cause a compression injury to the axillary nerve.

Other Trauma: Contusions in the shoulder region or injuries to the scapula may be accompanied by axillary nerve lesions. Because the nerve passes between the coracoid process of the scapula and the humerus, compression of these structures often results in an entrapment syndrome.

Effects of Injuries

Paralysis of the deltoid muscle with resultant atrophy causes a change in the contour of the shoulder; the shoulder becomes flattened and loses its normal rounded shape. There is a decreased ability to abduct, flex, and extend the arm at the glenohumeral joint. Paralysis of the teres minor muscle does not significantly affect function.

Special Tests

Muscle testing of the deltoid muscle, especially in the fully abducted position, reveals severe weakness. Confirmation of denervation of the teres minor muscle can be determined only through EMG because the infraspinatus muscle is also an external rotator of the arm.

MUSCULOCUTANEOUS NERVE
Course and Distribution

Muscles innervated by nerves are listed in italics.

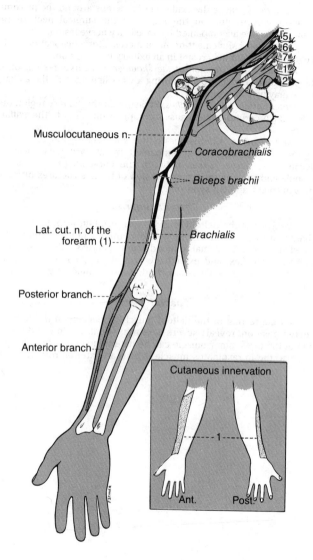

Musculocutaneous n.

Coracobrachialis

Biceps brachii

Lat. cut. n. of the forearm (1)

Brachialis

Posterior branch

Anterior branch

Cutaneous innervation

1

Ant.   Post.

Origin

The musculocutaneous nerve arises from the lateral cord of the brachial plexus from fibers originating at C5, C6, and C7.

Innervation

Motor

The musculocutaneous nerve innervates the coracobrachialis muscle, biceps brachii muscle, and most of the brachialis muscle.

Cutaneous and Joint

In the forearm, the musculocutaneous nerve gives rise to the lateral cutaneous nerve of the forearm that innervates the lateral forearm; the cutaneous division is also called the lateral antebrachial cutaneous nerve.

Common Injuries

Fractures or dislocations of the humerus can lead to lesions of the musculocutaneous nerve, as can open wounds (e.g., stab wounds). The nerve can also be entrapped by the coracobrachialis muscle or injured during surgery.

Effects of Injuries

Paralysis of the biceps brachii muscle and the brachialis muscle results in weak elbow flexion. The loss of the biceps is especially noticeable when elbow flexion is attempted with the forearm supinated. Weakness in supination occurs. Paralysis of the coracobrachialis muscle does not significantly affect function.

Special Tests

The examiner tests for the biceps brachii stretch reflex, for extreme weakness when the elbow flexors are muscle-tested with the forearm fully supinated, and for weakness when muscle-testing is performed for supination. Although EMG testing of the biceps brachii muscle, brachialis muscle, and the coracobrachialis muscle can show denervation, to determine specific nerve damage this should be accompanied by findings of impaired nerve conduction velocities.

Continued on following page

MUSCULOCUTANEOUS NERVE (Continued)

VALUES FOR ELECTRODIAGNOSTIC TESTING

Age (y)	Motor Nerve Conduction Between Erb's Point and Axilla					Orthodromic Sensory Nerve Conduction Between Erb's Point and Axilla				Orthodromic Sensory Nerve Conduction Between Axilla and Elbow		
	n*	Range of Conduction Velocities (m/s)	Range of Amplitudes (µV)			n*	Range of Conduction Velocities (m/s)	Range of Amplitudes (µV)	n*	Range of Conduction Velocities (m/s)	Range of Amplitudes (µV)
			Axilla	Erb's Point							
15–24	14	63–78	9–32	7–27		14	59–76	3.5–30	15	61–75	17–75
25–34	6	60–75	8–30	6–26		6	57–74	3–25	8	59–73	16–72
35–44	8	58–73	8–28	6–24		7	54–71	2.5–21	8	57–71	16–69
45–54	10	55–71	7–26	6–22		10	52–69	2–18	13	55–69	15–65
55–64	9	53–68	7–24	5–21		9	49–66	2–15	10	53–67	14–62
65–74	4	50–66	6–22	5–19		4	47–64	1.5–12	6	51–65	13–59

*Number of subjects tested to obtain values in the table.

From Trojaborg, W: Motor and sensory conduction in the musculocutaneous nerve. J Neurol Neurosurg Psychiatry 39:890, 1976, with permission.

LATERAL AND MEDIAL CUTANEOUS NERVES

				Latency			
				VALUES FOR ELECTRODIAGNOSTIC TESTING			
Nerve	Number of Patients Seen	Age (years) (mean)	Distance (cm)	Onset (ms)*	Peak (ms)*	Conduction Velocity (m/s)*	Amplitude (μV)*
Lateral cutaneous nerve	30	20–84 (35)	12	1.8 ± 0.1	2.3 ± 0.1	65 ± 4	24.0 ± 7.2
Lateral cutaneous nerve	154	17–80 (45)	14		2.8 ± 0.2	62 ± 4	18.9 ± 9.9
Medial cutaneous nerve	155	17–80 (45)	14		27. ± 0.2	63 ± 5	11.4 ± 5.2
Medial cutaneous nerve	30	23–60 (38)	18	2.7 ± 0.2	3.3 ± 0.2	66 ± 4	15.4 ± 4.1

* Mean ± SD.

From Kimura, J: Electrodiagnosis in Diseases of Nerve and Muscle: Principles and Practice, ed 2. FA Davis, Philadelphia, 1989, p 122, with permission.

319

MEDIAN NERVE

Course and Distribution

Muscles innervated by nerves are listed in italics.

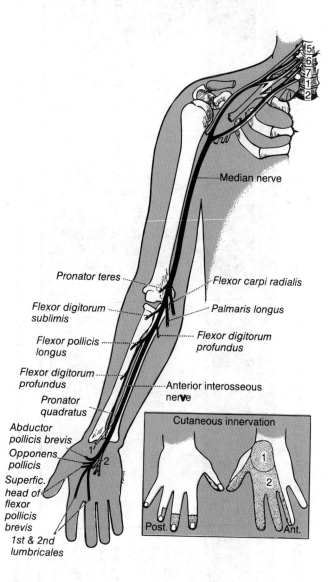

Median nerve

Pronator teres

Flexor carpi radialis

Flexor digitorum sublimis

Palmaris longus

Flexor pollicis longus

Flexor digitorum profundus

Flexor digitorum profundus

Anterior interosseous nerve

Pronator quadratus

Abductor pollicis brevis

Opponens pollicis

Superfic. head of flexor pollicis brevis

1st & 2nd lumbricales

Cutaneous innervation

Post.

Ant.

Origin

Portions of the medial and lateral cords of the brachial plexus join together to form the median nerve. These fibers, which originated at C6, C7, C8, and T1, pass through the anterior divisions of the upper, middle, and lower trunks of the brachial plexus. Sometimes fibers from C5 also are part of the median nerve.

Innervation

Motor

The median nerve supplies all the muscles in the anterior aspect of the forearm with the exception of the flexor carpi ulnaris muscle and the medial half of the flexor digitorum profundus muscle. The main trunk of the nerve supplies the pronator teres, flexor carpi radialis, palmaris longus, and the flexor digitorum superficialis muscles; the anterior osseous nerve (a pure motor nerve) innervates the flexor pollicis longus, the lateral half of the flexor digitorum profundus, and the pronator quadratus muscle before passing through the carpal tunnel to innervate lumbricals one and two. At the level of the distal carpal ligament, a recurrent (muscular) thenar branch is given off to innervate the abductor pollicis brevis, the lateral half of the flexor pollicis brevis, and the opponens pollicis muscle.

Cutaneous and Joint

The nerve supplies the skin over the lateral (radial) side of the palm and the palmar and dorsal (terminal parts) aspects of the lateral three-and-a-half digits.

Common Injuries

Entrapment syndromes: The median nerve can be entrapped at many points as it courses down the arm; often entrapment of the median nerve is also accompanied by entrapment of the ulnar nerve (see ulnar nerve).

Thoracic outlet syndrome: This is due to the scalenus-anticus syndrome, the presence of a cervical rib, or some other narrowing of the thoracic outlet where the median nerve can be compressed near its proximal origin.

Ligament of Struther's syndrome (supracondylar process syndrome): This is due to the presence of an anomalous ligament that forms a fibrous tunnel near the medial condyle of humerus, the median nerve can be compressed.

Pronator teres syndrome: The median nerve can be compressed as it passes between the deep and superficial heads of the pronator teres muscle. Trauma, fracture of the humerus, and hypertrophy of the pronator teres muscle can cause the entrapment; repetitive motion of the limb with the forearm in pronation and the fingers flexed (e.g., using a screwdriver) can also result in compression. An anomalous fibrous band connecting the pronator teres muscle to the flexor digitorum superficialis muscle can also compress the median nerve; compression may also occur if the nerve has an anomalous path that takes it behind both heads of the pronator teres muscle.

Anterior interosseous syndrome: As the median nerve gives

Continued on following page

rise to the anterior interosseous nerve (just below the level of the radial tuberosity), it can be compressed by several different anomalous structures, including fibrous sheaths, and the tendinous origin of the long flexors. Thrombosis of the vessels that are in close proximity with the nerve can cause entrapment, as can the presence of an accessory head of the flexor pollicis longus muscle. Forearm fractures and supracondylar fractures in children may also result in compression.

Carpal tunnel syndrome: As the median nerve enters the hand, it runs beneath a wide, fibrous ligamentous band that forms the *carpal tunnel*; this is a common site of median nerve compression. In women the syndrome may, in some cases, be caused by hormonal factors that occur with pregnancy or during the menstrual cycle; in addition, hypothyroidism has been thought to cause the syndrome. Inflammatory events that occur with tenosynovitis of the flexor tendons, rheumatoid arthritis, or overuse syndromes may also cause compression at the carpal tunnel. Moreover, congenital bony deformities, deformities secondary to fractures, or acromegaly may also cause the syndrome.

Digital nerve entrapment syndrome: The interdigital nerve that supplies the skin of the second and third digits and half of the fourth digit may be compressed against the edge of the deep transverse metacarpal ligament. This syndrome appears to be caused by trauma (such as phalangeal fractures), tumors, or inflammation of the MCP joints.

Trauma

In addition to causing compression syndromes, trauma may lead to direct injuries to the median nerve.

Humeral fractures: These fractures may lead to disruption of the median nerve above the elbow. This is especially true of supracondylar fractures.

Lacerations of the wrist: The superficial course of the median nerve at the wrist makes it vulnerable to damage from accidental lacerations (that occur with falls on sharp objects) or lacerations associated with suicide attempts.

Carpal bone injuries: Because the median nerve courses directly over the carpal bones, trauma to these bones often results in damage to the nerve. This damage may occur with fractures or dislocations or from direct trauma at the time the carpal bone was injured.

Effects of Injuries

The deficits associated with damage to the median nerve depend on the severity of the injury and the site of the lesion. To determine specific deficits for each syndrome and type of injury, the course of the nerve must be considered and the resultant loss of motor and sensory function distal to the site determined (see the listing of peripheral nerve entrapment syndromes for descriptions of the symptoms of some of the more common syndromes). Pain is a common feature of the entrapment syndromes; however, sensory effects can also include hypesthesia, paresthesia, and even complete sensory loss.

General Motor Defects with Median Nerve Lesions

Loss of opposition of the thumb, loss of ability to make a fist, and atrophy of the thenar eminence are common general motor defects.

Common deformities seen with median nerve lesions include:

Simian (ape) hand: occurs because of denervation and resultant atrophy of muscles in the thenar eminence. Opposition is lost. As a result of the atrophy and paralysis, the hand flattens.

Benediction sign: occurs because of paralysis to the flexors of the middle and ring fingers. When a person with a median nerve injury attempts to make a fist, these fingers do not fully flex, and they remain in a position similar to that used when clergy make a benediction.

Special Tests

Depending on the severity and site of the lesion, many different tests can be used to ascertain median nerve damage. General muscle and sensory testing can be used to indicate the level of the lesion by determining which portion of the nerve is damaged.

Motor

If, as part of general paralysis or weakness of all muscles innervated by the median nerve, muscles above the elbow are affected (e.g., flexor carpi radialis muscle and other long flexors), the main portion of the nerve must be injured. If the long flexors (those muscles first innervated by the nerve) are spared but there is isolated paralysis of the flexor pollicis longus muscle, the lateral half of the flexor digitorum profundus muscle, and the pronator quadratus muscle, damage to the anterior interosseous nerve is indicated. If paralysis or paresis is isolated to the abductor pollicis brevis, lateral half of the flexor pollicis brevis, and the opponens pollicis muscles, then damage to the thenar branch is indicated.

Cutaneous and Joint

Total sensory loss of the tip of the index finger and decreased sensation on the lateral (radial) side of the palm and the lateral three-and-a-half digits over their palmar aspects indicate interruption of the nerve at a level above the lower third of the forearm. Lesions distal to the origin of the palmar cutaneous branch (which arises proximal to the level of the wrist) result in preserved sensation of the more proximal portions of the dorsal surface of the hand, but loss of sensation in the most distal distribution of the median nerve (e.g., loss of sensation in the distal portion of the second and third fingers and some loss in the distal fourth finger).

Specific Tests

Adson's maneuver (test for thoracic outlet syndrome): The patient turns the head to the side of the suspected lesion, extends the neck fully, and takes and holds a deep breath while the examiner checks for a decreased radial pulse (in some patients the effect may be more

Continued on following page

noticeable if the patient turns the head away from the side of the suspected lesion). If the thoracic outlet is compromised, this maneuver further narrows the outlet and indicates whether the median nerve is likely to be compressed at this level.

Tests for compression by ligament of Struther's (supracondylar process syndrome): The examiner checks for decrease or absence of radial and/or ulnar pulses when the forearm is fully extended and supinated. The presence of weakness and EMG abnormalities of the pronator teres muscle indicates possible compression due to a ligament of Struthers (this muscle is usually not affected by the pronator teres syndrome); nerve conduction testing can also be used to determine blockage across the antecubital fossa.

Tests for pronator teres syndrome: Test for a pattern of weakness in the flexor carpi radialis muscle, flexor digitorum superficialis muscle, thenar muscles, and lumbricals one and two. Nerve conduction velocity testing indicates a slowing of velocity across the elbow, and there will be a diminished evoked response (see test for ligament of Struthers). The EMG shows denervation in affected muscles. Electrodiagnostic testing for pronator teres syndrome is usually not considered positive based on findings of abnormalities in the pronator teres because this muscle is usually spared in this syndrome. Phalen's sign and testing for normal conduction latencies are used to rule out carpal tunnel syndrome (see appropriate tests).

Tests for anterior interosseous syndrome: The patient is asked to make an "OK" sign (an *O* between the thumb and index finger) using the first two digits. The shape is observed. If there is damage to the interosseous nerve, a triangle (the "pinch sign") rather than a circle will be formed. Routine nerve conduction studies of the median nerve are normal with this syndrome, but slowed conduction velocities of the anterior interosseous nerve may be discerned by recording compound muscle action potentials from the pronator quadratus muscle after stimulation of the nerve at the elbow; EMG shows denervation in the flexor pollicis longus, flexor digitorum profundus (first and second fingers), and pronator quadratus muscles.

Tests for carpal tunnel syndrome: The examiner taps the patient's wrist over the carpal tunnel; if pain is felt in the cutaneous distribution of the median nerve (Tinel's sign), carpal tunnel syndrome is likely. The examiner can use Phalen's test by forcefully flexing the patient's wrist and holding it in that position for a minute; in this way the carpal tunnel is compressed and pain in the distribution of the median nerve is felt if carpal tunnel syndrome is present. In carpal tunnel syndrome, conduction abnormalities of sensory and motor fibers are usually seen in the wrist-to-palm segment of the median nerve with the distal segment of the nerve remaining relatively normal; EMG may be normal, or, in severe cases, signs of denervation may be seen in the median nerve-innervated lumbricals.

Observable signs: Look for the benediction sign or the appearance of a simian hand.

MEDIAN NERVE (Continued)

	VALUES FOR ELECTRODIAGNOSTIC TESTING[a]				
Site of Stimulation	Amplitude[b] Motor (mV) Sensory (μV)	Latency[c] to Recording Site (ms)	Difference Between Right and Left (ms)	Conduction Time Between Two Points (ms)	Conduction Velocity (m/s)
Motor Fibers					
Palm	6.9 ± 3.2 (3.5)[d]	1.86 ± 0.28 (2.4)[e]	0.19 ± 0.17 (0.5)[e]	1.65 ± 0.25 (2.2)[e]	48.8 ± 5.3 (38)[f]
Wrist	7.0 ± 3.0 (3.5)	3.49 ± 0.34 (4.2)	0.24 ± 0.22 (0.7)	3.92 ± 0.49 (4.9)	57.7 ± 4.9 (48)
Elbow	7.0 ± 2.7 (3.5)	7.39 ± 0.69 (8.8)	0.31 ± 0.24 (0.8)	2.42 ± 0.39 (3.2)	63.5 ± 6.2 (51)
Axilla	7.2 ± 2.9 (3.5)	9.81 ± 0.89 (11.6)	0.42 ± 0.33 (1.1)		58.8 ± 5.8 (47)
Sensory Fibers					
Digit	39.0 ± 16.8 (20)	1.37 ± 0.24 (1.9)	0.15 ± 0.11 (0.4)	1.37 ± 0.24 (1.9)	58.8 ± 5.8 (47)
Palm	38.5 ± 15.6 (19)	2.84 ± 0.34 (3.5)	0.18 ± 0.14 (0.5)	1.48 ± 0.18 (1.8)	56.2 ± 5.8 (44)
Wrist	32.0 ± 15.5 (16)	6.46 ± 0.71 (7.9)	0.29 ± 0.21 (0.7)	3.61 ± 0.48 (4.6)	61.9 ± 4.2 (53)

[a]Mean ± standard deviation (SD) in 122 nerves from 61 patients, 11–74 years of age (average, 40), with no apparent disease of the peripheral nerves.
[b]Amplitude of the evoked response, measured from the baseline to the negative peak.
[c]Latency, measured to the onset of the evoked response, with the cathode at the origin of the thenar nerve in the palm.
[d]Lower limits of normal, based on the distribution of the normative data.
[e]Upper limits of normal, calculated as the mean + 2 SD.
[f]Lower limits of normal, calculated as the mean − 2 SD.
From Kimura, J: Electrodiagnosis in Diseases of Nerve and Muscle: Principles and Practice, ed 2. FA Davis, Philadelphia, 1989, p 107, with permission.

325

ULNAR NERVE

Course and Distribution

Muscles innervated by nerves are listed in italics.

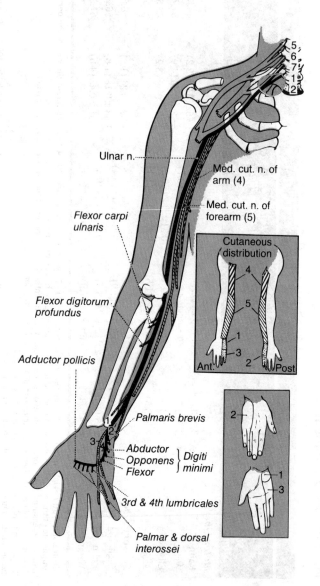

Ulnar n.

Med. cut. n. of arm (4)

Med. cut. n. of forearm (5)

Flexor carpi ulnaris

Flexor digitorum profundus

Adductor pollicis

Cutaneous distribution

Ant.   Post.

Palmaris brevis

Abductor
Opponens } *Digiti minimi*
Flexor

3rd & 4th lumbricales

Palmar & dorsal interossei

Origin

The medial cord of the brachial plexus gives rise to the ulnar nerve. Fibers originate in C8 and T1 and pass through the lower trunk of the brachial plexus and the anterior division before joining the medial cord.

Innervation

Motor

In the upper arm a branch of the ulnar nerve supplies the flexor carpi ulnaris muscle and the medial half of the flexor digitorum profundus muscle. In the hand a superficial branch is given off to supply the palmaris brevis muscle, while a deep branch innervates the hypothenar muscles, the opponens digiti minimi, abductor digiti minimi, and flexor digiti minimi muscles. After supplying innervation to the hypothenar muscles, the deep branch supplies interossei, third and fourth lumbricals, adductor pollicis muscle, and the deep head (or medial half) of the flexor pollicis brevis muscle.

Cutaneous and Joint

An articular branch is given off in the elbow region, where it innervates that joint. A dorsal branch (a pure cutaneous nerve) is given off in the forearm and continues down the forearm, winding around the ulna to supply the skin over the dorsal aspect of the hand and dorsal aspects of the medial one-and-a-half fingers (half of the fourth and all of the fifth digit). A superficial branch arises near the pisiform bone to innervate the volar aspects of the medial one-and-a-half fingers (half of the fourth and all of the fifth digit); a palmar branch also arises near the wrist to innervate the proximal hypothenar region.

Common Injuries

ENTRAPMENT SYNDROMES AND MONONEUROPATHIES. The ulnar nerve can be entrapped and damaged at many points as it courses down the arm. Often entrapment of the ulnar nerve is also accompanied by entrapment of the median nerve (see Median Nerve).

THORACIC OUTLET SYNDROME. The ulnar nerve, like the median nerve, may be compressed at the thoracic outlet (see thoracic outlet syndrome described under the Median Nerve).

INAPPROPRIATE USE OF CRUTCHES. Pressure on the axillary region, due to a patient leaning on crutches, can cause a compression injury to the ulnar nerve.

TARDY ULNAR PALSY AND CUBITAL TUNNEL SYNDROME. The term *tardy ulnar palsy* was once reserved for damage to the ulnar nerve secondary to trauma in the elbow region; now, however, the term is used to describe entrapment at the elbow due to traumatic and nontraumatic causes. This syndrome may occur in association with thoracic outlet syndrome (see thoracic outlet syndrome above and on page 321). The most common entrapment at the elbow is in the cubital tunnel, where the nerve is large and underlies the aponeurotic band between the two heads of the flexor carpi ulnaris muscle. Joint deformities, repetitive motion at the elbow, and inflammatory conditions

Continued on following page

may all cause entrapment at the tunnel, and trauma to the elbow is known to lead to ulnar nerve damage.

ANOMALOUS ANATOMIC FEATURES AT THE ELBOW. A ligament of Struthers, if present, may cause compression of the ulnar nerve similar to the way such a ligament affects the median nerve (see ligament of Struthers syndrome under the Median Nerve). The presence of an anomalous anconeus muscle (an epitrochleoanconeus muscle) can compress the ulnar nerve near the elbow; a hypertrophied flexor carpi ulnaris muscle may also press on the ulnar nerve.

COMPRESSION AT GUYON'S CANAL (ULNAR TUNNEL). The ulnar nerve can be entrapped as it crosses from the forearm into the hand through Guyon's canal (the ulnar tunnel). The tunnel is formed by the pisohamate ligament superficially, and the base of the tunnel is formed by the pisiform and the hamate bones; space-occupying lesions within the tunnel of the type that can occur with rheumatoid arthritis and ganglia can cause damage to the ulnar nerve. Persons who engage in activities that can traumatize the hypothenar region (e.g., persons who engage in karate or who have jobs requiring them to use the hypothenar portion of their hands to press or bang) are also at risk.

BICYCLE RIDER'S SYNDROME. Prolonged bicycle riding causes compression of the ulnar nerve in the hypothenar region; a similar compression injury may occur from pressing the hypothenar region on a crutch.

DIGITAL NERVE ENTRAPMENT SYNDROME. The digital nerves that supply the skin of the fifth digits and half of the fourth digit may be compressed against the edge of the deep transverse metacarpal ligament; this syndrome appears to be caused by trauma (such as phalangeal fractures), tumors, or inflammation of the MCP joints.

Effects of Injuries

The deficits associated with damage to the ulnar nerve depend on the severity of the injury to the nerve and the site of the lesion. To determine specific deficits for each syndrome and type of injury, the course of the nerve must be considered and the resultant loss of motor and sensory function distal to the site determined (see peripheral nerve entrapment syndromes for descriptions of the symptoms of some of the more common syndromes). Pain is a common feature of the entrapment syndromes; however, sensory effects can also include hypesthesia, paresthesia, and even complete sensory loss.

MOTOR DEFICITS AT THE HAND. Clawhand occurs with lesions to the ulnar nerve due to the unopposed action of the radial nerve–innervated extensor digitorum communis muscle in the fourth and fifth digits. The first phalanx is hyperextended and the distal two phalanges are flexed while the fifth finger remains abducted; there is an inability to abduct or adduct the fingers because of a loss of the interossei muscles. Flexion at the DIP joints of the fourth and fifth digits is lost because of denervation of the medial half of the flexor digitorum profundus muscle. Denervation of the adductor pollicis muscle results in weakened opposition of the thumb, and there is also a total loss of opposition by the fifth finger and an inability to abduct the little finger.

MOTOR DEFICITS AT THE WRIST. Resisted palmar flexion of the wrist results in deviation of the wrist to the radial side because of denervation of the flexor carpi ulnaris muscle.

Special Tests

ADSON'S MANEUVER (TEST FOR THORACIC OUTLET SYNDROME). The patient turns head to the side of the suspected lesion, extends neck fully, and takes and holds a deep breath while the examiner checks for a decreased radial pulse (in some patients the effect may be more noticeable if the patient turns head away from the side of the suspected lesion). If the thoracic outlet is compromised, this maneuver further narrows the outlet and indicates whether the ulnar nerve is likely to be compressed at this level.

TESTS FOR COMPRESSION BY LIGAMENT OF STRUTHERS (SUPRACONDYLAR PROCESS SYNDROME). The examiner checks for decrease or absence of radial and/or ulnar pulses when the forearm is fully extended and supinated.

FROMENT'S SIGN. The patient is asked to grasp a piece of paper between thumb and index finger; because of paralysis of the adductor pollicis muscle, the patient flexes the thumb. This flexion becomes more pronounced when the examiner pulls the paper away.

OBSERVABLE SIGNS. Guttering occurs between the fingers because of atrophy of the intrinsic muscles. There is flattening of the hypothenar eminence due to atrophy of the palmaris brevis muscle and the muscles of the fifth digit.

Continued on following page

ULNAR NERVE (Continued)

VALUES FOR ELECTRODIAGNOSTIC TESTING[a]

Site of Stimulation	Amplitude[b] Motor (mV) Sensory (μV)	Latency[c] to Recording Site (ms)	Difference Between Right and Left (ms)	Conduction Time Between Two Points (ms)	Conduction Velocity (m/s)
Motor Fibers					
Wrist	5.7 ± 2.0 (2.8)[d]	2.59 ± 0.39 (3.4)[e]	0.28 ± 0.27 (0.8)[e]		
Below elbow	5.5 ± 2.0 (2.7)	6.10 ± 0.69 (7.5)	0.29 ± 0.27 (0.8)	3.51 ± 0.51 (4.5)[e]	58.7 ± 5.1 (49)[f]
Above elbow	5.5 ± 1.9 (2.7)	8.04 ± 0.76 (9.6)	0.34 ± 0.28 (0.9)	1.94 ± 0.37 (2.7)	61.0 ± 5.5 (50)
Axilla	5.6 ± 2.1 (2.7)	9.90 ± 0.91 (11.7)	0.45 ± 0.39 (1.2)	1.88 ± 0.35 (2.6)	66.5 ± 6.3 (54)
Sensory Fibers					
Digit					
Wrist	35.0 ± 14.7 (18)	2.54 ± 0.29 (3.1)	0.18 ± 0.13 (0.4)	2.54 ± 0.29 (3.1)	54.8 ± 5.3 (44)
Below elbow	28.8 ± 12.2 (15)	5.67 ± 0.59 (6.9)	0.26 ± 0.21 (0.5)	3.22 ± 0.42 (4.1)	64.7 ± 5.4 (53)
Above elbow	28.3 ± 11.8 (14)	7.46 ± 0.64 (8.7)	0.28 ± 0.27 (0.8)	1.79 ± 0.30 (2.4)	66.7 ± 6.4 (54)

[a]Mean ± standard deviation (SD) in 130 nerves from 65 patients, 13–74 years of age (average, 39), with no apparent disease of the peripheral nerves.
[b]Amplitude of the evoked response, measured from the baseline to the negative peak.
[c]Latency, measured to the onset of the evoked response, with the cathode 3 cm above the distal crease in the wrist.
[d]Lower limits of normal, based on the distribution of the normative data.
[e]Upper limits of normal, calculated as the mean + 2 SD.
[f]Lower limits of normal, calculated as the mean − 2 SD.
From Kimura, J: Electrodiagnosis in Diseases of Nerve and Muscle: Principles and Practice, ed 2. FA Davis, Philadelphia, 1989, p 114, with permission.

RADIAL NERVE

Course and Distribution

Muscle innervated by nerves are listed in italics.

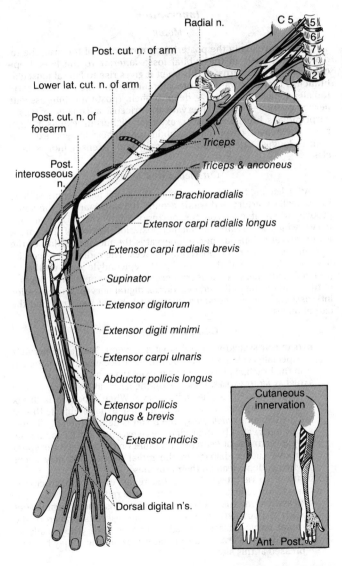

Radial n.

Post. cut. n. of arm

Lower lat. cut. n. of arm

Post. cut. n. of forearm

Post. interosseous n.

C 5

Triceps

Triceps & anconeus

Brachioradialis

Extensor carpi radialis longus

Extensor carpi radialis brevis

Supinator

Extensor digitorum

Extensor digiti minimi

Extensor carpi ulnaris

Abductor pollicis longus

Extensor pollicis longus & brevis

Extensor indicis

Dorsal digital n's.

Cutaneous innervation

Ant. Post.

Continued on following page

Origin

The radial nerve arises from the posterior cord of the brachial plexus. Fibers originating in C5, C6, C7, C8, and T1 pass through the posterior divisions of the upper, middle, and lower trunks to contribute to the radial nerve.

Innervation

Motor

After traveling in the posterior compartment of the arm, the radial nerve travels in the cubital fossa anterior to the lateral epicondyle of the humerus; at this point it gives rise to lateral muscular branches that innervate the brachioradialis, and the extensor carpi radialis longus muscles. A deep branch (posterior interosseous nerve) continues on to innervate the triceps, anconeus, extensor carpi radialis brevis, supinator, extensor digitorum, extensor digiti minimi, extensor carpi ulnaris, abductor pollicis longus, extensor pollicis longus, extensor pollicis brevis, and extensor indicis muscles.

Cutaneous and Joint

After leaving the brachial plexus, the radial nerve courses deep to the axillary artery and winds around the upper arm in the spiral groove, where it gives off the posterior (antebrachial) cutaneous nerve, which innervates the medial posterior portion of the arm. A lower lateral cutaneous nerve innervates the medial portion of the arm on the anterior and posterior surfaces. The radial nerve continues on in the arm and at the level of the epicondyle gives off the superficial radial nerve (a sensory nerve), which supplies the dorsum of the hand on the radial side via dorsal digital nerves. The posterior interosseous nerve innervates joint structures of the wrist and the carpal bones.

Common Injuries

ENTRAPMENT SYNDROMES AND MONONEUROPATHIES. The radial nerve is especially vulnerable to compression because of its location in the brachial plexus and its proximity to the humerus.

SATURDAY NIGHT PALSIES. Pressure on the nerve at the spiral groove causes damage to the radial nerve. When a person is drunk and falls asleep with an arm against a hard object, this is called *Saturday night palsy;* the result is denervation of all muscles innervated by the radial nerve except the triceps muscle.

INAPPROPRIATE USE OF CRUTCHES. Pressure on the nerve at the spiral groove causes damage to the radial nerve. This may occur when patients lean on their crutches.

SEQUELAE TO FRACTURES. During the repair of humeral fractures, newly formed callus may compress the radial nerve.

COMPRESSION AT THE ARCADE OF FROHSE (POSTERIOR INTEROSSEOUS NERVE ENTRAPMENT). The posterior interosseous branch of the radial nerve passes through a fibrous arch (the arcade of Frohse) at the level of the spinator muscle, and it may be compressed at this site.

TENNIS ELBOW. Compression of a branch of the radial nerve at the lateral epicondyle of the humerus may give rise to pain at the elbow. This form of tennis elbow may also involve entrapment of the deep branch of the nerve.

Trauma

Because the radial nerve runs superficially during part of its course and because it lies against the rigid spiral groove of the humerus, the nerve is very vulnerable to trauma. Shoulder dislocations, humeral fractures, and radial neck fractures can all cause damage to the radial nerve. The location of the radial nerve also makes it highly vulnerable to gunshot and stab wounds.

Effects of Injuries

The deficits associated with damage to the radial nerve depend on the severity of the injury to the nerve and the site of the lesion. To determine specific deficits for each syndrome and type of injury, the course of the nerve must be considered and the resultant loss of motor and sensory function distal to the site determined.

GENERAL MOTOR DEFECTS WITH RADIAL NERVE LESIONS. A lesion of the radial nerve above the innervation of the triceps muscle is possible, but quite rare; most lesions to the radial nerve affect all muscles innervated by the radial nerve except the triceps. The general findings with such lesions are an inability to extend the MCP joints, the wrist, and the thumb (tenodesis action may allow passive extension); inability to supinate unless the biceps muscle is used; weakness in palmar abduction of the thumb, although opposition is preserved; and paralysis of the brachioradialis muscle resulting in weakness of elbow flexors.

Special Tests

PALM-TO-PALM TEST (WRIST DROP). When separating hands that have been placed palm to palm, the hand of the affected side drops at the wrist. Wrist drop during functional activities is also an observable sign of radial nerve injury.

IMPAIRED GRIPPING. Patients have trouble gripping objects because of their inability to extend their wrists.

Continued on following page

RADIAL NERVE (Continued)

VALUES FOR ELECTRODIAGNOSTIC TESTING

Conduction	n*	Conduction Velocity (m/s) or Conduction Time (ms)†	Amplitude: Motor (mV) Sensory (μV)†	Distance (cm)†
Motor				
Axilla–elbow	8	69 ± 5.6	11 ± 7.0	15.7 ± 3.3
Elbow–forearm	10	62 ± 5.1	13 ± 8.2	18.1 ± 1.5
Forearm–muscle	10	2.4 ± 0.5	14 ± 8.8	6.2 ± 0.9
Sensory				
Axilla–elbow	16	71 ± 5.2	4 ± 1.4	18.0 ± 0.7
Elbow–wrist	20	69 ± 5.7	5 ± 2.6	20.0 ± 0.5
Wrist–thumb	23	58 ± 6.0	13 ± 7.5	13.8 ± 0.4

*Number of subjects tested to obtain values in the table.
†Mean ± SD.
Adapted from Trojaborg, W and Sindrup, EH: Motor and sensory conduction in different segments of the radial nerve in normal subjects. J Neurol Neurosurg Psychiatry 32:354–359, 1969, with permission.

LUMBAR PLEXUS

The lumbar plexus is formed from the anterior primary rami of L1, L2, and L3, with a contribution from L4. There is often a contribution from T12 (the subcostal nerve). The lower part of the plexus gives off the lumbosacral trunk, which contributes to the sacral plexus.

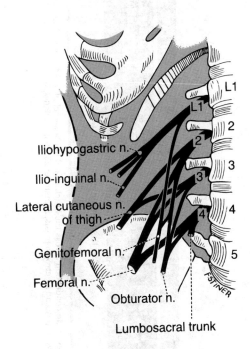

Anatomy

The lumbar plexus lies within the psoas major muscle and is composed of the anterior primary rami of L1, L2, and L3, with a contribution from L4. A contribution from T12 (the subcostal nerve) is quite common. Fibers from L4 contribute to the lumbosacral trunk, which forms part of the sacral plexus.

Injuries to the Lumbar Plexus

True lesions of the lumbar plexus are rare because the plexus lies deep within the abdomen. Damage to the plexus is often accompanied by fatal injuries. Fractures, dislocations, and space-occupying lesions (such as tumors), however, may occasionally damage the plexus. Stereotypical patterns of damage to the lumbar plexus are essentially nonexistent, although structures giving rise to the plexus may be associated with cauda equina lesions or spinal cord injuries.

Continued on following page

LUMBAR PLEXUS (Continued)

		LUMBAR PLEXUS LATENCY DETERMINATIONS FROM SPECIFIC NERVE ROOT STIMULATION	Latency Across Plexus (ms)	
Plexus	Site of Stimulation	Recording Site	Range	Mean ± SD
Lumbar	L2–L4 femoral nerve	Vastus medialis	2.0–4.4	3.4 ± 0.6

Based on MacLean, IC. Nerve root stimulation to evaluate conduction across the brachial and lumbosacral plexuses. Third Annual Continuing Education Course, American Association of Electromyography and Electrodiagnosis, September 25, 1980, Philadelphia.

ILIO-INGUINAL NERVE AND GENITOFEMORAL NERVE

Course and Distribution

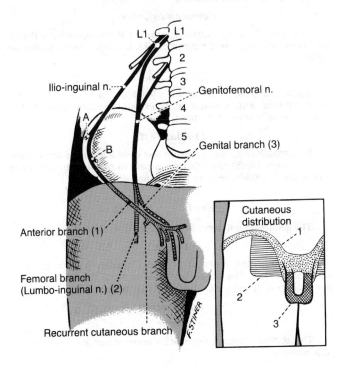

Ilio-inguinal n.

Genitofemoral n.

Genital branch (3)

Anterior branch (1)

Femoral branch (Lumbo-inguinal n.) (2)

Recurrent cutaneous branch

Cutaneous distribution

Ilio-Inguinal Nerve

Origin

The ilio-inguinal nerve is formed by fibers from L1, L2, L3, and L4. Although it is part of the lumbar plexus, it is functionally similar to the thoracic nerve because it innervates a segmental region.

Innervation

Motor

The nerve gives off segmental innervation to the obliquus internus abdominis and the transversus abdominis muscles.

Cutaneous and Joint

A cutaneous branch arises in the medial portion of the inguinal canal. An anterior branch innervates the anterior abdominal wall that overlies the pubic symphysis, the base and dorsum of the penis
Continued on following page

and the upper part of the scrotum in the male or the mons pubis and the labium majus in the female, and the thigh medial to the femoral triangle. A lateral recurrent branch innervates the skin over the thigh adjacent to the inguinal ligament.

Common Injuries

The nerve is rarely damaged; however, if it is injured, the deficit is manifest in a segmental pattern of loss. Damage may occur during surgery.

Effects of Injuries

Segmental deficits are of little clinical importance; however, some patients with ilio-inguinal neuropathies report pain in the groin, especially when they stand.

Special Tests

If an examiner applies pressure just medial to the anterior superior iliac spine (ASIS) and this causes pain to radiate into the crural region, there is evidence of an ilio-inguinal neuropathy.

Genitofemoral Nerve

The genitofemoral nerve is also called the genitocrural nerve.

Origin

Fibers from the roots of L1 and L2 unite to form the genitofemoral nerve. The nerve branches to form the lumboinguinal (femoral) branch and genital (external spermatic) branch.

Innervation

Motor

The genital (external spermatic) nerve innervates the cremasteric muscle.

Cutaneous and Joint

The genital (external spermatic) nerve innervates the skin of the inner aspect of the upper thigh and in males the scrotum and in females the labium; the lumboinguinal (femoral branch) nerve innervates the skin over the femoral triangle.

Common Injuries

Trauma to the groin may result in injury to the genitofemoral nerve; the nerve is sometimes injured during surgery or damaged by adhesions after surgery.

Effects of Injuries

With lesions, pain may be felt in the inguinal region; there is a loss of sensation over the femoral triangle, and in males the cremasteric reflex is absent.

Special Tests

To test the nerve in males the examiner strokes the inner aspect of the thigh, and the testicle elevates if the genitofemoral nerve is intact.

LATERAL CUTANEOUS NERVE OF THE THIGH AND OBTURATOR NERVE

Course and Distribution

Muscles innervated by nerves are listed in italics.

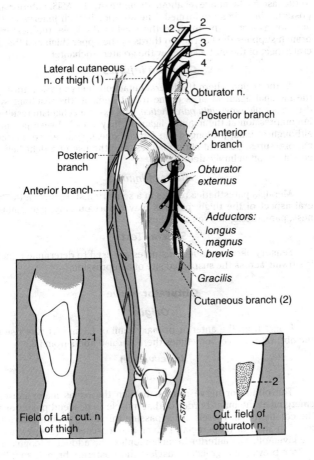

Field of Lat. cut. n of thigh

Cut. field of obturator n.

Lateral Cutaneous Nerve of the Thigh

Origin

The nerve is formed by contributions from L2 and L3.

Innervation

Motor

None.

Continued on following page

Cutaneous and Joint

After being formed by fibers from L2 and L3, the nerve penetrates the psoas major muscle, crosses the iliacus muscle, and then descends downward to pass below the inguinal ligament. The nerve moves from a position deep to the fascia lata to become superficial to the fascia lata; at a level about 10 cm below the ASIS, anterior and posterior branches are formed. The anterior branch innervates the anterior aspect of the thigh to the level of the knee; the posterior branch supplies the lateral two thirds of the upper thigh and the lateral aspect of the buttocks below the greater trochanter.

Common Injuries

In the region where the lateral cutaneous nerve passes through the inguinal ligament, it is prone to entrapment; the resultant syndrome is called *meralgia paresthetica*. The exact mechanism resulting in compression at the inguinal ligament may vary between persons, although trauma, prolonged hip flexion, obesity, increased abdominal pressures, postural abnormalities, and the use of a tight belt or corset are often implicated.

Effects of Injuries

Meralgia paresthetica results in a sensory disturbance in the lateral aspect of the thigh; patients may report burning, pain, numbness, paresthesia, or even anesthesia.

Special Tests

Sensory nerve conduction studies are used to determine if there is slowing across the suspected site of compression.

Obturator Nerve

Origin

Fibers from the anterior primary rami of L3 and L4 give rise to the obturator nerve. Sometimes there are also fibers from L2.

Innervation

Motor

The obturator nerve passes through the psoas major muscle, emerging at the inner border of that muscle to descend posterior to the common iliac vessels. After passing through the obturator foramen, an anterior (superficial) branch and a posterior (deep) branch are given off. The anterior branch supplies the adductor longus, adductor brevis, and gracilis muscles; the posterior branch supplies the obturator externus, part of the adductor magnus, and the adductor brevis muscles.

Cutaneous and Joint

The anterior branch gives rise to a cutaneous branch that innervates the medial aspect of the thigh and the hip joint.

Common Injuries

The obturator nerve may be damaged during labor or from the pressure caused by a gravid uterus. Pelvic fractures may also result in obturator nerve damage, as may surgical procedures designed to correct obturator hernias.

Effects of Injuries

Weakness of adduction, internal rotation, and external rotation of the thigh are seen with damage to the obturator nerve. With injuries to the nerve, pain in the groin may be felt to radiate along the medial aspect of the thigh.

Special Tests

The primary symptom of obturator nerve damage is the pain that radiates along the medial thigh. The pain may be greatest in the region of the knee.

3

FEMORAL NERVE

Course and Distribution

Muscles innervated by nerves are listed in italics.

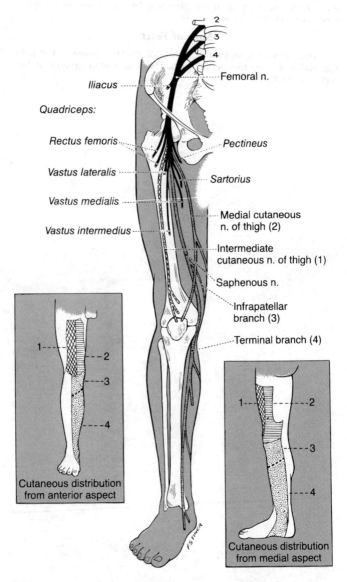

Iliacus

Quadriceps:

Rectus femoris

Vastus lateralis

Vastus medialis

Vastus intermedius

Femoral n.

Pectineus

Sartorius

Medial cutaneous n. of thigh (2)

Intermediate cutaneous n. of thigh (1)

Saphenous n.

Infrapatellar branch (3)

Terminal branch (4)

Cutaneous distribution from anterior aspect

Cutaneous distribution from medial aspect

Origin

Fibers from the anterior primary rami of L2, L3, and L4 give rise to the femoral nerve.

Innervation

Motor

The femoral nerve passes through the psoas major muscle and emerges from the lateral border before passing below the inguinal ligament and giving off a branch to innervate the iliacus muscle. After passing beneath the inguinal ligament to reach the thigh, the nerve innervates the pectineus, sartorius, and quadriceps femoris muscles.

Cutaneous and Joint

Below the inguinal ligament, the femoral nerve gives rise to sensory nerves; the anterior femoral cutaneous nerve supplies the anterior portion of the thigh while the saphenous nerve descends downward. The saphenous nerve, along with the femoral vessels, pass under the sartorius muscle (in the subsartorial canal); the saphenous nerve gives off an infrapatellar branch that supplies sensory innervation to the medial aspect of the knee. The main branch of the saphenous nerve continues down the leg to supply sensory innervation to the medial side of the leg and foot.

Common Injuries

The femoral nerve is vulnerable to compression as it passes through the pelvis; damage may be caused by tumors of the vertebrae, psoas abscesses, retroperitoneal lymphadenopathies, hematomas, and fractures of the pelvis and upper femur. Direct trauma to the nerve may occur with proximal femoral fractures or during cardiac catherization. Femoral neuropathies may also be caused by vascular compromise and secondary to diabetes. The saphenous portion of the femoral nerve may be compressed as it exits the subsartorial canal (in Hunter's canal); the compression may be due to obstructive vascular disease that causes the femoral artery to press on the nerve.

Effects of Injuries

The deficits associated with damage to the femoral nerve depend on the severity of the injury to the nerve and the site of the lesion. To determine specific deficits for each type of injury, the course of the nerve must be considered and the resultant loss of motor and sensory function distal to the site determined.

GENERAL MOTOR DEFICITS. If the lesion is above the innervation of the iliacus muscle, there is weakness in hip flexion. The nerve to the quadriceps muscle is the most often injured branch of the femoral nerve. Loss of innervation of the quadriceps results in difficulty in walking because of an inability to keep the knee from buckling; walking down stairs is especially difficult with paralysis of the quadriceps muscle.

GENERAL SENSORY DEFICITS. Sensory disturbances of the anterior thigh and medial side of leg and foot occur with lesions to the

Continued on following page

sensory portions of the femoral nerve. With saphenous nerve injuries, pain is felt in the medial aspect of the knee; this pain often radiates distally to the medial side of the foot.

Special Tests

Denervation of the quadriceps muscle results in weakness often requiring the patient to use a hand to steady the thigh; there is loss of the quadriceps reflex. With painful lesions to the saphenous nerve, the pain becomes worse with exercise and especially with stair climbing.

FEMORAL NERVE (Continued)

	VALUES FOR ELECTRODIAGNOSTIC TESTING				
Stimulation Point	Recording Site	n*	Age	Onset Latency (ms)†	Conduction Velocity (m/s)†
Just below inguinal ligament	14 cm from stimulus point	42	8–79	3.7 ± 0.45	70 ± 5.5 between the two recording sites
	30 cm from stimulus point	42	8–79	6.0 ± 0.60	

*Number of subjects tested to obtain values in the table.
†Mean ± SD.
Based on Gassel, MM: A study of femoral nerve conduction time. Arch Neurol 9:607, 1963.

SAPHENOUS NERVE

VALUES FOR ELECTRODIAGNOSTIC TESTING

Method	Age (yr)	n*	Inguinal Ligament—Knee Amplitude (μV)	Inguinal Ligament—Knee Conduction Velocity (m/s)	n*	Knee—Medial Malleolus Amplitude (μV)†	Knee—Medial Malleolus Conduction Velocity (m/s)†
Orthodromic	17–38	33	4.2 ± 2.3	59.6 ± 2.3	10	4.8 ± 2.4	52.3 ± 2.3
Orthodromic	<40	28	5.5 ± 2.6	58.9 ± 3.2	22	2.1 ± 1.1	51.2 ± 4.7
	>40	41	5.1 ± 2.7	57.9 ± 4.0	32	1.7 ± 0.8	50.2 ± 5.0
Antidromic	20–79			Peak latency of 3.6 ± 1.4 for 14 cm	80	9.0 ± 3.4	41.7 ± 3.4
Orthodromic	18–56	71					54.8 ± 1.9

*Number of subjects tested to obtain values in the table.
†Mean ± SD.
From Kimura, J: Electrodiagnosis in Diseases of Nerve and Muscle: Principles and Practice, ed 2. FA Davis, Philadelphia, 1989, p 134, with permission.

SACRAL PLEXUS

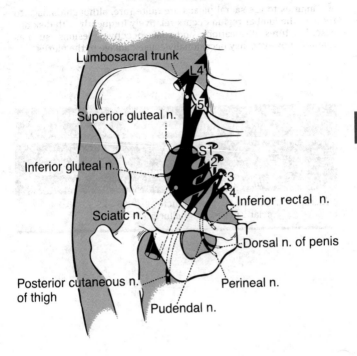

Lumbosacral trunk

L4

5

Superior gluteal n.

S1
2

Inferior gluteal n.

3
4

Inferior rectal n.

Sciatic n.

Dorsal n. of penis

Posterior cutaneous n. of thigh

Perineal n.

Pudendal n.

The sacral plexus is formed by the lumbosacral trunk, which comes from the lumbar plexus (L4), and the anterior primary rami of L5, S1, S2, and S3. Contributions may also come from S4.

Anatomy

The lumbosacral trunk from the lumbar plexus joins with fibers from the anterior primary rami of L4, L5, S1, S2, and S3 to form the sacral plexus. There may also be contributions from S4. The plexus lies in front of the sacroiliac joint.

Continued on following page

Injuries to the Sacral Plexus

Injuries to the sacral plexus are quite rare, although damage to roots of the lumbar region occurs relatively frequently with disk disease. Fractures, dislocations, and space-occupying lesions (such as tumors), however, may occasionally cause damage to the plexus.

			SACRAL PLEXUS LATENCY DETERMINATIONS FROM SPECIFIC NERVE ROOT STIMULATION	
			Latency Across Plexus (ms)	
Plexus	Site of Stimulation	Recording Site	Range	Mean ± SD
Sacral	L5 and S1 sciatic nerve	Abductor hallucis	2.5–4.9	3.9 ± 0.7

SCIATIC NERVE, TIBIAL NERVE, SURAL NERVE, AND COMMON PERONEAL NERVE

Course and Distribution

Muscles innervated by nerves are listed in italics.

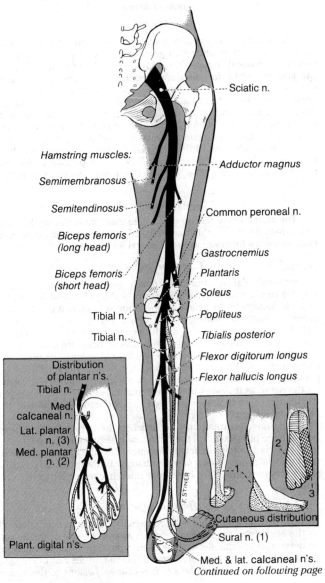

Sciatic n.

Hamstring muscles:

Adductor magnus

Semimembranosus

Semitendinosus

Common peroneal n.

Biceps femoris (long head)

Gastrocnemius

Plantaris

Biceps femoris (short head)

Soleus

Tibial n.

Popliteus

Tibial n.

Tibialis posterior

Flexor digitorum longus

Distribution of plantar n's.

Flexor hallucis longus

Tibial n.

Med. calcaneal n.

Lat. plantar n. (3)

Med. plantar n. (2)

2

1

3

Plant. digital n's.

Cutaneous distribution

Sural n. (1)

Med. & lat. calcaneal n's.

Continued on following page

F. STINER

Sciatic Nerve

Origin

The sciatic nerve is derived from fibers originating in the anterior primary rami of L4, L5, S1, S2, and S3.

Innervation

Motor

The sciatic nerve initially travels as one bundle but is actually made up of divisible units that give rise to the tibial nerve and the common peroneal nerve. The sciatic nerve leaves the pelvis via the greater sciatic foramen and courses under the gluteus maximus muscle to pass between the greater trochanter and the ischial tuberosity. In the thigh the nerve descends between the adductor magnus and the hamstring muscles. Rami from the tibial portion of the nerve innervate the long head of the biceps femoris, semitendinosus, semimembranosus, and adductor magnus muscles; in the thigh, rami of the peroneal portion innervate the short head of the biceps femoris muscle. Above the popliteal fossa the nerve divides, giving rise to the tibial and common peroneal nerves.

Cutaneous and Joint

The sciatic nerve has no direct cutaneous innervation; the tibial and peroneal nerves, which are derived from the sciatic nerve, provide cutaneous innervation to the lateral leg and foot.

Common Injuries

Intramuscular injections improperly given in the buttock region may injure the sciatic nerve. Fractures of the pelvis and femur may result in damage to the sciatic nerve. Wounds (stab and gunshot) are common causes of damage to the sciatic nerve, and it is often affected by tumors originating in the genitourinary tract or rectum. Compression of the nerve may also be due to pressure from a gravid uterus or from an abscess in the pelvic floor. A Baker's popliteal cyst may compress the lower portion of the sciatic nerve. Prolonged squatting can cause damage to the sciatic nerve owing to pressure on the nerve as it passes between ischial tuberosity and the greater trochanter or as it passes between the adductor magnus and the hamstring muscles.

Piriformis syndrome may occur when the nerve is compressed between the piriformis and the obturator internus muscles as it exits the pelvis in the greater sciatic foramen. Sustained contractions of the piriformis muscle and fibrotic changes in the piriformis muscle secondary to trauma have been implicated in causing piriformis syndrome.

Effects of Injuries

The deficits associated with damage to the sciatic nerve depend on the severity of the injury to the nerve and the site of the lesion. To determine specific deficits for each type of injury, the course of the nerve must be considered and the resultant loss of motor and sensory function distal to the site determined. Lesions to the sciatic nerve are always accompanied by loss of function of the common peroneal nerve, the tibial nerve, or both.

GENERAL MOTOR DEFICITS. With loss of the sciatic nerve, there is loss of voluntary flexion at the knee due to denervation of the hamstring muscles. Paralysis of all the muscles of the leg and foot leads to a steppage gait and an inability to run; footdrop is noticeable. With piriformis syndrome, there can be weakness of the hamstrings and all the muscles innervated by the peroneal and tibial nerve derivates.

GENERAL SENSORY DEFICITS. With lesions of the sciatic nerve, there is a loss of sensation on the lateral side of the leg and the foot; with piriformis syndrome, pain and/or diminished sensation may be felt on the posterior aspect of the leg and the plantar surface of the foot.

Special Tests

Loss of the Achilles reflex and the plantar reflex is seen with lesions of the sciatic nerve; there is an inability to stand on the toes or heels. If the nerve is damaged, placing the sciatic nerve on stretch by straight leg raising may evoke Lasègue's sign (pain along the distribution of the sciatic nerve). With sciatic nerve damage, joint position sense is lost for the foot and toes.

Tibial Nerve

Origin

The tibial nerve arises from sciatic nerve above the level of the popliteal fossa. It contains fibers from the anterior primary rami of L4, L5, S1, S2, and S3.

Innervation

Motor

The tibial nerve passes through the popliteal fossa and down the back of the leg and gives off branches that innervate both heads of the gastrocnemius, plantaris, soleus, popliteus, and the tibialis posterior muscles. The portion of nerve below the popliteal fossa was called the *posterior tibial nerve* but is now considered part of the tibial nerve. Below the popliteal fossa, the tibial nerve innervates the flexor digitorum longus and flexor hallucis longus muscles. After the tibial nerve passes the level of the heel, it divides into two terminal branches—the medial plantar nerve and the lateral plantar nerve.

The medial plantar nerve innervates the flexor digitorum brevis, abductor, hallucis, flexor hallucis brevis, and the first lumbrical muscles, and the lateral plantar nerve, which innervates the quadratus plantae, abductor digiti minimi, flexor digiti minimi brevis, opponens digit minimi, the plantar and dorsal interossei, and the second, third, and fourth lumbrical muscles.

Cutaneous and Joint

In the region of the popliteal fossa, the sural nerve, a cutaneous division of the tibial nerve, branches off and descends down the lateral leg; the sural nerve supplies innervation to the posterolateral
Continued on following page

leg and gives rise to the lateral calcaneal nerve at the level of the heel. The lateral calcaneal nerve innervates the posterolateral heel area; as the tibial nerve reaches the heel, it gives rise to the medial calcaneal nerve, which innervates the posteromedial heel area.

After the tibial nerve passes the level of the heel, it divides into two branches—the medial plantar nerve and the lateral plantar nerve. Digital branches from the medial plantar nerve innervate the medial plantar surface of the foot and the plantar surfaces of the medial three-and-a-half digits; digital branches from the lateral plantar nerve innervate the lateral portion of the plantar surface of the foot and the plantar surfaces of the lateral one-and-a-half toes.

Common Injuries

Damage to the sciatic nerve usually involves portions that form the tibial nerve. Isolated damage to the tibial nerve is usually due to an injury in or below the popliteal space; this region is particularly vulnerable to trauma. The tibial nerve is often compressed by the flexor retinaculum (the tarsal tunnel) as it passes behind and beneath the medial malleolus; this is called *tarsal tunnel syndrome* and is thought to occur as a result of trauma, tenosynovitis, or venous stasis of the posterior tibial vein.

The digital branches of the medial and lateral plantar nerves may be compressed under the metatarsal heads, giving rise to Morton's neuroma, a painful condition of the foot. Symptoms similar to those seen with Morton's neuroma are caused by other mechanical problems, such as irritation by ligaments placed on stretch due to the wearing of high-heeled shoes; hallux valgus, rheumatoid arthritis, congenital malformations, or trauma may also cause pain.

Effects of Injuries

The deficits associated with damage to the tibial nerve depend on the severity of the injury to the nerve and the site of the lesion. To determine specific deficits for each type of injury, the course of the nerve must be considered and the resultant loss of motor and sensory function distal to the site determined. With damage to the tibial nerve, there is an inability to plantar flex, adduct, and invert the foot and an inability to flex, abduct, and adduct the toes; patients are unable to stand on their toes and find walking fatiguing and even painful.

Tarsal tunnel syndrome results in pain and/or sensory loss on the plantar surface of the foot. This pain may be most severe after prolonged walking or standing; pain may be restricted to the area of the medial foot and the great toe.

Special Tests

With lesions of the tibial nerve, the Achilles reflex is lost. To test for tarsal tunnel syndrome, the examiner taps the medial malleolus just above the margin of the flexor retinaculum; paresthesias felt in the foot are indicative of tarsal tunnel syndrome.

Tibial Nerve (Continued)

		VALUES FOR ELECTRODIAGNOSTIC TESTING[a]			
Site of Stimulation	Amplitude[b] (mV)	Latency[c] to Recording Site (ms)	Difference Between Two Sides (ms)	Conduction Time Between Two Points (ms)	Conduction Velocity (m/s)
Ankle	5.8 ± 1.9 (2.9)[d]	3.96 ± 1.00 (6.0)[e]	0.66 ± 0.57 (1.8)[e]	8.09 ± 1.09 (10.3)[e]	48.5 ± 3.6 (41)[f]
Knee	5.1 ± 2.2 (2.5)	12.05 ± 1.53 (15.1)	0.79 ± 0.61 (2.0)		

[a]Mean ± standard deviation (SD) in 118 nerves from 59 patients, 11–78 years of age (average, 39), with no apparent disease of the peripheral nerves.
[b]Amplitude of the evoked response, measured from the baseline to the negative peak.
[c]Latency, measured to the onset of the evoked response, with a standard distance of 10 cm between the cathode and the recording electrode.
[d]Lower limits of normal, based on the distribution of the normative data.
[e]Upper limits of normal, calculated as the mean + 2 SD.
[f]Lower limits of normal, calculated as the mean − 2 SD.
From Kimura, J: Electrodiagnosis in Diseases of Nerve and Muscle: Principles and Practice, ed 2. FA Davis, Philadelphia, 1989, p 123, with permission.

Continued on following page

3

Tibial Nerve (Continued)

	LATENCY COMPARISON BETWEEN TWO NERVES IN THE SAME LIMB*		
Site of Stimulation	*Peroneal Nerve (ms)*	*Tibial Nerve (ms)*	*Difference (ms)*
Ankle	3.89 ± 0.87 (5.6)†	4.12 ± 1.06 (6.2)†	0.77 ± 0.65 (2.1)†
Knee	12.46 ± 1.38 (15.2)	12.13 ± 1.48 (15.1)	0.88 ± 0.71 (2.3)

From Kimura, J: Electrodiagnosis in Diseases of Nerve and Muscle: Principles and Practice, ed 2. FA Davis, Philadelphia, 1989, p 124, with permission.
*Mean ± standard deviation (SD) in 104 nerves from 52 patients, 17–86 years of age (average, 41), with no apparent disease of the peripheral nerve.
†Upper limits of normal, calculated as the mean + 2 SD.

Sural Nerve

VALUES FOR ELECTRODIAGNOSTIC TESTING

Stimulation Point	Recording Site	n*	Age (yr)	Amplitude (μV)†	Latency (ms)†	Conduction Velocity (m/s)†
Foot	High ankle	40	13–41	6.3 (1.9–17)		44.0 ± 4.7
Lower third of leg	Lateral malleolus	38	1–15	23.1 ± 4.4	1.46 ± 0.43	52.1 ± 5.1
		62	Over 15	23.7 ± 3.8	2.27 ± 0.43 (Peak)	46.2 ± 3.3
15 cm above lateral malleolus	Dorsal aspect of foot	71	15–30 40–65			51.2 ± 4.5 48.3 ± 5.3
14 cm above lateral malleolus	Lateral malleolus	101	13–66		3.50 ± 0.25 (Peak)	40.1
Lower third of leg	Lateral malleolus	80	20–79	18.9 ± 6.7	3.7 ± 0.3 (Peak)	41.0 ± 2.5
Distal 10 cm	Lateral malleolus	102				33.9 ± 3.25
Middle 10 cm		102				51.0 ± 3.8
Proximal 10 cm		102				51.6 ± 3.8
14 cm above lateral malleolus	Lateral malleolus	52	10–40 41–84	20.9 ± 8.0 17.2 ± 6.7	2.7 ± 0.3 2.8 ± 0.3 (Onset)	52.5 ± 5.6 51.1 ± 5.9

*Number of subjects tested to obtain values in the table.
†Mean ± SD.
From Kimura, J: Electrodiagnosis in Diseases of Nerve and Muscle: Principles and Practice, ed 2. FA Davis, Philadelphia, 1989, p 131, with permission.

355

Common Peroneal (Lateral Popliteal) Nerve

Origin

The common peroneal nerve arises from the sciatic nerve above the level of the popliteal fossa. It contains fibers from the anterior primary rami of L4, L5, S1, and S2.

Innervation

Motor

The common peroneal nerve arises from the sciatic nerve at the upper part of the popliteal fossa, descends along the posterior border of the biceps femoris muscle, and courses around the head of the fibula to the anterior compartment of the leg. Below the head of the fibula, it divides to form the deep peroneal nerve, which innervates the tibialis anterior, extensor digitorum longus, extensor hallucis longus, peroneus tertius, and extensor digitorum brevis muscles, and the superficial peroneal nerve, which innervates the peroneus longus and the peroneus brevis muscles.

Cutaneous and Joint

At the level of the popliteal fossa, the common peroneal nerve gives off the superior and inferior articular branches that innervate the knee joint. The lateral cutaneous nerve exits the common peroneal nerve above the head of the fibula (see figure on page 361 with superficial peroneal nerve); this branch innervates the lateral upper leg. Branches of the superficial peroneal nerve innervate the anterior portion of the leg, with the exception of the space between the great toe and the first toe, which is innervated by the deep peroneal nerve; the deep peroneal nerve also supplies the ankle joint, the inferior tibiofibular joint, and the joints of the toes.

Common Injuries

Damage to the sciatic nerve usually involves portions that form the common peroneal nerve. Because of the superficial course of the common peroneal nerve as it crosses by the head of the fibula, the nerve is more likely to be damaged than are either of its major branches. As a result of the firm attachment of the nerve to the fibular head, there is an additional predisposing factor to injury because the nerve cannot easily move when compressed.

Habitual sitting in a cross-legged position or prolonged squatting may compress the common peroneal nerve at the neck of the fibula; the nerve may also be injured at this site during sleep or anesthesia. Improper application of elastic bandages and plaster casts can damage the nerve near the fibula. Persons who are bedridden and allowed to maintain their legs in excessive external rotation are also prone to compression injuries of the common peroneal nerve.

Effects of Injuries

Complete lesions to the common peroneal nerve result in paralysis of the muscles of the anterior and lateral compartments of the leg; the subject cannot dorsiflex or evert the foot. Patients exhibit a steppage gait (e.g., to compensate for lack of dorsiflexion they use excessive hip flexion), and at heel strike the lateral border of the foot contacts the ground before the heel. Footdrop deformities commonly develop in patients who have lesions of the common peroneal nerve; sensation is lost in the lateral portion of the leg and in the dorsum of the foot with this lesion. Pain is a rare component of common peroneal injuries; when pain is present, it is quite mild.

Special Tests

Lesions to the common peroneal nerve can be differentiated from spinal root and sciatic nerve lesions because the Achilles reflex is preserved with the common peroneal nerve lesion and there is also normal inversion of the foot. Lesions of the common peroneal nerve are relatively apparent because of the pattern of motor loss and the footdrop that is not accompanied by symptoms of sciatic nerve damage.

Continued on following page

3

Peroneal Nerve (Continued)

			VALUES FOR ELECTRODIAGNOSTIC TESTING[a]			
Site of Stimulation	Amplitude[b] (mV)	Latency[c] to Recording Site (ms)	Difference Between Right and Left (ms)	Conduction Time Between Two Points (ms)	Conduction Velocity (m/s)
Ankle	5.1 ± 2.3 (2.5)[d]	3.77 ± 0.86 (5.5)[e]	0.62 ± 0.61 (1.8)[e]		
Below knee	5.1 ± 2.0 (2.5)	10.79 ± 1.06 (12.9)	0.65 ± 0.65 (2.0)	7.01 ± 0.89 (8.8)[e]	48.3 ± 3.9 (40)[f]
Above knee	5.1 ± 1.9 (2.5)	12.51 ± 1.17 (14.9)	0.65 ± 0.60 (1.9)	1.72 ± 0.40 (2.5)	52.0 ± 6.2 (40)

[a]Mean ± standard deviation (SD) in 120 nerves from 60 patients, 16–86 years of age (average, 41), with no apparent disease of the peripheral nerves.
[b]Amplitude of the evoked response, measured from the baseline to the negative peak.
[c]Latency, measured to the onset of the evoked response, with a standard distance of 7 cm between the cathode and the recording electrode.
[d]Lower limits of normal, based on the distribution of the normative data.
[e]Upper limits of normal, calculated as the mean + 2 SD.
[f]Lower limits of normal, calculated as the mean − 2 SD.
From Kimura, J: Electrodiagnosis in Diseases of Nerve and Muscle: Principles and Practice, ed 2. FA Davis, Philadelphia, 1989, p 126, with permission.

Deep Peroneal Nerve

Course and Distribution

Muscles innervated by nerves are listed in italics.

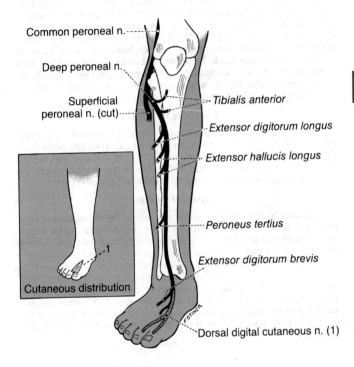

Common peroneal n.

Deep peroneal n.

Superficial peroneal n. (cut)

Tibialis anterior

Extensor digitorum longus

Extensor hallucis longus

Peroneus tertius

Extensor digitorum brevis

Cutaneous distribution

Dorsal digital cutaneous n. (1)

Origin

The deep peroneal nerve arises from the common peroneal nerve just below the head of the fibula. The fibers originated in L4, L5, and S1.

Innervation

Motor

The deep peroneal nerve arises below the neck of the fibula and then courses anteriorly down the leg along the interosseous membrane. As the nerve passes down the leg, it innervates the tibialis anterior, extensor digitorum longus, extensor hallucis longus, peroneus tertius, and extensor digitorum muscles.

Cutaneous and Joint

At the level of the foot, the deep peroneal nerve gives rise to a dorsal cutaneous branch that innervates the space between the

Continued on following page

great toe and the first toe; the deep peroneal nerve also supplies the ankle joint, the inferior tibiofibular joint, and the joints of the toes.

Common Injuries

Isolated injuries to the deep peroneal nerve are less likely than are injuries to the common peroneal nerve. With complete common peroneal nerve lesions, there is loss of innervation to all structures innervated by the deep peroneal nerve (see common peroneal nerve); lesions of the deep peroneal nerve, however, can occur in the region of the fibular neck. Increased pressure in the anterior compartment of the leg can lead to anterior compartment syndrome, where the vascular supply to muscles of the anterior leg is compromised and there is impairment of the deep peroneal nerve.

Effects of Injuries

After injury to the deep peroneal nerve, the patient cannot dorsiflex the foot. Patients exhibit a steppage gait (i.e., to compensate for lack of dorsiflexion, they use excessive hip flexion), and at heel strike the lateral border of the foot contacts the ground before the heel. Footdrop deformities commonly develop in these patients.

Special Tests

Lesions to the deep peroneal nerve can be differentiated from root and sciatic nerve lesions because the Achilles reflex is preserved with the deep peroneal nerve lesions and because there is also normal inversion of the foot. Lesions of the deep peroneal nerve are relatively apparent because of the pattern of motor loss and the footdrop that is not accompanied by symptoms of sciatic nerve damage. Lesions of the deep peroneal nerve can be differentiated from those of the common peroneal nerve because the cutaneous area supplied by the superficial peroneal nerve (the anterior leg) is not affected, but the space between the big toe and the first toe may lose sensation.

Superficial Peroneal Nerve

Course and Distribution

Muscles innervated by nerves are listed in italics.

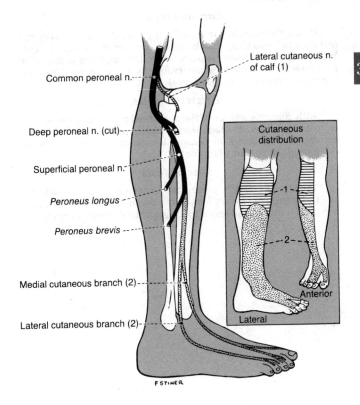

Origin

The superficial peroneal nerve is formed by the continuation of the common peroneal nerve in the lateral crural compartment after the deep peroneal nerve has branched off below the level of the fibular neck. The fibers originated in the L4, L5, and S1 roots.

Innervation

Motor

As the superficial peroneal nerve passes down the leg, it innervates the peroneus longus and the peroneus brevis muscles.

Continued on following page

Cutaneous and Joint

Above the ankle, medial and lateral cutaneous branches arise from the superficial peroneal nerve. These branches innervate the anterior portion of the leg and foot with the exception of the space between the great toe and the first toe, which is innervated by the deep peroneal nerve.

Common Injuries

Isolated injuries to the superficial peroneal nerve are very rare and are much less likely than injuries to the common peroneal nerve. With complete common peroneal nerve lesions, there is loss of innervation to all structures innervated by the superficial peroneal nerve (see common peroneal nerve).

Effects of Injuries

With complete lesions of the superficial peroneal nerve, there is an inability to evert the foot. Dorsiflexion is preserved but is always accompanied by inversion. Sensory loss is most notable on the medial part of the dorsum of the foot.

Special Tests

The loss of eversion, preservation of inversion and dorsiflexion, and the pattern of sensory loss on the dorsum of the foot are indicative of the rare isolated lesion to the superficial peroneal nerve.

Superficial Peroneal Nerve (Continued)

		VALUES FOR ELECTRODIAGNOSTIC TESTING			
Stimulation Point	Recording Site	n*	Age (y)	Amplitude (μV)†	Latency (ms)†	Conduction Velocity (m/s)†
5 cm above, 2 cm medial to lateral malleolus	Dorsum of foot	50	1–15	13.0 ± 4.6	1.22 ± 0.40 (Peak)	53.1 ± 5.3 (Distal segment)
	Medial border of lateral malleolus	50	Over 15	13.9 ± 4.0	2.24 ± 0.49 (Peak)	47.3 ± 3.4 (Distal segment)
Anterior edge of fibula, 12 cm above the active electrode		50	3–60	20.5 ± 6.1	2.9 ± 0.3 (Peak)	65.7 ± 3.7 (Proximal segment)
Anterolateral aspect of leg, 14 cm above active electrode	Medial border of lateral malleolus	80		18.3	2.8 ± 0.3 (Onset)	51.2 ± 5.7 (Proximal segment)

*Number of subjects tested to obtain values in the table.
†Mean ± SD.
From Kimura, J: Electrodiagnosis in Diseases of Nerve and Muscle: Principles and Practice, ed 2. FA Davis, Philadelphia, 1989, p 129, with permission.

3

CLASSIFICATION OF BRAIN TUMORS

Proposed Revision of 1979 World Health Organization Classification of Central Nervous System Tumors (1990)

Tumors of Neuroepithelial Tissue

- **Astrocytic:** astrocytomas, anaplastic astrocytomas, glioblastoma multiforme, pilocystic astrocytomas, pleomorphic xanthoastrocytomas, subependymal giant cell astrocytomas
- **Oligodendroglia:** oligodendrogliomas, anaplastic (malignant) oligodendrogliomas
- **Ependymal:** ependymomas, anaplastic (malignant) ependymomas, myxopapillary ependymomas, subependymomas
- **Mixed gliomas:** mixed oligoastrocytomas, anaplastic (malignant) oligoastrocytomas
- **Choroid plexus tumors:** choroid plexus papillomas, choroid plexus carcinomas
- **Neuroepithelial tumors of uncertain origin:** astroblastomas, polar spongioblastomas, gliomatosis cerebri
- **Neuronal and mixed neuronal glial tumors:** gangliocytomas, dysplastic gangliocytomas of the cerebellum, desmoplastic infantile gangliogliomas, dysembryoplastic neuroepithelial tumors, gangliogliomas, anaplastic (malignant) gangliogliomas
- **Pineal tumors:** pineocytomas, pineoblastomas
- **Embryonal tumors:** medulloepitheliomas, neuroblastomas (variant: ganglioneuroblastomas), ependymoblastomas, retinoblastomas, primitive neuroectodermal tumors (medulloblastomas, cerebral and spinal primitive neuroectodermal tumors)

Tumors of Cranial and Spinal Nerves

- **Schwannomas:** synonymous with neurilemmomas, neurinomas
- **Neurofibromas**
- **Malignant peripheral nerve sheath tumors**

Tumors of the Meninges

- Meningothelial cells:
  - meningiomas: (histologic types are meningothelial [syncytial], transitional/mixed, fibrous [fibroblastic], psammomatous, angiomatous, microcytic, secretory, clear cell, choroid, lymphoplasmacyte-rich, metaplastic variants [xanthomatous, myxoid, osseous, chondroid])
  - atypical meningiomas
  - anaplastic (malignant) meningiomas
- Mesenchymal, nonmeningothelial tumors:
  - benign: osseocartilaginous, lipomas, fibrous histiocytomas, others
  - malignant: mesenchymal chondrosarcomas, malignant fibrous histiocytomas, rhabdomyosarcomas, meningeal sarcomatosis, others

- Primary melanocytic lesions: diffuse melanosis, melanocytomas, malignant melanomas
- Tumors of uncertain origin: hemangiopericytomas, capillary hemangioblastomas

Hemopoietic Neoplasms

- Malignant lymphomas
- Plasmacytomas
- Granulocytic sarcomas
- Others

Germ Cell Tumors

- Germinomas
- Embryonal carcinomas
- Yolk sac tumors (endodermal sinus tumors)
- Choriocarcinomas
- Teratomas
- Mixed germ cell tumors

Cysts and Tumorlike Lesions

- Rathke's cleft-cysts
- Epidermoid cysts
- Dermoid cysts
- Colloid cysts of third ventricle
- Enterogenous cysts (neurenteric cysts)
- Neuroglial cysts
- Other cysts
- Lipomas
- Granular cell tumors (choriostomas, pituitcytomas)
- Hypothalamic neuronal hamartomas
- Nasal glial heterotopias

Tumors of the Anterior Pituitary

- Pituitary adenomas
- Pituitary carcinomas

Local Extensions from Regional Tumors

- Craniopharyngiomas (variants: adamantinomatous, squamous papillary)
- Paragangliomas (chemodectoma)
- Chordomas
- Chondrosarcomas
- Adenoid cystic carcinomas (cylindroma)
- Others

Continued on following page

Metastatic Tumors

Subcategorizations of metastatic tumors have not been attempted, primarily because of the large variety of tumors that can metastasize from the CNS. Most of these originate from breast and lung tissue, with many also originating from cutaneous malignant melanomas.

BASED ON

Gonzales, MF: Classification and pathogenesis of brain tumors. In Kaye, AH and Laws, ER (eds): Brain Tumors: An Encyclopedia Approach. Churchill Livingstone, New York, 1995, pp 31–45.

FACTS ABOUT TUMORS OF THE CENTRAL NERVOUS SYSTEM

- Approximately 15% of patients with CNS tumors have a family history of cancer.
- Anaplastic astrocytoma and glioblastoma multiforme are the most common brain tumors in adults.
- Brain tumors are the fourth most frequent cause of cancer-related deaths in middle-aged men and the second most common cause of cancer deaths in children.
- A relationship between oncogenes and CNS tumor type is emerging.

   Chemical and industrial agents associated with CNS tumors are aromatic hydrocarbons, hydrazines, bis(chloromethyl)ether, vinyl chloride, and acrylonitrile.

- Viruses associated with brain tumors are:

   Progressive multifocal leukoencephalopathy, leading to astrocytomas, Epstein-Barr virus, leading to primary CNS lymphoma.

Other factors associated with CNS tumors include hormones (meningiomas, particularly during pregnancy), alcohol, tobacco, radiation, and trauma.

FOR MORE INFORMATION

Fields, WS: Brain tumors: Morphological aspects and classification. Brain Pathol 3:251, 1993.

Kleihues, P: The new classification of brain tumors. Brain Pathol 3:225, 1993.

Salcman, M: Glioblastoma and malignant astrocytoma. In Kaye, AH and Laws, ER (eds): Brain Tumors: An Encyclopedic Approach. Churchill Livingstone, New York, 1995, pp 449–477.

REFLEX TESTING

MUSCLE STRETCH (DEEP TENDON) REFLEXES (listed in cephalad to caudal order)

Reflex	Stimulus	Response	Segmental Level and Nerve
Jaw (maxillary)	Tap mandible in half-open position.	Closure of jaw	Pons (trigeminal nerve)
Biceps	Tap biceps tendon.	Contraction of biceps	C5 and C6 (musculocutaneous nerve)
Brachioradialis (periosteoradial)	Tap styloid process of radius (insertion of brachioradialis).	Flexion of elbow and pronation of forearm	C5 and C6 (musculocutaneous nerve)
Triceps	Tap triceps tendon.	Extension of elbow	C6–C8 (radial nerve)
Wrist extension	Tap wrist extensor tendons.	Extension of wrist	C7 and C8 (radial nerve)
Wrist flexion	Tap wrist flexor tendons.	Flexion of wrist	C6–C8 (median nerve)
Patellar	Tap patellar tendon.	Extension of leg at knee	L2–L4 (femoral nerve)
Tendocalcaneus	Tap Achilles tendon.	Plantar flexion at ankle	S1 and S2 (tibial nerve)

3

Grading of Muscle Stretch (Deep Tendon) Reflexes

0	Areflexia
+	Hyporeflexia
1 to 3	Average
3+ to 4+	Hyperreflexia

MODIFIED ASHWORTH SCALE FOR GRADING SPASTICITY	
Grade	**Description**
0	No increase in muscle tone
1	Slight increase in muscle tone, manifested by a catch and release or by minimal resistance at the end of the ROM when the affected part(s) is moved in flexion or extension
1+	Slight increase in muscle tone, manifested by a catch, followed by minimal resistance throughout the remainder (less than half) of the ROM
2	More marked increase in muscle tone through most of the ROM, but affected part(s) easily moved
3	Considerable increase in muscle tone, passive movement difficult
4	Affected part(s) rigid in flexion or extension

ROM = range of motion.
Based on Ashworth, B: Preliminary trial of carisoprodol in multiple sclerosis. Practitioner 192:540, 1964.

DRUGS TO REDUCE UNWANTED MUSCLE ACTIVITY

Drug	Oral Dosage	Comments
Baclofen) (Lioresal)	*Adult:* 5 mg tid initially; increase by 15 mg/d at 3-d intervals as required; maximum recommended dosage is 80 mg/d	More effective in treating spasticity resulting from spinal cord lesions (versus cerebral lesions)
Dantrolene sodium (Dantrium)	*Adult:* 25 mg/d initially; increase up to 100 mg 2, 3, 4 times per day as needed; maximum recommended dose is 400 mg/d	Exerts an effect directly on the muscle cell; may cause generalized weakness in all skeletal musculature
	Children (older than 5 y of age): initially, 0.5 mg/kg body weight bid; increase total daily dosage by 0.5 mg/kg every 4–7 d as needed, and give total daily amount in 4 divided doses; maximum recommended dose in 400 mg/d	
Diazepam (Valium)	*Adult:* 2–10 mg tid or qid qid *Children* (older than 6 mo of age): 1.0–2.5 mg tid or qid (in both adults and children, begin at lower end of dosage range and increase gradually as tolerated and/or needed)	Produces sedation at dosages that decrease spasticity

From Ciccone, CD: Pharmacology in Rehabilitation, ed 2. FA Davis, Philadelphia, 1996, p 164, with permission.

3

SKELETAL MUSCLE RELAXANTS

Generic Name	Trade Name	Clinical Use	
		Reduction of Reflex Response	Muscle Spasms
Centrally Acting Relaxants			
Baclofen	Lioresal	X	
Carisoprodol	Soma, Rela, others		X
Chlorphenesin carbamate	Maolate		X
Chlorzoxazone	Parafon Forte, Paraflex		X
Cyclobenzaprine HCl	Flexeril		X
Diazepam	Valium	X	X
Metaxalone	Skelaxin		X
Methocarbamol	Robaxin, Robomol, others		X
Orphenadrine	Norflex, Norgesic, others		X
Direct-Acting Relaxants			
Dantrolene sodium	Dantrium	X	

X indicates clinical use.
From Ciccone, CD: Pharmacology in Rehabilitation, ed 2. FA Davis, Philadelphia, 1996, p 163, with permission.

DRUGS USED TO TREAT SKELETAL MUSCLE SPASMS

Drug	Usual Adult Oral Dosage (mg)	Onset of Action (min)	Duration of Action (h)
Carisoprodol (Soma, Rela)	350 tid and bedtime	30	4–6
Chlorphenesin carbamate (Maolate)	400 qid	—	—
Chlorzoxazone (Paraflex)	250–750 tid or qid	Within 60	3–4
Cyclobenzaprine HCl (Flexeril)	10 tid	60	12–24
Diazepam (Valium)	2–10 tid or qid	15–45	Variable
Metaxalone (Skelaxin)	800 tid or qid	60	4–6
Methocarbamol (Robaxin, Robomol)	1000 qid	Within 30	24
Orphenadrine (Norflex, Norgesic)	100 bid	Within 60	8

From Ciccone, CD: Pharmacology in Rehabilitation, ed 2. FA Davis, Philadelphia, 1996, p 170, with permission.

REFLEX TESTING (Continued)

MAJOR SUPERFICIAL REFLEXES (listed in cephalad to caudal order)			
Reflex	Stimulus	Response	Segmental Level
Corneal (conjunctival)	Touching cornea with hair or cotton wisp	Contraction of orbicularis oculi (closing the eye)	Pons (afferent: trigeminal nerve; efferent: facial nerve)
Nasal (sneeze)	Lightly touching nasal mucosa with cotton wisp	Sneezing	Pons and medulla (afferent: trigeminal nerve; efferent: trigeminal nerve, facial, glossopharyngeal, and vagus nerves)
Pharyngeal (gag)	Touching posterior wall of pharynx	Contraction of pharynx	Medulla (afferent: glossopharyngeal nerve; efferent: vagus nerve)
Palatal (uvular)	Touching soft palate	Elevation of palate	Medulla (afferent: glossopharyngeal nerve; efferent: vagus nerve)
Scapular (interscapular)	Stroking skin between scapulae	Contraction of scapular muscles	C5–T1
Epigastric	Stroking downward from the nipples	Dimpling of epigastrium ipsilaterally	T7–T9

Abdominal	Stroking beneath costal margins and above the inguinal ligament	Contraction of the abdominal muscles in the stimulated quadrant	T8–T12 (depending on the quadrant stimulated)
Cremasteric	Stroking medial surface of upper thigh	Ipsilateral elevation of testicle	L1 and L2 (afferent: femoral nerve; efferent: genitofemoral nerve)
Gluteal	Stroking skin of buttock	Contraction of glutei	L4 and L5 (superior gluteal nerve)
Bulbocavernosus	Pinching dorsum of glans of the penis	Contraction of the bulbous urethra	S3 and S4 (afferent: pudendal nerve; efferent: pelvic autonomic nerve)
Superficial anal	Pricking perineum	Contraction of rectal sphincters	S5 and coccygeal (pudendal nerves)
Plantar	Stroking sole of foot	Plantar flexion of toes (children may also retract foot)	S1 and S2 (tibial nerve)

FOR MORE INFORMATION

Alpers, BJ and Mancall, EL: Alpers and Mancall's Essentials of the Neurologic Examination, ed 2. FA Davis, Philadelphia, 1981.
Waxman, SG and deGroot, J: Correlative Neuroanatomy, ed 22. Appleton & Lange, Norwalk, CT, 1995.

3

REFLEX TESTING (Continued)

MAJOR VISCERAL REFLEXES (listed in cephalad to caudal order)

Reflex	Stimulus	Response	Segmental Level
Light reflex	Examiner projects light on the retina.	Constriction of pupil	Mesencephalon
Consensual light	Examiner projects light into the eye opposite the one being evaluated.	Constriction of the pupil in the eye not receiving the light	Commissural pathways in the pretectal area, as well as the same pathways used in the light reflex
Accommodation	Examiner asks the patient to look at a nearby object.	Convergence of eyes with constriction of the pupils	Occipital cortex (if light reflexes exist) and mesencephalon (afferent: optic nerve; efferent: oculomotor nerve)
Ciliospinal reflex	Examiner applies a painful stimulus to patient's neck (pinching).	Dilation of pupil	T1 and T2 for sympathetic portion (efferent) and whatever area is used for sensory

Blink reflex (of Descartes)	Unexpected movement of object near and toward eyes.	Closure of the eyes	Mesencephalon and occipital cortex (afferent: optic nerve; efferent: facial nerve)
Oculocardiac	Examiner applies pressure on eye.	Slowing of heart rate	Medulla (afferent: trigeminal nerve; efferent: vagus nerve)
Carotid sinus reflex	Examiner applies pressure over carotid sinus.	Slowing of heart rate and fall in blood pressure	Medulla (afferent: glossopharyngeal nerve; efferent: vagus nerve)

Based on Waxman, SG and deGroot, J: Correlative Neuroanatomy, ed 22. Appleton & Lange, Norwalk, CT, 1996.

MAJOR PATHOLOGIC REFLEXES

Reflexes That Indicate Pathology Affecting Corticospinal Systems

These reflexes can often be seen in healthy infants who are younger than 7 months of age.

MAJOR PATHOLOGIC REFLEXES: UPPER EXTREMITY (in alphabetical order)		
Reflex	**Stimulus**	**Response**
Bechterew's sign	Patient alternately flexes and relaxes the forearm.	If the sign is positive, the arm falls back into the extended position in a slow, jerky fashion.
Chaddock wrist sign	Examiner strokes the ulnar side of forearm (pressure on tendon of palmaris longus muscle).	Flexion of wrist with extension and possible fanning of fingers.
Clonus	Examiner rapidly extends the wrist.	Rapid reciprocal flexion and extension.
Extension-adduction (Dagnini reflex)	Examiner percusses the dorsum of hand on radial side.	Slight adduction and extension of wrist.
Finger flexion (Trömner's reflex)	Examiner taps the palmar surface or tips of the middle three fingers.	Flexion of the fingers.

Forced grasping	Examiner strokes the patient's palm in a radial direction.	Grasp reaction.
Gordon's sign	Examiner compresses the region of pisiform bone.	Extension of flexed fingers.
Hoffmann's sign	Examiner snaps the nail of the middle finger.	Flexion of fingers and thumb.
Kleist hooking sign	Examiner applies pressure against the surface of the finger tips.	Flexion of fingers.

Continued on following page

MAJOR PATHOLOGIC REFLEXES: UPPER EXTREMITY (in alphabetical order) (Continued)

Reflex	Stimulus	Response
Klippel and Weil thumb sign	Patient's flexed fingers are rapidly extended by the examiner.	Flexion and adduction of the thumb.
Leri's sign	Examiner forcefully flexes the wrist and fingers.	Absence of elbow flexion.
Mayer's sign	Examiner forcefully flexes the proximal phalanges of the supinated hand.	Absence of adduction and opposition of the thumb.
Mendel-Bechterew reflex of the hand	Examiner percusses the dorsal aspect of the carpals and metacarpals on the radial side.	Flexion of the fingers.
Palm-chin reflex (Marinesco-Radiovici)	Examiner stimulates the thenar eminence.	Contraction of muscles of chin and elevation of the corner of the mouth.
Rossolimo's sign of the hand	Examiner percusses the palmar aspect of the MCP joint.	Flexion of the fingers.
Souque's sign	Patient attempts to raise paretic arm.	Fingers adduct and extend.
Sterling's sign	Patient resists adduction of nonparetic arm.	Adduction of paretic arm.
Strümpell's pronation sign	Patient flexes the forearm.	The hand touches the shoulder (normally the palm should touch the shoulder).
Thumb-adductor reflex (Babinski of the hand or Marie-Foix of the hand)	Examiner strokes the hypothenar region.	Adduction and flexion of thumb, sometimes flexion of adjacent fingers with extension of the little finger.

MAJOR PATHOLOGIC REFLEXES: LOWER EXTREMITY (in alphabetical order)

Reflex	Stimulus	Response
Babinski's sign	Examiner strokes the outer edge of sole of foot.	Extension of the great toe, flexion of small toes, and spreading of small toes.
Bechterew-Mendel reflex	Examiner taps on the lateral surface of the dorsum of the foot.	Flexion of the toes.
Chaddock toe sign	Examiner strokes the lateral aspect of the dorsum of the foot and lateral malleolus.	Response similar to that seen with Babinski's sign (extension of great toe, flexion of small toes, and spreading of small toes).
Clonus	Examiner rapidly dorsiflexes the ankle.	Continued and prolonged reciprocal plantar flexion and dorsiflexion of the ankle.
Crossed extension	With the subject supine and both legs flexed at the hip, examiner stimulates the sole of the foot.	Extension of the contralateral extremity.
Extensor thrust	Examiner vigorously dorsiflexes the foot of a leg that has been flexed at the hip.	Extension of that entire lower extremity.
Gonda's sign	Examiner strongly flexes a toe and then rapidly releases it into extension (with a snap).	Extension of the big toe.

Continued on following page

3

379

	MAJOR PATHOLOGIC REFLEXES: LOWER EXTREMITY (in alphabetical order) (Continued)	
Reflex	**Stimulus**	**Response**
Gordon's leg sign	Examiner squeezes the calf.	Response similar to that seen with Babinski's sign (extension of great toe, flexion of small toes, and spreading of small toes).
Grasset-Gaussel phenomenon	Supine patient is asked to raise each leg and then both legs; if the paretic leg is raised, the examiner then passively raises the nonparetic leg.	A positive sign is when both legs cannot be raised together and the paretic limb falls back down if it is raised when the examiner lifts the nonparetic limb.
Hirschberg's sign	Examiner strokes the medial border of foot.	Adduction and internal rotation (inversion) of foot.
Hoover's sign	Examiner places palms under the heels of the supine patient and the patient is asked to press downward; the patient is then also asked to lift the nonparetic limb while the examiner resists the movement.	If there is true hemiplegia (nonhysterical), there will be no pressure felt under the heel of the paretic limb when the patient is asked to press down and no increased pressure when the patient is asked to move the nonparetic limb.
Huntington's sign	Patient coughs or strains.	The paretic limb will flex at the hip and there will be extension at the knee.
Marie-Foix	Examiner forcefully flexes the patient's toes.	There is flexion at the hip and knee.
Néri's sign	Supine patient attempts alternate straight leg raising.	Flexion at the knee on the paretic limb.

Oppenheim's reflex	Examiner strokes downward on the medial aspect of leg.	Response similar to that seen with Babinski's sign (extension of great toe, flexion of small toes, and spreading of small toes).
Patellar clonus (trepidation sign)	With the leg fully extended and relaxed, a downward movement of the patella is caused by the examiner.	Rapid up-and-down movements of the patella.
Ramiste's sign	Supine patient attempts either hip adduction or abduction of the nonparetic limb.	The paretic limb moves in the same way as the nonparetic limb (the effect is more dramatic if resistance is added to the nonparetic limb).
Rossolimo's sign	Examiner taps on balls of the patient's foot.	Flexion of toes.
Schäffer's reflex	Examiner squeezes the patient's Achilles tendon.	Response similar to that seen with Babinski's sign (extension of great toe, flexion of small toes, and spreading of small toes).
Stransky's sign	Patient abducts the small toe.	Extension of the great toe.
Strümpell's tibialis anterior sign	Patient flexes the hip.	Dorsiflexion and adduction of the foot (the effect is more dramatic if resistance is added to the hip flexion).

3

ADDITIONAL PATHOLOGICAL REFLEXES (in alphabetical order)

Name	Stimulus	Response
Babinski's platysma sign	Examiner resists neck flexion or mouth opening.	Normally the platysma on the nonparetic side contracts while the platysma on the paretic side does not contract.
Glabella (McCarthy's reflex)	Examiner taps the glabella.	The orbicularis oculi contract.
Snout reflex	Examiner taps middle of upper lip.	The upper lips move.

FOR MORE INFORMATION

Alpers, BJ and Mancall, EL: Alpers and Mancall's Essentials of the Neurologic Examination, ed 2. FA Davis, Philadelphia, 1981.

Waxman, SG and deGroot, J: Correlative Neuroanatomy, ed 22. Appleton & Lange, Norwalk, CT, 1995.

ELECTRODIAGNOSIS

Electrodes

The two types of electrodes used for clinical EMG are *surface* (or skin) electrodes and *percutaneous* (or indwelling) electrodes. The segment of the electrode that makes direct electrical contact with the tissue is referred to as the *detection surface*. Detection surfaces are used either singularly (*monopolar*) or in pairs (*bipolar*).

Surface Electrodes

Surface electrodes are applied to the overlying skin and can be used to record the global activity of evoked muscle and nerve action potentials and to stimulate peripheral nerves in nerve conduction tests. Recording electrodes can either be *passive,* wherein the detection surface senses the current on the skin through its skin-electrode interface, or *active,* wherein the input impedance of the electrode is greatly increased, rendering it less sensitive to the impedance of the electrode-skin interface. The chief advantage of surface electrodes is convenience, whereas the disadvantages are that they can only be used effectively with superficial muscles and that they cannot be easily used to detect signals selectively from small muscles.

Percutaneous Electrodes

For clinical purposes, the most commonly used percutaneous electrodes are needle electrodes, which are used to record from a single motor unit or just a few motor units. A wide variety of needle electrodes are available; however, the most common is the concentric electrode. The monopolar configuration of the concentric electrode contains one insulated wire in the cannula with the tip of the wire bared to act as a detection surface. The bipolar configuration of the concentric electrode contains a second wire in the cannula that provides a second detection surface. The main advantages of the needle electrode are its small pickup area (high selectivity) and the convenience with which new muscle territories can be explored by repositioning the needle.

Needle Electrode Configurations

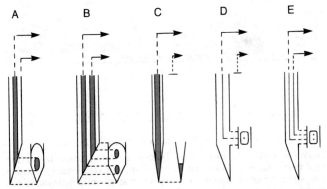

Schematic illustration of standard or coaxial bipolar (A), concentric bipolar (B), monopolar (C), and single fiber needles (D and E). Dimensions vary, but the diameters of the outside cannulas shown resemble 26-gauge hypodermic needles (460 μm) for A, D, and E, a 23-gauge needle (640 μm) for B, and a 28-gauge needle (360 μm) for C. The exposed-tip areas measure 150 by 300 μm, with spacing between wires of 200 μm center to center for B, 0.14 sq mm for C, and 25 μm in diameter for D and E. A flat-skin electrode completes the circuit with unipolar electrodes shown in C and D.

Clinical Electromyography: Typical Electromyographic Pattern

The figure shows the typical patterns of EMG activity of various diseases and lesions. *Insertional activity* is the electrical activity recorded when the needle is inserted or moved within the muscle. *Spontaneous activity* is the electrical activity recorded after the cessation of insertional activity in resting muscle. The *motor unit potential* is the compound electrical wave formed by the depolarization of

Continued on following page

the muscle fibers belonging to a motor unit. The size and shape of the potential are of diagnostic significance. The *interference pattern* is the electrical activity recorded from a muscle during maximal voluntary effort.

LESION EMG steps	NORMAL	NEUROGENIC LESION		MYOGENIC LESION		
		Motoneuron	CNS	Myopathy	Myotonia	Polymyositis
1 Insertional activity	Normal	Increased	Normal	Normal	Myotonic discharge	Increased
2 Spontaneous activity	—	Fibrillation / Positive wave	—	—	—	Fibrillation / Positive wave
3 Motor unit potential	0.5–1.0 mV / 5–10 ms	Large unit / Limited recruitment	Normal	Small unit / Early recruitment	Myotonic discharge	Small unit / Early recruitment
4 Interference pattern	Full	Reduced / Fast firing rate	Reduced / Slow firing rate	Full amplitude / Low	Full amplitude / Low	Full amplitude / Low

CLINICAL ELECTRICAL EVALUATION TESTS

Chronaxie Test: See *Strength-Duration Curve and Chronaxie Test.*

Galvanic Twitch-Tetanus Ratio Test: A test to characterize peripheral nerve degeneration that is based on the relationship between the intensity of DC required to obtain a single minimal-twitch contraction (rheobase or threshold current) and the intensity of DC required to elicit a sustained (tetanic) contraction. In the normally innervated muscle, the ratio of these two current intensities is usually 1:3.5–6.5. In a denervated muscle, the ratio approaches unity.

Nerve Excitability Test: A test of the responsiveness of a peripheral nerve to electrical stimulation. The test is typically performed serially to monitor changes in excitability and is based on the observation that the amplitude of a stimulus required to elicit a minimal response increases as the process of nerve degeneration progresses. The advantage of this test is that if performed early enough it can provide information on nerve status before total degeneration occurs. The test stimulus typically employs square-wave monophasic pulses (very short rise time) of 0.3- or 1.0-ms duration and an interpulse interval of 1 s.

Reaction of Degeneration Test: A gross screening procedure for assessment of problems that may involve lower (peripheral) motor neurons. A reaction to degeneration occurs when a muscle contracts in response to DC but not in response to AC. A response to DC stimulation in the absence of a response to AC stimulation indicates that the muscle is denervated, because muscle tissue is less excitable than nerve tissue. DC stimulation provides a more prolonged duration of current flow than AC stimulation and is therefore able to produce a contraction that is characteristically slow and wormlike.

rheobase: See *Strength-Duration Curve and Chronaxie Test.*

Strength-Duration (S-D) Curve and Chronaxie Test: A once widely used test that has sharply declined in use since the development of nerve conduction testing and electromyography. The test is intended for electrodiagnosis of peripheral nervous system disorders, particularly peripheral nerve injuries. The two parameters of stimulation that determine tissue excitability, the stimulus intensity and stimulus pulse duration, are plotted against each other to depict the combination of these two parameters needed to produce just measurable evoked neural responses in a nerve. A third factor, the manner in which the stimulus is applied, is implicit to all strength-duration curves and is typically evoked by rectangular pulses or sine waves. Chronaxie and rheobase are determined from the S-D curve. *Rheobase* (described in units of current, i.e., milliamps) refers to the minimal intensity of stimulus amplitude required to elicit a minimally perceptible muscle contraction for a stimulus of infinite pulse duration (by convention, infinite pulse duration is specified as 300 ms). *Chronaxie* (described in units of time, i.e., milliseconds) is the minimum pulse duration needed to stimulate a muscle at twice the current intensity of the rheobase current. The chronaxie for nerve is short, usually less than 1 ms, whereas the chronaxie for muscle is much larger, usually greater than 10 ms.

CLINICAL ELECTRICAL EVALUATION TESTS (Continued)

| | ELECTRICAL TEST FOR REACTION OF DEGENERATION | |
| | I | II |
Status of Muscle Innervation	*Muscle Response Elicited with a Series of Short-Duration Pulses (<1 ms) Applied Continuously at Frequency ≥ 20–50 Hz (Usually Biphasic or AC Pulses)*	*Muscle Response Elicited with Individual 100-ms Pulses (Usually Monophasic or Interrupted DC Pulses)*
Normal peripheral nerve innervation	Smooth, continuous isotonic (tetanic) contraction	Brisk, individual twitch contraction
Partial RD: degeneration of part of nerve fibers	Partial or diminished tetanic contraction	Partial or diminished, sluggish individual contraction
Complete RD: degeneration of all nerve fibers; muscle tissue retains contractile elements	No contraction	Very slow, sluggish individual contraction
Absolute RD: degeneration of all nerve fibers; muscle tissue severely atrophic, fibrotic, or noncontractile	No contraction	No contraction

RD = reaction of degeneration.
From Gersh, MR: Electrotherapy in Rehabilitation. FA Davis, Philadelphia, 1992, p 103, with permission.

AAEE GLOSSARY OF TERMS IN CLINICAL ELECTROMYOGRAPHY*

A wave: A compound action potential evoked consistently from a muscle by submaximal electric stimuli to the nerve and frequently abolished by supramaximal stimuli. The amplitude of the A wave is similar to that of the F wave, but the latency is more constant. The A wave usually occurs before the F wave, but may occur afterwards. The A wave is due to normal or pathologic axonal branching.

absolute refractory period: See *refractory period.*

accommodation: True accommodation in neuronal physiology is a rise in the threshold transmembrane depolarization required to initiate a spike when depolarization is slow or a subthreshold depolarization is maintained. In the older literature, accommodation described the observation that the final intensity of current applied in a slowly rising fashion to stimulate a nerve was greater than the intensity of a pulse of current required to stimulate the same nerve. The latter may largely be an artifact of the nerve sheath and bears little relation to true accommodation as measured intracellularly.

accommodation curve: See *strength-duration curve.*

action current: The electric currents associated with an *action potential.*

action potential (AP): The brief regenerative electric potential that propagates along a single axon or muscle fiber membrane. The action potential is an all-or-none phenomenon; whenever the stimulus is at or above threshold, the action potential generated has a constant size and configuration. See also *compound action potential, motor unit action potential.*

active electrode: Synonymous with *exploring electrode.* Also refers to a surface EMG electrode with high input impedance. See *recording electrode.*

adaptation: A decline in the frequency of the spike discharge as typically recorded from sensory axons in response to a maintained stimulus.

AEPs: See *auditory evoked potentials.*

afterdischarge: The continuation of an impulse train in a neuron, axon, or muscle fiber following the termination of an applied stimulus. The number of extra impulses and their periodicity in the train may vary depending on the circumstances.

afterpotential: The membrane potential between the end of the spike and the time when the membrane potential is restored to its

Continued on following page

---

* Reprinted with permission from AAEM. Compiled by the Nomenclature Committee of the American Association of Electrodiagnostic Medicine (formerly American Association of Electromyography and Electrodiagnosis): AAEE's Glossary of Terms in Clinical Electromyography. Muscle & Nerve 10:G1–G20, 1987. Approval for inclusion of the glossary in this book in no way implies review or endorsement by the AAEM of material contained in this book.

resting value. The membrane during this period may be depolarized or hyperpolarized.

amplitude: With reference to an *action potential*, the maximum voltage difference between two points, usually baseline to peak or peak to peak. By convention, the amplitude of the *compound muscle action potential* is measured from the baseline to the most negative peak. In contrast, the amplitude of a *compound sensory nerve action potential, motor unit potential, fibrillation potential, positive sharp wave, fasciculation potential,* and most other *action potentials* is measured from the most positive peak to the most negative peak.

anodal block: A local block of nerve conduction caused by *hyperpolarization* of the nerve cell membrane by an electric stimulus. See *stimulating electrode.*

anode: The positive terminal of a source of electric current.

antidromic: Propagation of an impulse in the direction opposite to physiologic conduction; e.g., conduction along motor nerve fibers away from the muscle and conduction along sensory fibers away from the spinal cord. Contrast with *orthodromic.*

AP: See *action potential.*

artifact (also artefact): A voltage change generated by a biologic or nonbiologic source other than the ones of interest. The *stimulus artifact* is the potential recorded at the time the stimulus is applied and includes the *electric* or *shock artifact*, which represents cutaneous spread of stimulating current to the recording electrode. The stimulus and shock artifacts usually precede the activity of interest. A *movement artifact* refers to a change in the recorded activity caused by movement of the recording electrodes.

auditory evoked potentials (AEPs): Electric waveforms of biologic origin elicited in response to sound stimuli. AEPs are classified by their latency as short-latency brainstem AEPs (BAEPs) with a latency of up to 10 ms, middle-latency AEPs with a latency of 10–50 ms, and long-latency AEPs with a latency of over 50 ms. See *brainstem auditory evoked potentials.*

axon reflex: Use of term discouraged as it is incorrect. No reflex is considered to be involved. See preferred term, *A wave.*

axon response: See preferred term, *A wave.*

axon wave: See *A wave.*

axonotmesis: Nerve injury characterized by distribution of the axon and myelin sheath, but with preservation of the supporting connective tissue, resulting in axonal degeneration distal to the injury site.

backfiring: Discharge of an antidromically activated motor neuron.

BAEPs: See *brainstem auditory evoked potentials.*

BAERs: Abbreviation for *brainstem auditory evoked responses.* See preferred term, *brainstem auditory evoked potentials.*

baseline: The potential recorded from a biologic system while the system is at rest.

benign fasciculation: Use of term discouraged to describe a firing pattern of fasciculation potentials. The term has been used to describe a clinical syndrome and/or the presence of fasciculations in nonprogressive neuromuscular disorders. See *fasciculation potential.*

BERs: Abbreviation for *brainstem auditory evoked responses.* See preferred term, *brainstem auditory evoked potentials.*

bifilar needle recording electrode: *Recording electrode* that measures variations in voltage between the bare tips of two insulated wires cemented side by side in a steel cannula. The bare tips of the electrodes are flush with the level of the cannula. The latter may be grounded.

biphasic action potential: An *action potential* with two phases.

biphasic end-plate activity: See *end-plate activity (biphasic).*

bipolar needle recording electrode: See preferred term, *bifilar needle recording electrode.*

bipolar stimulating electrode: See *stimulating electrode.*

bizarre high-frequency discharge: See preferred term, *complex repetitive discharge.*

bizarre repetitive discharge: See preferred term, *complex repetitive discharge.*

bizarre repetitive potential: See preferred term, *complex repetitive discharge.*

blink reflex: See *blink responses.*

blink response: Strictly defined, one of the *blink responses.* See *blink responses.*

blink responses: *Compound muscle action potentials* evoked from orbicularis oculi muscles as a result of brief electric or mechanical stimuli to the cutaneous area innervated by the supraorbital (or less commonly, the infraorbital) branch of the trigeminal nerve. Typically, there is an early compound muscle action potential (*R1 wave*) ipsilateral to the stimulation site with a latency of about 10 ms and a bilateral late compound muscle action potential (*R2 wave*) with a latency of approximately 30 ms. Generally, only the *R2 wave* is associated with a visible twitch of the orbicularis oculi. The configuration, amplitude, duration, and latency of the two components, along with the sites of recording and the sites of stimulation, should be specified. *R1* and *R2 waves* are probably oligosynaptic and polysynaptic brainstem reflexes, respectively, together called the *blink reflex*, with the afferent arc provided by the sensory branches of the trigeminal nerve and the efferent are provided by the facial nerve motor fibers.

brainstem auditory evoked potentials (BAEPs): Electric waveforms of biologic origin elicited in response to sound stimuli. The normal BAEP consists of a sequence of up to seven waves, named I to VII, which occur during the first 10 ms after the onset of the stimulus and have positive polarity at the vertex of the head.

brainstem auditory evoked responses (BAERs, BERs): See preferred term, *brainstem auditory evoked potentials.*

BSAPs: Abbreviation for brief, small, abundant potentials. Use of term is discouraged. It is used to describe a recruitment pattern of brief-duration, small-amplitude, overly abundant motor unit action

Continued on following page

3

potentials. Quantitative measurements of motor unit potential duration, amplitude, numbers of phases, and recruitment frequency are to be preferred to qualitative descriptions such as this. See *motor unit action potential.*

BSAPPs: Abbreviation for brief, small abundant, polyphasic potentials. Use of term is discouraged. It is used to describe a recruitment pattern of brief-duration, small-amplitude, overly abundant, polyphasic motor unit action potentials. Quantitative measurements of motor unit potential duration, amplitude, numbers of phases, and recruitment frequency are to be preferred to qualitative descriptions such as this. See *motor unit action potential.*

cathode: The negative terminal of a source of electric current.

central electromyography (central EMG): Use of electromyographic recording techniques to study reflexes and the control of movement by the spinal cord and brain.

chronaxie (also chronaxy): See *strength-duration curve.*

clinical electromyography: Synonymous with *electroneuromyography.* Used to refer to all electrodiagnostic studies of human peripheral nerves and muscle. See also *electromyography* and *nerve conduction studies.*

coaxial needle electrode: See synonym, *concentric needle electrode.*

collision: When used with reference to nerve conduction studies, the interaction of two action potentials propagated toward each other from opposite directions on the same nerve fiber so that the refractory periods of the two potentials prevent propagation past each other.

complex action potential: See preferred term, *serrated action potential.*

complex motor unit action potential: A *motor unit action potential* that is polyphasic or serrated. See preferred terms, *polyphasic action potential or serrated action potential.*

complex repetitive discharge: Polyphasic or serrated action potentials that may begin spontaneously or after a needle movement. They have a uniform frequency, shape, and amplitude, with abrupt onset, cessation, or change in configuration. Amplitude ranges from 100 μV to 1 mV and frequency of discharge from 5 to 100 Hz. This term is preferred to *bizarre high-frequency discharge, bizarre repetitive discharge, bizarre repetitive potential, near constant frequency trains, pseudomyotonic discharge,* and *synchronized fibrillation.*

compound action potential: See *compound mixed nerve action potential, compound motor nerve action potential, compound nerve action potential, compound sensory nerve action potential,* and *compound muscle action potential.*

compound mixed nerve action potential (compound mixed NAP): A compound nerve action potential is considered to have been evoked from afferent and efferent fibers if the recording electrodes detect activity on a mixed nerve with the electric stimulus applied to a segment of the nerve that contains both afferent and efferent fibers. The amplitude, latency, duration, and phases should be noted.

compound motor nerve action potential (compound motor NAP): A compound nerve action potential is considered to have been evoked from efferent fibers to a muscle if the recording electrodes detect activity only in a motor nerve or a motor branch of a mixed nerve, or if the electric stimulus is applied only to such a nerve or a ventral root. The amplitude, latency, duration, and phases should be noted. See *compound nerve action potential.*

compound muscle action potential (CMAP): The summation of nearly synchronous muscle fiber action potentials recorded from a muscle commonly produced by stimulation of the nerve supplying the muscle either directly or indirectly. Baseline-to-peak amplitude, duration, and latency of the negative phase should be noted, along with details of the method of stimulation and recording. Use of specific named potentials is recommended, e.g., *M wave, F wave, H wave, T wave, A wave* and *R1 wave* or *R2 wave (blink responses).*

compound nerve action potential (compound NAP): The summation of nearly synchronous nerve fiber action potentials recorded from a nerve trunk, commonly produced by stimulation of the nerve directly or indirectly. Details of the method of stimulation and recording should be specified, together with the fiber type (sensory, motor, or mixed).

compound sensory nerve action potential (compound SNAP): A compound nerve action potential is considered to have been evoked from afferent fibers if the recording electrodes detect activity only in a sensory nerve or in a sensory branch of a mixed nerve, or if the electric stimulus is applied to a sensory nerve or a dorsal nerve root, or an adequate stimulus is applied synchronously to sensory receptors. The amplitude, latency, duration, and configuration should be noted. Generally, the amplitude is measured as the maximum peak-to-peak voltage, the latency as either the *latency* to the initial deflection or the *peak latency* to the negative peak, and the duration as the interval from the first deflection of the waveform from the baseline to its final return to the baseline. The compound sensory nerve action potential has been referred to as the *sensory response* or *sensory potential.*

concentric needle electrode: *Recording electrode* that measures an electric potential difference between the bare tip of an insulated wire, usually stainless steel, silver, or platinum, and the bare shaft of a steel cannula through which it is inserted. The bare tip of the central wire (*exploring electrode*) is flush with the level of the cannula (*reference electrode*).

conditioning stimulus: See *paired stimuli.*

conduction block: Failure of an action potential to be conducted past a particular point in the nervous system whereas conduction is possible below the point of the block. Conduction block is documented by demonstration of a reduction in the area of an evoked potential greater than that normally seen with electric stimulation at two different points on a nerve trunk; anatomic variations of nerve pathways and technical factors related to nerve stimulation must be excluded as the cause of the reduction in area.

conduction distance: See *conduction velocity.*

Continued on following page

conduction time: See *conduction velocity.*

conduction velocity (CV): Speed of propagation of an *action potential* along a nerve or muscle fiber. The nerve fibers studied (motor, sensory, autonomic, or mixed) should be specified. For a nerve trunk, the maximum conduction velocity is calculated from the *latency* of the evoked potential (muscle or nerve) at maximal or supramaximal intensity of stimulation at two different points. The distance between the two points (*conduction distance*) is divided by the difference between the corresponding latencies (*conduction time*). The calculated velocity represents the conduction velocity of the fastest fibers and is expressed as meters per second (m/s). As commonly used, the term *conduction velocity* refers to the maximum conduction velocity. By specialized techniques, the conduction velocity of other fibers can be determined as well and should be specified, e.g., minimum conduction velocity.

contraction: A voluntary or involuntary reversible muscle shortening that may or may not be accompanied by *action potentials* from muscle. This term is to be contrasted with the term *contracture*, which refers to a condition of fixed muscle shortening.

contraction fasciculation: Rhythmic, visible twitching of a muscle with weak voluntary or postural contraction. The phenomenon occurs in neuromuscular disorders in which the motor unit territory is enlarged and the tissue covering the muscle is thin.

contracture: The term is used to refer to immobility of a joint due to fixed muscle shortening. Contrast *contraction.* The term has also been used to refer to an electrically silent, involuntary state of maintained muscle contraction, as seen in phosphorylase deficiency, for which the preferred term is *muscle cramp.*

coupled discharge: See preferred term, *satellite potential.*

cps (also c/s): See *cycles per second.*

cramp discharge: Involuntary repetitive firing of *motor unit action potentials* at a high frequency (up to 150 Hz) in a large area of muscles, usually associated with painful muscle contraction. Both the discharge frequency and the number of *motor unit action potentials* firing increase gradually during development and both subside gradually with cessation. See *muscle cramp.*

c/s (also cps): See *cycles per second.*

CV: See *conduction velocity.*

cycles per second: Unit of frequency. (cps or c/s). See also *hertz* (Hz).

decremental response: See preferred term, *decrementing response.*

decrementing response: A reproducible decline in the amplitude and/or area of the *M wave* of successive responses to *repetitive nerve stimulation.* The rate of stimulation and the total number of stimuli should be specified. Decrementing responses with disorders of neuromuscular transmission are most reliably seen with slow rates (2–5 Hz) of nerve stimulation. A decrementing response with repetitive nerve stimulation commonly occurs in disorders of neuromuscular transmission but can also be seen in some neuropathies, myopathies, and motor neuron disease. An artifact resembling a decrementing response can result from movement of the stimulating or recording electrodes during repetitive nerve stimulation. Contrast with *incrementing response*.

delay: As originally used in clinical electromyography, delay referred to the time between the beginning of the horizontal sweep of the oscilloscope and the onset of an applied stimulus. The term is also used to refer to an information storage device (delay line) used to display events occurring before a trigger signal.

denervation potential: The term has been used to describe a *fibrillation potential*. The use of this term is discouraged because fibrillation potentials may occur in settings where transient muscle membrane instability occurs in the absence of denervation, e.g., hyperkalemia periodic paralysis. See preferred term, *fibrillation potential*.

depolarization: See *polarization*.

depolarization block: Failure of an excitable cell to respond to a stimulus because of depolarization of the cell membrane.

discharge: Refers to the firing of one or more excitable elements (neurons, axons, or muscle fibers) and as conventionally applied refers to the all-or-none potentials only. Synonymous with *action potential*.

discharge frequency: The rate of repetition of potentials. When potentials occur in groups, the rate of recurrence of the group and the rate of repetition of the individual components in the groups should be specified. See also *firing rate*.

discrete activity: See *interference pattern*.

distal latency: See *motor latency* and *sensory latency*.

double discharge: Two action potentials (*motor unit action potential, fibrillation potential*) of the same form and nearly the same amplitude, occurring consistently in the same relationship to one another at intervals of 2 to 20 ms. Contrast with *paired discharge*.

doublet: Synonymous with *double discharge*.

duration: The time during which something exists or acts. (1) The total duration of individual potential *waveforms* is defined as the interval from the beginning of the first deflection from the baseline to its final return to the baseline, unless otherwise specified. For example, the duration of the *M wave* may refer to the interval from the deflection of the first negative phase from the baseline to its return to the baseline. (2) The duration of a single electric stimulus refers to the interval of the applied current or voltage. (3) The duration of recurring stimuli or action potentials refers to the interval from the beginning to the end of the series.

earth electrode: Synonymous with *ground electrode*.

EDX: See *electrodiagnosis*.

electric artifact: See *artifact*.

electric inactivity: Absence of identifiable electric activity in a structure or organ under investigation. See preferred term, *electric silence*.

electric silence: The absence of measurable electric activity due to

Continued on following page

biologic or nonbiologic sources. The sensitivity and signal-to-noise level of the recording system should be specified.

electrode: A conducting device used to record an electric potential (*recording electrode*) or to apply an electric current (*stimulating electrode*). In addition to the *ground electrode* used in clinical recording, two electrodes are always required either to record an electric potential or to apply an electric current. Depending on the relative size and location of the electrodes, however, the stimulating or recording condition may be referred to as *monopolar* or *unipolar*. See *ground electrode, recording electrode,* and *stimulating electrode*. Also see specific needle electrode configurations: *monopolar, unipolar, concentric, bifilar recording, bipolar stimulating, multilead, single fiber,* and *macro-EMG needle electrodes*.

electrodiagnosis (EDX): The recording and analysis of responses of nerves and muscles to electric stimulation and the identification of patterns of insertion, spontaneous, involuntary and voluntary action potentials in muscle and nerve tissue. See also *electromyography, electroneurography, electroneuromyography,* and *evoked potential studies*.

electrodiagnostic medicine: A specific area of medical practice in which a physician uses information from the clinical history, observations from the physical examination, and the techniques of *electrodiagnosis* to diagnose and treat neuromuscular disorders. See *electrodiagnosis*.

electromyelography: The recording and study of electric activity from the spinal cord and/or from the cauda equina.

electromyogram: The record obtained by *electromyography*.

electromyograph: Equipment used to activate, record, process, and display nerve and muscle action potentials for the purpose of evaluating nerve and muscle function.

electromyography (EMG): Strictly defined, the recording and study of insertion, spontaneous, and voluntary electric activity of muscle. It is commonly used to refer to nerve conduction studies as well. See also *clinical electromyography* and *electroneuromyography*.

electroneurography (ENG): The recording and study of the action potentials of peripheral nerves. Synonymous with *nerve conduction studies*.

electroneuromyography (ENMG): The combined studies of *electromyography* and *electroneurography*. Synonymous with *clinical electromyography*.

EMG: See *electromyography*.

end-plate activity: Spontaneous electric activity recorded with a needle electrode close to muscle end-plates. May be either of two forms:
1. *Monophasic:* Low-amplitude (10–20 μV), short-duration (0.5–1 ms), monophasic (negative) potentials that occur in a dense, steady pattern and are restricted to a localized area of the muscle. Because of the multitude of different potentials occurring, the exact frequency, although appearing to be high, cannot be defined. These nonpropagated potentials are probably miniature end-plate potentials recorded extracellu-

larly. This form of end-plate activity has been referred to as *end-plate noise* or *sea shell sound (sea shell noise* or *roar).*

2. *Biphasic:* Moderate-amplitude (100–300 μV), short-duration (2–4 ms), biphasic (negative-positive) spike potentials that occur irregularly in short bursts with a high frequency (50–100 Hz), restricted to a localized area within the muscle. These propagated potentials are generated by muscle fibers excited by activity in nerve terminals. These potentials have been referred to as *biphasic spike potentials, end-plate spikes,* and, incorrectly, *nerve potentials.*

end-plate noise: See *end-plate activity (monophasic).*

end-plate potential (EPP): The graded nonpropagated membrane potential induced in the postsynaptic membrane of the muscle fiber by the action of acetylcholine released in response to an action potential in the presynaptic axon terminal.

end-plate spike: See *end-plate activity (biphasic).*

end-plate zone: The region in a muscle where the neuromuscular junctions of the skeletal muscle fibers are concentrated.

ENG: See *electroneurography.*

ENMG: See *electroneuromyography.*

EPP: See *end-plate potential.*

EPSP: See *excitatory postsynaptic potential.*

evoked compound muscle action potential: See *compound muscle action potential.*

evoked potential: Electric waveform elicited by and temporally related to a stimulus, most commonly an electric stimulus delivered to a sensory receptor or nerve, or applied directly to a discrete area of the brain, spinal cord, or muscle. See *auditory evoked potential, brainstem auditory evoked potential, spinal evoked potential, somatosensory evoked potential, visual evoked potential, compound muscle action potential,* and *compound sensory nerve action potential.*

evoked potential studies: Recording and analysis of electric waveforms of biologic origin elicited in response to electric or physiologic stimuli. Generally used to refer to studies of waveforms generated in the peripheral and central nervous system, whereas *nerve conduction studies* refers to studies of waveforms generated in the peripheral nervous system. There are two systems for naming complex waveforms in which multiple components can be distinguished. In the first system, the different components are labeled PI or NI for the initial positive and negative potentials, respectively, and PII, NII, PIII, NIII, and so on, for subsequent positive and negative potentials. In the second system, the components are specified by polarity and average peak latency in normal subjects to the nearest millisecond. The first nomenclature principle has been used in an abbreviated form to identify the seven positive components (I–VII) of the normal *brainstem auditory evoked potential.* The second nomenclature principle has been used to identify the positive and negative components of *visual evoked potentials* (N$\overline{75}$, P$\overline{100}$) and *somatosensory evoked potentials* (P$\overline{9}$, P$\overline{11}$, P$\overline{13}$, P$\overline{14}$, N$\overline{20}$, P$\overline{23}$). Regardless of the nomenclature system, it is possible

Continued on following page

under standardized conditions to establish normal ranges of amplitude, duration, and latency of the individual components of these *evoked potentials*. The difficulty with the second system is that the latencies of components of evoked potentials depend upon the length of the pathways in the neural tissues. Thus the components of an SEP recorded in a child have different average latencies from the same components of an SEP recorded in an adult. Despite this problem, there is no better system available for naming these components at this time. See *auditory evoked potentials, brainstem auditory evoked potentials, visual evoked potentials, somatosensory evoked potentials.*

evoked response: Tautology. Use of term discouraged. See preferred term, *evoked potential.*

excitability: Capacity to be activated by or react to a stimulus.

excitatory postsynaptic potential (EPSP): A local, graded depolarization of a neuron in response to activation by a nerve terminal of a synapse. Contrast with *inhibitory postsynaptic potential.*

exploring electrode: Synonymous with *active electrode.* See *recording electrode.*

F reflex: See preferred term, *F wave.*

F response: Synonymous with *F wave.* See preferred term, *F wave.*

F wave: A *compound action potential* evoked intermittently from a muscle by a supramaximal electric stimulus to the nerve. Compared with the maximal amplitude *M wave* of the same muscle, the F wave has a smaller amplitude (1–5% of the *M wave*), variable configuration and a longer, more variable latency. The F wave can be found in many muscles of the upper and lower extremities, and the latency is longer with more distal sites of stimulation. The F wave is due to antidromic activation of motor neurons. It was named by Magladery and McDougal in 1950. Compare to the *H wave* and the *A wave.*

facilitation: Improvement of neuromuscular transmission that results in the activation of previously inactive muscle fibers. Facilitation may be identified in several ways:

1. *Incrementing response:* A reproducible increase in the amplitude associated with an increase in the area of successive electric responses (*M waves*) during *repetitive nerve stimulation.*
2. *Postactivation* or *posttetanic facilitation:* Nerve stimulation studies performed within a few seconds after a brief period (2–15 s) of nerve stimulation producing *tetanus* or after a strong voluntary contraction may show changes in the configuration of the *M wave(s)* compared to the results of identical studies of the rested neuromuscular junction as follows:
   a. *Repair of the decrement:* A diminution of the decrementing response seen with slow rates (2–5 Hz) of *repetitive nerve stimulation.*
   b. *Increment after exercise:* An increase in the amplitude associated with an increase in the area of the M wave elicited by a single supramaximal stimulus. *Facilitation* should be distinguished from pseudofacilitation. *Pseudofacilitation* occurs in normal subjects with *repetitive nerve stimulation* at high (20–50 Hz) rates or after strong volitional contraction, and probably reflects a reduction in the temporal dispersion of the summa-

tion of a constant number of muscle fiber action potentials. *Pseudofacilitation* produces a response characterized by an increase in the amplitude of the successive M waves with a corresponding decrease in the duration of the M wave, resulting in no change in the area of the negative phase of the successive M waves.

far-field potential: Electric activity of biologic origin generated at a considerable distance from the recording electrodes. Use of the terms *near-field potential* and *far-field potential* is discouraged because all potentials in clinical neurophysiology are recorded at some distance from the generator and there is no consistent distinction between the two terms.

fasciculation: The random, spontaneous twitching of a group of muscle fibers or a motor unit. This twitch may produce movement of the overlying skin (limb), mucous membrane (tongue), or digits. The electric activity associated with the spontaneous contraction is called the *fasciculation potential*. See also *myokymia*. Historically the term *fibrillation* has been used to describe fine twitching of muscle fibers visible through the skin or mucous membrane, but this usage is no longer acceptable.

fasciculation potential: The electric potential often associated with a visible *fasciculation* which has the configuration of a *motor unit action potential* but which occurs spontaneously. Most commonly these potentials occur sporadically and are termed "single fasciculation potentials." Occasionally, the potentials occur as a grouped discharge and are termed a "brief repetitive discharge." The occurrence of repetitive firing of adjacent fasciculation potentials, when numerous, may produce an undulating movement of muscle (see *myokymia*). Use of the terms *benign fasciculation* and *malignant fasciculation* is discouraged. Instead, the configuration of the potentials, peak-to-peak amplitude, duration, number of phases, and stability of configuration, in addition to frequency of occurrence, should be specified.

fatigue: Generally, a state of depressed responsiveness resulting from protracted activity and requiring an appreciable recovery time. Muscle fatigue is a reduction in the force of contraction of muscle fibers and follows repeated voluntary contraction or direct electric stimulation of the muscle.

fiber density: (1) Anatomically, fiber density is a measure of the number of muscle or nerve fibers per unit area. (2) In *single fiber electromyography*, the fiber density is the mean number of *muscle fiber action potentials* fulfilling amplitude and rise time criteria belonging to one motor unit within the recording area of the *single fiber needle electrode* encountered during a systematic search in the weakly, voluntarily contracted muscle. See also *single fiber electromyography, single fiber needle electrode.*

fibrillation: The spontaneous contractions of individual muscle fibers that are not visible through the skin. This term has been used loosely in electromyography for the preferred term, *fibrillation potential.*

fibrillation potential: The electric activity associated with a sponta-
Continued on following page

neously contracting (fibrillating) muscle fiber. It is the action potential of a single muscle fiber. The action potentials may occur spontaneously or after movement of the needle electrode. The potentials usually fire at a constant rate, although a small proportion fire irregularly. Classically, the potentials are biphasic spikes of short duration (usually less than 5 ms) with an initial positive phase and a peak-to-peak amplitude of less than 1 mV. When recorded with concentric or monopolar needle electrodes, the firing rate has a wide range (1–50 Hz) and often decreases just before cessation of an individual discharge. A high-pitched regular sound is associated with the discharge of fibrillation potentials and has been described in the old literature as "rain on a tin roof." In addition to this classic form of fibrillation potentials, *positive sharp waves* may also be recorded from fibrillating muscle fibers when the potential arises from an area immediately adjacent to the needle electrode.

firing pattern: Qualitative and quantitative descriptions of the sequence of discharge of potential waveforms recorded from muscle or nerve.

firing rate: Frequency of repetition of a potential. The relationship of the frequency to the occurrence of other potentials and the force of muscle contraction may be described. See also *discharge frequency.*

frequency: Number of complete cycles of a repetitive waveform in one second. Measured in *hertz* (Hz) or *cycles per second* (cps or c/s).

frequency analysis: Determination of the range of frequencies composing a potential waveform, with a measurement of the absolute or relative amplitude of each component frequency.

full interference pattern: See *interference pattern.*

functional refractory period: See *refractory period.*

G1, G2: Synonymous with *Grid 1, Grid 2,* and newer terms, *Input Terminal 1, Input Terminal 2.* See *recording electrode.*

"giant" motor unit action potential: Use of term discouraged. It refers to a *motor unit action potential* with a peak-to-peak amplitude and duration much greater than the range recorded in corresponding muscles in normal subjects of similar age. Quantitative measurements of amplitude and duration are preferable.

Grid 1: Synonymous with *G1, Input Terminal 1,* or *active* or *exploring electrode.* See *recording electrode.*

Grid 2: Synonymous with *G2, Input Terminal 2,* or *reference electrode.* See *recording electrode.*

ground electrode: An electrode connected to the patient and to a large conducting body (such as the earth) used as a common return for an electric circuit and as an arbitrary zero potential reference point.

grouped discharge: The term has been used historically to describe three phenomena: (1) irregular, voluntary grouping of *motor unit action potentials* as seen in a tremulous muscular contraction, (2) involuntary grouping of *motor unit action potentials* as seen in *myokymia,* (3) general term to describe repeated firing of *motor unit action potentials.* See preferred term, *repetitive discharge.*

H reflex: Abbreviation for Hoffmann reflex. See *H wave*.

H response: See preferred term *H wave*.

H wave: A compound muscle action potential having a consistent latency evoked regularly, when present, from a muscle by an electric stimulus to the nerve. It is regularly found only in a limited group of physiologic extensors, particularly the calf muscles. The H wave is most easily obtained with the cathode positioned proximal to the anode. Compared with the maximum amplitude *M wave* of the same muscle, the H wave has a smaller amplitude, a longer latency, and a lower optimal stimulus intensity. The latency is longer with more distal sites of stimulation. A stimulus intensity sufficient to elicit a maximal amplitude M wave reduces or abolishes the H wave. The H wave is thought to be due to a spinal reflex, the Hoffmann reflex, with electric stimulation of afferent fibers in the mixed nerve to the muscle and activation of motor neurons to the muscle through a monosynaptic connection in the spinal cord. The reflex and wave are named in honor of Hoffmann's description (1918). Compare the *F wave*.

habituation: Decrease in size of a reflex motor response to an afferent stimulus when the latter is repeated, especially at regular and recurring short intervals.

hertz: (Hz) Unit of frequency equal to *cycles per second*.

Hoffmann reflex: See *H wave*.

hyperpolarization: See *polarization*.

Hz: See *hertz*.

increased insertion activity: See *insertion activity*.

increment after exercise: See *facilitation*.

incremental response: See preferred term, *incrementing response*.

incrementing response: A reproducible increase in amplitude and/or area of successive responses (M wave) to *repetitive nerve stimulation*. The rate of stimulation and the number of stimuli should be specified. An incrementing response is commonly seen in two situations. First, in normal subjects the configuration of the M wave may change with repetitive nerve stimulation so that the amplitude progressively increases as the duration decreases, but the area of the M wave remains the same. This phenomenon is termed *pseudofacilitation*. Second, in disorders of neuromuscular transmission, the configuration of the M wave may change with repetitive nerve stimulation so that the amplitude progressively increases as the duration remains the same or increases, and the area of the M wave increases. This phenomenon is termed *facilitation*. Contrast with *decrementing response*.

indifferent electrode: Synonymous with *reference electrode*. Use of term discouraged. See *recording electrode*.

inhibitory postsynaptic potential (IPSP): A local graded hyperpolarization of a neuron in response to activation at a synapse by a nerve terminal. Contrast with *excitatory postsynaptic potential*.

injury potential: The potential difference between a normal region of the surface of a nerve or muscle and a region that has been injured;

Continued on following page

also called a "demarcation potential." The injury potential approximates the potential across the membrane because the injured surface is almost at the potential of the inside of the cell.

Input Terminal 1: The input terminal of the differential amplifier at which negativity, relative to the other input terminal, produces an upward deflection on the graphic display. Synonymous with *active* or *exploring electrode* (or older term, *Grid 1*). See *recording electrode*.

Input Terminal 2: The input terminal of the differential amplifier at which negativity, relative to the other input terminal, produces a downward deflection on the graphic display. Synonymous with *reference electrode* (or older term, *Grid 2*). See *recording electrode*.

insertion activity: Electric activity caused by insertion or movement of a needle electrode. The amount of the activity may be described as normal, reduced, increased (prolonged), with a description of the waveform and repetitive rate.

interdischarge interval: Time between consecutive discharges of the same potential. Measurement should be made between the corresponding points on each waveform.

interference: Unwanted electric activity arising outside the system being studied.

interference pattern: Electric activity recorded from a muscle with a needle electrode during maximal voluntary effort. A *full interference pattern* implies that no individual *motor unit action potentials* can be clearly identified. A *reduced interference pattern (intermediate interference pattern)* is one in which some of the individual MUAPs may be identified while other individual MUAPs cannot be identified because of overlap. The term *discrete activity* is used to describe the electric activity recorded when each of several different MUAPs can be identified. The term *single unit pattern* is used to describe a single MUAP, firing at a rapid rate (should be specified) during maximum voluntary effort. The force of contraction associated with the interference pattern should be specified. See also *recruitment pattern*.

intermediate interference pattern: See *interference pattern*.

International 10–20 System: A system of electrode placement on the scalp in which electrodes are placed either 10% or 20% of the total distance between the nasion and inion in the sagittal plane, and between right and left preauricular points in the coronal plane.

interpeak interval: Difference between the peak latencies of two components of a waveform.

interpotential interval: Time between two different potentials. Measurement should be made between the corresponding parts on each waveform.

involuntary activity: *Motor unit potentials* that are not under voluntary control. The condition under which they occur would be described, for example, spontaneous or reflex potentials and, if elicited by a stimulus, the nature of the stimulus. Contrast with *spontaneous activity*.

IPSP: See *inhibitory postsynaptic potential*.

irregular potential: See preferred term, *serrated action potential*.

iterative discharge: See preferred term, *repetitive discharge.*

jitter: Synonymous with "single fiber electromyographic jitter." Jitter is the variability with consecutive discharges of the *interpotential interval* between two muscle fiber action potentials belonging to the same motor unit. It is usually expressed quantitatively as the mean value of the difference between the interpotential intervals of successive discharges (the mean consecutive difference, MCD). Under certain conditions, jitter is expressed as the mean value of the difference between interpotential intervals arranged in the order of decreasing interdischarge intervals (the mean sorted difference, MSD).

Jolly test: A technique described by Jolly (1895), who applied an electric current to excite a motor nerve while recording the force of muscle contraction. Harvey and Masland (1941) refined the technique by recording the M wave evoked by repetitive, supramaximal nerve stimulation to detect a defect of neuromuscular transmission. Use of the term is discouraged. See preferred term, *repetitive nerve stimulation.*

late component (of a motor unit action potential): See preferred term, *satellite potential.*

late response: A general term used to describe an evoked potential having a longer latency than the *M wave.* See *A wave, F wave, H wave, T wave.*

latency: Interval between the onset of a stimulus and the onset of a response. Thus the term *onset latency* is a tautology and should not be used. The *peak latency* is the interval between the onset of a stimulus and a specified peak of the evoked potential.

latency of activation: The time required for an electric stimulus to depolarize a nerve fiber (or bundle of fibers as in a nerve trunk) beyond threshold and to initiate a regenerative action potential in the fiber(s). This time is usually on the order of 0.1 ms or less. An equivalent term now rarely used in the literature is the "utilization time."

latent period: See synonym, *latency.*

linked potential: See preferred term, *satellite potential.*

long-latency SEP: That portion of a *somatosensory evoked potential* normally occurring at a time greater than 100 ms after stimulation of a nerve in the upper extremity at the wrist or the lower extremity at the knee or ankle.

M response: See synonym, *M wave.*

M wave: A *compound action potential* evoked from a muscle by a single electric stimulus to its motor nerve. By convention, the M wave elicited by supramaximal stimulation is used for motor nerve conduction studies. Ideally, the recording electrodes should be placed so that the initial deflection of the evoked potential is negative. The *latency,* commonly called the *motor latency,* is the latency (ms) to the onset of the first phase (positive or negative) of the M wave. The amplitude (MV) is the baseline-to-peak amplitude of the first negative phase, unless otherwise specified. The *duration* (ms) refers to the duration of the first negative phase, unless otherwise specified. Normally, the configuration of the M wave (usually biphasic) is quite sta-

Continued on following page

ble with repeated stimuli at slow rates (1–15 Hz). See *repetitive nerve stimulation.*

macro motor unit action potential (macro MUAP): The average electric activity of that part of an anatomic motor unit that is within the recording range of a *macro-EMG electrode.* The potential is characterized by its consistent appearance when the small recording surface of the macro-EMG electrode is positioned to record action potentials from one muscle fiber. The following parameters can be specified quantitatively: (1) maximal peak-to-peak amplitude, (2) area contained under the waveform, (3) number of phases.

macro MUAP: See *macro motor unit action potential.*

macroelectromyography (macro-EMG): General term referring to the technique and conditions that approximate recording of all *muscle fiber action potentials* arising from the same motor unit.

macro-EMG: See *macroelectromyography.*

macro-EMG needle electrode: A modified *single fiber electromyography* electrode insulated to within 15 mm from the tip and with a small recording surface (25 μm in diameter) 7.5 mm from the tip.

malignant fasciculation: Use of term discouraged to describe a firing pattern of fasciculation potentials. Historically, the term was used to describe large, polyphasic fasciculation potentials firing at a slow rate. This pattern has been seen in progressive motor neuron disease, but the relationship is not exclusive. See *fasciculation potential.*

maximal stimulus: See *stimulus.*

maximum conduction velocity: See *conduction velocity.*

MCD: Abbreviation for mean consecutive difference. See *jitter.*

mean consecutive difference (MCD): See *jitter.*

membrane instability: Tendency of a cell membrane to depolarize spontaneously, with mechanical irritation, or after voluntary activation.

MEPP: Miniature end-plate potential.

microneurography: The technique of recording peripheral nerve action potentials in man by means of intraneural electrodes.

midlatency SEP: That portion of the waveforms of a *somatosensory evoked potential* normally occurring within 25–100 ms after stimulation of a nerve in the upper extremity at the wrist, within 40–100 ms after stimulation of a nerve in the lower extremity at the knee, and within 50–100 ms after stimulation of a nerve in the lower extremity at the ankle.

miniature end-plate potential (MEPP): The postsynaptic muscle fiber potentials produced through the spontaneous release of individual quanta of acetylcholine from the presynaptic axon terminals. As recorded with conventional concentric needle electrodes inserted in the end-plate zone, such potentials are characteristically monophasic, negative, or relatively short duration (less than 5 ms) and generally less than 20 μV in amplitude.

MNCV: Abbreviation for *motor nerve conduction velocity.* See *conduction velocity.*

monophasic action potential: See *action potential* with one phase.

monophasic end-plate activity: See *end-plate activity (monophasic)*.

monopolar needle recording electrode: A solid wire, usually stainless steel, usually coated, except at its tip, with an insulating material. Variations in voltage between the tip of the needle (active or exploring electrode) positioned in a muscle and a conductive plate on the skin surface or a bare needle in subcutaneous tissue (reference electrode) are measured. By convention, this recording condition is referred to as a monopolar needle electrode recording. It should be emphasized, however, that potential differences are always recorded between two electrodes.

motor latency: Interval between the onset of a stimulus and the onset of the resultant *compound muscle action potential (M wave)*. The term may be qualified, as "proximal motor latency" or "distal motor latency," depending on the relative position of the stimulus.

motor nerve conduction velocity (MNCV): See *conduction velocity*.

motor point: The point over a muscle where a contraction of a muscle may be elicited by a minimal-intensity, short-duration electric stimulus. The motor point corresponds anatomically to the location of the terminal portion of the motor nerve fibers (end-plate zone).

motor response: (1) The compound muscle action potential (*M wave*) recorded over a muscle with stimulation of the nerve to the muscle, (2) the muscle twitch or contraction elicited by stimulation of the nerve to a muscle, (3) the muscle twitch elicited by the muscle stretch reflex.

motor unit: The anatomic unit of an anterior horn cell, its axon, the neuromuscular junctions, and all of the muscle fibers innervated by the axon.

motor unit action potential (MUAP): Action potential reflecting the electric activity of a single anatomic motor unit. It is the compound action potential of those muscle fibers within the recording range of an electrode. With voluntary muscle contraction, the action potential is characterized by its consistent appearance with, and relationship to, the force of contraction. The following parameters should be specified, quantitatively if possible, after the recording electrode is placed so as to minimize the *rise time* (which by convention should be less than 0.5 ms):
1. Configuration
   a. *Amplitude,* peak-to-peak (μv or mV).
   b. *Duration,* total (ms).
   c. Number of *phases* (monophasic, biphasic, triphasic, tetraphasic, polyphasic).
   d. Sign of each *phase* (negative, positive).
   e. Number of *turns*.
   f. Variation of shape, if any, with consecutive discharges.
   g. Presence of *satellite* (linked) *potentials*, if any.
2. *Recruitment* characteristics
   a. Threshold of activation (first recruited, low threshold, high threshold).
   b. *Onset frequency* (Hz).

Continued on following page

> c. *Recruitment frequency* (Hz) or *recruitment interval* (ms) of individual potentials.

Descriptive terms implying diagnostic significance are not recommended, e.g., "myopathic," "neuropathic," "regeneration," "nascent," "giant," *BSAP,* and *BSAPP.* See *polyphasic action potential, serrated action potential.*

motor unit fraction: See *scanning EMG.*

motor unit potential (MUP): See synonym, *motor unit action potential.*

motor unit territory: The area in a muscle over which the muscle fibers belonging to an individual motor unit are distributed.

movement artifact: See *artifact.*

MSD: Abbreviation for mean sorted difference. See *jitter.*

MUAP: See *motor unit action potential.*

multielectrode: See *multilead electrode.*

multilead electrode: Three or more insulated wires inserted through a common metal cannula with their bared tips at an aperture in the cannula and flush with the outer circumference of the cannula. The arrangement of the bare tips relative to the axis of the cannula and the distance between each tip should be specified.

multiple discharge: Four or more *motor unit action potentials* of the same form and nearly the same amplitude occurring consistently in the same relationship to one another and generated by this same axon or muscle fiber. See *double* and *triple discharge.*

multiplet: See *multiple discharge.*

MUP: Abbreviation for *motor unit potential.* See preferred term, *motor unit action potential.*

muscle action potential: Term commonly used to refer to a *compound muscle action potential.*

muscle cramp: Most commonly, an involuntary, painful muscle *contraction* associated with electric activity (see *cramp discharge*). Muscle cramps may be accompanied by other types of *repetitive discharges,* and in some metabolic myopathies (McArdle's disease) the painful, contracted muscles may show *electric silence.*

muscle fiber action potential: Action potential recorded from a single muscle fiber.

muscle fiber conduction velocity: The speed of propagation of a single *muscle fiber action potential,* usually expressed as meters per second. The muscle fiber conduction velocity is usually less than most nerve conduction velocities, varies with the rate of discharge of the muscle fiber, and requires special techniques for measurement.

muscle stretch reflex: Activation of a muscle follows stretch of the muscle, for example, by percussion of a muscle tendon.

myoedema: Focal muscle contraction produced by muscle percussion and not associated with propagated electric activity; may be seen in hypothyroidism (myxedema) and chronic malnutrition.

myokymia: Continuous quivering or undulating movement of surface and overlying skin and mucous membrane associated with spontaneous, repetitive discharge of *motor unit potentials.* See *myokymic discharge, fasciculation,* and *fasciculation potential.*

myokymic discharge: *Motor unit action potentials* that fire repetitively and may be associated with clinical myokymia. Two firing patterns have been described. Commonly, the discharge is a brief, repetitive firing of single units for a short period (up to a few seconds) at a uniform rate (2–60 Hz) followed by a short period (up to a few seconds) of silence, with repetition of the same sequence for a particular potential. Less commonly, the potential recurs continuously at a fairly uniform firing rate (1–15 Hz). Myokymic discharges are a subclass of *grouped discharges* and *repetitive discharges.*

myopathic motor unit potential: Use of term discouraged. It has been used to refer to low-amplitude, short-duration, polyphasic *motor unit action potentials.* The term incorrectly implies specific diagnostic significance of a motor unit potential configuration. See *motor unit action potential.*

myopathic recruitment: Use of term discouraged. It has been used to describe an increase in the number of and firing rate of *motor unit action potentials* compared with normal for the strength of muscle contraction.

myotonia: The clinical observation of delayed relaxation of muscle after voluntary contraction or percussion. The delayed relaxation may be electrically silent, or accompanied by propagated electric activity, such as *myotonic discharge, complex repetitive discharge,* or *neuromyotonid discharge.*

myotonic discharge: Repetitive discharge at rates of 20–80 Hz are of two types: (1) biphasic (positive-negative) spike potentials less than 5 ms in duration resembling *fibrillation potentials.* (2) positive waves of 5–20 ms in duration resembling *positive sharp waves.* Both potential forms are recorded after needle insertion, after voluntary muscle contraction or after muscle percussion, and are due to independent, repetitive discharges of single muscle fibers. The amplitude and frequency of the potentials must both wax and wane to be identified as myotonic discharges. This change produces a characteristic musical sound in the audio display of the electromyograph due to the corresponding change in pitch, which has been likened to the sound of a dive bomber. Contrast with *waning discharge.*

myotonic potential: See preferred term, *myotonic discharge.*

NAP: Abbreviation for nerve action potential. See *compound nerve action potential.*

nascent motor unit potential: From the Latin "nascens," to be born. Use of term is discouraged as it incorrectly implies diagnostic significance of a motor unit potential configuration. Term has been used to refer to very-low-amplitude, long-duration, highly polyphasic motor unit potentials observed during early stages of reinnervation of muscle. See *motor unit action potential.*

NCS: See *nerve conduction studies.*

NCV: Abbreviation for *nerve conduction velocity.* See *conduction velocity.*

Continued on following page

near constant frequency trains: See preferred term, *complex repetitive discharge.*

near-field potential: Electric activity of biologic origin generated near the recording electrodes. Use of the terms *near-field potential* and *far-field potential* is discouraged because all potentials in clinical neurophysiology are recorded at some distance from the generator and there is no consistent distinction between the two terms.

needle electrode: An electrode for recording or stimulating, shaped like a needle. See specific electrodes: *bifilar (bipolar) needle recording electrode, concentric needle electrode, macro-EMG needle electrode, monopolar needle recording electrode, multilead electrode, single fiber needle electrode,* and *stimulating electrode.*

nerve action potential (NAP): Strictly defined, refers to an action potential recorded from a single nerve fiber. The term is commonly used to refer to the compound nerve action potential. See *compound nerve action potential.*

nerve conduction studies (NCS): Synonymous with *electroneurography.* Recording and analysis of electric *waveforms* of biologic origin elicited in response to electric or physiologic *stimuli.* Generally *nerve conduction studies* refers to studies of waveforms generated in the peripheral nervous system, whereas *evoked potential studies* refers to studies of waveforms generated in both the peripheral and central nervous system. The waveforms recorded in *nerve conduction studies* are *compound sensory nerve action potentials.* The *compound sensory nerve action potentials* are generally referred to as *sensory nerve action potentials.* The *compound muscle action potentials* are generally referred to by letters that have historical origins: *M wave, F wave, H wave, T wave, A wave, R1 wave,* and *R2 wave.* It is possible under standardized conditions to establish normal ranges of amplitude, duration, and latencies of these *evoked potentials* and to calculate the maximum conduction velocity of sensory and motor nerves.

nerve conduction velocity (NCV): Loosely used to refer to the maximum nerve conduction velocity. See *conduction velocity.*

nerve fiber action potential: Action potential recorded from a single nerve fiber.

nerve potential: Equivalent to *nerve action potential.* Also commonly, but inaccurately, used to refer to the biphasic form of *endplate activity.* The latter use is incorrect because muscle fibers, not nerve fibers, are the source of these potentials.

nerve trunk action potential: See preferred term, *compound nerve action potential.*

neurapraxia: Failure of nerve conduction, usually reversible, due to metabolic or microstructural abnormalities without disruption of the axon. See preferred electrodiagnostic term, *conduction block.*

neuromyotonia: Clinical syndrome of continuous muscle fiber activity manifested as continuous muscle rippling and stiffness. The accompanying electric activity may be intermittent or continuous. Terms used to describe related clinical syndromes are continuous muscle fiber activity, Isaac syndrome, Isaac-Merton syndrome, quantal squander syndrome, generalized myokymia, pseudomyotonia, normocalcemic tetany, and neurotonia.

neuromyotonic discharge: Bursts of *motor unit action potentials* which originate in the motor axons firing at high rates (150–300 Hz) for a few seconds, and which often start and stop abruptly. The amplitude of the response typically wanes. Discharges may occur spontaneously or be initiated by needle movement, voluntary effort and ischemia, or percussion of a nerve. These discharges should be distinguished from *myotonic discharges* and *complex repetitive discharges*.

neuropathic motor unit potential: Use of term discouraged. It was used to refer to abnormally high-amplitude, long-duration, polyphasic *motor unit action potentials*. The term incorrectly implies a specific diagnostic significance of a motor unit potential configuration. See *motor unit action potential*.

neuropathic recruitment: Use of term discouraged. It has been used to describe a recruitment pattern with a decreased number of *motor unit action potentials* firing at a rapid rate. See preferred terms, *reduced interference pattern, discrete activity, single unit pattern*.

neurotmesis: Partial or complete severance of a nerve, with disruption of the axons, their myelin sheaths, and the supporting connective tissue, resulting in degeneration of the axons distal to the injury site.

noise: Strictly defined, potentials produced by electrodes, cables, amplifier, or storage media and unrelated to the potentials of biologic origin. The term has been used loosely to refer to one form of *end-plate activity*.

onset frequency: The lowest stable frequency of firing for a single *motor unit action potential* that can be voluntarily maintained by a subject.

onset latency: Tautology. See *latency*.

order of activation: The sequence of appearance of different *motor unit action potentials* with increasing strength of voluntary contraction. See *recruitment*.

orthodromic: Propagation of an impulse in the direction the same as physiologic conduction, for instance, conduction along motor nerve fibers towards the muscle and conduction along sensory nerve fibers towards the spinal cord. Contrast with *antidromic*.

paired discharge: Two action potentials occurring consistently in the same relationship with each other. Contrast with *double discharge*.

paired response: Use of term discouraged. See preferred term, *paired discharge*.

paired stimuli: Two consecutive stimuli. The time interval between the two stimuli and the intensity of each stimulus should be specified. The first stimulus is called the *conditioning stimulus* and the second stimulus is the *test stimulus*. The *conditioning stimulus* may modify the tissue excitability, which can then be evaluated by the response to the *test stimulus*.

Continued on following page

parasite potential: See preferred term, *satellite potential.*

peak latency: Interval between the onset of a stimulus and a specified peak of the evoked potential.

phase: That portion of a *wave* between the departure from, and the return to, the *baseline.*

polarization: As used in neurophysiology, the presence of an electric potential difference across an excitable cell membrane. The potential across the membrane of a cell when it is not excited by an input or spontaneously active is termed the *resting potential*; it is at a stationary nonequilibrium state with regard to the electric potential difference across the membrane. *Depolarization* describes a reduction in the magnitude of the polarization toward the zero potential while *hyperpolarization* refers to an increase in the magnitude of the polarization relative to the resting potential. *Repolarization* describes an increase in polarization from the depolarized state toward, but not above, the normal resting potential.

polyphasic action potential: An *action potential* having five or more phases. See *phase*. Contrast with *serrated action potential.*

positive sharp wave: A biphasic, positive-negative *action potential* initiated by needle movement and recurring in a uniform, regular pattern at a rate of 1–50 Hz; the discharge frequency may decrease slightly just before cessation of discharge. The initial positive deflection is rapid (< 1 ms), its duration is usually less than 5 ms, and the amplitude is up to 1 mv. The negative phase is of low amplitude, with a duration of 10–100 ms. A sequence of positive sharp waves is commonly referred to as a *train of positive sharp waves.* Positive sharp waves can be recorded from the damaged area of fibrillating muscle fibers. Its configuration may result from the position of the needle electrode which is felt to be adjacent to the depolarized segment of a muscle fiber injured by the electrode. Note that the positive sharp waveform is not specific for muscle fiber damage. *Motor unit action potentials* and potentials in *myotonic discharges* may have the configuration of positive sharp waves.

positive wave: Loosely defined, the term refers to a positive sharp wave. See *positive sharp wave.*

postactivation depression: A descriptive term indicating a reduction in the amplitude associated with a reduction in the area of the M wave(s) in response to a single *stimulus* or *train of stimuli* which occurs a few minutes after a brief (30–60 s), strong voluntary contraction or a period of *repetitive nerve stimulation* that produces *tetanus*. *Postactivation exhaustion* refers to the cellular mechanisms responsible for the observed phenomenon of *postactivation depression.*

postactivation exhaustion: A reduction in the safety factor (margin) of neuromuscular transmission after sustained activity of the neuromuscular junction. The changes in the configuration of the M wave due to *postactivation exhaustion* are referred to as *postactivation depression.*

postactivation facilitation: See *facilitation.*

postactivation potentiation: Refers to the increase in the force of contraction (mechanical response) after *tetanus* or strong voluntary contraction. Contrast *postactivation facilitation.*

posttetanic facilitation: See *facilitation.*

posttetanic potentiation: The incrementing mechanical response of muscle during and after *repetitive nerve stimulation* without a change in the amplitude of the action potential. In spinal cord physiology, the term has been used to describe enhancement of excitability or reflex outflow of the central nervous system following a long period of high-frequency stimulation. This phenomenon has been described in the mammalian spinal cord, where it lasts minutes or even hours.

potential: A physical variable created by differences in charges, measurable in volts, that exists between two points. Most biologically produced potentials arise from the difference in charge between two sides of a cell membrane. See *polarization.*

potentiation: Physiologically, the enhancement of a response. Some authors use the term *potentiation* to describe the incrementing mechanical response of muscle elicited by *repetitive nerve stimulation,* that is, *posttetanic potentiation,* and the term *facilitation* to describe the incrementing electric response elicited by *repetitive nerve stimulation,* that is, *postactivation facilitation.*

prolonged insertion activity: See *insertion activity.*

propagation velocity of a muscle fiber: The speed of transmission of a muscle fiber action potential.

proximal latency: See *motor latency* and *sensory latency.*

pseudofacilitation: See *facilitation.*

pseudomyotonic discharge: Use of term discouraged. It has been used to refer to different phenomena, including (1) *complex repetitive discharges,* and (2) *repetitive discharges* that do not wax or wane in both frequency and amplitude, and end abruptly. These latter discharges may be seen in disorders such as polymyositis in addition to disorders with *myotonic discharges.* See preferred term, *waning discharge.*

pseudopolyphasic action potential: Use of term discouraged. See preferred term, *serrated action potential.*

R1, R2 waves: See *blink responses.*

recording electrode: Device used to record electric potential difference. All electric recordings require at least two *electrodes.* The recording electrode close to the source of the activity to be recorded is called the *active* or *exploring electrode,* and the other recording electrode is called the *reference electrode.* Active electrode is synonymous with *Input Terminal 1* (or older terms *Grid 1* and *G1*) and the reference electrode with *Input Terminal 2* (or older terms *Grid 2* and *G2*).

In some recordings, it is not certain which electrode is closer to the source of the biologic activity, that is, recording with a *bifilar (bipolar) needle recording electrode.* In this situation, it is convenient to refer to one electrode as Input Electrode 1 and the other electrode as Input Electrode 2.

By present convention, a potential difference that is negative at
Continued on following page

the active electrode (Input Terminal 1) relative to the reference electrode (Input Terminal 2) causes an upward deflection on the oscilloscope screen. The term "monopolar recording" is not recommended, because all recording requires two electrodes; however, it is commonly used to describe the use of an intramuscular needle exploring electrode in combination with a surface disk or subcutaneous needle reference electrode. A similar combination of needle electrodes has been used to record nerve activity and also has been referred to as "monopolar recording."

recruitment: The successive activation of the same and additional motor units with increasing strength of voluntary muscle contraction. See *motor unit action potential.*

recruitment frequency: Firing rate of a *motor unit action potential (MUAP)* when a different MUAP first appears with gradually increasing strength of voluntary muscle contraction. This parameter is essential to assessment of *recruitment pattern.*

recruitment interval: The *interdischarge interval* between two consecutive discharges of a *motor unit action potential (MUAP)* when a different MUAP first appears with gradually increasing strength of voluntary muscle contraction. The reciprocal of the recruitment interval is the *recruitment frequency.*

recruitment pattern: A qualitative and/or quantitative description of the sequence of appearance of *motor unit action potentials* with increasing strength of voluntary muscle contraction. The *recruitment frequency* and *recruitment interval* are two quantitative measures commonly used. See *interference pattern* for qualitative terms commonly used.

reduced insertion activity: See *insertion activity.*

reduced interference pattern: See *interference pattern.*

reference electrode: See *recording electrode.*

reflex: A stereotyped *motor response* elicited by a sensory *stimulus.*

refractory period: The *absolute refractory period* is the period following an *action potential* during which no stimulus, however strong, evokes a further response. The *relative refractory period* is the period following an *action potential* during which a stimulus must be abnormally large to evoke a second response. The *functional refractory period* is the period following an *action potential* during which a second *action potential* cannot yet excite the given region.

regeneration motor unit potential: Use of term discouraged. See *motor unit action potential.*

relative refractory period: See *refractory period.*

repair of the decrement: See *facilitation.*

repetitive discharge: General term for the recurrence of an *action potential* with the same or nearly the same form. The term may refer to recurring potentials recorded in muscle at rest, during voluntary contraction, or in response to single nerve stimulus. See *double discharge, triple discharge, multiple discharge, myokymic discharge, myotonic discharge, complex repetitive discharge.*

repetitive nerve stimulation: The technique of repeated supramaximal stimulations of a nerve while recording M waves from muscles innervated by the nerve. The number of stimuli and the frequency of stimulation should be specified. Activation procedures performed prior to the test should be specified, for example, sustained voluntary contraction or contraction induced by nerve stimulation. If the test was performed after an activation procedure, the time elapsed after the activation procedure was completed should also be specified. The technique is commonly used to assess the integrity of neuromuscular transmission. For a description of specific patterns of responses, see the terms *incrementing response, decrementing response, facilitation*, and *postactivation depression*.

repolarization: See *polarization.*

residual latency: Refers to the calculated time difference between the measured distal latency of a motor nerve and the expected distal latency, calculated by dividing the distance between the stimulus cathode and the active recording electrode by the maximum conduction velocity measured in a more proximal segment of a nerve. The residual latency is due in part to neuromuscular transmission time and to slowing of conduction in terminal axons due to decreasing diameter and the presence of unmyelinated segments.

response: Used to describe an activity elicited by a *stimulus.*

resting membrane potential: Voltage across the membrane of an excitable cell at rest. See *polarization.*

rheobase: See *strength-duration curve.*

rise time: The interval from the onset of a change of a potential to its peak. The method of measurement should be specified.

satellite potential: A small action potential separated from the main MUAP by an isoelectric interval and firing in a time-locked relationship to the main *action potential.* These potentials usually follow, but may precede, the main action potential. Also called *late component, parasite potential, linked potential*, and *coupled discharge* (less preferred terms).

scanning EMG: A technique by which an electromyographic electrode is advanced in defined steps through muscle while a separate *SFEMG* electrode is used to trigger both the oscilloscope sweep and the advancement device. This recording technique provides temporal and spatial information about the motor unit. Distinct maxima in the recorded activity are considered to be generated by muscle fibers innervated by a common branch of the axon. These groups of fibers form a *motor unit fraction.*

sea shell sound (sea shell roar or noise): Use of term discouraged. See *end-plate activity, monophasic.*

sensory delay: See preferred terms, *sensory latency* and *sensory peak latency.*

sensory latency: Interval between the onset of a stimulus and the onset of the *compound sensory nerve action potential.* This term has been loosely used to refer to the *sensory peak latency.* The term may be qualified as "proximal sensory latency" or "distal sensory latency," depending on the relative position of the stimulus.

Continued on following page

sensory nerve action potential (SNAP): See *compound sensory nerve action potential.*

sensory nerve conduction velocity: See *conduction velocity.*

sensory peak latency: Interval between the onset of a *stimulus* and the peak of the negative phase of the *compound sensory nerve action potential.* Note that the term *latency* refers to the interval between the onset of a stimulus and the onset of a response.

sensory potential: Used to refer to the compound sensory nerve action potential. See *compound sensory nerve action potential.*

sensory response: Used to refer to a sensory evoked potential, for example, *compound sensory nerve action potential.*

SEP: See *somatosensory evoked potential.*

serrated action potential: An action potential waveform with several changes in direction (*turns*) which do not cross the baseline. This term is preferred to the terms *complex action potential* and *pseudopolyphasic action potential.* See also *turn* and *polyphasic action potential.*

SFEMG: See *single fiber electromyography.*

shock artifact: See *artifact.*

short-latency somatosensory evoked potential (SSEP): That portion of the waveforms of a *somatosensory evoked potential* normally occurring within 25 ms after stimulation of the median nerve in the upper extremity at the wrist, 40 ms after stimulation of the common peroneal nerve in the lower extremity at the knee, and 50 ms after stimulation of the posterior tibial nerve in the lower extremity at the ankle.

> **Median nerve SSEPs:** Normal short-latency response components to median nerve stimulation are designated $P\overline{9}$, $P\overline{11}$, $P\overline{13}$, $P\overline{14}$, $N\overline{20}$, and $P\overline{23}$ in records taken between scalp and noncephalic reference electrodes, and $N\overline{9}$, $N\overline{11}$, $N\overline{13}$, and $N\overline{14}$ in cervical spine-scalp derivation. It should be emphasized that potentials having opposite polarity but similar latency in spine-scalp and scalp-noncephalic reference derivations do not necessarily have identical generator sources.

> **Common peroneal nerve SSEPs:** Normal short-latency response components to common peroneal stimulation are designated $P\overline{27}$ and $N\overline{35}$ in records taken between scalp and noncephalic reference electrodes, and L3 and T12 from a cervical spine-scalp derivation.

> **Posterior tibial nerve SSEPs:** Normal short-latency response components to posterior tibial nerve stimulation are designated as the PF potential in the popliteal fossa, $P\overline{37}$ and $N\overline{45}$ waves in records taken between scalp and noncephalic reference electrode, and L3 and T12 potentials from a cervical spine-scalp derivation.

silent period: A pause in the electric activity of a muscle such as that seen after rapid unloading of a muscle.

single fiber electromyography (SFEMG): General term referring to the technique and conditions that permit recording of a single *muscle fiber action potential.* See *single fiber needle electrode* and *jitter.*

single fiber EMG: See *single fiber electromyography.*

single fiber needle electrode: A needle *electrode* with a small recording surface (usually 25 μm in diameter) permitting the recording of single muscle fiber action potentials between the active recording surface and the cannula. See *single fiber electromyography.*

single unit pattern: See *interference pattern.*

SNAP: Abbreviation for *sensory nerve action potential.* See *compound sensory nerve action potential.*

somatosensory evoked potentials (SEPs): Electric waveforms of biologic origin elicited by electric stimulation or physiologic activation of peripheral sensory fibers, for example, the median nerve, common peroneal nerve, or posterior tibial nerve. The normal SEP is a complex waveform with several components that are specified by polarity and average peak latency. The polarity and latency of individual components depend upon (1) subject variables, such as age, sex, (2) stimulus characteristics, such as intensity, rate of stimulation, and (3) recording parameters, such as amplifier time constants, electrode placement, electrode combinations. See *short-latency somatosensory evoked potentials.*

spike: (1) In cellular neurophysiology, a short-lived (usually in the range of 1–3 ms), all-or-none change in membrane potential that arises when a graded response passes a threshold. (2) The electric record of a nerve impulse or similar event in muscle or elsewhere. (3) In clinical EEG recordings, a wave with duration less than 80 ms (usually 15–80 ms).

spinal evoked potential: Electrical waveforms of biologic origin recorded over the sacral, lumbar, thoracic, or cervical spine in response to electric stimulation or physiologic activation of peripheral sensory fibers. See preferred term, *somatosensory evoked potential.*

spontaneous activity: Electric activity recorded from muscle or nerve at rest after insertion activity has subsided and when there is no voluntary contraction or external stimulus. Compare with *involuntary activity.*

SSEP: See *short-latency somatosensory evoked potential.*

staircase phenomenon: The progressive increase in the force of a muscle contraction observed in response to continued low rates of direct or indirect muscle stimulation.

stigmatic electrode: Of historic interest. Used by Sherrington for *active* or *exploring electrode.*

stimulating electrode: Device used to apply electric current. All electric stimulation requires two electrodes; the negative terminal is termed the *cathode* and the positive terminal, the *anode.* By convention, the stimulating electrodes are called "bipolar" if they are encased or attached together. Stimulating electrodes are called "monopolar" if they are not encased or attached together. Electric stimulation for *nerve conduction studies* generally requires application of the cathode to produce depolarization of the nerve trunk fibers. If the anode is inadvertently placed between the cathode and the recording electrodes, a focal block of nerve conduction (*anodal block*) may occur and cause a technically unsatisfactory study.

Continued on following page

stimulus: Any external agent, state, or change that is capable of influencing the activity of a cell, tissue, or organism. In clinical *nerve conduction studies*, an electric stimulus is generally applied to a nerve or muscle. The electric stimulus may be described in absolute terms or with respect to the evoked potential of the nerve or muscle. In absolute terms, the electric stimulus is defined by a duration (ms), a waveform (square, exponential, linear, etc.) and a strength or intensity measured in voltage (V) or current (mA). With respect to the evoked potential, the stimulus may be graded as subthreshold, threshold, submaximal, maximal, or supramaximal. A *threshold stimulus* is that stimulus just sufficient to produce a detectable response. Stimuli less than the threshold stimulus are termed *subthreshold*. The *maximal stimulus* is the stimulus intensity after which a further increase in the stimulus intensity causes no increase in the amplitude of the evoked potential. Stimuli of intensity below this level but above threshold are *submaximal*. Stimuli of intensity greater than the maximal stimulus are termed *supramaximal*. Ordinarily, supramaximal stimuli are used for nerve conduction studies. By convention, an electric stimulus of approximately 20 percent greater voltage/current than required for the maximal stimulus may be used for supramaximal stimulation. The frequency, number, and duration of a series of stimuli should be specified.

stimulus artifact: See *artifact*.

strength-duration curve: Graphic presentation of the relationship between the intensity (Y axis) and various durations (X axis) of the threshold electric stimulus for a muscle with the stimulating cathode positioned over the *motor point*. The *rheobase* is the intensity of an electric current of infinite duration necessary to produce a minimal visible twitch of a muscle when applied to the motor point. In clinical practice, a duration of 300 ms is used to determine the rheobase. The *chronaxie* is the time required for an electric current twice the *rheobase* to elicit the first visible muscle twitch.

submaximal stimulus: See *stimulus*.

subthreshold stimulus: See *stimulus*.

supramaximal stimulus: See *stimulus*.

surface electrode: Conducting device for stimulating or recording placed on a skin surface. The material (metal, fabric), configuration (disk, ring), size, and separation should be specified. See *electrode (ground, recording, stimulating)*.

synchronized fibrillation: See preferred term, *complex repetitive discharge*.

T wave: A compound action potential evoked from a muscle by rapid stretch of its tendon, as part of the muscle stretch reflex.

temporal dispersion: Relative desynchronization of components of a compound action potential due to different rates of conduction of each synchronously evoked component from the stimulation point to the recording electrode.

terminal latency: Synonymous with preferred term, *distal latency*. See *motor latency*, and *sensory latency*.

test stimulus: See *paired stimuli*.

tetanic contraction: The contraction produced in a muscle through repetitive maximal direct or indirect stimulation at a sufficiently high frequency to produce a smooth summation of successive maximum twitches. The term may also be applied to maximum voluntary contractions in which the firing frequencies of most or all of the component motor units are sufficiently high that successive twitches of individual motor units fuse smoothly. Their tensions all combine to produce a steady, smooth maximum contraction of the whole muscle.

tetanus: The continuous contraction of muscle caused by repetitive stimulation or discharge of nerve or muscle. Contrast *tetany*.

tetany: A clinical syndrome manifested by muscle twitching, cramps, and carpal and pedal spasm. These clinical signs are manifestations of peripheral and central nervous system nerve irritability from several causes. In these conditions, *repetitive discharges (double discharge, triple discharge, multiple discharge)* occur frequently with voluntary activation of *motor unit action potentials* or may appear as *spontaneous activity* and are enhanced by systemic alkalosis or local ischemia.

tetraphasic action potential: *Action potential* with four phases.

threshold: The level at which a clear and abrupt transition occurs from one state to another. The term is generally used to refer to the voltage level at which an *action potential* is initiated in a single axon or a group of axons. It is also operationally defined as the intensity that produced a response in about 50 percent of equivalent trials.

threshold stimulus: See *stimulus*.

train of positive sharp waves: See *positive sharp wave*.

train of stimuli: A group of stimuli. The duration of the group or the number of stimuli and the frequency of the stimuli should be specified.

triphasic action potential: *Action potential* with three phases.

triple discharge: Three *motor unit action potentials* of the same form and nearly the same amplitude, occurring consistently in the same relationship to one another and generated by this same axon or muscle fiber. The interval between the second and the third action potential often exceeds that between the first two, and both are usually in the range of 2–20 ms.

triplet: See *triple discharge*.

turn: Point of change in direction in the waveform and the magnitude of the voltage change following the turning point. It is not necessary that the voltage change passes through the baseline. The minimal excursion required to constitute a change should be specified.

unipolar needle electrode: See synonym, *monopolar needle recording electrode*.

utilization time: See preferred term, *latency of activation*.

VEPs: See *visual evoked potentials*.

VERs: Abbreviation for *visual evoked responses*. See *visual evoked potentials*.

Continued on following page

visual evoked potentials (VEPs): Electric waveforms of biologic origin are recorded over the cerebrum and elicited by light stimuli. VEPs are classified by stimulus rate as transient or steady state VEPs, and can be further divided by presentation mode. The normal transient VEP to checkerboard pattern reversal or shift has a major positive occipital peak at about 100 ms (P$\overline{100}$), often preceded by a negative peak (N$\overline{75}$). The precise range of normal values for the latency and amplitude of P$\overline{100}$ depends on several factors: (1) subject variables, such as age, sex, and visual acuity, (2) stimulus characteristics, such as type of stimulator, full-field or half-field stimulation, check size, contrast, and luminescence, and (3) recording parameters, such as placement and combination of recording electrodes.

visual evoked responses (VERs): See *visual evoked potentials*.

volitional activity: See *voluntary activity*.

voltage: Potential difference between two recording sites.

volume conduction: Spread of current from a potential source through a conducting medium, such as the body tissues.

voluntary activity: In electromyography, the electric activity recorded from a muscle with consciously controlled muscle contraction. The effort made to contract the muscle should be specified relative to that of a corresponding normal muscle, for example, minimal, moderate, or maximal. If the recording remains isoelectric during the attempted contraction of the muscle and artifacts have been excluded, it can be concluded that there is no voluntary activity.

waning discharge: General term referring to a *repetitive discharge* that gradually decreases in frequency or amplitude before cessation. Contrast with *myotonic discharge*.

wave: An undulating line constituting a graphic representation of a change, for instance, a changing electric potential difference. See *A wave*, *F wave*, *H wave*, and *M wave*.

waveform: The shape of a *wave*. The term is often used synonymously with wave.

FROM

Compiled by the Nomenclature Committee of the American Association of Electrodiagnostic Medicine (formerly American Association of Electromyography and Electrodiagnosis): AAEE's Glossary of Terms in Clinical Electromyography. Muscle & Nerve 10:G1–G20, 1987, with permission. Approval for inclusion of the glossary in this book in no way implies review or endorsement by the AAEM of material contained in the book.

ELECTROENCEPHALOGRAPHS

Electroencephalogram Patterns

The figure on page 418 shows representative patterns of EEG activity for a variety of disorders.

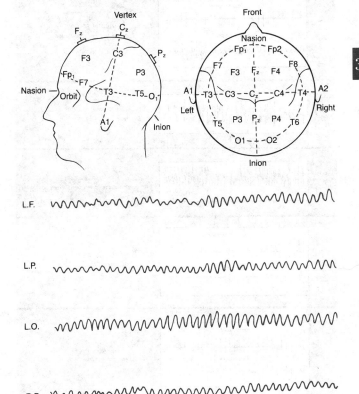

The upper figure shows the placement of EEG electrodes and the names used for each electrode. The lower figure shows a normal EEG with a normal 8 to 10 per sec rhythm. In the lower figure, L represents left and R represents right; F means the recording was from the frontal lobe, and P represents parietal and O, occipital.

Abnormal EEG Patterns

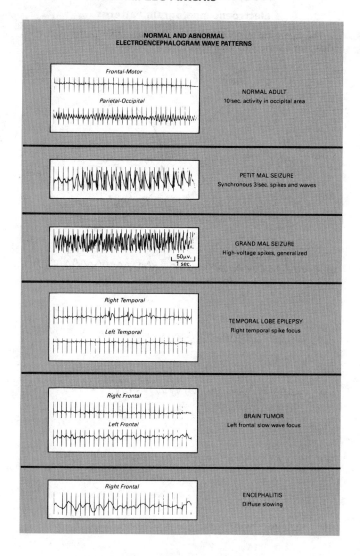

NORMAL AND ABNORMAL ELECTROENCEPHALOGRAM WAVE PATTERNS

Frontal-Motor

Parietal-Occipital

NORMAL ADULT
10/sec. activity in occipital area

PETIT MAL SEIZURE
Synchronous 3/sec. spikes and waves

50μv.
1 sec.

GRAND MAL SEIZURE
High-voltage spikes, generalized

Right Temporal

Left Temporal

TEMPORAL LOBE EPILEPSY
Right temporal spike focus

Right Frontal

Left Frontal

BRAIN TUMOR
Left frontal slow wave focus

Right Frontal

ENCEPHALITIS
Diffuse slowing

EPILEPTIC SEIZURES

Categories of Epilepsy and Seizures
(in alphabetical order)

grand mal (tonic-clonic) seizure: A common type of seizure with sudden onset of unconsciousness, tonic contraction of muscles, loss of postural control, and a cry produced by the respiratory muscles causing a forced expiration. This is followed by generalized contraction of the muscles of the extremities. The seizure is often preceded by an aura. Two to five minutes after consciousness has been lost and contractions have subsided, consciousness is gradually regained. Fecal and urinary incontinence may occur, as well as biting of the tongue. There is postictal amnesia for the time of the seizure. Complete functional recovery from the seizure may take several days.

Jacksonian (focal) epilepsy: With this type of epilepsy, there is a localized seizure with spasms confined to one part of the body or one group of muscles. The spasm may spread to involve adjacent areas of the body.

petit mal (absence) seizures: Seizures in which there is a sudden brief cessation of activity (this may last a few seconds or a few minutes). During the seizure, postural maintenance is not lost, and there are no convulsive muscle contractions. Seizures may occur very frequently (as many as a 100 times a day).

psychomotor (temporal lobe) epilepsy: Seizures that are not grand mal, petit mal, or Jacksonian. Psychomotor seizures are characterized by automatisms. The seizure often begins with an aura. The seizure progresses to include motor symptoms that are often associated with emotional or behavioral states. The movements are stereotypical and nonpurposeful (e.g., lip smacking, leg kicking, picking at clothing, chewing). The movements will be similar during subsequent seizures. With temporal lobe lesions, cognitive and emotional functions are often altered. Hallucinations may occur, as well as sexual arousal and a feeling of déjà vu. The person may feel violent, depressed, or fearful. Postictally there is amnesia for the time of the seizure, with some drowsiness and confusion.

status epilepticus: A state in which there are prolonged seizures with short periods of recovery between attacks. When these seizures are tonic-clonic, they may be life threatening.

FOR MORE INFORMATION

Strub, RL and Black, FW: Neurobehavioral Disorders: A Clinical Approach. FA Davis, Philadelphia, 1988.

International Classification of Epileptic Seizures

I. Partial or focal seizures (seizures beginning locally)
  A. Simple partial seizures (usually without impairment of consciousness)
    1. With motor symptoms
      a. Focal motor
      b. Jacksonian (seizures due to focal irritation of a portion of the motor cortex; motor involvement starts in areas associated with the damaged region of the cortex and may spread to other areas)
      c. Versive
      d. Postural
      e. Somatic inhibitory
      f. Aphasic

Continued on following page

       g. Phonatory (vocalization and arrest of speech)

   2. With special sensory or somatosensory symptoms

      a. Somatosensory

      b. Visual

      c. Auditory

      d. Olfactory

      e. Gustatory

      f. Vertiginous

   3. With autonomic symptoms

   4. Compound forms (includes psychic symptoms)

B. Complex partial (psychomotor or temporal lobe) seizures (usually with impairment of consciousness)

   1. With only impaired consciousness

   2. With cognitive symptoms

      a. With dysmnesic disturbance (impairment of memory)

      b. With ideational disturbances

   3. With affective symptoms

   4. With psychosensory symptoms

      a. Illusions

      b. Hallucinations

   5. With psychomotor symptoms (automatisms)

   6. Compound forms

C. Partial seizures secondarily generalized

II. Generalized seizures (bilaterally symmetric without local onset)

A. Absences (petit mal)

   1. Simple absences with impairment of consciousness only

   2. Complex absences with other associated phenomena

      a. With mild clonic components (myoclonic)

      b. With increase of postural tone (retropulsive)

      c. With diminution or abolition of postural tone (atonic)

      d. With automatisms

      e. With automatic phenomena (e.g., enuresis)

      f. Mixed forms

B. Bilateral massive epileptic mycolonus (myoclonic jerks)

C. Infantile spasms

D. Clonic seizures

E. Tonic seizures

F. Tonic-clonic seizures (grand mal seizures)

G. Atonic seizures

   1. Very brief in duration (drop attacks)

   2. Longer in duration (including atonic absences)

III. Unilateral or predominantly unilateral seizures

IV. Unclassified epileptic seizures (seizures that cannot be classified because of a lack of data)

CHEMICAL CLASSIFICATION AND ACTIONS OF ANTIEPILEPTIC AGENTS

Chemical Class	Possible Mechanism of Action

Barbiturates
    Mephobarbital (Mebaral)
    Phenobarbital (Solfoton)
    Primidone (Mysoline)
	Potentiate inhibitory effects of GABA; may also block excitatory effects of glutamate.

Benzodiazepines
    Clonazepam (Klonopin)
    Clorazepate (Tranxene; others)
    Diazepam (Valium; Vazepam)
    Lorazepam (Alzapam; Ativan)
	Potentiate inhibitory effects of GABA.

Carboxylic acids Valproic acid (Depakene; others)	Unclear; may hyperpolarize membrane through an effect on potassium channels; higher concentrations increase CNS GABA concentrations.
Dicarbamates Felbamate (Felbatol)	Unclear; may block excitatory effects of glutamate in CNS.

Hydantoins
    Ethotoin (Peganone)
    Mephenytoin (Mesantoin)
    Phenacemide (Phenurone)
    Phenytoin (Dilantin)
	Primary effect is to stabilize membrane by blocking sodium channels in repetitive-firing neurons; higher concentrations may also influence concentrations of other neurotransmitters (GABA, norepinephrine, others).

Iminostilbenes Carbamazepine (Tegretol)	Similar to hydantoins.

Oxazolidinediones
    Paramethadione (Paradione)
    Trimethadione (Tridione)
	Affect calcium channels; appear to inhibit spontaneous firing in thalamic neurons by limiting calcium entry.

Succinimides
    Ethosuximide (Zarontin)
    Methsuximide (Celontin)
    Phensuximide (Milontin)
	Similar to oxazolidinediones.

3

GABA = γ-aminobutyric acid.
From Ciccone, CD: Pharmacology in Rehabilitation, ed 2. FA Davis, Philadelphia, 1996, p 110, with permission.

COMMON METHODS OF TREATING SEIZURES

Seizure Type	Primary Agents	Alternative Agents
Generalized tonic-clonic and simple partial seizures	Carbamazepine, phenytoin	Phenobarbital, primidone, valproic acid
Absence	Ethosuximide, valproic acid	Clonazepam
Complex partial	Carbamazepine, phenytoin, valproic acid	Phenobarbital, primidone
Myoclonic	Valproic acid	Clonazepam

From Ciccone, CD: Pharmacology in Rehabilitation, ed 2. FA Davis, Philadelphia, 1996, p 113, with permission.

PHARMACOLOGIC VARIABLES OF COMMON ANTIEPILEPTIC DRUGS

Drug	Absorption	HalfLife (h)	Time to Reach Steady State (d)	Therapeutic Range (μg/ml)
Phenytoin	Slow	10–40	5–7	10–20
Carbamazepine	Slow to moderate	8–20	3–5	4–10
Valproic acid	Rapid	8–12	2–3	50–100
Phenobarbital	Moderate	50–150	2–3 wk	10–45
Primidone	Slow to moderate	6–18	2–3	5–15
Ethosuximide	Rapid	20–60	4–10	50–100

From Bruni, J: Epilepsy in adolescents and adults. In Rakel, RE (ed): Conn's Current Therapy. WB Saunders, Philadelphia, 1993, p 854, with permission.

IMPAIRED CONSCIOUSNESS

Causes of Coma

MANIFESTATIONS OF COMMON CAUSES OF UNCONSCIOUSNESS	
Condition	*Manifestations*
Acute alcoholism	Alcoholic breath; patient usually stuporous, not comatose, responds to noxious stimuli; face and conjunctivae hyperemic; normal or subnormal temperature; moderately dilated, equal pupils react to light; respirations deep and noisy, not stertorous; blood alcohol > 200 mg/dl
Cranial trauma	Coma onset sudden or gradual; often local evidence or history of injury (eg, scalp edema over fractures; bleeding from ear, nose, or throat); temperature normal or elevated; pupils usually unequal and sluggish or inactive; respirations vary (often slow or irregular); pulse variable (rapid initially, then slow); BP variable; reflexes often altered, often with incontinence and paralysis; CT or MRI reveals intracranial hemorrhage or skull fracture
Stroke (brainstem ischemia or acute brain hemorrhage)	Age > 40; with cardiovascular disease or hypertension; sudden onset, with signs of brain stem dysfunction; face often asymmetric; TPR variable; pupils usually unequal and inactive; focal neurologic signs common, including hemiplegia. MRI or CT reveals intracranial hemorrhage; if negative, diagnostic LP indicated
Epilepsy	History of "fits"; sudden, convulsive onset; incontinence common; TPR usually normal (possibly elevated after repeated convulsions); pupils reactive; tongue bitten or scarred from prior attacks
Diabetic acidosis	Onset gradual; skin dry, face flushed; breath odor fruity; temperature often subnormal; eyeballs may be soft; hyperventilation; glucosuria, ketonuria, hyperglycemia; metabolic acidosis in blood
Hypoglycemia	Onset may be acute with convulsions, usually preceded by lightheadedness, sweating, nausea, vomiting, palpitations, headache, abdominal pain, hunger; skin moist and

MANIFESTATIONS OF COMMON CAUSES OF UNCONSCIOUSNESS	
Condition	*Manifestations*
	pale; hypothermia; pupils reactive; deep reflexes exaggerated; positive Babinski's sign; hypoglycemia during attack
Syncope	Onset sudden, often associated with emotional crisis or heart block; coma seldom deep or prolonged; pallor; pulse slow at onset, later rapid and weak; prompt awakening if supine
Drugs	Cause of 70%–80% of acute coma of unknown cause

BP = blood pressure; CT = computed tomography; LP = lumbar puncture; MRI = magnetic resonance imaging; TPR = temperature, pulse, respirations.
From The Merck Manual, ed 16. Merck & Co, Rahway, NJ, 1992, p 1401, with permission.

IMPAIRED CONSCIOUSNESS (Continued)

Glasgow Coma Scale*

The Glasgow Coma Scale (see table that follows) is used to reflect changes in a patient's consciousness.* The scale can be used to quantify the degree of coma. Three indicators of consciousness are used: the stimulus needed to elicit eye opening, the type of verbal response, and the type of motor response. A score of 7 or less means that the patient is in coma, whereas a score of 9 or greater excludes the diagnosis of coma.

Eye Opening	Points	Best Verbal Response	Points	Best Motor Response	Points
Spontaneous Indicates arousal mechanisms in brain stem are active	4	**Oriented** Patient knows who and where he is, and the year, season, and month	5	**Obey Commands** Do not classify a grasp reflex or a change in posture as a response	6
To Sound Eyes open to any sound stimulus	3	**Confused** Responses to questions indicate varying degrees of confusion and disorientation	4	**Localized** Moves a limb to attempt to remove stimulus	5
To Pain Apply stimulus to limbs, not to face	2			**Flexor: Normal** Entire shoulder or arm is flexed in response to painful stimuli	4

Never	1	Inappropriate	3	Flexion: Abnormal	3
		Speech is intelligible but sustained conversation is not possible		Slow stereotyped assumption of decorticate rigidity posture in response to painful stimuli	
		Incomprehensible	2	Extension	2
		Unintelligible sounds such as moans and groans are made		Abnormal with adduction and internal rotation of the shoulder and pronation of the forearm	
		None	1	None	1
				Be certain that a lack of response is not due to a spinal cord injury	

*This scale, originally described in 1974 and further discussed in 1979 by Teasdale and his associates is widely used in assessing head injury patients, both at the time of the injury and as the patient is followed. The score is recorded every 2–3 d.

From Teasdale, G and Jennett, B: Assessment of coma and impaired consciousness: A practical scale. Lancet 2:81, 1974; and Teasdale, G et al: Adding up the Glasgow coma score. ACTA Neurochir (Suppl) 28:13, 1979.

DIAGNOSTIC FEATURES OF COMALIKE STATES

Diagnosis	Level of Consciousness	Voluntary Movement	Speech	Eye Responses	Limb Tone	Reflexes
Akinetic mute (apathetic—midbrain)	Lethargy	Little and infrequent; but when sufficiently stimulated, can move *all* extremities purposefully	With stimulation can produce normal, short phrases	Open when stimulated. Usually good eye contact	Usually normal; sometimes slight increase	Can be normal. Occasionally asymmetrical with pathologic reflexes
Akinetic mute (coma—vigil—septal)	Wakeful, with occasional outbursts. Some patients are somnolent	Little but purposeful; arms usually move much better than legs	Little; can occasionally produce normal phrases. Also, can have outbursts of unintelligible utterances	Open during much of the day in most patients. Eye contact variable	Often increased in legs	Frequently have increased leg reflexes. Babinski signs, snout, grasp often present

Apallic state (decorticate)	Awake; no meaningful interaction with environment	No or little purposeful movement; mostly reflex or mass movements	None or occasional grunting	Open, searching, but no real eye contact	Increased in all extremities. Extremities often in flexion	Increased in all extremities with pathologic reflexes
Persistent vegetative state	Awake; no or little interaction with environment	Usually little or none, depending upon areas of brain damaged. Mostly primitive postural reflexes	None or occasional grunts or groans. Some patients produce a few words	Open, searching, but no real eye contact	Variable, usually increased. Extremities often in flexion	Variable, usually increased with pathologic reflexes
Locked-in syndrome	Awake and alert; able to communicate meaningfully with examiners by eye movement	None or slight, except for eye movement	None	Open, with normal following and good eye contact. Some patients have restricted lateral gaze	Increased	Increased in all extremities

From Strub, RL and Black, FW: The Mental Status Examination in Neurology, ed 3. FA Davis, Philadelphia, 1993, p 38, with permission.

HYDROCEPHALUS

Classification of Chronic Hydrocephalus

Chronic hydrocephalus may produce dementia or mental retardation. The syndrome of acute hydrocephalus is a neurologic emergency and does not manifest itself as a dementia.

Nonobstructive (Ex Vacuo or Compensatory) Hydrocephalus

Nonobstructive hydrocephalus is due to degeneration or destruction of cerebral tissue with secondary increase in ventricular size. There is an increase in the volume of the cerebrospinal fluid (CSF) as a compensation for cerebral atrophy due to primary CNS disease. Nonobstructive hydrocephalus is seen with the following disorders:

1. Alzheimer's disease
2. Pick's disease
3. Multiple cerebral infarctions
4. Huntington's disease

FOR MORE INFORMATION

Samuels, MA: Manual of Neurologic Therapeutics, ed 5. Little, Brown, Boston, 1995.

Obstructive Hydrocephalus

Obstructive hydrocephalus is classified according to the site of the CSF blockage.

1. Communicating (normal pressure, low pressure, tension): Blockage is outside of the ventricular system; there is free communication between the ventricles and the subarachnoid space. Communicating hydrocephalus is seen with the following disorders:
   a. Postsubarachnoid hemorrhage
   b. Postmeningitis
   c. Idiopathic
2. Noncommunicating (internal): Blockage is within the ventricular system so that there is no flow between the ventricular system and the subarachnoid space. Noncommunicating hydrocephalus is seen with the following conditions:
   a. Aqueductal stenosis
   b. Masses compressing the fourth ventricle (e.g., cerebellar tumors)
   c. Malformation at the foramen magnum (e.g., Arnold-Chiari malformation and Dandy-Walker malformation)

SHUNTING PROCEDURES FOR HYDROCEPHALUS

Intracranial Shunts

In selected cases of noncommunicating hydrocephalus, an intracranial shunt may be used to divert CSF from the obstructed segment of the ventricular system to the subarachnoid space beyond the block. This procedure is usually reserved for cases in which the ventricular obstruction is not amenable to direct operation (e.g., pineal tumor) and in which the subarachnoid space is competent.

Features

1. Re-establishes a normal route for CSF flow and absorption
2. Performed with a minimal number of mechanical devices
3. Rarely requires revision to accommodate somatic growth

Procedures

1. **Third ventriculostomy shunt:** Establishment of a permanent fistula between the third ventricle and the basilar cistern. The most common technique employs the subfrontal approach.
2. **Ventriculocisternostomy (Torkildsen) shunt:** Diverting CSF from one lateral ventricle to the cisterna magna by means of a rubber tube or catheter. It is technically simpler than the third ventriculostomy shunt and can be used in cases in which the third ventricle is not grossly dilated or when the ventricle is directly involved by tumor.

Extracranial Shunts

These shunts divert CSF to the bloodstream or the body cavity. This procedure is the preferred method of treating most cases of communicating hydrocephalus that are not amenable to direct operations or intracranial shunts. Repeated revisions are usually required to accommodate somatic growth, and procedures are often associated with mechanical obstruction or infections.

Features

The majority of shunting devices consist of three integrated components:
1. Ventricular catheter
2. Connecting flush pump
3. Distal catheter

Procedures

1. **Ventriculoperitoneal shunt:** Diversion of CSF from one lateral ventricle to the peritoneal cavity. Considered safer and simpler than ventriculoatrial shunt and usually performed as the initial shunting procedure, particularly when somatic growth is a factor.
2. **Ventriculoatrial shunt:** Diversion of CSF from one lateral ventricle to the right atrium of the heart by means of a valve-regulated shunt. A catheter is introduced to the atrium via the facial or jugular vein. This procedure is considered to be the procedure of choice for patients with hydrocephalus not amenable to direct operation or intracranial shunting in whom somatic growth is complete.
3 **Direct cardiac shunt:** Direct implantation of ventricular shunt to the right atrium of the heart. It is a newly developed procedure that allows for somatic growth and holds promise as a single-stage operation.
4. Miscellaneous procedures:

Continued on following page

a. **Ventriculopleural shunt:** Useful alternative shunt in older children, particularly when objective proof of a functioning shunt is required and when atrial and peritoneal routes are unavailable.

b. **Lumbar subarachnoid-peritoneal shunt:** Procedure of choice in patients with pseudotumor cerebri requiring prolonged CSF drainage. Scoliosis can be a late complication.

c. **Lumbar subarachnoid-ureteral shunt:** Procedure requires removal of one kidney and is indicated only for cases of communicating hydrocephalus as a last resort.

FOR MORE INFORMATION

Milhorat, TH: Pediatric Neurosurgery. FA Davis, Philadelphia, 1978.

INNERVATION OF THE URINARY BLADDER AND RECTUM

Peripheral Nervous System for Voluntary Control

pudendal nerve (S2, S3, S4): Supplies the voluntary muscles of the external and urethral sphincters, which provide a means for voluntary control over these orifices. Sensory fibers to the mucosa of the anal canal and to the urethra are also supplied.

Autonomic Nervous System

sympathetic fibers: Reach the rectum by both the inferior mesenteric and the inferior hypogastric plexuses, and the urinary bladder through the inferior hypogastric plexus. Preganglionic fibers originate from the upper lumbar area. The afferents associated with the sympathetic system are associated with painful sensations (e.g., overdistension) from the bladder and rectum. The sympathetic efferents cause contraction of the internal anal and vesical sphincters, with relaxation of the muscular walls of these organs.

parasympathetic fibers: Reach the rectum and urinary bladder from the inferior hypogastric plexus. Preganglionic fibers enter this plexus by the pelvic splanchnic nerves. The afferents associated with the parasympathetic system carry information regarding normal sensations of bladder and rectal distension. The parasympathetic efferents supply the urinary bladder and the rectal muscle for micturition and defecation.

FOR MORE INFORMATION

Gilman, S and Newman, SW: Manter and Gatz's Essentials of Clinical Neuroanatomy and Neurophysiology, ed 9. FA Davis, Philadelphia, 1996.

INNERVATION OF THE BLADDER

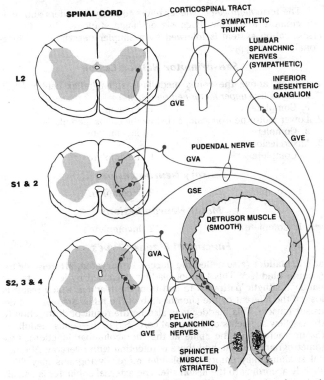

Autonomic innervation of the urinary bladder and associated somatic innervation of the sphincter.

THE NEUROGENIC BLADDER

Classification of Neurogenic Bladders

The term *neurogenic bladder* refers to many disorders and does not connote a specific diagnosis or single etiology. The following classification system is followed by a simpler description of functional bladder types.

Sensorimotor Neuron Lesion

1. Lesions above the conus medullaris spinal reflex center (commonly called *upper motor neuron lesions*)
   a. Complete   b. Incomplete
2. Lower motor neuron lesions (below the conus medullaris)
   a. Complete   b. Incomplete
3. Mixed lesions
   a. Complete   b. Incomplete

Sensory Neuron Lesions

1. Complete   2. Incomplete

Motor Neuron Lesions

1. Complete   2. Incomplete

Functional Bladder Types

atonic bladder (also called the flaccid, denervated, afferent, or hypotonic bladder): This type of bladder is caused by lesions to the parasympathetic pathways to and from the bladder, which result in loss of the afferent or the efferent limb of the reflex arc from the detrusor muscle. This bladder may also be the result of destruction to the last few segments of the spinal cord (S3) in the conus medullaris (as in fractures of the spine at the thoracolumbar junction). Cystometrograms are flat, and there is retention with overflow. Abdominal straining may empty the bladder more. Cystograms may differ slightly according to the lesion site. The external sphincter is usually tonically active for the denervated bladder, whereas for lesions of the sacral portion of the cord, the external sphincter is usually flaccid.

spastic bladder (also called the reflex or efferent neurogenic bladder): This type of bladder is caused by lesions of the higher pathways to and from the cortex, with preservation of the spinal sacral segments and their innervation. This bladder is commonly associated with disorders of the pyramidal tracts, as in gunshot wounds, multiple sclerosis, whiplash injuries, or transverse myelitis. The cystometrogram is "jumpy," showing many uninhibited contractions without the patient feeling the need to void. Bladder capacity is reduced, and the residual urine further decreases the true capacity. Incontinence, dribbling, and residual urine are often present with this type of bladder, even with training and medication.

FOR MORE INFORMATION

John Blandy, Lecture Notes on Urology, Blackford Scientific Publications, Oxford, 1976.

CYSTOMETROGRAMS

Cystometry is a urodynamic study used to assess bladder function. The resultant cystometrograph (CMG) reflects the contractility of the detrusor muscle and the bladder's ability to respond to changes in volume. The bladder's responsiveness to stretch is also evaluated. The patient's report of fullness, desire to void, and reports of pain are noted on the CMG.

The CMG is performed by introducing a catheter into the bladder of the recumbent patient in order to completely empty the bladder. Sterile water (at 37°C) or carbon dioxide is then introduced into the bladder as pressure is recorded by use of a manometer. Patients report any sensations of fullness and indicate when they feel the need to void. Patients are then instructed to void; during voiding, patients are asked to cease voiding.

During a normal cystometrogram, pressure within the bladder remains below 20 cm water until the urge to void occurs between 350 and 500 ml. At that point, pressure rises to 60–80 cm water. Uninhibited bladder contractions are absent during bladder filling. Bladder capacity is 350–600 ml with no residual urine.

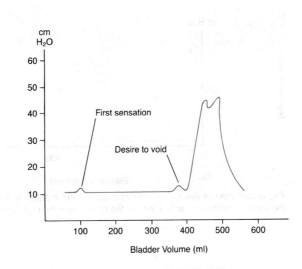

NORMAL CYSTOMETROGRAM

Continued on following page

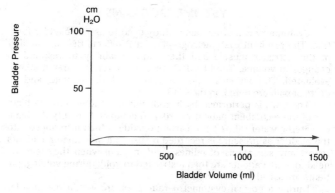

DENERVATED BLADDER

The denervated bladder resulting from injury to the parasympathetic pathways.

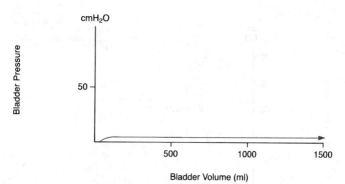

Bladder Volume (ml)

The destruction of the spinal reflex center for the bladder will result in the same condition as will injury of the parasympathetic pathways.

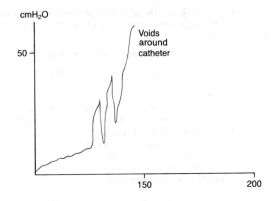

Cortical inhibition cut off by an upper-motor-neuron lesion.

FOR MORE INFORMATION

Blandy, J: Lecture Notes on Urology. Blackford Scientific Publications, Oxford, 1976.

Kottke, F and Lehman, J: Krusen's Handbook of Physical Medicine and Rehabilitation, ed 4. WB Saunders, Philadelphia, 1990.

BOWEL INCONTINENCE

Fecal continence is primarily dependent on two mechanisms:
1. The reflex action of the external anal sphincter initiated by contraction of the rectum.
2. The reservoir capability of the colon independent of sphincteric action *(reservoir continence)*

Effects of Spinal Cord Lesions on the Bowel

spinal shock: Fecal retention and paralysis of peristalsis is the immediate effect of spinal cord transection at any level. After the phase of spinal shock, one of the following conditions may occur, depending on the type of lesion.

Automatic Reflex Activity

For lesions above the thoracolumbar junction:
1. Peristalsis, bowel sounds, anal and bulbocavernosus reflexes return after spinal shock.
2. Intermittent automatic reflex defecation occurs following the return of reflex activity and peristalsis.
3. Greatly increased tone of the external anal sphincter (during the stage of hyperreflexia) results in increased resistance to the expulsive function of sigmoid and rectum.

Continued on following page

For lesions above T6, hyperreflexive abdominal muscles may interfere with the propulsive activity of the various compartments of the intestinal tract.

Autonomous Function

For lesions resulting in destruction of the lumbosacral or spinal roots, there is:

1. Lower motor neuron type paralysis (flaccid, denervation) with loss of normal response of sigmoid and rectum to distension.
2. Loss of tone (reflexes) of the external sphincter.
3. Impaired function of the levator ani.
4. Progressive accumulation of feces leading to impaction and fecal incontinence. The patient is usually dependent on digital evacuation aided by increased intra-abdominal pressure, suppositories, and enemas.

FOR MORE INFORMATION

Guttmann, L: Spinal Cord Injuries Comprehensive Management and Research, ed 2. Blackwell Scientific Publications, London, 1976.

MUSCULAR DYSTROPHY

Classification of Muscular Dystrophies

The following classification of muscular dystrophies is based on genetic criteria and distribution of muscle degeneration. Each category is followed by a list of characteristic features.

Duchenne Muscular Dystrophy
(Pseudohypertrophic Muscular Dystrophy)

- It is inherited as an X-linked recessive gene (passed to boys by their relatively unaffected mothers).
- Diagnosis is rarely made before 3 years.
- It is characterized by late onset of sitting, walking, and running.
- Waddling lordotic gait, difficulty in climbing stairs, and hypertrophy of calf muscles are typical.
- Deltoid, brachioradialis, and tongue may also be hypertrophied.
- Moderately severe form demonstrates Gowers' sign.
- Moderate to slight mental retardation is common (IQ is 85 on average).
- Majority develop cardiomyopathy; death occurs in 75% of patients before 20 years of age.

Becker Muscular Dystrophy
(Slowly Progressive Muscular Dystrophy)

- It is an X-linked recessive dystrophy resembling Duchenne's variety but less severe, with later onset, and survival is prolonged until middle adult life.
- It is characterized by proximal weakness of upper and lower extremities and pseudohypertrophy.
- Patient initially develops difficulty in gait, climbing stairs, and rising from the floor.
- Patient eventually develops contractures and skeletal deformi-

ties, but these are less conspicuous than with Duchenne's variety; early myocardial disease may develop.
- Mental retardation is less common than in Duchenne's variety.

Facioscapulohumeral Dystrophy
(of Landouzy-Déjérine)

- It is inherited as an autosomal dominant trait; it affects both sexes equally.
- It is characterized by rather benign and slowly progressive weakness of the face, shoulder, and upper arm.
- Onset is typically toward the end of the first decade or beginning of second.
- Less classical forms of this dystrophy type include infantile facioscapulohumeral dystrophy, facioscapulohumeral dystrophy with late exacerbation, and a form that is concurrent with Coats' syndrome.

Limb-Girdle Dystrophy

- It probably includes a group of disorders with progressive weakness of the hip and shoulder muscles.
- There is variety in the inheritance, age of onset, progression of the illness, and distribution and severity of weakness.
- Patients may eventually be confined to a wheelchair, but skeletal deformities are not frequent.
- Death may occur from cardiopulmonary complications and terminal pneumonia.

Humeroperoneal Muscular Dystrophy
(Emery-Dreifuss Disease)

- It is an X-linked recessive disorder.
- It is present during first decade of life; tendency to walk on toes and the development of elbow contractures are among the first manifestations.
- Patients develop wasting and weakness of scapulohumeroperoneal distribution that is very slowly progressive.
- Patients may develop cardiac conduction abnormalities that are threatening to life.

Scapuloperoneal Dystrophy

- It may be a variety of facioscapulohumeral dystrophy.
- It is often inherited as autosomal dominant, but an X-linked recessive pattern has also been described.
- Peroneal and anterior tibial muscle groups are involved early, followed by shoulder muscle weakness; patients may also have facial weakness.

Hereditary Distal Myopathy

- It is common in Sweden but less frequent elsewhere.
- Inheritance is autosomal dominant with onset between 40 and 60 years of age.
- It begins with clumsiness in the hands and then slowly pro-

Continued on following page

gresses and involves the feet and anterior compartment muscles of the leg.
- Typically it does not progress to total incapacity.

Ocular Myopathies

- Three types include ocular dystrophy, oculopharyngeal dystrophy, and oculocraniosomatic neuromuscular disease.
- Controversy exists as to whether these ocular diseases are true myopathies.

	FUNCTIONAL STAGES OF DUCHENNE MUSCULAR DYSTROPHY
Stage	Description
I	Walks and climbs stairs without assistance
II	Walks and climbs stairs with the aid of railings
III	Walks and climbs stairs slowly with the aid of railings (greater than 25 s for eight standard steps)
IV	Walks unassisted and rises from chair but cannot climb stairs
V	Walks unassisted but cannot rise from chair or climb stairs
VI	Walks only with assistance or walks independently with long-leg braces
VII	Walks in long-leg braces but requires assistance for balance
VIII	Stands in long-leg braces but unable to walk, even with assistance
IX	Remains in a wheelchair or bed

FOR MORE INFORMATION

Brooke, MH: A Clinician's View of Neuromuscular Diseases, ed 2. Williams & Wilkins, Baltimore, 1986.
Molnar, GE (ed): Pediatric Rehabilitation, ed 2. Williams & Wilkins, Baltimore, 1992.

COMMUNICATION DISORDERS

Aphasia

Aphasia is a disturbance to language caused by focal or diffuse damage to the language areas of the brain. Aphasia results in linguistic errors in word choice, comprehension, or syntax rather than in problems of articulation or pronunciation. The term *aphasia* encompasses a variety of syndromes that are described below.

Types of Aphasia

anomic aphasia: Nominal or amnesia aphasia; characterized by difficulty in naming objects and by word-finding problems. Reading, writing, and comprehension are usually unimpaired. A variety of lesions in the dominant hemisphere can result in anomia. The most severe forms usually involve the second and third temporal gyri and the parietotemporal area.

Broca's aphasia: Expressive aphasia; characterized by severe difficulty in verbal expression and mild difficulty in understanding complex syntax. Comprehension of both spoken and written language is excellent; verbal output is telegraphic or agrammatic. Patients are also impaired in object naming and in writing abilities. Most patients with Broca's aphasia are right hemiplegics with large, deep lesions affecting the inferior frontal lobe (this includes Broca's area 44). Language recovery is slow, with fluency and grammatical complexity often permanently impaired.

conduction aphasia: Aphasia characterized by deficits in the repetition of spoken language, halting speech with word-finding pauses, and literal paraphasia (letter or whole-word substitutions). Comprehension and reading are not usually impaired, but there may be errors in object naming and writing. Lesions causing this type of aphasia are usually in the areas of the supramarginal gyrus and arcuate fasciculus or the insula and auditory cortex

crossed aphasia: A transient aphasia that often occurs in right-handed patients with a right-hemisphere lesion and no history of left-hemisphere damage or familial left-handedness. Patients are often agrammatic with decreased comprehension. Naming abilities are preserved. Reading and writing are rarely impaired.

global aphasia: The most common and severe form of aphasia, it is characterized by spontaneous speech that is either absent or reduced to a few stereotyped words or sounds. Comprehension is reduced or absent. Repetition, reading, and writing are impaired to the same level as spontaneous speech. Lesions are usually large, involving the entire perisylvian area of the frontal, temporal, and parietal lobes. An occlusion of the internal carotid area or the middle cerebral artery at its origin is the most common cause. Prognosis for the recovery of speech is poor.

subcortical (thalamic) aphasia: Aphasia is associated with vascular lesions of the thalamus, putamen, caudate, or internal capsule. Patients are dysarthric and have mild anomia and comprehension deficits.

transcortical aphasia: The linguistic opposite of conduction aphasia. Patients with transcortical motor aphasia are able to repeat, comprehend, and read well but have restricted spontaneous speech. Patients with transcortical sensory aphasia can repeat words but do not comprehend the meaning of the words. Spontaneous speech and naming are fluent but paraphasic (letter or whole-word substitutions). Some patients have combined motor and sensory transcortical aphasia. Patients with the complete syndrome can only repeat and tend to echo what they hear (echolalia). Lesions are extensive.

Continued on following page

Wernicke's aphasia: The linguistic opposite of Broca's aphasia, characterized by fluent, effortless, well-articulated speech that is frequently out of context and containing many paraphasias (letter or whole-word substitutions). There are severe disturbances of auditory comprehension resulting in inappropriate responses to questions. Reading, writing, and repetition of words are also impaired, and naming is paraphasic. Patients are often mistakenly thought to have psychotic illnesses. The lesion is in the posterior language area (area 1) and usually includes the superior temporal gyrus (area 22), where auditory comprehension is processed.

Agraphia

A syndrome in which writing ability is disturbed by an acquired brain lesion. Agraphia is not an abnormality in writing mechanics. With the exception of patients with pure word deafness, all aphasic patients have some degree of agraphia. Lesions in the posterior language area (where the message is translated into visual symbols) or the frontal language area (for motor processing) cause agraphia. There are rare instances in which isolated pure agraphia has been seen.

Aprosody

A syndrome in which the melodic qualities of language are disturbed by an acquired brain lesion. A dramatic change is heard in the intonation patterns of expressive language that results in a monotonal delivery of speech. Perisylvian lesions and anterior lesions can result in aprosody. Patients with a posterior lesion cannot comprehend the prosodic qualities of language but can express themselves with proper intonation.

Dysarthria (Articulation Disturbances)

Speech disorders that result from loss of control of the muscles of articulation. These disturbances may be due to a variety of diseases. Among the structures that can be implicated in lesions causing dysarthria are the cortical motor area, basal ganglia, corticobulbar tract, motoneurons of the 9th, 10th, and 12th cranial nerves, and the muscles used for articulation.

FOR MORE INFORMATION

Goodglass, H and Kaplan, E: Assessment of Aphasia and Related Disorders. Lea & Febiger, Philadelphia, 1972.

TESTS OF LANGUAGE PERFORMANCE

Comprehensive Aphasia Batteries

aphasia language performance scales: A 30-minute test of communicative ability designed to determine whether a patient is suitable for speech therapy.

Boston Diagnostic Aphasia Examination: Assesses all areas of language in a systematic fashion. The test is used for describing aphasic disorders, planning treatment, and research.

Communication Abilities in Daily Living: A test for functional communication ability in aphasic adults, primarily used by speech therapists to identify which aspects of communication should be treated.

Multilingual Aphasia Examination: A research-derived examination that evaluates the major components of speech and language. Subtests can be administered independently.

Neurosensory Center Comprehensive Examination for Aphasia: Assesses 20 different components of language and includes tests for tactile and visual functioning. It is oriented to neurolinguistic research.

Porch Index of Communicative Ability (PICA): A psychometrically oriented test battery used to quantify verbal, gestural, and graphic language abilities, as well as a variety of other communicative functions. It is most frequently used by speech pathologists to establish baseline levels, predict possible recovery, and to measure treatment outcome or spontaneous recovery.

Western Aphasia Battery: An adaptation and standardization of the Boston Diagnostic Aphasia Examination, it assesses a number of functions related to communication, such as arithmetic, praxis, constructional ability, and Raven's Matrices. This relatively new test has not been fully evaluated for clinical and research applications.

Tests of Language Abilities

Boston Naming Test: A test of single-word expressive vocabulary or naming ability that is the reciprocal of the Peabody Picture Vocabulary Test–Revised (PPVT-R). It requires the patient to name a 60-item series of pictured objects ordered in increasing difficulty. If the patient is unable to name an item, the examiner first provides a categorical cue and then a phonemic cue. Provisional norms are provided for children, normal adults, and aphasic adults.

Peabody Picture Vocabulary Test—Revised (PPVT-R): A recently revised and standardized test of single-word vocabulary comprehension. It contains two equivalent sets of stimuli plates that contain four pictures. There are also two associated lists of 175 words that are ordered in ascending difficulty. The patient must indicate which of each set of four pictures is most like the word provided by the examiner. Norms are provided for subjects between 2½ and 41 years of age.

Sentence Repetition Tests: The Spreen-Benton Sentence Repetition Test and the Sentence Repetition Test are the two most widely used sentence repetition tests. Both tests evaluate the patient's ability to repeat immediately a series of sentences of increasing length and semantic complexity. Normative data are available for normal and neurologically impaired adults.

Token Tests: Simple-to-administer tests of language comprehension. Plastic tokens are manipulated by the patient in response to a series of hierarchically ordered verbal commands. Comprehension is there-

Continued on following page

fore tested at several levels of difficulty. It is useful in the assessment of the aphasic patient, as well as patients with comprehension deficits secondary to dementia or other neurologic conditions.

verbal fluency tests: Verbal fluency—the ability to produce spontaneous speech fluently without undue word-finding difficulty—is typically evaluated by tabulating the number of words the patient produces within a restricted category and time limit (usually 60 s). Two easily and commonly administered tests are the Animal Naming Test and Controlled Oral Word Association Test. There are normative data for both tests.

FROM

Lezak, MD: Neuropsychological Assessment, ed 5. Oxford University Press, New York, 1995, with permission.

COMMON PERCEPTUAL AND COMMUNICATION PROBLEMS IN PERSONS WITH HEMIPLEGIA

Clinical Problem	Examples of Functional Deficits
LESION: LEFT HEMISPHERE	
Aphasias	Lacks functional speech
Ideomotor and ideational apraxias	Cannot plan and execute serial steps in performances
Number alexia	Cannot recognize symbols to do simple computations
Right-left discrimination	Unable to distinguish right from left on self or reverse on others
Slow in organization and performance	Cannot remember what he or she intended to do next
LESION: RIGHT HEMISPHERE	
Visuospatial	Cannot orient self to changes in environment while going from one treatment area to another
Left unilateral neglect of self	Generally unaware of objects to left and propels wheelchair into them
Body image	Distorted awareness and impression of self
Dressing apraxia	Applies sweater to right side, but unable to do left-side application
Constructional apraxia	Unable to transpose two-dimensional instructions into three-dimensional structure, as per "do-it-yourself" kits
Illusions of shortening of time	Arrives extremely early for appointments
Number concepts—spatial type	Unable to align columns and rows of digits
Rapid organization and performance	Makes errors from haste; may cause accidents
Depth of language skills	May mention task related to prestroke occupation, but cannot go into details of it

3

PARKINSON'S DISEASE

PROGNOSTIC CLASSIFICATION OF PARKINSON'S DISEASE

	Schwab Classification of Progression*		Hoehn and Yahr Classification of Disability†	
Grade	Chronology of Disease Manifestations	Comments	Stage	Character of Disability
1	Symptoms generally remain stable for at least 5 y after diagnosis.	Diagnosis may be uncertain. Minimal therapy is required. Ability to live independently is usually not threatened.	I	Minimal or absent; unilateral if present.
2	Some evidence of progression may be observed after 5 y. Disease may remain unilateral.	With appropriate pharmacotherapy, most patients can remain independent.	II	Minimal bilateral or midline involvement. Balance not impaired.
3	Marked progression is observed after 3–5 y. Disease may remain unilateral.	Partial incapacitation is likely, but most patients are still able to live independently 10 y after diagnosis.	III	Impaired righting reflexes. Unsteadiness when turning or rising from chair. Some activities are restricted, but patient can live independently and continue some forms of employment.

| 4 | Disease progresses to severe tremor and rigidity after 3–5 y. Manifestations are usually bilateral after 8–10 y. | Patient may remain ambulatory, but serious disability may supervene. | IV | All symptoms present and severe. Requires help with some activities of daily living. |
| 5 | Onset of disease is abrupt. Severe bilateral tremor, rigidity, and akinesia are present within a few months. Marked incapacity and motor deficiency are present within 1 y. | Outlook is for severe or total disability. | V | Confined to bed or wheelchair unless aided. |

*From Schwab, RS: Progression and prognosis in Parkinson's disease. J Nerv Ment Dis 130:556, 1960.
†From Hoehn, MM and Yahr, MD: Parkinsonism: Onset, progression, and mortality. Neurology 17:427, 1967.

Continued on following page

OVERVIEW OF DRUG THERAPY IN PARKINSON'S DISEASE

Drug	Mechanism of Action	Special Comments
Levodopa	Resolves dopamine deficiency by being converted to dopamine after crossing blood-brain barrier	Still the best drug for resolving parkinsonian symptoms; long-term use limited by side effects and decreased efficiency
Dopamine agonists (bromocriptine, pergolide)	Directly stimulate dopamine receptors in basal ganglia	Often used in combination with levodopa to get optimal benefits with lower dose of each drug
Anticholinergics	Inhibit excessive acetylcholine influence caused by dopamine deficiency	Use in Parkinson's disease limited by frequent side effects
Amantadine	Unclear; may stimulate release of remaining dopamine	May be used alone during early/mild stages or added to drug regimen when levodopa loses effectiveness
Selegiline	Inhibits the enzyme that breaks down dopamine in the basal ganglia; enables dopamine to remain active for longer periods of time	May also have neuroprotective effects; can delay the degeneration of dopaminergic neurons

From Ciccone, CD: Pharmacology in Rehabilitation, ed 2. FA Davis, Philadelphia, 1996, p 122, with permission.

ANTICHOLINERGIC DRUGS USED IN TREATING PARKINSONISM

Generic Name	Trade Name	Usual Daily Dose (mg)
Benztropine mesylate	Cogentin	0.5–6.0
Biperiden	Akineton	6.0–8.0
Ethopropazine	Parsidol	50–600
Procyclidine	Kemadrin	7.5–20.0
Trihexyphenidyl	Artane	6.0–10.0
Orphenadrine	Disipal	150–250
Diphenhydramine*	Benadryl	75–200

*Antihistamine drugs with anticholinergic properties.
From Ciccone, CD: Pharmacology in Rehabilitation, ed 2. FA Davis, Philadelphia, 1996, p 129, with permission.

MANIFESTATIONS OF PARKINSON'S DISEASE

Cardinal Manifestations of Parkinson's Disease

Tremor

Rigidity

Bradykinesia

Postural instability

Secondary Manifestations of Parkinson's Disease

Incoordination	Edema
Micrographia	Scoliosis
Blurred vision	Kyphosis
Impaired upgaze	Pain and sensory symptoms
Blepharospasm	Seborrhea
Glabellar reflex	Constipation
Dysarthria	Urinary urgency, hesitancy, and frequency
Dysphagia reflex	Loss of libido
Sialorrhea	Impotence
Masked facies	Freezing
Hand and foot deformities	Dementia
Dystonia	Depression

From Stern, M and Hurtig, H: The Comprehensive Management of Parkinson's Disease. PMA, New York, 1988, p 4, with permission.

COGNITIVE FUNCTIONING

Rancho Los Amigos Cognitive Functioning Scale

I–**No response** Patient appears to be in a deep sleep and is completely unresponsive to any stimuli.

II–**Generalized response** Patient reacts inconsistently and nonpurposefully to stimuli in a nonspecific manner. Responses are limited and often the same regardless of stimulus presented. Responses may be physiologic changes, gross body movements, and/or vocalization.

III–**Localized responses** Patient reacts specifically but inconsistently to stimuli. Responses are directly related to the type of stimulus presented. May follow simple commands in an inconsistent, delayed manner, such as closing eyes or squeezing hand.

IV–**Confused-agitated** Patient is in heightened state of activity. Behavior is bizarre and nonpurposeful relative to immediate environment. Does not discriminate among persons or objects; is unable to cooperate directly with treatment efforts. Verbalizations frequently are incoherent and/or inappropriate to the environment; confabulation may be present. Gross attention to environment is very brief; selective attention is often nonexistent. Patient lacks short-term and long-term recall.

V–**Confused-inappropriate** Patient is able to respond to simple commands fairly consistently. However, with increased complexity of commands or lack of any external structure, responses are nonpurposeful, random, or fragmented. Demonstrates gross attention to the environment but is highly distractible and lacks ability to focus attention on a specific task. With structure, may be able to converse on a social automatic level for short periods of time. Verbalization is often inappropriate and confabulatory. Memory is severely impaired; often shows inappropriate use of objects; may perform previously learned tasks with structure but is unable to learn new information.

VI–**Confused-appropriate** Patient shows goal-directed behavior but is dependent on external input or direction. Follows simple directions consistently and shows carry-over for relearned problems but appropriate to the situation; past memories show more depth and detail than recent memory.

VII–**Automatic-appropriate** Patient appears appropriate and oriented within hospital and home settings: goes through daily routine automatically, but frequently robotlike with minimal to absent confusion and has shallow recall of activities. Shows carry-over for new learning but a decreased rate. With structure is able to initiate social or recreational activities; judgment remains impaired.

VIII–**Purposeful and appropriate** Patient is able to recall and to integrate past and recent events and is aware of and responsive to environment. Shows carry-over for new learning and needs no supervision once activities are learned. May continue to show a decreased ability relative to premorbid abilities, abstract reasoning, tolerance for stress, and judgment in emergencies or unusual circumstances.

FROM

Rehabilitation of the Head Injured Adult: Comprehensive Physical Management. Professional Staff Association, Rancho Los Amigos Hospital, Downey, CA, 1979, with permission.

BRAINTREE HOSPITAL COGNITIVE CONTINUUM	
Level	*Description*
1 Arousal	The patient has difficulty initiating attention to purposeful tasks. The patient's behavior is purposeless, reflexive, inconsistent, and dependent in all functional areas. They may show some visual tracking and are usually not vocal.
2 Attention	
Low Level	The patient initiates attention but has difficulty sustaining attention. Patient is able to follow one-step commands but inconsistently. The patient may function automatically in overlearned behaviors. Patient does not initiate activities and may wander if left unsupervised.
High Level	The patient's main deficit area is in sustaining and switching attention. The patient is distractible and perseverative. He or she may recall pieces of information but is unable to integrate information.
3 Discrimination	Patient is able to sustain and to switch attention sufficiently to integrate small amounts of information. Patient initiates activities but may still show some perseveration and impulsivity. Behavior can be partly modified by feedback. Recall over time is improved.
4 Organization	
Low Level	Patient can integrate multiple pieces of information for a task but tends to be concrete and have difficulty sequencing the task. Patient can begin simple problem solving.

Continued on following page

Level	Description
High Level	Patient can use selective attention to perceive stimuli or task elements accurately, select a strategy, and reach a solution. Patient continues to be concrete, has trouble generalizing and carrying over learning from one setting to another. In stressful situations, shows breakdown in cognitive function.
5 Higher-level cognitive function	The patient is able to do complex problem solving but is limited owing to limited flexibility, insight, social behavior, and endurance. The patient is susceptible to breakdown of behavior outside of a structured setting (e.g., school or work). In stressful situations, shows preserved cognitive functions. Cognitive processing is slow.

From Braintree Hospital Cognitive Continuum, Braintree, MA, with permission.

COORDINATION

COORDINATION TESTS (in alphabetical order*)

Test	Description
Alternate heel to knee; heel to toe	From a supine position, the patient is asked to touch his knee and big toe alternately with the heel of the opposite extremity.
Alternate nose to finger	The patient alternately touches the tip of his nose and the tip of the therapist's finger with the index finger. The position of the therapist's finger may be altered during testing to assess ability to change distance, direction, and force of movement.
Drawing a circle	The patient draws an imaginary circle in the air with either upper or lower extremity (a table or the floor also may be used). This also may be done using a figure-eight pattern. This test may be performed in the supine position for lower extremity assessment.
Finger to finger	Both shoulders are abducted to 90° with the elbows extended. The patient is asked to bring both hands toward the midline and approximate the index fingers from opposing hands.
Finger to nose	The shoulder is abducted to 90° with the elbow extended. The patient is asked to bring the tip of the index finger to the tip of the nose. Alterations may be made in the initial starting position to assess performance from different planes of motion.
Finger opposition	The patient touches the tip of the thumb to the tip of each finger in sequence. Speed may be gradually increased.

Continued on following page

3

453

COORDINATION (Continued)

COORDINATION TESTS (in alphabetical order* (Continued)

Test	Description
Finger to therapist's finger	The patient and therapist sit opposite each other. The therapist's index finger is held in front of the patient. The patient is asked to touch the tip of the index finger to the therapist's index finger. The position of the therapist's finger may be altered during testing to assess ability to change distance, direction, and force of movement.
Fixation or position holding	Upper extremity: The patient holds arms horizontally in front. Lower extremity: The patient is asked to hold the knee in an extended position.
Heel on shin	From the supine position, patient slides the heel of one foot up and down the shin of the opposite lower extremity.
Mass grasp	An alternation is made between opening and closing fist (from finger flexion to full extension). Speed may be gradually increased.
Pointing and past-pointing	The patient and therapist are opposite each other, either sitting or standing. Both patient and therapist bring shoulders to a horizontal position of 90° of flexion with elbows extended. Index fingers are touching, or the patient's finger may rest lightly on the therapist's. The patient is asked to fully flex the shoulder (fingers will be pointing toward ceiling) and then return to the horizontal position such that index fingers will again approximate. Both arms should be tested, either separately or simultaneously. A normal response consists of an accurate return to the starting position. In an abnormal response, there is typically a "past-pointing," or movement beyond the target. Several variations to this test include movements in other directions such as toward 90° of shoulder abduction or toward 0° of shoulder flexion (finger will point toward floor).

	Following each movement, the patient is asked to return to the initial horizontal starting position.
Pronation/supination	With elbows flexed to 90° and held close to body, the patient alternately turns his palms up and down. This test also may be performed with shoulders flexed to 90° and elbows extended. Speed may be gradually increased. The ability to reverse movements between opposing muscle groups can be assessed at many joints. Examples include active alternation between flexion and extension of the knee, ankle, elbow, fingers, and so forth.
Rebound test	The patient is positioned with the elbow flexed. The therapist applies sufficient manual resistance to produce an isometric contraction of biceps. Resistance is suddenly released. Normally, the opposing muscle group (triceps) will contract and "check" movement of the limb. Many other muscle groups can be tested for this phenomenon, such as the shoulder abductors or flexors, and elbow extensors.
Tapping (foot)	The patient is asked to "tap" the ball of one foot on the floor without raising the knee; heel maintains contact with floor.
Tapping (hand)	With the elbow flexed and the forearm pronated, the patient is asked to "tap" his hand on the knee.
Toe to examiner's finger	From a supine position, the patient is instructed to touch his great toe to the examiner's finger. The position of finger may be altered during testing to assess ability to change distance, direction, and force of movement.

*Tests should be performed first with eyes open and then with eyes closed. Abnormal responses include a gradual deviation from the "holding" position and/or a diminished quality of response with vision occluded. Unless otherwise indicated, tests are performed with the patient in a sitting position.

From O'Sullivan, SB and Schmitz, TJ: Physical Rehabilitation: Assessment and Treatment, ed 3. FA Davis, Philadelphia, 1994, p 102, with permission.

TESTS FOR COMMON DISTURBANCES THAT AFFECT COORDINATION (in alphabetical order)

Deficit	Sample Test
Asthenia	Fixation or position holding (upper and lower extremity) Application of manual resistance to assess muscle strength
Bradykinesia	Walking, observation of arm swing Walking, alterations in speed and direction Request that a movement or gait activity be stopped abruptly Observation of functional activities
Disturbances of gait	Walk along a straight line Walk sideways, backward March in place Alter speed of ambulatory activities Walk in a circle
Disturbances of posture	Fixation or position holding (upper and lower extremity) Displacement of balance unexpectedly in sitting or standing Standing, alterations in base of support Standing, one foot directly in front of the other Standing on one foot
Dysdiadochokinesia	Finger to nose Alternate nose to finger Pronation/supination Knee flexion/extension Walking with alternations in speed
Dysmetria	Pointing and past-pointing Drawing a circle or figure eight Heel on shin Placing feet on floor markers while walking
Hypotonia	Passive movement Deep tendon reflexes
Movement decomposition	Finger to nose Finger to therapist's finger Alternate heel to knee Toe to examiner's finger
Rigidity	Passive movement Observation during functional activities Observation of resting posture(s)

TESTS FOR COMMON DISTURBANCES THAT AFFECT COORDINATION (in alphabetical order)	
Deficit	**Sample Test**
Tremor (intention)	Observation during functional activities (tremor will typically increase as target is approached or when the patient attempts to hold a position)
	Alternate nose to finger
	Finger to finger
	Finger to therapist's finger
	Toe to examiner's finger
Tremor (postural)	Observation of normal standing posture
Tremor (resting)	Observation of patient at rest
	Observation during functional activities (tremor will diminish significantly or disappear)

3

SENSORY ORGANIZATION TEST
FOR POSTURAL CONTROL

1. Normal vision, fixed support

2. Absent vision, fixed support

3. Sway-referenced vision, fixed support

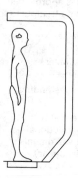
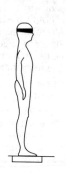
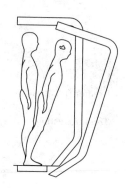

4. Normal vision, sway referenced support

5. Absent vision, sway referenced support

6. Sway referenced vision and support

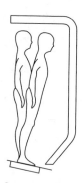
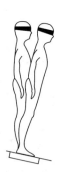
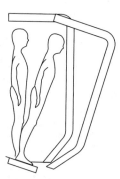

Sensory Organization Test on Equitest device. Upper row—fixed surface support—and lower row—sway-referenced support—under conditions of normal vision (left column), no vision (center column), and sway-referenced vision (right column). These six tests provide informatioin for assessing visual, somatosensory, and vestibular contributions to postural stability.

FOR MORE INFORMATION

Shumway-Cook, A and Wollacott, M: Control of posture and balance. In Shumway-Cook, A and Wollacott, M (eds): Motor Control. Williams & Wilkins, Baltimore, 1995, pp 119–142.

STANCE PHASE

Deviation	Cause
Ankle and Foot	
Equinus gait	Excessive activity of the gastrocnemius muscle.
	Plantar flexion contracture.
Varus foot	Excessive activity of the tibialis anterior, tibialis posterior, or toe flexor muscles causes the foot to come down on the lateral surface at heel strike.
Painful short steps	Contraction of the toe flexors causes excessive pressure on the toes and results in the patient taking short steps to minimize stance time and rollover.
Excessive flexion	Flexion contracture.
	Excessive dorsiflexion.
	Poor position sense.
	Weak knee quadriceps.
Hyperextension	Plantar flexion contracture.
	Poor position sense.
	Excessive activity of the quadriceps muscles.
	Compensatory locking of the knee to adjust for weak knee extensors (patient leans forward to mechanically lock the knee).
Lateral (Trendelenburg or gluteus medius) limb	Weak hip abductors.
Scissoring	Excessive activity of the adductors.
Improper positioning of the hip	Weakness of hip girdle.
	Poor position sense.

Continued on following page

COMMON GAIT DEVIATIONS SEEN IN PATIENTS WITH HEMIPLEGIA (Continued)

STANCE PHASE

Deviation	Cause
Trunk and Pelvis	
Flexed trunk	Compensation for weak knee flexors (the patient brings center of gravity forward).
	Weak hip extensors.
Improper positioning	Poor position sense.
Lack of pelvic rotation	Weakness and lack of control of pelvic girdle muscle.

SWING PHASE

Deviation	Cause
Ankle and Foot	
Equinus gait	Excessive activity of the gastrocnemius.
	Plantar flexion contracture.
	Weak dorsiflexors.
Varus foot	Excessive activity of the tibialis anterior.
	Weakness of peroneals and toe extensors.
Equinovarus	Excessive activity of the triceps surae.
Excessive dorsiflexion	Part of powerful flexor synergy pattern.

Based on O'Sullivan, SB and Schmitz, TJ: Physical Rehabilitation: Assessment and Treatment, ed 3. FA Davis, Philadelphia, 1994, p 342.

PRINCIPLES IN TEACHING MOTOR SKILLS: A STRATEGY FOR TASK ANALYSIS

1. Identify the task(s) and specify the goal and subgoals.
2. Amass information concerning:
   a. The *action*, including classification of the function of the action and movement.
   b. The *environment*, including the influence of both direct and indirect conditions.
   c. The *mover/patient*, including his/her characteristics, abilities, and whether the minimal prerequisite skills for success are present.
   d. The *prerequisite skills* required of the client.
   e. The *expectations* of outcome and movement outcomes.
3. Develop a strategy to make up for any deficits identified in #2.
4. Plan the intervention strategy based upon the preceding information concerning the individual-task-environment interaction.
   a. With the broader context in mind, systematically plan the action-goal-task encounter and include an observational strategy focusing upon the critical aspects of the action and outcomes that can be used for patient feedback and evaluation of the effectiveness of the strategy.
   b. Structure the environment for appropriate task-action encounter, including attention to the broadest range of conditions possible.
   c. Clarify the goal and subgoals.
5. Effect the strategy.
   a. Observe the performance of the mover.
   b. Record *what happened:* what was the outcome, and what was the approach and effect of the movement solution?
6. Evaluate the observations.
   a. Compare *expectations* and *what happened.*
   b. Provide feedback based on the comparison above and assist the mover/learner in making decisions about the next encounter.
   c. With the mover, plan the next intervention/task-action encounter.

Based on Arend, S and Higgins, JR: A strategy for the classification, subjective analysis and observation of human movement. J Human Movement Studies 2:36, 1976. As appearing in Craik, RA and Otis, CA: Gait Analysis: Theory and Application. Mosby Year Book, St. Louis, 1995, p 70, with permission.

PRINCIPLES IN TEACHING MOTOR SKILLS: SUBSTRATE CATEGORIES FOR IDENTIFICATION OF PREREQUISITE SKILLS

1. **Postural control:** appropriate integration of body and limb orientation for stability and transport.

2. **Dynamic equilibrium:** maintaining balance during all forms of movement, including stopping, initiating, and maintaining locomotion.

3. **Exploratory movements:** informing the mover about the environment and physical world; functionally incorporated into ongoing actions in order to support perceptual processes.

4. **Independent arm use:** allows mover to manipulate devices in the service of locomotion or to simultaneously engage in two tasks (dual task condition).

5. **Integration of postural control and limb manipulation:** progressively larger and more efficient and successful action units are incorporated into functionally larger and more appropriate units.

6. **Symmetric and asymmetric use of torso and/or limbs:** reciprocal and symmetric arm swing or asymmetric arm use when carrying an object during locomotion.

7. **Differential relaxation:** absence or presence of efficient use of muscle tensions in producing the movement required for the realization of the action.

8. **Use of momentum:** incorporating the motion already in effect into the ongoing movement or action; the use of existing internal or external force in the service of the ongoing action in order to minimize the energy production needs of the muscle.

9. **Generation of force:** identify what force problems are to be solved for any task and what is required by the mover to generate the appropriate force.

10. **Absorbing force:** task constraint requiring absorption of force generated either internally or externally; going down a ramp or stairs as contrasted with ascending same.

Based on Arend, S and Higgins, JR: A strategy for the classification, subjective analysis and observation of human movement. J Human Movement Studies 2:36, 1976. As appearing in Craik, RA and Otis, CA: Gait Analysis: Theory and Application. Mosby Year Book, St. Louis, 1995, p 73, with permission.

PRINCIPLES IN TEACHING MOTOR SKILLS: PRACTITIONER'S ROLE IN INSTRUCTION AND PRACTICE

1. Facilitate the development of motor skills.
2. Provide a nurturing, safe, supportive, and facilitory environment for bringing about change in functional movements.
3. Analyze tasks.
4. Identify prerequisite skills required of task(s) and compensate deficits identified.
5. Clarify the goal of the movement and minimize goal confusion.
6. Establish appropriate conditions for understanding task and task conditions:
   - Observation
   - Demonstration
   - Functional problem solution
   - Clarification of perceptual demands and relevant environmental features
7. Identify the critical features of the movement for both observation and for instruction and practice.
8. Select tasks requiring a variety of locomotion strategies that incorporate dual task and varied environmental conditions.
9. Capitalize on learner's successes and failures.
10. Provide feedback appropriate to task and skill level of learner.
11. Employ appropriate motivational strategies.

From Craik, RA and Otis, CA: Gait Analysis: Theory and Application. Mosby Year Book, St. Louis, 1995, p 74, with permission.

BRUNNSTROM'S SIX STAGES OF RECOVERY FROM HEMIPLEGIA

Stage	Movement	Spasticity	Evaluation Method
One	None	Absent	No voluntary movement is present; little or no resistance to passive movement.
Two	Weak associated movements in synergy; little or no active finger flexion	Developing	When movement is attempted, there are associated movements in synergy (in the upper extremity seen first with flexion).
Three	All movements are in synergy; mass grasp in hand	Marked	Full upper extremity synergy; hip, knee, and ankle flexion are coupled in either sitting or standing.
Four	Some deviation from synergies; lateral prehension and semivoluntary finger extension	Decrease	The patient in this stage can: (1) place his hand behind his back; (2) flex at the glenohumeral joint with his elbow extended; (3) pronate and supinate his forearm while the elbow is flexed to 90°; (4) sit and dorsiflex his foot while keeping the foot on the floor; (5) sit and slide his foot on the floor by flexing his knee past 90°.

| Five | Almost free from synergies; palmar prehension and voluntary mass extension of digits | Further decrease from stage four | The patient in this stage can perform the tests for stage four with greater ease and: (1) abduct at the glenohumeral joint with the elbow extended; (2) flex at the shoulder joint past 90° with the elbow extended; (3) pronate and supinate the forearm with the elbow extended, especially with abduction at the glenohumeral joint; (4) stand non-weight-bearing with the affected limb, flex the knee, and extend at the hip; (5) stand with the heel forward, knee extended, and dorsiflex the ankle. |
| Six | Free of synergy, slightly awkward; all types of prehension (grasps) can be controlled; individual finger movements present | Present only during active rapid movements | The patient in this stage can: perform the test for stage five with greater ease and: (1) stand and abduct the hip; (2) sit, reciprocally contract the medial and lateral hamstring muscles, causing inversion and eversion. |

Continued on following page

3

Based on Brunnstrom, S: Movement Therapy in Hemiplegia. Harper & Row, New York, 1970.

Brunnstrom's Classification of Synergies

The following tables present Signe Brunnstrom's descriptions of hemiplegic synergy patterns. For both the upper and lower extremities, the flexion and extension synergies are listed. Brunnstrom states that, when a person is dominated by a synergy, all of the movements in either the flexion or extension columns occur together.

UPPER EXTREMITY SYNERGIES*		
Joint	**Flexion**	**Extension**
Scapulothoracic	Retraction and/or elevation	Protraction
Glenohumeral	− Abduction to 90°†	+ Adduction‡
	− External rotation†	+ Internal rotation‡
Elbow	+ Flexion‡	− Extension†
Radioulnar	Supination	+ Pronation‡
Wrist	Flexion	− Extension‡
Fingers	Flexion	Flexion†

*Although Brunnstrom states that the upper extremity flexion synergy dominates in hemiplegia, she believes that a typical posture for the patient includes the strongest component of each synergy, that is, glenohumeral internal rotation, elbow flexion, radioulnar pronation, and wrist and finger flexion with the thumb in the palm.

† − indicates a weak component of a synergy.

‡ + indicates a strong component of a synergy.

Based on Brunnstrom, S: Movement Therapy in Hemiplegia. Harper & Row, New York, 1970.

LOWER EXTREMITY SYNERGIES*		
Joint	**Flexion**	**Extension**
Hip	+ Flexion, abduction, external rotation†	− Extension (limited to the neutral or 0° position),‡ + adduction, − internal rotation
Knee	Flexion to 90°	+ Extension†
Ankle	+ Dorsiflexion†	+ Plantar flexion†
Subtalar	Inversion	+ Inversion†
Toes	Dorsiflexion (extension)	Plantar flexion (flexion), great toe may extend

*In the lower extremity, the extensor synergy dominates.

† + indicates a strong component of a synergy.

‡ − indicates a weak component of a synergy.

Based on Brunnstrom, S: Movement Therapy in Hemiplegia. Harper & Row, New York, 1970.

PROPRIOCEPTIVE NEUROMUSCULAR FACILITATION

Proprioceptive Neuromuscular Facilitation Terms and Techniques (in alphabetical order)

The definitions presented are those of Knott and Voss. The definitions include a statement explaining the intent of the techniques.

approximation: Joint compression for the purpose of stimulating afferent nerve endings.

contract-relax: Alternating muscle activity that occurs when a limb is passively moved to its point of limitation in the range of motion and then the patient contracts the muscles to be stretched. The therapist resists all movement from this contraction except rotation. The patient is then asked to relax, and the therapist moves the limb in the opposite direction to the motion that would have been caused by the contraction. This is a proprioceptive neuromuscular facilitation (PNF) relaxation technique designed to increase motion of the agonist; also see *hold-relax* and *slow-reversal–hold–relax*.

hold-relax: Alternating muscle activity that is similar to contract-relax, except that, when the patient contracts, no motion, not even rotation, is allowed to occur and following the isometric contraction the patient's own contraction causes movement to take place. This is a PNF relaxation technique designed to increase motion of the agonist; also see *contract-relax* and *slow reversal–hold–relax*.

manual contact: Deep, painless pressure through the therapist's contact for the purpose of stimulating muscle, tendon, and joint afferents.

maximal resistance: Resistance to stronger muscles to obtain "overflow" to weaker muscles.

reinforcement: Use of major muscle groups, or other body parts, in a coordinated fashion to bring about a desired movement pattern.

repeated contractions: An isometric contraction anywhere in the range of motion that is followed by an isotonic contraction for the purpose of facilitating the agonist and relaxing the antagonist.

rhythmic initiation: Passive motion, then assistive motion, and then resistive motion for the purpose of increasing a patient's ability to move.

rhythmic stabilization: Alternating isometric contractions of the agonist and antagonist muscles for the purpose of stimulating movement of the agonist, developing stability, and relaxing the antagonist.

slow reversal: Alternation of activity of opposing muscle groups to stimulate active motion of the agonist, relaxation of the antagonist, and coordination between agonist and antagonist patterns.

slow reversal–hold: Alternation of activity of opposing muscle groups with a pause between reversals to achieve relaxation of the antagonist and to stimulate the agonist.

slow reversal–hold–relax: The patient actively brings the extremity to the point of limitation and then reverses the direction of the motion, while the therapist resists rotation and prevents all other motions. In practice this means that, after movement into rotation, the

Text continued on page 470; PNF continued on page 468

Proprioceptive Neuromuscular Facilitation Diagonals According to Knott and Voss

PNF diagonals are named according to the movement that will take place. To place a limb in the starting position for a diagonal, the limb is positioned so that maximum movement will take place. For example, D1 flexion starts with the humerus internally rotated, abducted, and extended at the shoulder. The movement is then into external rotation, adduction, and flexion.

UPPER EXTREMITY DIAGONALS

Joint (Proximal to Distal)	Diagonal One (D1)		Diagonal Two (D2)	
	Flexion	Extension	Flexion	Extension
Scapulothoracic	Rotation, abduction, anterior elevation	Rotation, adduction, posterior depression	Rotation, adduction, posterior elevation	Rotation, abduction, anterior depression
Glenohumeral	External rotation, adduction, flexion	Internal rotation, abduction, extension	External rotation, abduction, flexion	Internal rotation, adduction, extension
Elbow (may be kept flexed or extended)	Flexion	Extension	Flexion	Extension
Radioulnar	Supination	Pronation	Supination	Pronation

Joint (Proximal to Distal)	Diagonal One (D1)		Diagonal Two (D2)	
	Flexion	Extension	Flexion	Extension
Wrist	Flexion, radial deviation	Extension, ulnar deviation	Extension, radial deviation	Flexion, ulnar deviation
Fingers	Flexion, adduction to the radial side	Extension, abduction to the ulnar side	Extension, abduction to the radial side	Flexion, adduction to the ulnar side
Thumb	Flexion, abduction	Extension, abduction	Extension, adduction	Flexion, abduction

LOWER EXTREMITY DIAGONALS

Joint (Proximal to Distal)	Diagonal One (D1)		Diagonal Two (D2)	
	Flexion	Extension	Flexion	Extension
Hip	External rotation, adduction, flexion	Internal rotation, abduction, extension	Internal rotation, abduction, flexion	External rotation, adduction, extension
Knee (may be kept flexed or extended)	Flexion or extension	Extension or flexion	Flexion or extension	Extension or flexion
Ankle	Dorsiflexion	Plantar flexion	Dorsiflexion	Plantar flexion
Subtalar	Inversion	Eversion	Eversion	Inversion
Toes	Extension, abduction to the tibial side	Flexion, adduction to the fibular side	Extension, abduction to the tibial side	Flexion, adduction to the tibial side

Based on Voss, DE, Ionta, MK, and Meyers, BJ: Proprioceptive Neuromuscular Facilitation, ed 3. Harper & Row, New York, 1985.

Proprioceptive Neuromuscular Terms and Techniques
(Continued from page 467)

therapist is resisting an isometric contraction of the shortened muscle. After the isometric contraction, the patient is told to relax and then to move the limb in the direction in which it was limited. The procedure is then repeated. This is a PNF relaxation technique designed to increase motion of the agonist; also see *contract-relax* and *hold-relax.*

timing for emphasis: Maximal resistance of more powerful muscle groups to obtain "overflow" to weaker muscle groups.

traction: Force used to separate joint surfaces by manual contact. The stated purpose is to make joint motion less painful and presumably to stimulate stretch receptors.

BASED ON

Voss, DE, Ionta, MK, and Meyers, BJ: Proprioceptive Neuromuscular Facilitation, ed 3. Harper & Row, Philadelphia, 1985.

SPINAL CORD INJURY

Modified Frankel Classification Scale
for Spinal Cord Damage

Grade A: complete motor and sensory involvement
Grade B: complete motor involvement, some sensory sparing including sacral sparing
Grade C: motor sparing that is not functional
Grade D: motor sparing that is functional
Grade E: no neurologic involvement

BASED ON

Blauvet, CT and Nelson, FRT: A Manual of Orthopaedic Terminology, ed 5. CV Mosby, St. Louis, 1994.

Spinal cord injury continued on pages 472–480.

3

SPINAL CORD INJURY (Continued)

	FUNCTIONAL EXPECTATIONS FOR PATIENTS WITH SPINAL CORD INJURIES*		
Most Distal Nerve Root Segments Innervated and Key Muscles	Available Movements	Functional Capabilities (Assistive Equipment May Be Required)	Equipment and Assistance Required
C1, C2, C3 Face and neck muscles (cranial innervation)	Talking Mastication Sipping Blowing	1. Total dependence in ADLs Activation of light switches, page turners, call buttons, electrical appliances, and speaker phones 2. Locomotion	Respirator dependent; may use phrenic nerve stimulator during the day. Full-time attendant required. Environmental control units. Electric wheelchair (typical components include a high, electrically controlled reclining back, a seat belt and trunk support); a portable respirator may be attached; microswitch or sip-and-puff controls may be used.
C4 Diaphragm Trapezius	Respiration Scapular elevation	1. ADLs a. Limited self-feeding	Mobile arm supports (possibly with powered elbow orthosis), powered flexor hinge hand splint.

472

	Adapted eating equipment (long straws, built-up handles on utensils, plate guards, and so forth).
b. Typing	Plexiglas lapboard. Electric typewriter using head or mouth stick or sip-and-puff controls: another option is a rubber-tipped stick held in hand by a splint (in combination with mobile arm supports and powered splints).
c. Page turning	Head or mouth stick. Environmental control unit for powered page turner.
d. Activation of light switches, call buttons, electrical appliances, and speaker phone	Environmental control units.
2. Locomotion	Electric wheelchair with mouth, chin, breath, or sip-and-puff controls.
3. Pressure relief	Electric reclining back on wheelchair.
4. Transfers and bed mobility	Dependent

Continued on following page

3

SPINAL CORD INJURY (Continued)

FUNCTIONAL EXPECTATIONS FOR PATIENTS WITH SPINAL CORD INJURIES* (Continued)			
Most Distal Nerve Root Segments Innervated and Key Muscles	Available Movements	Functional Capabilities (Assistive Equipment May Be Required)	Equipment and Assistance Required
		5. Skin inspection	Dependent.
		6. Cough with glossopharangeal breathing	Dependent.
		7. Recreation	
		a. Table games such as cards or checkers	Head or mouth stick. Built-up playing pieces.
		b. Painting and drawing	Full-time attendant required.
C5 Biceps Brachialis Brachioradialis	Elbow flexion and supination Shoulder external rotation	1. ADLs: able to accomplish all activities of a C4 quadriplegic with less adaptive equipment and more skill	Assistance is required in setting up patient with necessary equipment; patient can then accomplish activity independently.
Deltoid Infraspinatus Rhomboid (major and minor)	Shoulder abduction to 90° Limited shoulder flexion	a. Self-feeding	Mobile arm supports. Adapted utensils.

474

Supinator

b. Typing
Electric typewriter.
Hand splints.
Adapted typing sticks.
Some patients may require mobile arm supports or slings.

c. Page turning

d. Limited upper extremity dressing
Same as above.
Assistance required.

e. Limited self-care (i.e., washing, brushing teeth, and grooming)
Hand splints.
Adapted equipment (wash mitt, adapted toothbrush, and so forth).

2. Locomotion
Manual wheelchair with hand-rim projections.
Electric wheelchair with joystick or adapted upper extremity controls.

3. Transfer activities
Overhead swivel bar.
Sliding board.
Dependent.

4. Skin inspection and pressure relief
Dependent.

5. Cough with manual pressure to diaphragm
Assistance required.

Continued on following page

3

SPINAL CORD INJURY (Continued)

	FUNCTIONAL EXPECTATIONS FOR PATIENTS WITH SPINAL CORD INJURIES* (Continued)		
Most Distal Nerve Root Segments Innervated and Key Muscles	*Available Movements*	*Functional Capabilities (Assistive Equipment May Be Required)*	*Equipment and Assistance Required*
		6. Driving	Van with hand controls. Part-time attendant required.
C6 Extensor carpi radialis Infraspinatus Latissimus dorsi	Shoulder flexion, extension, internal rotation, and adduction	1. ADLs a. Self-feeding	Universal cuff. Intertwine utensils in fingers. Adapted utensils.
Pectoralis major (clavicular portion) Pronator teres Serratus anterior Teres minor	Scapular abduction and upward rotation Forearm pronation Wrist extension (tenodesis grasp)	b. Dressing	Utilizes momentum, button hooks, zipper pulls, or other clothing adaptations; dependent on momentum to extend limbs. Cannot tie shoes. Flexor hinge splint.
		c. Self-care	Universal cuff. Adaptive equipment. Independent.
		d. Bed mobility	
		2. Locomotion	Manual wheelchair with projection or friction surface hand rims.
		3. Transfer activities	Independent with sliding board.

C7		
Extensor pollicus longus and brevis		
Extrinsic finger extensors		
Flexor carpi radialis		
Triceps	Elbow extension	
	Wrist flexion	
	Finger extension	
	4. Skin inspection and pressure relief	Independent.
	5. Bowel and bladder care	Can be independent, depending on bowel and bladder routine.
	6. Cough with application of pressure to abdomen	Independent.
	7. Driving	Automobile with hand controls and U-shaped cuff attached to steering wheel. Usually requires assistance in getting wheelchair into car. Limited participation.
	8. Wheelchair sports	
	1. ADLs	
	a. Self-feeding	Independent.
	b. Dressing	Independent.
		Button hook may be required.
	c. Self-care	Shower chair. Adapted hand shower nozzle. Adapted handles on bathroom items may be required.
	2. Locomotion	Manual wheelchair with friction surface hand rims.
	3. Transfers	Independent (usually without sliding board).

Continued on following page

SPINAL CORD INJURY (Continued)

	FUNCTIONAL EXPECTATIONS FOR PATIENTS WITH SPINAL CORD INJURIES* (Continued)	
Most Distal Nerve Root Segments Innervated and Key Muscles	*Available Movements*	*Functional Capabilities (Assistive Equipment May Be Required)*	*Equipment and Assistance Required*
		4. Bowel and bladder care	Independent with appropriate equipment (digital stimulator, suppositories, raised toilet seat, urinary drainage device, and so forth).
		5. Manual cough	Independent.
		6. Housekeeping	Light kitchen activities. Requires wheelchair-accessible kitchen and living environment. Adapted kitchen tools.
		7. Driving	Automobile with hand controls. Able to get wheelchair in and out of car.
C8–T1 Extrinsic finger flexors Flexor carpi ulnaris Flexor pollicis longus and brevis Intrinsic finger flexors	Full innervation of upper extremity muscles	1. ADLs	Independent in all self-care and personal hygiene. Some adaptive equipment may be required (e.g., tub seat, grab bars, and so forth).
		2. Locomotion	Manual wheelchair with standard hand rims.

		3. Housekeeping	Independent in light housekeeping and meal preparation. Some adaptive equipment may be required (e.g., reachers). Requires a wheelchair-accessible living environment.
		4. Driving	Automobile with hand controls.
		5. Employment	Able to work in a building free of architectural barriers.
T4–T6 Top half of intercostals Long muscles of back (sacrospinalis and semispinalis)	Improved trunk control Increased respiratory reserve	1. ADLs 2. Physiologic standing (not practical for functional ambulation)	Independent in all areas. Standing table. Bilateral knee-ankle orthoses with spinal attachment. Some patients may be able to ambulate for short distances with assistance.
		3. Housekeeping	Independent with routine activities. Requires a wheelchair-accessible living environment.
		4. Curb climbing in wheelchair 5. Wheelchair sports	Able to negotiate curbs using a "wheelie" technique. Full participation.
T9–T12 Lower abdominals All intercostals	Improved trunk control Increased endurance	1. Household ambulation	Bilateral knee-ankle orthoses and crutches or walker (high energy consumption for ambulation)

Continued on following page

3

479

SPINAL CORD INJURY (Continued)

FUNCTIONAL EXPECTATIONS FOR PATIENTS WITH SPINAL CORD INJURIES* (Continued)

Most Distal Nerve Root Segments Innervated and Key Muscles	Available Movements	Functional Capabilities (Assistive Equipment May Be Required)	Equipment and Assistance Required
		2. Locomotion	Wheelchair used for energy conservation.
L2, L3, L4 Gracilis Iliopsoas Quadratus lumborum Rectus femoris Sartorious	Hip flexion Hip adduction Knee extension	1. Functional ambulation 2. Locomotion	Bilateral knee-ankle orthoses and crutches. Wheelchair used for convenience and energy conservation.
L4, L5 Extensor digitorum Low back muscles Medial hamstrings (weak) Posterior tibialis Quadriceps Tibialis anterior Posterior tibialis Quadriceps Tibialis anterior	Strong hip flexion Strong knee extension Weak knee flexion Improved trunk control	1. Functional ambulation 2. Locomotion	Bilateral ankle-foot orthoses and crutches or canes. Wheelchair used for convenience and energy conservation.

*This table presents general functional expectations at various lesion levels. Each progressively lower segment includes the muscles from the previous levels. Although the key muscles listed frequently receive innervation from several nerve root segments, they are listed here at the neurologic levels where they add to functional outcomes.

ADLs = activities of daily living.

From O'Sullivan, SB and Schmitz, TJ: Physical Rehabilitation: Assessment and Treatment, ed 3. FA Davis, Philadelphia, 1994, pp 554–556, with permission

ACUPUNCTURE POINTS

Acupuncture is a technique that has been part of traditional Chinese medicine for the last 5000 y. Needles are used to stimulate specific points along defined meridians. There are approximately 1000 acupuncture points located on 12 paired and 2 unpaired meridians. According to traditional Chinese medical theory, the meridians are associated with body organs and areas of the external body.

The following table is a key to the abbreviations used on the acupuncture charts. The numbers identify the specific points on a meridian. For example, Gb20 indicates that it is point number 20 on the gallbladder meridian.

Twelve Paired Meridians

B	Bladder channel (urinary bladder channel)
Gb	Gallbladder channel
H	Heart channel
K	Kidney channel
Li	Large intestine channel
Liv	Liver channel
Lu	Lung channel
P	Pericardium channel (heart constrictor channel)
Si	Small intestine channel
Sj	Sanjiao channel
Sp	Spleen channel
St	Stomach channel

Two Unpaired Meridians

Gv	Governor vessel (Du Mo) (back midline)
Vc	Vessel of conception (Ren Mo) (front midline)

Extra Points

Ex	Extraordinary points
Ah Shi	Any tender points

Acupuncture Points:
Ventral View

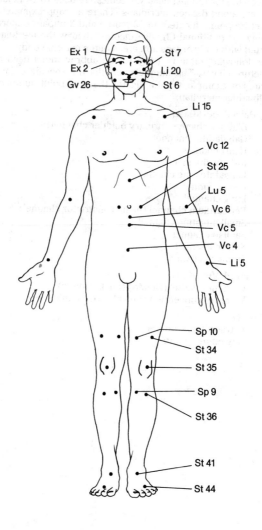

Acupuncture Points:
Dorsal and Lateral Views

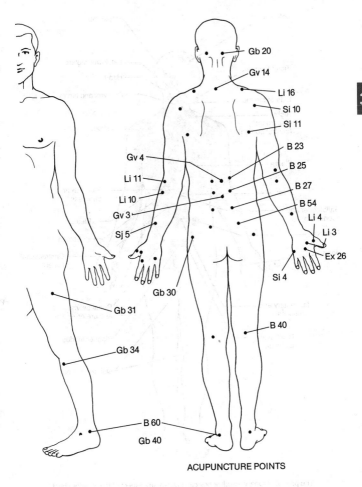

Gb 20
Gv 14
Li 16
Si 10
Si 11
B 23
B 25
B 27
B 54
Li 4
Li 3
Ex 26
Si 4
Gv 4
Li 11
Li 10
Gv 3
Sj 5
Gb 30
Gb 31
Gb 34
B 40
B 60
Gb 40

ACUPUNCTURE POINTS

3

PAIN REFERRED FROM VISCERA

Anterior View

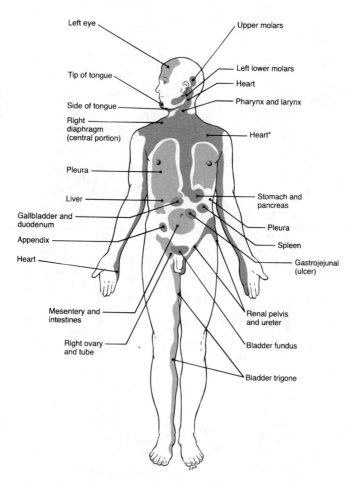

*The pain of coronary insufficiency can involve any aspect of the anterior chest but is more common in the substernal region.

Posterior View

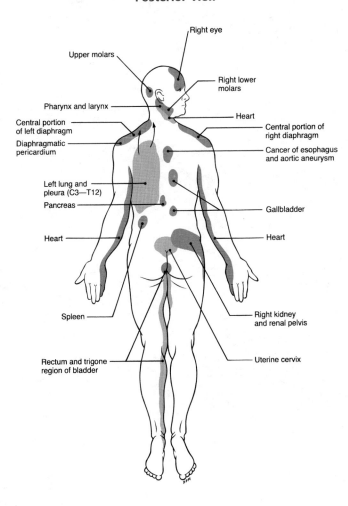

- Right eye
- Upper molars
- Right lower molars
- Pharynx and larynx
- Heart
- Central portion of left diaphragm
- Central portion of right diaphragm
- Diaphragmatic pericardium
- Cancer of esophagus and aortic aneurysm
- Left lung and pleura (C3—T12)
- Pancreas
- Gallbladder
- Heart
- Heart
- Spleen
- Right kidney and renal pelvis
- Rectum and trigone region of bladder
- Uterine cervix

General and Visceral Anatomy

4

PLANES OF THE BODY

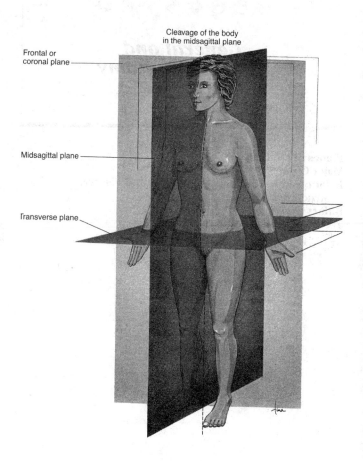

Cleavage of the body
in the midsagittal plane

Frontal or
coronal plane

Midsagittal plane

Transverse plane

MAJOR ORGANS IN SITU

This figure shows major organs of the body as viewed from the front with part of the lungs, small intestine, and colon removed to allow a view of surrounding and underlying structures.

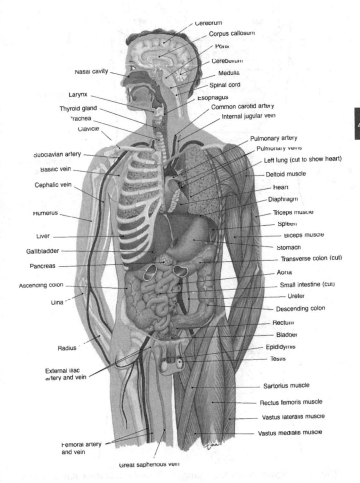

RELATIONSHIP OF SURFACE TOPOGRAPHY (PLANES) AND VISCERAL STRUCTURES

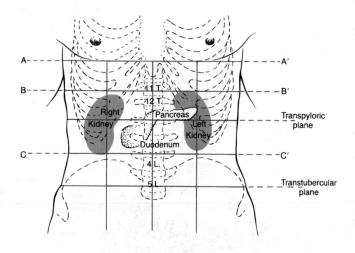

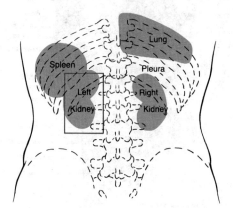

The upper figure shows the transpyloric and transtubercular planes in relationship to underlying skeletal structures. Plane A-A' is through the intersection of the xiphoid and body of the sternum. Plane B-B' is midway between plane A-A' and the transpyloric plane. Plane C-C' is midway between the transpyloric and transtubercular planes. The lower figure shows the surface anatomy from behind in relationship to the position of the kidneys.

THE BILIARY SYSTEM

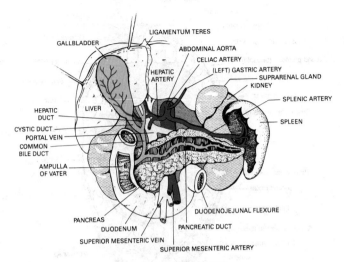

BILIARY TRACT (IN RELATION TO LIVER, PANCREAS, AND DUODENUM)

TEETH AND STRUCTURES OF THE MOUTH

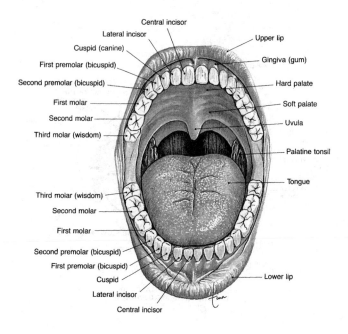

Central incisor

Lateral incisor

Cuspid (canine)

First premolar (bicuspid)

Second premolar (bicuspid)

First molar

Second molar

Third molar (wisdom)

Upper lip

Gingiva (gum)

Hard palate

Soft palate

Uvula

Palatine tonsil

Tongue

Third molar (wisdom)

Second molar

First molar

Second premolar (bicuspid)

First premolar (bicuspid)

Cuspid

Lateral incisor

Central incisor

Lower lip

SECTION 5

Pulmonary Anatomy and Pulmonary Therapy

5

LUNGS—EXTERNAL ANATOMY
Anterior View

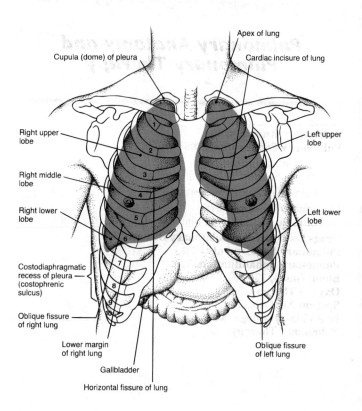

Cupula (dome) of pleura

Apex of lung

Cardiac incisure of lung

Right upper lobe

Left upper lobe

Right middle lobe

Right lower lobe

Left lower lobe

Costodiaphragmatic recess of pleura (costophrenic sulcus)

Oblique fissure of right lung

Left lower lobe

Oblique fissure of left lung

Lower margin of right lung

Gallbladder

Horizontal fissure of lung

LUNGS—EXTERNAL ANATOMY
Posterior View

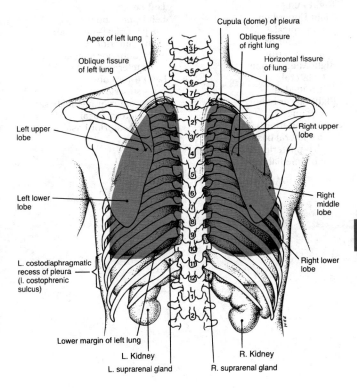

Cupula (dome) of pleura

Apex of left lung

Oblique fissure of right lung

Oblique fissure of left lung

Horizontal fissure of lung

Left upper lobe

Right upper lobe

Left lower lobe

Right middle lobe

L. costodiaphragmatic recess of pleura (l. costophrenic sulcus)

Right lower lobe

Lower margin of left lung

L. Kidney

R. Kidney

L. suprarenal gland

R. suprarenal gland

5

KEY TO FIGURE OF THE BRONCHOPULMONARY TREE

Right Lung
Right Upper Lobe
   ap = apical
   an = anterior
   p = posterior
Right Middle Lobe
   l = lateral
   m = medial
Right Lower Lobe
   s = superior
   ab = anterior basal
   lb = lateral basal
   pb = posterior basal
   mb = medial basal

Left Lung
Left Upper Lobe
   a-p = apical–posterior
   an = anterior
   sl = superior lingula
   il = inferior lingula
Left Lower Lobe
   s = superior
   ab = anterior medial basal
   lb = lateral basal
   pb = posterior basal

ANATOMY OF THE BRONCHOPULMONARY TREE

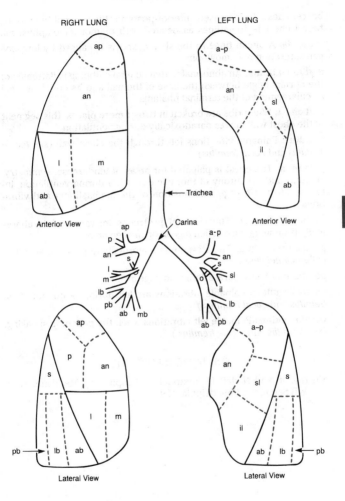

RIGHT LUNG

LEFT LUNG

Anterior View

Anterior View

Trachea

Carina

Lateral View

Lateral View

PHYSICAL EXAMINATION OF THE PULMONARY SYSTEM

Terms Associated with the Evaluation of the Pulmonary System

barrel chest: An increased anterior-posterior diameter of the thorax, barrel chest is sometimes associated with pulmonary emphysema.

cyanosis: A bluish tinge to the skin, cyanosis is caused by low oxygen saturation of hemoglobin.

digital clubbing: An abnormal finding, digital clubbing is flattening of the normal angle between the base of the nail and its cuticle as well as enlargement of the terminal phalanx.

flail chest: When ribs are broken in two or more places, this segment of the chest wall moves paradoxically during ventilation.

fremitus: Palpable vibrations felt through the chest wall (see *tactile fremitus* and *vocal fremitus*).

palpation: The chest is palpated for areas of tenderness, symmetry, amount, and synchrony of thoracic excursion during ventilation, integrity of the rib cage, and position of the mediastinum and vibrations.

pectus carinatum: The sternum protrudes forward and is abnormally prominent; also called *pigeon* or *chicken breast*.

pectus excavatum: The sternum is abnormally depressed; also it is called *funnel chest*.

percussion: See separate listing on page 500.

tactile fremitus: Palpable vibrations are felt during ventilation. (See *fremitus* and *vocal fremitus*.)

vocal fremitus: Palpable felt vibrations when the patient is speaking. (See *fremitus* and *tactile fremitus*.)

FOR MORE INFORMATION

Murray, JF and Nadel, JA: Textbook of Respiratory Medicine, ed 2. WB Saunders, Philadelphia, 1994.

TERMS USED TO DESCRIBE BREATHING

Term	Explanation
Apnea	Absence of breathing
Apneusis	Cessation of respiration in the inspiratory position
Biot's breathing	Several short breaths or gasps followed by irregular periods of apnea
Bradypnea	Abnormally slow rate
Cheyne-Stokes respiration	Cycles of gradual increase in rate and depth of respiration with apneic pauses between cycles
Dyspnea	Complaint of shortness of breath
Eupnea	Normal rate and rhythm
Hyperpnea	Increased breathing; increased depth with or without increased rate
Hyperventilation	Increased ventilation; technically a decrease in Pa_{CO_2}
Hypoventilation	Decreased ventilation; technically an increase in Pa_{CO_2}
Kussmaul's breathing	Deep gasping respirations associated with diabetic acidosis and coma ("air hunger")
Orthopnea	Dyspnea that occurs when patient assumes recumbent position
Paroxysmal nocturnal dyspnea	Dyspnea that comes on at night and suddenly awakens the patient
Tachypnea	Abnormally rapid rate

5

AUSCULTATION

Breath sounds are classified as normal or abnormal and with or without accompaniments (adventitious breath sounds). Normal breath sounds vary, depending on what area is being auscultated.

Location of Normal Breath Sounds

Definitions of breath sounds are on the following pages.

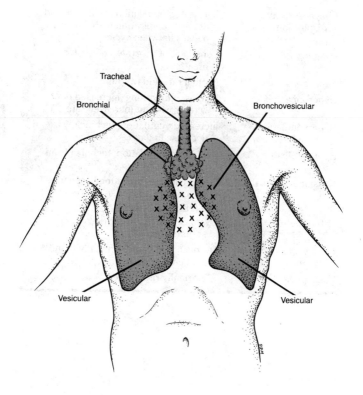

PERCUSSION OF THE PULMONARY SYSTEM

percussion: An evaluation technique where the examiner strikes the distal end of the middle finger of one hand over the middle finger of the other hand, which is placed firmly over the chest wall. The resonance created by this maneuver has a variable pitch and feel, depending on the density of the underlying tissue. Four different percussion notes are described.

PERCUSSION SOUNDS

Note (Sound)	Characteristics of Normal Location	Underlying Tissue
Flat	Muscle on extremity	No underlying air
Dull	Liver, heart, viscera	Primarily soft tissue, some air
Normal resonance	Lung	Air and soft tissue
Hyper-resonant (tympanic)	Stomach	Primarily air

NORMAL BREATH SOUNDS

Type	Location Auscultated	Description of Sound
Tracheal	Trachea	Inspiration and expiration are equal in duration; loud, high pitched, and hollow; short pause between inspiration and expiration
Bronchial	Over manubrium, between clavicles, or between scapulae	Inspiration shorter than expiration; loud, high pitched, short pause between inspiration and expiration
Bronchovesicular	Over large airways near sternum and between scapulae	Inspiration should equal expiration in duration, lower intensity than bronchial; medium pitched, no pause between inspiration and expiration
Vesicular	Over peripheral lung tissue	Long inspiration with short expiration; relatively faint and low pitched; no pause between inspiration and expiration

Abnormal Breath Sounds

When tracheal, bronchial, or bronchovesicular breath sounds are auscultated over a lung that should sound vesicular, the breath sound is abnormal. Sound is transmitted better through solid or consolidated lung tissue, and increased transmission is indicative of pathology. Sometimes these abnormal breath sounds are termed *tubular*. An abnormal intensity of a breath sound is also noted when present.

bronchophony: Abnormal transmission of spoken words. Typically, the patient is asked to say the letter *E* or *99*; with bronchophony, the *E* will sound like an *A* and is sometimes noted as "E to A change."

egophony: The nasal, bleating sound of spoken or whispered words auscultated over consolidated lung tissue.

pectoriloquy: Abnormal transmission of whispered syllables that normally cannot be heard distinctly. Examining for pectoriloquy usually involves asking the patient to whisper, "One, two, three."

Adventitious Breath Sounds

Adventitious breath sounds are accompaniments to normal or abnormal breath sounds. Adventitious breath sounds are always abnormal and should be described by name and by when they are heard during respiration (inspiration, expiration, early, late, etc.). They are further classified into three major categories: continuous and noncontinuous breath sounds and rubs.

continuous breath sounds: Most prominent during expiration, they are thought to be caused by the vibrations of air passing through airways narrowed by inflammation, bronchospasm, or secretions. Frequently they are present in asthma and chronic bronchitis. The noises of wheezes are described as squeaky, snoring, or groaning.

wheezes: High-pitched, sibilant, and musical.

rhonchi: Low-pitched and sonorous.

noncontinuous breath sounds: Most common during inspiration, they are thought to be caused by the sound of gas bubbling through secretions or by the opening of alveoli and small airways that have collapsed because of fluid, poor aeration, or inflammation. These sounds are frequently associated with congestive heart failure, atelectasis, and pulmonary fibrosis. Noncontinuous breath sounds are described as sounding like soda pop fizzing or hair rubbed through the fingers next to the ear. They should be called *crackles*; other terms used are *rales* and *crepitations*. Descriptive terms used with crackles are *fine* or *coarse*.

friction rub: Caused by the rubbing of pleural surfaces against one another, usually as a result of inflammation or neoplastic processes. A friction rub sounds similar to footsteps on packed snow or creaking old leather and is more commonly heard during inspiration, but this can be highly variable. A friction rub may be accompanied by pain during inspiration.

TERMS USED IN PULMONARY FUNCTION TESTING

PULMONARY FUNCTION ABBREVIATIONS

Abbreviation	Term
$A\text{-}aD_{O_2}$	Alevolar-arterial O_2 difference (gradient)
C_{STAT}	Static lung compliance
D_{LCO}	Diffusing capacity for CO (mL/min/mm Hg)
ERV	Expiratory reserve volume
$FEF_{25\%-75\%}$	Mean forced expiratory flow during the middle of FVC
$FEV_1(L)$	Forced expiratory volume in 1 s, in liters
FEV_1 %FVC	Forced expiratory volume in 1 s as percentage of FVC
FI_{O_2}	Percentage of inspired O_2
FRC	Functional residual capacity
FVC	Forced vital capacity
$[H^+]$	Hydrogen ion concentration (nanomole/L)
MEF 50%VC	Mid-expiratory flow at 50% of FVC
MEP	Maximal expiratory pressure (cm H_2O)
MIF 50%VC	Mid-inspiratory flow at 50% of FVC
MIP	Maximal inspiratory pressure (cm H_2O)
MVV	Maximal voluntary ventilation
$P_{A_{O_2}}$	Partial pressure of alveolar O_2
$P_{A_{CO_2}}$	Partial pressure of alveolar CO_2
Pa_{O_2}	Partial pressure of arterial O_2
Pa_{CO_2}	Partial pressure of arterial CO_2
P_B	Barometric pressure
P_{CO_2}	Partial pressure of CO_2
$P_{ET_{CO_2}}$	Partial pressure of end tidal CO_2
PEF	Peak expiratory flow (L/min)
PI_{O_2}	Partial pressure of inspired O_2
P_{O_2}	Partial pressure of O_2
$P\bar{v}$	Partial pressure of mixed venous (pulmonary arterial) blood
$P_{v_{O_2}}$	Partial pressure of mixed venous O_2
$P\dot{v}_{CO_2}$	Partial pressure of mixed venous CO_2
$\dot{Q}$	Perfusion (L/min)

Continued on following page

PULMONARY FUNCTION ABBREVIATIONS (Continued)	
Abbreviation	*Term*
Raw	Airways resistance
RV	Residual volume
TLC	Total lung capacity
VC	Vital capacity
$\dot{V}$	Ventilation (L/min)
$\dot{V}_A$	Alveolar ventilation (L/min)
$\dot{V}_{CO_2}$	CO_2 production (L/min)
$\dot{V}_{O_2}$	O_2 consumption (L/min)

From the Merck Manual, ed 16. Merck & Co, Rahway, NJ, 1992, p 608, with permission.

COMMON PULMONARY FUNCTION TESTS

spirometry: Measures lung volumes and capacities (with the exception of RV and TLC), flow rates, and the MVV; used as a general screening test for detection of abnormal breathing patterns, lung obstruction and/or restriction, efficacy of medication (bronchodilation), estimate ventilatory reserve, and patient compliance.

Spirograms and Lung Volumes

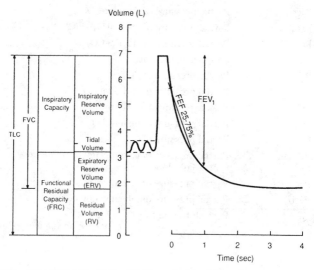

$FRC = RV + ERV$. $VC = TLC - RV$. Normal: $RV \approx 25\%$ of TLC; $FRC \approx 40\%$ of TLC; $FEV_1 \geq 75\%$ of FVC.   From Berkow, R (ed): The Merck Manual of Diagnosis and Therapy, ed 16. Merck & Co, Rahway, NJ, 1992, p 609, with permission.

Restrictive Disease

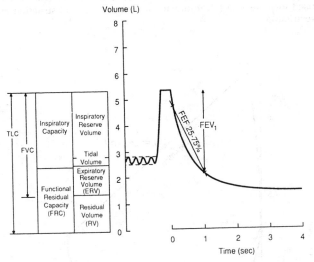

Lung volumes are all diminished, the RV less so than the FRC, FVC, and TLC. FEV_1 %FVC is normal or greater than normal. Tidal breathing is rapid and shallow. From Berkow, R (ed): The Merck Manual of Diagnosis and Therapy, ed 16. Merck & Co, Rahway, NJ, 1992, p 609, with permission.

Obstructive Disease

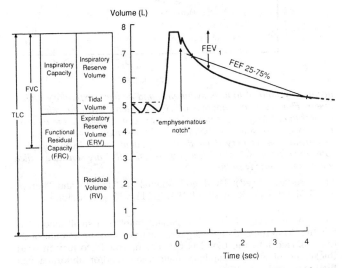

RV and FRC are increased. TLC is also increased but to a lesser degree, so that VC is decreased. Expiration is prolonged. $FEV_1 \leq 75\%$ of FVC. Note the "emphysematous notch." From Berkow, R (ed): The Merck Manual of Diagnosis and Therapy, ed 16. Merck & Co, Rahway, NJ, 1992, p 610, with permission.

flow-volume loops: Graphically plot maximal inspiratory and expiratory volumes and flows; visual examination of the shape of the loop used for detecting intrathoracic and extrathoracic obstruction and restriction.

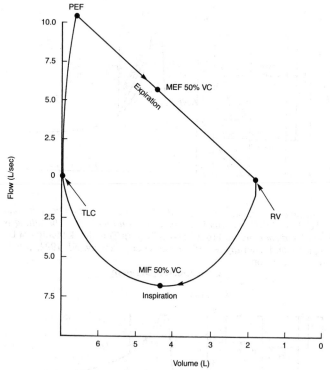

Inspiratory limb of loop is symmetric and convex. Expiratory limb is linear. Flow rates at midpoint of VC are often measured. MIF$_{50\%VC}$ is greater than MEF$_{50\%VC}$ because of dynamic compression of the airways. Peak expiratory flow is sometimes used to estimate degree of airways' obstruction but is very dependent on patient effort. Expiratory flow rates over lower 50% of VC (i.e., approaching RV) are sensitive indicators of small airway status.

From Berkow, R (ed): The Merck Manual of Diagnosis and Therapy, ed 16. Merck & Co, Rahway, NJ, 1992, p 611, with permission.

diffusing capacity (DLco): The patient inspires a small amount of CO; the CO in the end-expired gas is analyzed and the amount of CO that diffused into the blood is calculated. Low DLco may indicate thickening of alveolar-capillary membranes and/or abnormal ventilation-perfusion relationships.

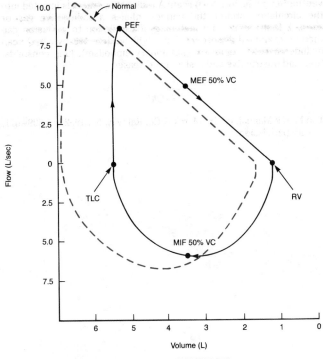

FLOW-VOLUME LOOPS

Restrictive disease (e.g., sarcoidosis, kyphoscoliosis). Configuration of loop is narrowed because of diminished lung volumes. Flow rates are normal (actually greater than normal at comparable lung volumes because increased elastic recoil of lungs and/or chest wall holds airways open).

From Berkow, R (ed): The Merck Manual of Diagnosis and Therapy, ed 16. Merck & Co, Rahway, NJ, 1992, p 611, with permission.

body plethysmography: Measures total lung capacity and airway resistance. It allows the RV to be accurately determined and is most useful for diagnosing obstructive disorders.

nitrogen washout test: Measures the distribution of ventilation and closing volume (the volume during expiration when small airways collapse). Concentration of N_2 is measured over complete expiration after breathing 100% O_2. An abnormal curve of N_2 concentration reflects asynchronous alveolar emptying and small airway closure, characteristic of obstructive disorders.

ventilation-perfusion ($\dot{V}/\dot{Q}$) scan: A radioactive tracer is injected into the circulation and/or the patient inhales a radioactive gas or aerosol. Distribution and matching of ventilation to perfusion can then be examined. Disorders that might be detected by a $\dot{V}/\dot{Q}$ scan include vascular occlusion (pulmonary embolism), lung consolidation, and obstructive and restrictive diseases.

FROM

The Merck Manual, ed 16. Merck & Co, Rahway, NJ, 1992, pp 609–611, with permission.

LUNG VOLUMES AND CAPACITIES

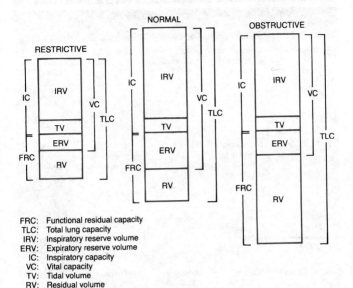

FRC: Functional residual capacity
TLC: Total lung capacity
IRV: Inspiratory reserve volume
ERV: Expiratory reserve volume
 IC: Inspiratory capacity
 VC: Vital capacity
 TV: Tidal volume
 RV: Residual volume

FOR MORE INFORMATION

Brannon, FJ, et al: Cardiopulmonary Rehabilitation: Basic Theory and Application, ed 2. FA Davis, Philadelphia, 1993, pp 33–62.

TYPICAL SIGNS AND SYMPTOMS OF PULMONARY DISEASES

Pathologic Process	Chest Wall Movement	Mediastinal Position	Percussion Note	Breath Sounds
Atelectasis	Reduced on affected side	Shifted toward affected side	Dull or flat	Decreased or absent
Asthma	Normal or symmetrically decreased	Midline	Normal or hyper-resonant	Vesicular with prolonged expiration
Chronic or acute bronchitis	Normal or symmetrically decreased	Midline	Normal	Vesicular with prolonged expiration
Bronchiectasis	May be reduced over affected area	Midline or toward affected area	Abnormal, may be dull or hyperresonant	Bronchial or broncho-vesicular
Pulmonary effusion or empyema	Reduced or absent on affected side	Away from affected side	Dull or flat	Decreased or absent; high-pitched bronchial may be present
Pneumonia (lung consolidation)	Reduced on affected side	Midline	Dull	Broncho-vesicular, bronchial
Lung abcess, cavitation	Normal or reduced on affected side	Normal or toward affected side	Abnormal (dull or hyperresonant	Bronchial, amphoric

Vocal Sounds	Adventitious Sounds	Cough—Sputum	Miscellaneous
Reduced or absent with large area collapsed; egophony and whispering pectoriloquy with smaller collapse	None or coarse rales	None, hacking or productive, particularly if atelectasis is due to mucous plugging	May have fever; may have pain
Normal or diminished	Wheezing cough	Dry or productive of tenacious mucoid sputum with plugs	Anxiety, severe bronchospasm may restrict air flow to the extent that no wheezing is heard
Normal	Wheezing and rhonchi	Productive of mucoid or purulent sputum with infection	May have fever
Increased	Coarse rales, rhonchi	Usually copious amounts of purulent sputum; possibly foul-smelling; hemoptysis may occur	Physical exam depends on amount of fluid ectatic areas
Reduced or absent	May have pleural rub	Absent or nonproductive	
Egophony, whispering pectoriloquy	Fine rales early; coarse later	Dry, hacking, or productive; sputum may be purulent, bloody	Fever; may have pleuritic pain
Increased, egophony, whispering pectoriloquy	Coarse rales	Productive of purulent, foul-smelling sputum	Physical exam depends on amount of fluid in affected area; abscess may develop distal to bronchial obstruction; lung cancer should be ruled out; may have fever

Continued on following page

Pathologic Process	Chest Wall Movement	Mediastinal Position	Percussion Note	Breath Sounds
Emphysema	Normal or symmetrically decreased	Midline	Normal or hyperresonant	Harsh vesicular with prolonged expiration; may be decreased or distant
Pulmonary edema	Normal or symmetrically reduced	Midline	Normal, may be dull at lung bases	Vesicular
Pulmonary embolism	Reduced on affected side	Midline	Normal or dull	May be reduced
Cystic fibrosis	Normal or reduced	Midline	Normal, dull or hyper-resonant	Vesicular, broncho-vesicular, bronchial
Pneumothorax	Reduced on affected side (but hemi-thorax may be enlarged)	Away from affected side	Hyper-resonant, tympanic	Decreased, distant, or absent
Laryngo-tracheo-bronchitis (Croup)	Retractions	Midline	Normal	Vesicular, prolonged inspiration
Bronchiolitis	Retractions	Midline	Hyper-resonant	Vesicular, prolonged expiration

URI = upper respiratory infection.

Vocal Sounds	Adventitious Sounds	Cough—Sputum	Miscellaneous
Normal or reduced	None, rhonchi, rales	Variable	
Normal	Rales, generally symmetric	Irritating, frothy white or pink sputum	
Normal	Rales, wheezing, pleural friction rub	Dry, hacking, or productive; may have hemoptysis	May have pleuritic pain, apprehension
May have egophony	Rales, wheezing	Productive of large amounts of tenacious mucoid, muco-purulent, or purulent sputum; may have hemoptysis	Physical exam depends on extent of disease and amount of retained secretions
Decreased	None	Dry	May have local or referred pain
Normal	Stridor, wheezing, rales	Barking, productive of viscous sputum	Low-grade fever
Normal	Wheezing, rales	Hacking, productive of mucoid to purulent sputum	Typically follows a URI

5

FOR MORE INFORMATION

Seidel, HM, et al: Mosby's Guide to Physical Examination, ed 3. CV Mosby, St. Louis, 1995.

Feature	DIFFERENTIAL FEATURES OF CHRONIC OBSTRUCTIVE PULMONARY DISEASE		
	Emphysema	Chronic Bronchitis	Asthma
Family history	Occasional (α_1 antitrypsin deficiency)	Occasional (cystic fibrosis)	Frequent
Atopy	Absent	Absent	Frequent
Smoking history	Usual	Usual	Infrequent
Sputum character	Absent or mucoid	Predominantly neutrophilic	Predominantly eosinophilic
Chest x-ray	Useful if bullae, hyperinflation, or loss of peripheral vascular markings are present	Often normal; occasional hyperinflation	Often normal; hyperinflation during acute attack
Spirometry	Obstructive pattern unimproved with bronchodilator	Obstructive pattern improved with bronchodilator	Obstructive pattern usually shows good response to bronchodilator

STAGES OF CHRONIC OBSTRUCTIVE PULMONARY DISEASE

Stage	Signs
Early	Examination may be negative or show only slight prolongation of forced expiration (which can be timed while ausculating over the trachea—normally 3 s or less); slight diminution of breath sounds at the apices or bases; scattered rhonchi or wheezes, especially on expiration, often best heard over the hila anteriorly. The rhonchi often clear after cough.
Moderate	Above signs are usually present and more pronounced, often with decreased rib expansion; in addition there is: Use of the accessory muscles of respiration. Retraction of the Supraclavicular fossae in inspiration. Generalized hyper-resonance. Decreased area of cardiac dullness. Diminished heart sounds at base. Increased anteroposterior distance of the chest.*
Advanced	Examination usually shows the above findings to a greater degree and often shows: Evidence of weight loss. Depression of the liver. Hyperpnea and tachycardia with mild exertion. Low and relatively immobile diaphragm. Contraction of abdominal muscles on inspiration. Inaudible heart sounds, except in the xiphoid area cyanosis.
Cor pulmonale	Increased pulmonic second sound and close splitting. Right-sided diastolic gallop. Left parasternal heave (right ventricular overactivity). Early systolic pulmonary ejection click, with or without systolic ejection murmur. With failure, there is: Distended neck veins, functional tricuspid insufficiency. V waves, and hepatojugular reflux. Hepatomegaly. Peripheral edema.

5

*Misplaced confidence may be placed in relating the shape of the thorax to the presence or absence of obstructive lung disease. It has been shown that the classic "barrel chest" with poor rib separation may be due solely or largely to dorsal kyphosis. In such patients, ventilatory function may nonetheless be normal because of good diaphragmatic motion.

DRUGS USED TO TREAT PULMONARY DISEASE

ANTIHISTAMINES

Generic Name	Trade Name(s)	Dosage*	Sedation Potential†
Astemizole	Hismanal	10 mg once a day	Low
Azatadine	Optimine	1–2 mg every 8–12 h	Low
Brompheniramine	Bromphen, Dimetane, others	4 mg every 4–6 h	Low
Carbinoxamine	Clistin	4–8 mg every 6–8 h	Low to moderate
Cetirizine	Reactine	5–10 mg once a day	Low
Chlorpheniramine	Chlor-Trimeton, Phenetron, others	4 mg every 4–6 h	Low
Clemastine	Tavist	1.34 mg twice daily or 2.68 mg 1–3 times daily	Low
Cyproheptadine	Periactin	4 mg every 6–8 h	Moderate
Dexchlorpheniramine	Polaramine	2 mg every 4–6 h	Low
Dimenhydrinate	Dramamine, others	50–100 mg every 4 h	High

516

Diphenhydramine	Allerdryl, Benadryl, others	25–50 mg every 4–6 h	High
Diphenylpyraline	Hispril	5 mg every 12 hr	High
Doxylamine	Unisom Nighttime Sleep-Aid	12.5–25 mg every 4–6 h	High
Hydroxyzine	Atarax, others	25–100 mg 3–4 times a day	Moderate
Loratadine	Claritin	10 mg once a day	Low
Phenindamine	Nolahist	25 mg every 4–6 h	Low
Pyrilamine	Nisaval	25–50 mg every 8 h	Moderate
Terfenadine	Seldane	60 mg every 8–12 h	Low
Tripelennamine	PBZ	25–50 mg every 4–6 h	Moderate
Triprolidine	Actidil, others	2.5 mg every 6–8 h	Low

*Normal adult dosage when taken orally for antihistamine effects.
†Sedation potential is based on comparison to other antihistamines and may vary considerably from person to person.
From Ciccone, CD: Pharmacology in Rehabilitation, ed 2. FA Davis, Philadelphia, 1996, p 372, with permission.

5

β-ADRENERGIC BRONCHODILATORS					
Drug	Primary Receptor	Route of Administration	Onset of Action (min)	Time to Peak Effect (h)	Duration of Action (h)
Albuterol	β_2	Inhalation	5–15	1–1.5	3–6
		Oral	15–30	2–3	8 or more
Bitolterol	β_2	Inhalation	3–4	0.5–1	5–8
Ephedrine	$\alpha, \beta_{1,2}$	Oral	15–60	—	3–5
		Intramuscular	10–20	—	0.5–1
		Subcutaneous	—	—	0.5–1
Epinephrine	$\alpha, \beta_{1,2}$	Inhalation	3–5	—	1–3
		Intramuscular	Variable	—	<1–4
		Subcutaneous	6–15	0.3	<1–4
Ethylnorepinephrine	$\beta_{1,2}$	Intramuscular	6–12	—	1–2
		Subcutaneous	6–12	—	1–2

Drug	Receptor	Route	Onset	Peak	Duration
Fenoterol	β_2	Inhalation	5	0.5–1	2–3
		Oral	30–60	2–3	6–8
Isoetharine	β_2	Inhalation	1–6	0.25–1	1–4
Isoproterenol	$\beta_{1,2}$	Inhalation	2–5	—	0.5–2
		Intravenous	Immediate	—	<1
		Sublingual	15–30	—	1–2
Metaproterenol	β_2	Inhalation (aerosol)	Within 1	1	1–5
		Oral	Within 15–30	Within 1	Up to 4
Pirbuterol	β_2	Inhalation	Within 5	0.5–1	5
Procaterol	β_2	Inhalation	Within 5	1.5	6–8
Terbutaline	β_2	Inhalation	15–30	1–2	3–6
		Oral	Within 60–120	Within 2–3	4–8
		Parenteral	Within 15	Within 0.5–1	1.5–4

From Ciccone, CD: Pharmacology in Rehabilitation, ed 2. FA Davis, Philadelphia, 1996, p 375, with permission.

XANTHINE DERIVATIVE BRONCHODILATORS

Drug	Common Trade Names	Dosage Forms
Aminophylline	Palaron, Phyllocontin	Oral, extended-release oral, rectal, injection
Dyphylline	Dilor, Lufyllin, Neothylline, others	Oral, injection
Oxtriphylline	Choledyl, Novotriphyl	Oral, extended-release oral
Theophylline	Aerolate, Quibron, Theo-Dur, many others	Oral, extended-release oral, injection

From Ciccone, CD: Pharmacology in Rehabilitation, ed 2. FA Davis, Philadelphia, 1996, p 378, with permission.

CORTICOSTEROIDS USED IN OBSTRUCTIVE PULMONARY DISEASE

Generic Name	Trade Name(s)	Dosage Forms
Beclomethasone	Beclovent, Vanceril	Inhalation
Dexamethasone	Decadron	Inhalation
Flunisolide	AeroBid	Inhalation
Methylprednisolone	Medrol	Intravenous injection
Prednisolone	Hydeltrasol	Intravenous or intramuscular injection
Triamcinolone	Azmacort	Inhalation

From Ciccone, CD: Pharmacology in Rehabilitation, ed 2. FA Davis, Philadelphia, 1996, p 380, with permission.

CLASSIFICATION OF PULMONARY IMPAIRMENTS

restrictive: Characterized by a decreased VC with normal expiratory air flows.

obstructive: Characterized by reductions in air flows with or without reductions in the VC.

	SEVERITY OF PULMONARY IMPAIRMENTS (percent of predicted normal)					
Severity	VC	FEV[1]	FEV[1]/FVC	MEF	TLC	DLco
Normal	>80	>80	>70	>65	>80	>80
Mild	66–80	66–80	60–70	50–65	66–80	61–80
Moderate	50–65	50–65	45–59	35–49	50–65	40–60
Severe	<50	<50	<45	<35	<50	<40

FOR MORE INFORMATION

Murray, JF and Nadel, JA: Textbook of Respiratory Medicine, ed 2. WB Saunders, Philadelphia, 1994.

5

521

CLASSES OF RESPIRATORY IMPAIRMENT

	Class 1 0% Impairment	Class 2 20%–30% Impairment	Class 3 40%–50% Impairment	Class 4 60%–90% Impairment
Roentgenographic appearance	Usually normal but there may be evidence of healed or inactive chest disease including, for example, minimal nodular silicosis or pleural scars	May be normal or abnormal	May be normal but usually is not	Usually is abnormal
Dyspnea	When it occurs, it is consistent with the circumstances of activity	Does not occur at rest and seldom occurs during the performance of the usual activities of daily living. The patient can keep pace with persons of same age and body build on the level without breathlessness but not on hills or stairs	Does not occur at rest but does occur during the usual activities of daily living. However, the patient can walk a mile at his own pace without dyspnea although he cannot keep pace on the level with others of the same age and body build	Occurs during such activities as climbing one flight of stairs or walking 100 yd on the level, on less exertion, or even at rest

Tests of ventilatory function (at least two should be performed)			
FEV FVC	Not <85% of predicted	70%–85% of predicted	55%–70% predicted	<55% of predicted
Arterial oxygen saturation	Not applicable	Not applicable	Usually 88%* or greater at rest and after exercise	Usually <88% at rest and after exercise

*Eighty-eight percent saturation corresponds to an arterial PO$_2$ of 58 mm, assuming the arterial pH is in the normal range. From Guides to the Evaluator of Permanent Impairment—The Respiratory System. JAMA 194:919, 1965.

5

EXERCISE TESTING THE PATIENT WITH PULMONARY DISEASE

Mode	Author	Protocol
PROTOCOLS USED FOR EXERCISE TESTING THE PATIENT WITH PULMONARY DISEASE		
Walk test	Cooper	Ambulate as far as possible in 12 min.
	Guyatt et al.	Ambulate as far as possible in 6 min.
Cycle test	Jones	Begin with 100 kpm (17 W), increase 100 kpm every minute.
	Berman and Sutton	Begin with 100 kpm/min, increase 100 kpm/min every minute or 50 kpm/min every minute when $FEV_1 < 1$ L/s.
	Mass. Respiratory Hospital	Begin at 25 W, increase 10 W every 20 s or 5 W every 20 s when $FEV_1 < 1$ L/s.
Treadmill tests	Naughton et al.	2 mph constant 0 grade. 3.5% grade every 3 min.
	Balke and Ware	3.3 mph constant 0 grade. 3.5% grade every 2 min.
	Mass. Respiratory Hospital	1.5 mph constant 0 grade. 4% grade every 2 min. 2% grade every 2 min if $FEV_1 < 1$ L/s.

Data from Cooper, K: A means of assessing maximal oxygen intake: Correlation between field and treadmill walking. JAMA 203:201, 1968; Guyatt, G, Berman, L, and Townsend, M: Long-term outcome after respiratory rehabilitation. Can Med Assoc J 137:1089, 1987; Jones, N: Exercise testing in pulmonary evaluation: Rationale, methods and the normal respiratory response to exercise. N Eng J Med 293:541, 1975; Berman, L and Sutton, J: Exercise for the pulmonary patient. J Cardiopulmonary Rehabilitation 6:55, 1986; Massachusetts Respiratory Hospital, Exercise Testing Protocol, Braintree, MA; Naughton, J, Balke, B and Poarch, R: Modified work capacity studies in individuals with and without coronary artery disease. J Sports Med 4:208, 1964; Balke, B and Ware, R: An experimental study of physical fitness of Air Force personnel. US Armed Forces Med J 10:675, 1959.

FOR MORE INFORMATION

American Thoracic Society: Evaluation of impairment secondary to respiratory disease. Am Rev Respir Dis 126:945, 1982.

Weber, K and Janicki, J: Cardiopulmonary Exercise Testing. WB Saunders, Philadelphia, 1986.

Zadai, C: Rehabilitation of the patient with chronic obstructive pulmonary disease. In Irwin, S and Tecklin, J (eds): Cardiopulmonary Physical Therapy. CV Mosby, St. Louis, 1985.

DEFINITIONS FOR A TEN-POINT PERCEIVED SHORTNESS OF BREATH SCALE

Score	Activity	Perceived Shortness of Breath
1	Rest	Not short of breath
2	Minimal activity	Minimally short of breath
3	Very light activity	Slightly short of breath
4	Light activity	Mildly short of breath
5	Somewhat hard activity	Mildly to moderately short of breath
6	Hard activity	Moderately short of breath
7		Moderately to severely short of breath
8	Very hard activity	Severely short of breath
9		Breathing not in control
10	Very, very hard activity	Maximally short of breath

Based on Pulmonary Rehabilitation Program, Massachusetts Respiratory Hospital, Braintree, MA.

ARTERIAL BLOOD GASES AND OXYGENATION

arterial blood gas (ABG) studies: Provide information about how well the lungs are functioning to provide oxygen, eliminate carbon dioxide, and, with the kidneys, regulate the blood's acid-base balance. Serious consequences can result from abnormal ABGs.

FOR MORE INFORMATION

West, JB: Respiratory Physiology—The Essentials, ed 5. Williams & Wilkins, Baltimore, 1995.

NORMAL ARTERIAL BLOOD GAS VALUES

Arterial	Premature	Term Infant	Child	Adult
pH	7.35–7.39	7.26–7.41	7.35–7.45	7.35–7.45
$PaCO_2$	38–44 mm Hg	34–54 mm Hg	35–45 mm Hg	35–45 mm Hg
PaO_2	65–80 mm Hg	60 mm Hg	75–100 mm Hg	75–100 mm Hg
O_2 sat	40%–90%	40%–95%	95%–98%	95%–98%
CO_2 content	19–27 mEq/L	20–28 mEq/L	18–27 mEq/L	23–29 mEq/L
Base excess	–1 to –2 mEq/L	–7 to –1 mEq/L	–4 to +2 mEq/L	–2 to +2 mEq/L

5

GAS PRESSURE (mm Hg)					
Gas	Dry Air	Moist Tracheal Air	Alveolar Gas	Arterial Blood	Mixed Venous Blood
PO_2	159.1	149.2	104	100	40
PCO_2	0.3	0.3	40	40	46
PH_2O	0.0	47.0	47	47	47
PN_2	600.6	563.5	569	573	573
P_{TOTAL}	760	760	760	760	706

INTERPRETATION OF ABNORMAL ACID-BASE BALANCE

Type	pH	$PaCO_2$	CO_2	Causes	Signs and Symptoms
Respiratory alkalosis	↑	↓	WNL	Alveolar hyperventilation	Dizziness, syncopy, tingling, numbness, early tetany
Respiratory acidosis	↓	↑	WNL	Alveolar hypoventilation	Early: anxiety, restlessness, dyspnea, headache; late: confusion, somnolence, coma
Metabolic alkalosis	↑	WNL	↑	Bicarbonate ingestion, vomiting, diuretics, steroids, adrenal disease	Vague symptoms: weakness, mental dullness, possibly early tetany
Metabolic acidosis	↓	WNL	↓	Diabetic, lactic, or uremic acidosis, prolonged diarrhea	Secondary hyperventilation (Kussmaul's breathing), nausea and vomiting, cardiac dysrhythmias, lethargy, and coma

↑ = increase; ↓ = decrease; WNL = within normal limits.

FOR MORE INFORMATION

West, JB: Respiratory Physiology—The Essentials, ed 5. Williams & Wilkins, Baltimore, 1995.

5

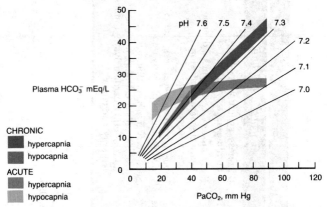

RESPIRATORY ALTERATIONS IN ACID-BASE BALANCE

This nomogram, adapted from McLean, relates the values of the pH, PCO_2, and bicarbonate concentration in the plasma of arterial blood. If two of these are known, a line drawn through the corresponding points will intersect the third column at the point of the desired value. The values shown are only approximate because there are normal differences between men and women and because variations in the levels of hematocrit, blood buffer base, oxygen saturation of the blood, and temperature at which the determinations are made also affect these relationships.

OXYGENATION

The PaO_2 and the hemoglobin oxygen saturation (O_2 sat) provide information about how well the lungs are functioning as an oxygenator.

hypoxemia: An abnormally low amount of oxygen in the blood.

hypoxia: Refers to a low amount of oxygen, usually at the tissue level.

NONINVASIVE OXYGEN MONITORING

Ear oximetry is useful for monitoring oxygen saturation during exercise. Capillary oxygen saturation is measured by spectrophotometry using a device that attaches to the ear. Transcutaneous skin electrodes are also used to assess oxygen saturation in pediatric patients; transcutaneous oxygen pressure (TCO_2) correlates well with the PaO_2, although the TCO_2 value tends to be lower.

CAUSES OF HYPOXEMIA

Type	Description	Causes
Hypoventilation	Low level of ventilation causes increase in Pa_{CO_2} with concomitant decrease in Pa_{O_2}.	Drug overdose, anesthesia, pathology of medulla, abnormalities of spinal pathways, poliomyelitis, diseases and pathology of respiratory muscles, chest wall trauma, kyphoscoliosis, upper airway obstruction
Diffusion impairment	Blood-gas barrier is thickened.	Asbestosis, sarcoidosis, interstitial fibrosis, collagen diseases, alveolar cell carcinoma
Shunt	Blood reaches arterial system without passing through ventilated regions of the lungs; can be anatomic or physiologic.	Congenital cardiac defects, infectious and inflammatory processes
$\dot{V}/\dot{Q}$ inequality	Mismatching of ventilation to blood flow.	Chronic obstructive lung disease, interstitial lung disease, vascular disorders
Decreased inspired oxygen	Partial pressure of oxygen lowers as barometric pressure decreases	High altitudes

5

OXYGEN THERAPY

high-flow: All of the gas the patient breathes is delivered by a mask or tube, which allows for precise control of FiO_2. Venturi or "Venti" masks are high-flow systems that mix room air with oxygen to provide a precise FiO_2.

low-flow: This system provides only part of the patient's minute volume and uses masks, nasal cannula, or prongs. The tidal volume should be between 300 and 700 ml and the ventilatory rate below 25 per minute to use a low-flow system. Due to variability in ventilation, the FiO_2 can only be estimated.

ESTIMATED FRACTION OF INSPIRED OXYGEN WITH LOW-FLOW DEVICES	
Low-Flow Device	*Estimated FiO_2 (%)*
Room air	21
Nasal prongs	
1 L/min	24
3 L/min	28
3 L/min	32
4 L/min	36
5 L/min	40
6 L/min	44
Oxygen mask	
5–6 L/min	40
6–7 L/min	50
7–8 L/min	60
Mask with reservoir bag	
6 L/min	60
7 L/min	70
8 L/min	80
9 L/min	90
10 L/min	99+

SPUTUM ANALYSIS

Sputum is described in terms of quantity, viscosity, color, and odor. The frequency, time of day, and ease of expectoration is also noted. Laboratory analysis is necessary to establish a definitive diagnosis. These tests include Gram's stain for bacteria, culture and sensitivity for infectious agent, and appropriate antibiotic, acid-fast bacillus stain to detect the tuberculosis bacillus, and cytology to examine for cellular constituents and malignancy.

SPUTUM	
Term	*Description*
Fetid	Foul-smelling, typical of anaerobic infection; typically occurs with bronchiectasis, lung abscess, or cystic fibrosis
Frothy	White or pink-tinged, foamy, thin sputum associated with pulmonary edema
Hemoptysis	Expectoration of blood or bloody sputum; amount may range from blood-streaked to massive hemorrhage and is present in a variety of pathologies
Mucoid	White or clear, not generally associated with bronchopulmonary infection but is present with chronic cough (acute or chronic bronchitis, cystic fibrosis)
Mucopurulent	Mixture of mucoid sputum and pus, yellow to pale green, associated with infection
Purulent	Pus, yellow or greenish sputum, often copious and thick, common with acute and chronic infection
Rusty	Descriptive of the color of sputum; classic for pneumococcal pneumonia (also called *prune juice*)
Tenacious	Thick, sticky sputum

FOR MORE INFORMATION

Irwin, S and Tecklin, JS: Cardiopulmonary Physical Therapy, ed 3. CV Mosby, St. Louis, 1995.

BRONCHIAL DRAINAGE

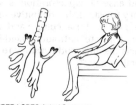

UPPER LOBES Apical Segments

Bed or drainage table flat.

Patient leans back on pillow at 30° angle against therapist.

Therapist claps with markedly cupped hand over area between clavicle and top of scapula on each side.

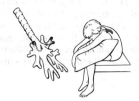

UPPER LOBES Posterior Segments

Bed or drainage table flat.

Patient leans over folder pillow at 30° angle.

Therapist stands behind and claps over upper back on both sides.

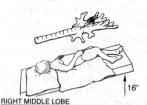

RIGHT MIDDLE LOBE

Foot of table or bed elevated 16 inches.

Patient lies head down on left side and rotates ¼ turn backward. Pillow may be placed behind from shoulder to hip. Knees should be flexed.

Therapist claps over right nipple area. In females with breast development or tenderness, use cupped hand with heel of hand under armpit and fingers extending forward beneath the breast.

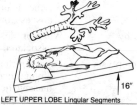

LEFT UPPER LOBE Lingular Segments

Foot of table or bed elevated 16 inches.

Patient lies head down on right side and rotates ¼ turn backward. Pillow may be placed behind from shoulder to hip. Knees should be flexed.

Therapist claps with moderately cupped hand over left nipple area. In females with breast development or tenderness, use cupped hand with heel of hand under armpit and fingers extending forward beneath the breast.

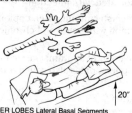

LOWER LOBES Lateral Basal Segments

Foot of table or bed elevated 20 inches.

Patient lies on abdomen, head down, then rotates ¼ turn upward. Upper leg is flexed over a pillow for support.

Therapist claps over uppermost portion of lower ribs. (Position shown is for drainage of right lateral basal segment, patient should lie on his right side in the same posture).

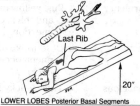

LOWER LOBES Posterior Basal Segments

Foot of table or bed elevated 20 inches.

Patient lies on abdomen, head down, with pillow under hips. Therapist claps over lower ribs close to spine on each side.

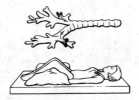

UPPER LOBES Anterior Segments

Bed or drainage table flat.

Patient lies on back with pillow under knees.

Therapist claps between clavicle and nipple on each side.

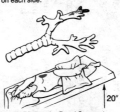

20″

LOWER LOBES Anterior Basal Segments

Foot of table or bed elevated 20 inches.

Patient lies on side, head down, pillow under knees.

Therapist claps with slightly cupped hand over lower ribs. (Position shown is for drainage of left anterior basal segment. To drain the right anterior basal segment, patient should lie on his left side in same posture).

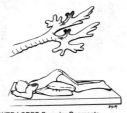

LOWER LOBES Superior Segments

Bed or table flat.

Patient lies on abdomen with two pillows under hips.

Therapist claps over middle of back at tip of scapula on either side of spine.

ESSENTIALS OF PULMONARY THERAPY

Treatment Components	Purpose	How to Perform	When to Use	Things to Avoid	Important Details to Remember
Postural drainage	Mobilize retained secretions through assistance of gravity	Patient positioned so that involved segmental bronchus is uppermost.	When coughing or suctioning, breathing exercises, and patient mobilization are not adequate to clear retained secretions	Avoid significant changes in patient's vital signs, increase in intracranial pressure, and stress to intravascular lines and indwelling tubes.	Patient must be properly positioned for bronchial drainage of lung segment involved; this can be attained despite the presence of multiple injuries, monitoring equipment, and lines.
Percussion	As an adjunct to postural drainage for mobilization of secretions	Rhythmic clapping of cupped hands over bare skin or thin material covering area of lung involvement; performed during inspiration and expiration.	Same as above	Avoid redness or petechiae of skin (indicates improper hand positioning by therapist, or patient coagulopathy).	May be performed in the presence of rib fractures, chest tubes and subcutaneous emphysema; should produce a hollow sound; should not cause

| Vibration | As an adjunct to postural drainage for mobilization of secretions | Intermittent chest wall compression over area of lung involvement; performed during expiration only. | Same as above | Avoid pinching or shearing of soft tissue and digging of fingers into soft tissue. |

undue pain; does not need to be forceful to be effective if performed properly.

Should not be performed over rib fractures or unstable thoracic spine injuries; be sure to vibrate chest wall, not just shake soft tissue; forcefulness should vary according to patient's needs and tolerance.

Continued on following page

5

ESSENTIALS OF PULMONARY THERAPY (Continued)

Treatment Components	Purpose	How to Perform	When to Use	Things to Avoid	Important Details to Remember
Breathing exercises	Assistance in removal of secretions; relaxation; and to increase thoracic cage mobility and tidal volume	Patient taught to produce a full inspiration followed by a controlled expiration; use hand placement for sensory feedback; for diaphragmatic, costal excursion, and lateral costal excursion techniques.	For use with spontaneously breathing patients	Avoid use of accessory muscles of respiration.	May be used independently or in conjunction with other chest therapy techniques; with practice, breathing exercises lead to increased chest expansion; breathing exercises should promote relaxation, not increase the work of breathing.
Coughing	Removal of secretions from the larger airways	Steps: 1. Inspiratory gasp. 2. Closing of the glottis. 3. Contraction of expiratory muscles.	For use with spontaneously breathing patients	Avoid bronchospasm induced by repetitive coughing.	Coughing is less effective in tracheally intubated patients; coughing ability can be improved by manual support

4. Opening of the glottis.

of the patient's incision; stomas following tracheal tube removal should be covered with an airtight dressing to improve cough efficiency; an effective cough must be preceded by a large inspiration; methods of cough stimulation, including "huffing," vibration, summed breathing, external tracheal compression and oral pharyngeal stimulation, are used.

Continued on following page

	ESSENTIALS OF PULMONARY THERAPY (Continued)			
Treatment Components	Purpose	How to Perform	When to Use	Important Details to Remember
Suctioning	Removal of secretions from the larger airways	Use aseptic technique. Steps: 1. Provide supplemental oxygen. 2. Insert suction catheter without applying suction, as fully as possible; be gentle. 3. Apply suction while withdrawing catheter. 4. Re-expand lung with mechanical ventilator or manual inflation by resuscitator bag attached to tracheal tube.	Tracheal suctioning for use only with patients who have an artificial airway in place	Avoid hypoxemia (cyanosis and significant changes in vital signs) and cardiac dysrhythmias, mechanical trauma and bacterial contamination of tracheo-bronchial tree, and increase in intracranial pressure.	In intubated patients, suctioning is performed routinely and is an integral part of chest therapy; frequency of suctioning is determined by the quantity of secretions; the suctioning procedure should be limited to a total of 15 s; the suction catheter can reach only to the level of the main-stem bronchus; it is more difficult to cannulate the left main-stem bronchus than the

Bagging	Provide artificial ventilation; restore oxygen and re-expand the lungs after suctioning	Coordinate with patient's breathing pattern. Steps: 1. Attach manual resuscitator bag to oxygen source. 2. Connect manual resuscitator bag to tracheal tube. 3. Squeeze bag rhythmically to deliver volume of air to patient. 4. Patient expires passively.	Before and after suctioning patients who are not mechanically ventilated and who cannot be mechanically sighed	Avoid barotrauma.	right; nasotracheal suctioning should be avoided. Bagging can be used in conjunction with vibration when treating patients not breathing deeply; hyperinflation can produce alterations in cardiac output.
Patient mobilization	To prevent the detrimental sequelae of bedrest and immobilization; to decrease	Turning and passively positioning the patient; appropriate splint usage; passive	Used to some degree with every patient according to patient's diagnosis and	Avoid stress to intravascular lines and indwelling tubes, orthostatic	Mobilization is possible to some degree for every patient; minimal supplies are needed for mobilization;

Continued on following page

5

		ESSENTIALS OF PULMONARY THERAPY (Continued)		
Treatment Components	Purpose	How to Perform	When to Use	Things to Avoid	Important Details to Remember
	rehabilitation time	and active range of motion; active and resistive exercises; sitting, standing, and ambulating the patient.	tolerance	hypotension, significant changes in vital signs, and dyspnea.	emphasis should be placed on functional activities; proper positioning may decrease spasticity in patients with head injuries; ECG leads and arterial and central venous pressure lines should be temporarily disconnected from the recording module during ambulation; at the physician's discretion, chest tubes and abdominal sumps may be disconnected from wall suction to allow ambulation.

ECG = electrocardiograph.

Vascular Anatomy, Cardiology, and Cardiac Rehabilitation

6

BRANCHES OF THE AORTA

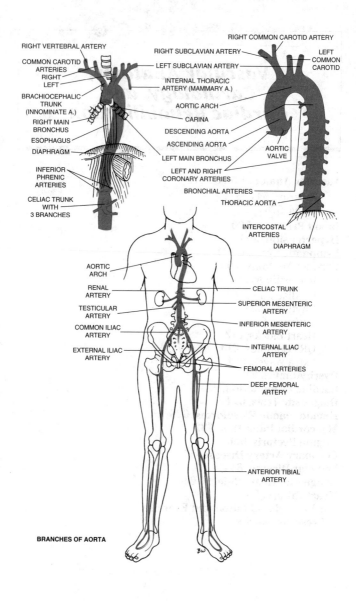

RIGHT VERTEBRAL ARTERY

COMMON CAROTID ARTERIES
RIGHT
LEFT

BRACHIOCEPHALIC TRUNK (INNOMINATE A.)

RIGHT MAIN BRONCHUS

ESOPHAGUS

DIAPHRAGM

INFERIOR PHRENIC ARTERIES

CELIAC TRUNK WITH 3 BRANCHES

RIGHT COMMON CAROTID ARTERY

RIGHT SUBCLAVIAN ARTERY

LEFT SUBCLAVIAN ARTERY

INTERNAL THORACIC ARTERY (MAMMARY A.)

AORTIC ARCH

CARINA

DESCENDING AORTA

ASCENDING AORTA

LEFT MAIN BRONCHUS

LEFT AND RIGHT CORONARY ARTERIES

BRONCHIAL ARTERIES

THORACIC AORTA

LEFT COMMON CAROTID

AORTIC VALVE

INTERCOSTAL ARTERIES

DIAPHRAGM

AORTIC ARCH

RENAL ARTERY

TESTICULAR ARTERY

COMMON ILIAC ARTERY

EXTERNAL ILIAC ARTERY

CELIAC TRUNK

SUPERIOR MESENTERIC ARTERY

INFERIOR MESENTERIC ARTERY

INTERNAL ILIAC ARTERY

FEMORAL ARTERIES

DEEP FEMORAL ARTERY

ANTERIOR TIBIAL ARTERY

BRANCHES OF AORTA

BRANCHES OF THE AORTA

Location	Name	Status
Thorax		
Ascending aorta	Right and left coronary arteries	One pair
Aortic arch	Brachiocephalic trunk	Unpaired
	Right subclavian	
	Right common carotid	
	Left common carotid	Unpaired
	Left subclavian	Unpaired
Descending aorta	Visceral branches	Unpaired
	Esophageal	
	Left upper and lower bronchial	
	Right bronchial	
	Pericardial	
	Mediastinal	
	Parietal branches	Paired
	Posterior intercostal (T3–T11)	
	Subcostal (T12)	
	Superior phrenic	
Abdominal	Visceral branches	Unpaired
	Celiac	
	Superior mesenteric	
	Inferior mesenteric	
	Glandular/visceral branches	Paired
	Suprarenal	
	Renal	
	Testicular (ovarian)	
	Parietal branches	
	Inferior phrenic	Paired
	Lumbar (L1–L4)	Paired
	Median sacral	Unpaired

6

ARTERIES OF THE BODY

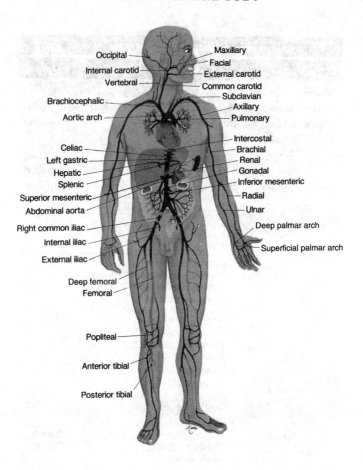

Occipital
Internal carotid
Vertebral
Brachiocephalic
Aortic arch
Celiac
Left gastric
Hepatic
Splenic
Superior mesenteric
Abdominal aorta
Right common iliac
Internal iliac
External iliac
Deep femoral
Femoral
Popliteal
Anterior tibial
Posterior tibial

Maxillary
Facial
External carotid
Common carotid
Subclavian
Axillary
Pulmonary
Intercostal
Brachial
Renal
Gonadal
Inferior mesenteric
Radial
Ulnar
Deep palmar arch
Superficial palmar arch

ARTERIES OF THE PELVIS AND PERINEUM

Parent Vessel	Primary Branch	Secondary Branches	Anastomoses	Area Supplied
Internal iliac (visceral)	Umbilical	Superior vesical	Artery of ductus Deferens to testicular	Bladder
		Ductus deferens	Testicular	Ductus deferens
		Middle vesical	Branches from the opposite side	Fundus of bladder, seminal vesicles
	Inferior vesicular		Branches from opposite side	
	Middle rectal		Inferior vesical, superior and inferior rectal	
	Uterine		Ovarian	
		Vaginal	Inferior vesical	
Internal iliac (anterior parietal)	Obturator			
		Iliac	Iliolumbar	Iliacus muscle
		Vesical		Bladder
		Pubic	Inferior epigastric, and its opposite side	

Continued on following page

ARTERIES OF THE PELVIS AND PERINEUM (Continued)

Parent Vessel	Primary Branch	Secondary Branches	Anastomoses	Area Supplied
		Anterior	Posterior branch, femoral circumflex	Obturator externus, pectineus, gracilis, and adductor muscles
		Posterior	Anterior branch, inferior gluteal	Hip joint, buttocks
	Internal pudendal (Listings here are for the male; in the female the artery is smaller and supplies homologous structures.)	Muscular	Inferior gluteal	Levator ani, obturator internus, piriformis, coccygeus, and gluteus maximus muscles and other lateral rotators
		Inferior rectal	Perineal, superior and middle rectal, and vessels on the opposite side	Muscles and integument of the anal region
		Perineal	Inferior rectal and vessels on the opposite side	Bulbospongiosus, ischiocavernosus, scrotum
		Artery of the bulb of the penis		Bulb of the penis

		Urethral		Urethra
		Deep artery of the penis	Terminal branch of internal pudendal	Erectile tissue
		Dorsal artery of the penis	Deep artery of the penis	Glans, prepuce
Internal iliac (posterior parietal)	Iliolumbar	Lumbar	Last lumbar	Psoas major and quadratus lumborum muscles
		Iliac	Iliac of obturator, superior gluteal, iliac circumflex, lateral femoral circumflex	Iliacus and gluteal and abdominal muscles
	Lateral sacral	Superior	Middle sacral, superior gluteal	Skin and muscles on the dorsum of the sacrum
		Inferior	Middle sacral and opposite branch of the lateral sacral	Skin and muscles on the dorsum of the sacrum

Continued on following page

6

Parent Vessel	Primary Branch	Secondary Branches	Anastomoses	Area Supplied
	Superior gluteal	Superficial	Inferior gluteal, posterior branches of lateral sacral	Gluteus maximus, skin over the dorsal sacrum
		Deep	Deep iliac circumflex, ascending branch of lateral femoral circumflex	Gluteal muscles, hip joint
	Inferior gluteal	Muscular	Superior gluteal, internal pudendal, posterior branch of obturator, medial femoral circumflex	Gluteus maximus, lateral rotator muscles, upper part of hamstring muscles
		Coccygeal	Medial and lateral circumflex	Gluteus maximus and skin over the coccyx
		Artery of sciatic nerve		Artery that runs in the sciatic nerve and supplies that nerve
		Articular	Obturator	Capsule of the hip joint
		Cutaneous		Skin of buttock and posterior thigh

External iliac	Inferior epigastric			
			Superior epigastric of internal thoracic, lower intercostals	Cremaster muscle
		Cremasteric (in males)	Testicular, external pudendal, perineal	Round ligament
		Artery of the round ligament (in females)	(Corresponds to cremasteric in women)	
		Pubic	Obturator	
		Muscular	Iliac circumflex, lumbar, superficial epigastric of femoral	Abdominal muscles
		Deep iliac circumflex	Ascending branch of lateral femoral circumflex, iliolumbar, superior gluteal, lumbar, inferior epigastric	

ARTERIES OF THE TRUNK

Parent Vessel	Primary Branch	Secondary Branches	Anastomoses	Area Supplied
Thoracic aorta (visceral)	Pericardial		Pericardiophrenic of internal thoracic	Pericardium, pleura, diaphragm
	Bronchial			Bronchial tubes, areolar tissue of lung, bronchial lymph nodes
	Esophageal		Esophageal branches of inferior thyroid, ascending branches of left inferior phrenic and left gastric	
	Mediastinal			Lymph nodes, vessels, nerve and loose areolar tissue in the posterior mediastinum
Thoracic aorta (parietal)	Posterior intercostal	Dorsal branch		Muscles of the back, dorsal ramus of the spinal nerve

		Collateral intercostal	Internal thoracic	Intercostal, pectoral, and serratus anterior muscles
		Muscular	Highest and lateral thoracic of axillary	Skin and superficial fascia overlying the intercostal space
		Lateral cutaneous		Breasts
		Mammary	Superior epigastric, caudal intercostal, and lumbar	
	Subcostal		Musculophrenic and pericardiophrenic	Dorsal part of the upper surface of the diaphragm
	Superior phrenic			
Abdominal aorta (visceral)	Celiac	Left gastric	Dorsal branch with right gastric; cardioesophageal branch with esophageals	Cardiac portion of the stomach, lower esophagus, stomach

Continued on following page

6

553

Parent Vessel	Primary Branch	Secondary Branches	Anastomoses	Area Supplied
		Common hepatic (branches listed below)		
		Gastroduodenal	Vessels to stomach and pancreas from superior mesenteric	Pylorus, pancreas, duodenum
		Right gastric	Dorsal branch of left gastric	Pylorus, stomach
		Right hepatic		Liver and via the cystic artery to the gallbladder
		Left hepatic		Capsule of the liver, caudate lobe of the liver
		Middle hepatic		Quadrate lobe of liver
	Splenic (lienal)	Pancreatic	Gastroduodenal, inferior pancreaticoduodenal of superior mesenteric	Pancreas
		Left gastroepiploic	Gastric and epiploic branches of the right gastroepiploic	Stomach

	Short gastrics	Left gastric, left gastroepiploic, inferior phrenic	Fundus and cardia of stomach
	Splenic	Other splenic branches	Spleen
Superior mesenteric	Inferior pancreatico-duodenal	Superior and posterior branches of the pancreaticoduodenal of celiac	Pancreas, duodenum
	Intestinal (jejunal and ileal)		Small intestine
	Ileocolic	End of superior mesenteric and right colic	Ascending colon, cecum, appendix, termination of ileum
	Right colic	Ileocolic, middle colic	Ascending colon
	Middle colic	Right colic, left colic of inferior mesenteric	Transverse colon
Inferior mesenteric			Left half of transverse colon and descending colon
	Left colic	Middle colic, highest sigmoid	Descending colon, left part of transverse colon

Continued on following page

6

ARTERIES OF THE TRUNK (Continued)

Parent Vessel	Primary Branch	Secondary Branches	Anastomoses	Area Supplied
		Sigmoid	Left colic and superior rectal	Caudal part of descending colon, sigmoid colon
		Superior rectal	Middle rectal branches of internal iliac; inferior rectal branches of internal pudendal	Rectum
	Middle suprarenal		Suprarenal branches of inferior phrenic and renals	Suprarenal glands
	Renal			Kidneys
	Testicular (ovarian)		Artery of ductus deferens (ovarian: uterine of internal iliac)	Epididymis (ovaries, round ligament, skin of inguinal region, labia majora)

Abdominal aorta (parietal)	Inferior phrenic	Medial branch	Medial branch of opposite side, musculophrenic, pericardiophrenic	Inferior vena cava, esophagus
		Lateral branch	Lower intercostals, musculophrenic	
	Lumbar		Lower intercostals, subcostal, iliolumbar, deep iliac circumflex, inferior epigastric	Muscles and skin of the back
	Middle sacral		Lumbar branch of iliolumbar, lateral sacral	
Abdominal aorta (terminal branch)	Common iliacs (see Arteries of the Pelvis and Perineum, page 547)			

6

ARTERIES OF THE HEAD AND UPPER EXTREMITY

Parent Vessel	Primary Branch	Secondary Branches	Anastomoses	Area Supplied by Secondary Branches
Subclavian	Vertebral	Spinal	Other spinal arteries	Periosteum and bodies of vertebrae
		Muscular	Occipital, ascending and deep cervical arteries	Deep muscles of neck
		Meningeal	Small branches	Falx cerebelli
		Posterior spinal	Vessels on opposite side	
		Anterior spinal	Inferior thyroid, intercostals, lumbar, iliolumbar, and lateral sacral	Pia mater and spinal cord
		Posterior inferior cerebellar	Anterior inferior cerebellar, superior cerebellar of basilar	Medulla and choroid plexus of fourth ventricle, inferior surface of the cerebellum to the lateral border

Basilar	Pontine		Pons and midbrain
	Labyrinthine (internal auditory)		Internal ear
	Anterior inferior cerebellar		Lateral aspect of the pons, anterolateral and anteromedial parts of the inferior surface of the cerebellum
	Superior cerebellar		Superior surface of the cerebellum, midbrain, pineal body, anterior medullary velum, tela choroidea of the third ventricle
	Posterior cerebral		Temporal and occipital lobes
Thyrocervical trunk	Inferior thyroid	Inferior thyroid on the opposite side	Inferior part of thyroid gland

Continued on following page

6

ARTERIES OF THE HEAD AND UPPER EXTREMITY (Continued)

Parent Vessel	Primary Branch	Secondary Branches	Anastomoses	Area Supplied by Secondary Branches
		Suprascapular	Scapular circumflex, descending scapular, thoracoacromial, and subscapular	Supraspinatus and infraspinatus muscles and sternocleidomastoid and surrounding muscles, skin of anterior superior chest, and structures of the shoulder joint, clavicle, and scapular
		Transverse cervical	Descending branch of occipital, subscapular, suprascapular, circumflex scapular, and, through its descending scapular branch, with posterior intercostals	Trapezius, levator scapulae and deep cervical muscles, rhomboid and serratus posterior superior, subscapularis, supraspinatus, and infraspinatus muscles

Internal thoracic	Pericardiophrenic	Musculophrenic and inferior phrenic	Pleura and pericardium
	Mediastinal		Lymph nodes and areolar tissue in the anterior mediastinum
	Thymic		Thymus
	Sternal	Intercostal and bronchial	Transversus thoracis muscle and posterior surface of the sternum
	Anterior intercostals	Posterior intercostals	Intercostal muscles
	Musculophrenic	Pericardiophrenic, mediastinal, intercostals	Diaphragm, abdominal muscles
	Superior epigastric	Superior epigastric on opposite side,	Abdominal muscles and overlying skin

Continued on following page

6

ARTERIES OF THE HEAD AND UPPER EXTREMITY (Continued)

Parent Vessel	Primary Branch	Secondary Branches	Anastomoses	Area Supplied by Secondary Branches
			inferior epigastric; the right superior epigastric connects with the hepatic	
	Costocervical trunk	Highest (supreme) intercostal	Second intercostal	
		Deep cervical	Vertebral, descending occipital	Semispinalis capitis, cervicis and adjacent muscles
		Descending scapular	(Variable artery; when found, its distribution is similar to the deep branch of the transverse cervical)	
Axillary	Highest thoracic		Internal thoracic, intercostals	Pectoral muscles
	Thoracoacromial	Pectoral	Internal and lateral thoracic, intercostals	Pectoral muscles and breast

	Acromial	Suprascapular, thoracoacromial, posterior humeral circumflex	Deltoid muscle
	Clavicular		Pectoralis major and deltoid muscle
	Deltoid		Sternoclavicular joint and subclavius muscles
	Suprascapular		Serratus anterior, pectoral, and subscapularis, and axillary lymph nodes
Lateral thoracic		Internal thoracic, subscapular, intercostal, pectoral branch of thoracoacromial	
Subscapular	Scapular circumflex	Suprascapular, descending scapular	Infraspinatus, teres major and minor muscles, long head of the triceps and deltoid muscles

Continued on following page

ARTERIES OF THE HEAD AND UPPER EXTREMITY (Continued)

Parent Vessel	Primary Branch	Secondary Branches	Anastomoses	Area Supplied by Secondary Branches
		Thoracodorsal	Circumflex scapular, descending scapular, intercostal, lateral thoracic, thoracoacromial	Subscapularis, latissimus dorsi, serratus anterior, and intercostal muscles
	Posterior humeral circumflex		Anterior humeral circumflex, deep brachial	Deltoid muscle and shoulder joint
	Anterior humeral circumflex		Posterior humeral circumflex	Head of humerus and shoulder joint
Brachial	Deep brachial	Radial collateral	Posterior humeral circumflex, radial recurrent of radial	
		Middle collateral	Interosseous recurrent	
		Deltoid (ascending)	Posterior humeral circumflex	Brachialis and deltoid muscles
	Principal nutrient of the humerus	Nutrient		Humerus
				Humerus

	Branch	Anastomoses	Supplies
	Superior ulnar collateral	Posterior ulnar recurrent, inferior ulnar collateral	
	Inferior ulnar collateral	Anterior ulnar recurrent, superior ulnar collateral, posterior ulnar recurrent	
	Muscular		Coracobrachialis, biceps brachii, and brachialis muscles
Radial	Radial recurrent	Radial collateral of deep brachial	Supinator, brachioradialis and brachialis muscles, elbow joint
	Muscular		Brachioradialis and pronator teres muscles

Continued on following page

6

Parent Vessel	Primary Branch	Secondary Branches	Anastomoses	Area Supplied by Secondary Branches
	Palmar carpal		Palmar carpal of ulnar, palmar interosseous, deep palmar arch	Carpal bones
	Superficial palmar		Terminal ulnar branches	Muscles of the thenar eminence
	Dorsal carpal		Dorsal carpal branch of ulnar, palmar interosseous, and dorsal interosseous	Fingers
	First dorsal metacarpal			Thumb and index finger
	Princeps pollicis		Proper digital, princeps pollicis	Skin and subcutaneous tissue of the thumb
	Radial indicis		Deep palmar arch of ulnar	Ulnar aspect of the index finger
	Deep palmar arch		Common digital branches of the superficial palmar arch	
	Palmar metacarpal			

	Perforating		Dorsal metacarpal	Intercarpal articulations
	Recurrent		Palmar carpal network	
	Anterior ulnar recurrent		Superior and inferior ulnar collaterals	Brachialis and pronator teres muscles
	Posterior ulnar recurrent		Superior and inferior ulnar collaterals, interosseous recurrents	Elbow joint and muscles near the elbow joint
	Common interosseus	Palmar (anterior) interosseous	Dorsal interosseous	Flexor digitorum profundus and flexor pollicis longus muscles, radius and ulna
		Dorsal (posterior) interosseous	Palmar interosseous, dorsal carpal network	Superficial and deep muscles of the posterior compartment of the forearm
Ulnar				

Continued on following page

6

Parent Vessel	Primary Branch	Secondary Branches	Anastomoses	Area Supplied by Secondary Branches
	Muscular			Superficial and deep flexors of the finger and muscles on the ulnar aspect of the forearm
	Palmar carpal		Corresponding palmar carpal branch of the radial	
	Dorsal carpal		Corresponding dorsal carpal branch of the radial	Ulnar aspect of dorsal surface of the little finger
	Deep palmar		Radial to complete the deep palmar arch	
	Superficial palmar arch		Superficial palmar branch of the radial	
	Common palmar digital		Dorsal digital	Soft parts on the dorsum of the middle and distal phalanges
		Proper palmar digital	Dorsal branches to dorsal digital	

ARTERIES OF THE LOWER EXTREMITY

Parent Vessel	Primary Branch	Secondary Branches	Anastomoses	Area Supplied
Femoral	Superficial epigastric		Inferior epigastric and superficial epigastric on the opposite side	Superficial subinguinal lymph nodes
	Superficial iliac circumflex		Deep circumflex iliac, superior gluteal, lateral femoral circumflex	Skin of the groin and superficial subinguinal lymph nodes
	Superficial external pudendal		Internal pudendal	Skin of the lower part of the abdomen, scrotum, and penis (labia majora in female)
	Deep external pudendal		Posterior scrotal (labial), branches of the perineal	Skin of the scrotum (labia majora in female)
	Muscular			Sartorius, vastus medialis, adductor muscles
	Deep femoral	Medial femoral circumflex	Ascending branch with obturator; superficial branch with inferior	Ascending to adductor muscles, gracilis and obturator externus

Continued on following page

ARTERIES OF THE LOWER EXTREMITY (Continued)

Parent Vessel	Primary Branch	Secondary Branches	Anastomoses	Area Supplied
			gluteal, lateral femoral circumflex, first perforating; deep branch with gluteals; acetabular branch with obturator	muscles; transverse branch to the adductor magnus and brevis muscles; acetabular branch to the fat in the acetabular fossa
		Lateral femoral circumflex	Ascending branch with superior gluteal and deep iliac circumflex; descending branch with superior lateral genicular branch of popliteal; transverse branch with medial femoral circumflex, inferior gluteal, first perforating	
		Perforating	First perforating with inferior gluteal, medial and lateral femoral circumflex, and second perforating; second with first and third perforating; third with second perforating, deep	First perforating to adductor brevis and magnus muscles, biceps femoris and gluteus maximus muscles; second perforating to

Descending genicular		femoral terminal branches and popliteal	posterior femoral muscles
	Muscular	Medial femoral circumflex, superior branches of popliteal	Adductor muscles, hamstring muscles
	Saphenous	Medial inferior genicular	Skin on the upper and medial leg
	Articular branch	Medial superior genicular and anterior recurrent tibial	Knee joint
Popliteal			
Superior muscular		Terminals of deep femoral	Lower parts of the adductor magnus and hamstring muscles
Sural			Gastrocnemius, soleus, and plantaris muscles
Cutaneous			Skin on the back of the leg
Superior genicular	Medial superior genicular	Descending and medial inferior geniculars, lateral superior genicular	Vastus medialis muscle, femur, knee joint

Continued on following page

Parent Vessel	Primary Branch	Secondary Branches	Anastomoses	Area Supplied
		Lateral superior genicular (superficial and deep branches)	Descending branch of lateral femoral circumflex and lateral inferior genicular	Vastus lateralis muscle, femur, knee joint
	Middle genicular			Ligaments and synovial membrane of the knee joint
	Inferior genicular	Medial inferior genicular	Lateral inferior and medial superior geniculars	Popliteus muscle, upper end of tibia, knee joint
		Lateral inferior genicular	Medial inferior and lateral superior geniculars, anterior and posterior recurrents of tibial, circumflex fibular	
Anterior tibial	Posterior tibial recurrent		Inferior genicular of popliteal	Popliteus muscle
	Anterior tibial recurrent		Genicular branches of popliteal, circumflex fibular, and descending genicular	
	Muscular		Posterior tibial and peroneal	Muscles along the vessel
	Anterior medial malleolar		Posterior tibial, medial plantar	

Artery	Branch	Branches	Description	Distribution
Dorsal pedis	Anterior lateral malleolar			Lateral aspect of the ankle
	Lateral tarsal	Arcuate, anterior lateral malleolar, lateral plantar, peroneal	Perforating branch of the peroneal and lateral tarsal	Extensor digitorum brevis muscle
	Medial tarsal		Medial malleolar network	
	Arcuate		Lateral tarsal and plantars to yield the second through fourth dorsal metatarsals and two dorsal digital arteries	
	First dorsal metatarsal			Medial border of the great toe
	Deep plantar		Unites with terminals of lateral plantar to complete plantar arch; produces first plantar metarsal artery	
Posterior tibial	Circumflex fibular		Vessels around knee joint	Soleus and peroneal muscles

Continued on following page

6

573

ARTERIES OF THE LOWER EXTREMITY (Continued)

Parent Vessel	Primary Branch	Secondary Branches	Anastomoses	Area Supplied
	Peroneal			
		Muscular		Soleus, tibialis posterior, flexor hallucis longus, and peroneal muscles
		Nutrient (fibular)		Fibular
		Perforating	Anterior lateral malleolar, lateral metatarsal	Tarsal bone
		Communicating	Communicating of posterior tibial	
		Lateral malleolar	Lateral malleolar network	
		Lateral calcaneal	Anterior lateral malleolar, medial calcaneal	
	Nutrient (tibial)			Tibialis posterior muscle, tibia
	Muscular			Soleus and deep muscles along the back of the leg

Medial malleolar		Medial malleolar network	
Communicating		Artery that joins communicating branch of the peroneal	
Medial calcaneal		Peroneal, medial malleolar, lateral calcaneal	Muscles on the tibial side of the sole of the foot
Medial plantar		First dorsal or plantar metatarsal	
Lateral plantar	Perforating	Dorsal metatarsals to yield plantar digital arteries; anterior perforating branch to join dorsal metatarsal	Digits

6

VEINS OF THE BODY

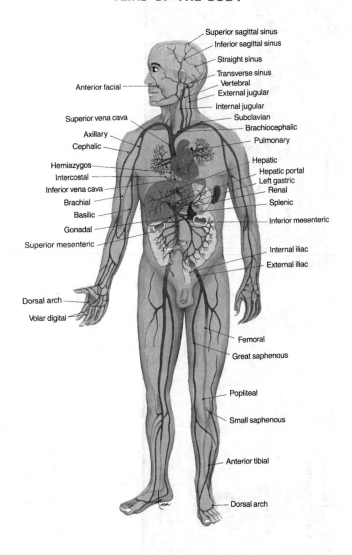

Superior sagittal sinus
Inferior sagittal sinus
Straight sinus
Transverse sinus
Vertebral
External jugular
Internal jugular
Subclavian
Brachiocephalic
Pulmonary
Hepatic
Hepatic portal
Left gastric
Renal
Splenic
Inferior mesenteric
Internal iliac
External iliac

Anterior facial
Superior vena cava
Axillary
Cephalic
Hemiazygos
Intercostal
Inferior vena cava
Brachial
Basilic
Gonadal
Superior mesenteric
Dorsal arch
Volar digital

Femoral
Great saphenous
Popliteal
Small saphenous
Anterior tibial
Dorsal arch

VENOUS SYSTEM

VENOUS DRAINAGE FROM THE LUNGS

Vein	Primary Tributary	Area Drained
Right pulmonary veins (2)	Right superior pulmonary	Right superior and middle lobes
	Apical segmental	Apex and anterior segments
	Posterior segmental	Posterior middle and superior lobes
	Anterior segmental	Right superior lobe
	Right middle lobe	Middle lobe
	Right inferior pulmonary	Right inferior hilum
	Superior segmental	Medial middle lobe
	Common basal	Anterior basal, lateral basal, and posterior basal segments
Left pulmonary veins (2)	Left superior pulmonary	Apicoposterior, anterior segments
	Apicoposterior segmental	Apicoposterior segments
	Posterior segmental	Intrasegmental and intersegmental areas
	Lingular division	Superior and inferior lingular segments
	Left inferior pulmonary	Intrasegmental and intersegmental areas
	Superior basal	Anterior basal segments
	Inferior basal	Posterior and lateral basal segments

6

VENOUS DRAINAGE OF THE HEART

Vein	Primary Tributary	Area Drained
Coronary sinus	Great cardiac	Left atrium, both ventricles
	Small cardiac	Posterior right atrium and ventricles
	Middle cardiac	Both ventricles
	Posterior vein of left ventricle	Left ventricle
	Oblique vein of left atrium	Left atrium
Anterior cardiac		Anterior right ventricle
Small cardiac (thebesian)		Both atria

VENOUS DRAINAGE OF THE FACE—DEEP

Vein	Primary Tributary	Area Drained
Maxillary	Confluence of veins of pterygoid plexus	Cavernous sinus
Pterygoid plexus	Veins accompanying maxillary artery	Muscles of mastication

VENOUS DRAINAGE OF THE FACE—SUPERFICIAL

Vein	Primary Tributary	Area Drained
Facial	Angular, which is formed by the following:	
	Frontal	Anterior scalp
	Supraorbital	Forehead
	Deep facial	Muscles of facial expression
	Superficial temporal	Vertex and side of head
	Posterior auricular	Back of ear
	Occipital	Superior sagittal and transverse sinuses
	Retromandibular	Parotid gland and masseter

VENOUS DRAINAGE OF THE CRANIUM—THE BRAIN		
Vein	**Primary Tributary**	**Area Drained**
External cerebral	Superior cerebral (8–12 veins)	Superior, lateral, and medial surfaces of hemisphere and opens into the superior sagittal sinus
	Middle cerebral	Lateral hemispheric surfaces into cavernous and sphenoparietal sinuses
	Inferior cerebral	Inferior hemispheric surfaces into superior sagittal sinus
Internal cerebral	Great cerebral (Galen's)	Interior of hemispheres into inferior sagittal sinus
	Internal cerebral, which is formed by the following:	
	Thalamostriate	Corpus striatum, thalamus
	Choroid	Choroid plexus, hippocampus, fornix, corpus callosum
	Basal	Insula, corpus striatum
Cerebellar	Superior cerebellar	Superior vermis into the straight sinus
	Inferior cerebellar	Lower cerebellum into transverse, occipital, and superior petrosal sinuses

6

VENOUS DRAINAGE OF THE CRANIUM— SINUSES OF THE DURA MATER

Vein	Primary Tributary	Area Drained
Posterior superior sinuses	Superior sagittal sinus	Superior cerebral veins, dura mater
	Inferior sagittal sinus	Falx cerebri and medial surfaces of the hemispheres
	Straight sinus	Inferior sagittal sinus, great cerebral vein
	Transverse sinuses	Right drains superior sagittal and the left straight sinuses; also receives blood from the superior petrosal sinuses
	Sigmoid sinuses	Transverse sinuses
	Occipital sinus	Posterior internal vertebral venous plexus into the confluence of sinuses
	Confluence of sinuses	Superior sagittal, straight, occipital, and both transverse sinuses
Anterior inferior sinuses	Cavernous sinus	Superior and inferior ophthalmic veins, some cerebral veins, sphenoparietal sinus
	Superior ophthalmic vein	Corresponding branches of ophthalmic artery
	Inferior ophthalmic vein	Muscles of eye movements
	Intercavernous sinuses	Connects the two cavernous sinuses across the midline
	Superior petrosal sinus	Cerebellar and inferior cerebral

Vein	Primary Tributary	Area Drained
		veins, veins from tympanic cavity; connects cavernous and transverse sinuses
	Inferior petrosal sinus	Internal auditory veins, veins from medulla, pons, and inferior surface of cerebellum; drains into the internal jugular bulb
	Basilar plexus	Connects inferior petrosal sinuses

VENOUS DRAINAGE OF THE CRANIUM—
DIPLOIC AND EMISSARY VEINS

Vein	Primary Tributary	Area Drained
Diploic	Frontal	Communicates with supraorbital vein and superior sagittal sinus
	Anterior temporal	Temporal communicates with the sphenoparietal sinus and the deep temporal veins
	Posterior temporal	Transverse sinus
	Occipital	Occipital vein, transverse sinus, or confluence of sinuses
Emissary	Mastoid	Connects transverse sinus with the posterior auricular or occipital veins
	Parietal	Connects superior sagittal sinus with veins of the scalp

Continued on following page

Vein	Primary Tributary	Area Drained
	Rete hypoglossal canal	Joins transverse sinus with vertebral vein and deep veins of the neck
	Rete foramen ovalis	Connects cavernous sinus with pterygoid plexus through foramen ovale
	Internal carotid plexus	Connects cavernous sinus and internal jugular vein via carotid canal
	Vein of foramen cecum	Connects superior sagittal sinus with veins of nasal cavity

VENOUS DRAINAGE OF THE NECK

Vein	Primary Tributary	Area Drained
External jugular	Posterior external jugular	Skin and superficial muscles in cranium and posterior neck
	Anterior jugular	Inferior thyroid veins by way of jugular venous arch, internal jugular
	Transverse cervical	Trapezius and surrounding muscles
	Suprascapular	Supraspinatus and feeds into the external jugular near the subclavian
Internal jugular	Inferior petrosal sinus	Internal auditory veins and veins of brain stem
	Lingual	Tongue
	Pharyngeal	Pharynx and vein of pterygoid canal
	Superior thyroid	Thyroid gland and receives superior laryngeal and cricothyroid veins

Vein	Primary Tributary	Area Drained
	Middle thyroid	Inferior thyroid gland
Vertebral	Anterior vertebral	Upper cervical vertebrae
	Accessory vertebral	Cervical vertebrae
	Deep cervical	Suboccipital muscles and cervical vertebrae

VENOUS DRAINAGE OF THE THORAX		
Vein	**Primary Tributary**	**Area Drained**
Azygos	Posterior intercostals	Dorsal spinal musculature and thoracic vertebrae
	Subcostal	Musculature about the 12th rib and thoracic vertebrae
	Hemiazygos	Four or five intercostal veins, left subcostal vein, some esophageal and mediastinal veins
	Accessory hemiazygos	Intercostal veins on the left side
	Bronchial	Bronchi of lungs
Brachiocephalic	Right brachiocephalic	Right vertebral, internal thoracic, inferior thyroid, and first intercostal veins
	Left brachiocephalic	Same as right brachiocephalic, except it drains left side
Internal thoracic		Drainage corresponds to arterial blood supply of internal thoracic
Inferior thyroid		Lower portion of thyroid gland and receives esophageal,

Continued on following page

Vein	Primary Tributary	Area Drained
		tracheal, and inferior laryngeal veins
Highest intercostal		Upper two or three intercostal spaces; right drains into azygos and left into brachiocephalic
Veins of vertebral column	External vertebral venous plexus	Mostly cervical vertebrae and connects with vertebral, occipital, and deep cervical veins
	Internal vertebral venous plexus	Posterior aspects of vertebrae, including ligaments and arches and connects with vertebral veins, occipital sinus, and basilar plexus
	Basivertebral	Foramina of dorsal vertebral bodies and communicates with anterior external vertebral plexuses
	Intervertebral	Internal and external vertebral plexuses and ends in vertebral, intercostal, lumbar, and lateral sacral veins
	Veins of spinal cord	Spinal cord into vertebral veins

VENOUS DRAINAGE OF THE ABDOMEN		
Vein	Primary Tributary	Area Drained
Inferior vena cava	Lumbar	Posterior wall muscles, vertebral plexuses, and into azygos system via ascending lumbar veins

Vein	Primary Tributary	Area Drained
	Testicular (in males)	Epididymis, testis, spermatic cord; right testicular enters the inferior vena cava and left into the renal vein
	Ovarian (in females)	Ovaries, broad ligament; right enters the inferior vena cava and left into the renal vein
	Renal	Kidneys and receives left testicular (or ovarian), inferior phrenic, and suprarenal veins
	Suprarenal	Suprarenal glands
	Inferior phrenic	Undersurface of diaphragm and ending in renal or suprarenal vein on left and inferior vena cava on right
	Hepatic	Liver

6

VENOUS DRAINAGE OF THE LIVER—PORTAL VENOUS DRAINAGE

Vein	Primary Tributary	Area Drained
Portal	Lienal (splenic)	Spleen and entering superior mesenteric vein to form the portal vein
	Branches: Short gastric	Greater curvature of the stomach
	Left gastro-epiploic	Stomach and greater omentum
	Pancreatic	Body and tail of pancreas
	Inferior mesenteric	Rectum, sigmoid and descending colon and receives sigmoid, and inferior rectal veins
	Superior mesenteric	Small intestine, cecum, ascending and transverse colon

Continued on following page

Vein	Primary Tributary	Area Drained
	Branches:	
	Right gastroepiploic	Stomach and greater omentum
	Pancreatico-duodenal	Pancreas and duodenum
	Coronary	Stomach and its lesser curvature, lesser omentum ending in portal vein
	Pyloric	Pyloric portion of lesser curvature of stomach and ending in portal vein
	Cystic	Gallbladder ending in right branch of portal vein
	Paraumbilical	Ligamentum teres of liver and connecting veins of anterior abdominal wall to portal, internal, and common iliac veins

VENOUS DRAINAGE OF THE PELVIS AND PERINEUM

Vein	Primary Tributary	Area Drained
Common iliac	Iliolumbar	Posterior pelvis and lumbar vertebrae
	Lateral sacral	Anterior sacrum
	Middle sacral	Additional sacral drainage to left common iliac vein
Internal iliac	Superior gluteal	Buttocks
	Inferior gluteal	Posterior thigh and buttocks
	Internal pudendal	Penis, urethral bulb
	Obturator	Adductor region of the thigh
	Lateral sacral	Anterior surface of sacrum
	Middle rectal	Rectal plexus, bladder, prostate, seminal vesicle, and levator ani
	Inferior rectal	Lower rectum draining into the internal pudendal vein

Vein	Primary Tributary	Area Drained
	Dorsal vein of penis	Superficial vein drains prepuce and skin while deep vein drains glans penis, corpora cavernosa
	Vesical	Bladder and base of prostate
	Uterine	Uterus
	Vaginal	Vagina

VENOUS DRAINAGE OF THE LOWER EXTREMITY—
BOUNDARY OF ABDOMEN AND LOWER EXTREMITY

Vein	Primary Tributary	Area Drained
External iliac	Inferior epigastric	Internal surface of lower abdominal wall
	Deep iliac circumflex	Deep tissue around anterior superior iliac spine and inner pelvic brim
	Superficial external pudendal	Superficial lower abdomen, scrotum, and labia and upper thigh

6

VENOUS DRAINAGE OF THE LOWER
EXTREMITY—SUPERFICIAL

Vein	Primary Tributary	Area Drained
Great saphenous		Medial aspect of leg from ankle upward across medial knee and thigh to enter femoral vein at femoral ring
	Accessory saphenous	Medial and posterior thigh
Small saphenous		Lateral to Achilles tendon up posterior leg to popliteal vein

Continued on following page

Vein	Primary Tributary	Area Drained
VENOUS DRAINAGE OF THE LOWER EXTREMITY—SUPERFICIAL (Continued)		
Dorsal digital		Clefts between toes
Intercapitular		From short common digital veins to produce dorsal venous arch
Plantar cutaneous venous arch		Sole of the foot

Vein	Primary Tributary	Area Drained
VENOUS DRAINAGE OF THE LOWER EXTREMITY—DEEP		
Plantar digital		Plantar surface of toes of foot to drain into plantar metatarsal veins
Plantar metatarsal		Along metatarsal bones to ankle and contributing to deep plantar venous arch
Medial plantar		Medial aspect of sole of foot and upward to form posterior tibial vein
Lateral plantar		Lateral aspect of sole of foot and upward to form posterior tibial vein
Posterior tibial		Medial portion of deep muscles of leg and draining into popliteal vein
Peroneal		Venous plexus of heel along lateral leg to drain into posterior tibial vein
Anterior tibial		Anterior compartment of leg to drain into popliteal vein
Popliteal		Posteromedial muscles of thigh to become femoral vein
Femoral		Anterior compartment of thigh to drain into external iliac
Femoral profunda		Deep muscles of anterior, anteromedial, and anterolateral thigh to drain into femoral vein

VENOUS DRAINAGE OF THE UPPER EXTREMITY—SUPERFICIAL

Vein	Primary Tributary	Area Drained
Palmar digital		Palmar surface of digits and connected to dorsal digital veins by oblique intercapitular veins
Dorsal digital venous network		Tissues of fingers and along fingers dorsally to back of hand
Medial ante-brachial		Superficial veins of hand up forearm to basilic vein below elbow
Basilic		Back of hand to anterior surface of arm above elbow to upper third of arm, draining into brachial vein
Accessory cephalic		Ulnar side of dorsal venous network to cephalic at elbow
Cephalic		Drainage of hand, forearm, and arm by extending up lateral aspect of arm to axillary vein near clavicle

6

VENOUS DRAINAGE OF THE UPPER EXTREMITY—DEEP

Vein	Primary Tributary	Area Drained
Superficial and deep palmar venous arches		Fingers
Palmar and dorsal metacarpal		Metacarpals
Brachial		From the elbow on each side of forearm, draining deep tissues to form the axillary in the arm
Axillary		Axillary and clavicular join to drain into subclavian vein

Continued on following page

VENOUS DRAINAGE OF THE UPPER EXTREMITY—DEEP
(Continued)

Vein	Primary Tributary	Area Drained
Subclavian		Drains external jugular and anterior jugular and enters the internal jugular vein, along with thoracic duct on left and right lymphatic duct on right

BLOOD PRESSURE

Systole

Systole is the period of cardiac contraction.

Diastole

Diastole is the period of cardiac relaxation, or cardiac filling.

Procedure for Measuring Blood Pressure

The cuff is placed 1–2 in above the antecubital fossa, inflated until no radial pulse is palpable, and then the brachial artery is auscultated over the fossa during deflation of the cuff. The sounds heard vary in intensity and quality during deflation and are called *Korotkoff's sounds*. Five phases of Korotkoff's sounds are described.

phase 1: First sounds that are heard, clear tapping sounds that increase in intensity. Systolic blood pressure is when rhythmic tapping is first heard.

phase 2: The clear tapping sound of phase 1 is replaced with a softer muffled sound or murmur.

phase 3: A less clear but louder and crisper tapping sound replaces the muffled sound of phase 2.

phase 4: Tapping of phase 3 changes to muffled, soft blowing sound. This is sometimes called the *first diastolic pressure.*

phase 5: Disappearance of all sounds. Diastolic blood pressure generally measured as this phase if only two values are recorded. If three pressures are recorded, phase 5 is the *second diastolic pressure.*

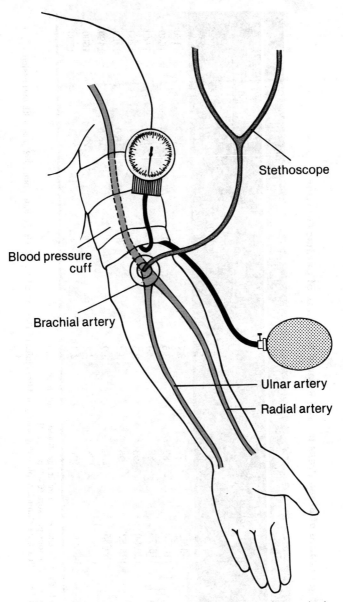

Stethoscope

Blood pressure
cuff

Brachial artery

Ulnar artery

Radial artery

6

Placement of the blood pressure cuff and stethoscope for monitoring brachial artery pressure.

Clinical Significance of Blood Pressure and Related Measures of Cardiac Function

CHANGES IN BLOOD PRESSURE, CARDIAC OUTPUT, AND PERIPHERAL VASCULAR RESISTANCE WITH AGE

Age (y)	Blood Pressure (mm Hg)		Blood Flow		Peripheral Vascular Resistance†	
	Systolic/ Diastolic	Mean	Cardiac Index* ($L \cdot min^{-1} \cdot m^{-2}$)	Cardiac Output (L/min)	$mm\,Hg \cdot L^{-1} min^{-1}$	$dyne \cdot s \cdot cm^{-1}$
10	90/60	70	3.7	4.4	14.7	1180
20	110/70	83	3.5	6.0	13.0	1040
30	115/75	88	3.4	5.8	14.3	1140
40	120/80	93	3.3	5.6	15.7	1260
50	125/82	96	3.2	5.4	16.9	1350
60	130/85	100	3.0	5.1	18.6	1480
70	135/88	104	2.9	4.9	20.2	1600
80	140/90	107	2.8	4.8	21.3	1700

*Assuming a body surface area of 1.2 m^2 at age 10 and 1.7 m^2 thereafter.
†Assuming a central venous pressure (CVP) of 5 mm Hg.
From Wilson, RF: Critical Care Manual: Applied Physiology and Principles of Therapy, ed 2. FA Davis, Philadelphia, 1992, p 24, with permission.

CLASSIFICATION OF BLOOD PRESSURES*

Category	Range (mm Hg)
Normal BP	Systolic < 140; diastolic < 85
High-normal BP	Diastolic 85–89
Mild hypertension	Diastolic 90–104
Moderate hypertension	Diastolic 105–114
Severe hypertension	Diastolic ≥ 115
Borderline isolated systolic hypertension	Systolic 140–159; diastolic < 90
Isolated systolic hypertension	Systolic ≥ 160; diastolic < 90

*The diastolic pressure is the primary value used to make a diagnosis of mild, moderate, or severe hypertension. "Isolated" hypertension indicates an increase in only the systolic value, with the diastolic pressure remaining relatively normal.
BP = blood pressure.
From Joint National Committee on Detection, Evaluation, and Treatment of High Blood Pressure: The 1984 report. Arch Intern Med 144:1047, 1984, with permission.

CLASSIFICATION OF HYPERTENSION IN THE YOUNG BY AGE GROUP

6

Age Group	≥ 95th Percentile (mm Hg)	≥ 99th Percentile (mm Hg)
Newborns		
7 d	SBP ≥ 96	SBP ≥ 106
8–30 d	SBP ≥104	SBP ≥ 110
Infants	SBP ≥ 112	SBP ≥ 118
(≤ 2 y)	DBP ≥ 74	DBP ≥ 82
Children	SBP ≥ 116	SBP ≥ 124
(3–5 y)	DBP ≥ 76	DBP ≥ 84
Children	SBP ≥ 122	SBP ≥ 130
(6–9 y)	DBP ≥ 78	DBP ≥ 86
Children	SBP ≥ 126	SBP ≥ 134
(10–12 y)	DBP ≥ 82	DBP ≥ 90
Adolescents	SBP ≥ 136	SBP ≥ 144
(13–15 y)	DBP ≥ 86	DBP ≥ 92
Adolescents	SBP ≥ 142	SBP ≥ 150
(16–18 y)	DBP ≥ 92	DBP ≥ 98

SBP = systolic blood pressure; DBP = diastolic blood pressure.
From Report of the second task force on blood pressure control in children— 1987. Pediatrics 79(1):1–25, 1987; reproduced by permission of Pediatrics.

HYPERTENSION* PREVALENCE RATES BY GENDER, RACE, AND AGE (18–74 YEARS) IN THE CIVILIAN, NONINSTITUTIONALIZED POPULATION, 1976–1980†

Age (y)	Men			Women			Both Sexes		
	Whites (%)	Blacks (%)	All races (%)	Whites (%)	Blacks (%)	All races (%)	Whites (%)	Blacks (%)	All races (%)
18–74	32.6	37.9	33.0	25.3	38.6	26.8	28.8	38.2	29.8
18–24	16.2	10.9	15.2	2.3	9.6	3.5	9.1	10.2	9.2
25–34	21.1	23.2	20.9	5.7	15.3	6.9	13.3	18.8	13.7
35–44	26.4	44.2	28.4	16.6	37.0	19.3	21.3	40.1	23.7
45–54	42.6	55.2	43.7	36.3	67.4	39.1	39.4	61.7	41.3
55–64	51.4	66.3	52.6	50.0	74.3	52.6	50.6	70.7	52.6
65–74	59.2	67.1	60.2	66.2	82.9	67.5	63.1	76.1	64.3

*Defined as the average of three blood pressure measurements 140 mm Hg or greater systolic and/or 90 mm Hg or greater diastolic on a single occasion or those reported to be taking antihypertensive medication.
†Data obtained from the 1976–1980 National Health and Nutrition Examination Survey.
From American Heart Association, Inc.: Hypertension prevalence and the status of awareness, treatment, and control in the United States. Final report of the Subcommittee on Definition and Prevalence of the Joint National Committee. Hypertension 7:457–468, 1985; by permission of the American Heart Association, Inc.

RECOMMENDATIONS FOR FOLLOW-UP BASED ON INITIAL BLOOD PRESSURE MEASUREMENTS FOR ADULTS AGE 18 AND OVER

Initial Screening Blood Pressure (mm Hg)*		Follow-Up Recommended†
Systolic	Diastolic	
<130	<85	Recheck in 2 y.
130–139	85–89	Recheck in 1 y.‡
140–159	90–99	Confirm within 2 mo.
160–179	100–109	Evaluate or refer to source of care within 1 mo.
180–209	110–119	Evaluate or refer to source of care within 1 wk.
≥210	≥120	Evaluate or refer to source of care immediately.

*If the systolic and diastolic categories are different, follow recommendations for the shorter time follow-up (e.g., 160/85 mm Hg should be evaluated or referred to source of care within 1 mo).

†The scheduling of follow-ups should be modified by reliable information about past blood pressure measurements, other cardiovascular risk factors, or target-organ disease.

‡Consider providing advice about lifestyle modifications.

From Joint National Committee on Detection, Evaluation, and Treatment of High Blood Pressure: The fifth report of the Joint National Committee on Detection, Evaluation, and Treatment of High Blood Pressure. Arch Intern Med 153:154, 1993, with permission.

6

DRUG TREATMENT FOR HYPERTENSION AND CARDIAC DISEASE: STEPPED-CARE APPROACH TO HYPERTENSION

STEP 1: In patients with mild hypertension, drug therapy is usually initiated with a single agent (monotherapy) from one of the following classes: a diuretic, a β-blocker, an ACE inhibitor, or a calcium channel blocker.

STEP 2: If a single drug is unsuccessful in reducing blood pressure, a second agent is added. The second drug can be from one of the initial classes not used in step 1, or it can be from a second group that includes the centrally acting agents (clonidine, guanabenz), presynaptic adrenergic inhibitors (reserpine, guanethidine), α_1 blockers (prazocin, doxazosin), and vasodilators (hydralazine, minoxidil).

STEP 3: A third agent is added, usually from one of the classes listed in step 2 that has not already been used. Three different agents from three different classes are often administered concurrently in this step.

STEP 4: A fourth drug is added from still another class.

ACE = angiotensin-converting enzyme.
From Ciccone, CD: Pharmacology in Rehabilitation, ed 2. FA Davis, Philadelphia, 1996, p 303, with permission.

ANTIHYPERTENSIVE DRUG CATEGORIES

Category	Primary Site(s) of Action	Primary Antihypertensive Effect(s)
Diuretics	Kidneys	Decrease plasma fluid volume.
Sympatholytics	Various sites within the sympathetic division of the autonomic nervous system	Decrease sympathetic influence on the heart and/or peripheral vasculature.
Vasodilators	Peripheral vasculature	Lower vascular resistance by directly vasodilating peripheral vessels.
Angiotensin-converting enzyme inhibitors	Angiotensin-converting enzyme located in the lungs and other tissues	Prevent the conversion of angiotensin I to angiotensin II (angiotensin II is a potent vasoconstrictor).
Calcium channel blockers	Limit calcium entry into vascular smooth muscle and cardiac muscle	Decrease vascular smooth-muscle contraction; decrease myocardial force and rate of contraction.

From Ciccone, CD: Pharmacology in Rehabilitation, ed 2. FA Davis, Philadelphia, 1996, p 293, with permission.

6

SYMPATHOLYTIC DRUGS

β-Blockers
Acebutolol (Sectral)
Atenolol (Tenormin)
Betaxolol (Kerlone)
Bisoprolol (Zebeta)
Carteolol (Cartrol)
Labetalol (Normodyne; Trandate)
Metoprolol (Lopressor)
Nadolol (Corgard)
Oxprenolol (Trasicor)
Penbutolol (Levatol)
Pindolol (Visken)
Propranolol (Inderal)
Sotalol (Betapace)
Timolol (Blocadren)

α-Blockers
Doxazosin (Cardura)
Phenoxybenzamine (Dibenzyline)
Prazocin (Minipress)
Terazosin (Hytrin)

Presynaptic Adrenergic Inhibitors
Guanadrel (Hylorel)
Guanethidine (Ismelin)
Reserpine (Serpalan, others)

Centrally Acting Agents
Clonidine (Catapres)
Guanabenz (Wytensin)
Guanfacine (Tenex)
Methyldopa (Aldomet)

Ganglionic Blockers
Mecamylamine (Inversine)
Trimethaphan (Arfonad)

From Ciccone, CD: Pharmacology in Rehabilitation, ed 2. FA Davis, Philadelphia, 1996, p 295, with permission.

ANTIHYPERTENSIVE VASODILATORS, ANGIOTENSIN-CONVERTING ENZYME INHIBITORS, AND CALCIUM CHANNEL BLOCKERS

VASODILATORS

Diazoxide (Hyperstat)	Minoxidil (Loniten)
Hydralazine (Apresoline)	Nitroprusside (Nipride, Nitropress)

ACE INHIBITORS

Benazepril (Lotensin)	Lisinopril (Prinivil, Zestril)
Captopril (Capoten)	Quinapril (Accupril)
Enalapril (Vasotec)	Ramipril (Altace)
Fosinopril (Monopril)	

CALCIUM CHANNEL BLOCKERS

Diltiazem (Cardizem)	Nicardipine (Cardene)
Felodipine (Plendil)	Nifedipine (Adalat, Procardia)
Isradipine (DynaCirc)	Verapamil (Calan, Isoptin)

ACE = angiotensin-converting enzyme.
From Ciccone, CD: Pharmacology in Rehabilitation, ed 2. FA Davis, Philadelphia, 1996, p 299, with permission.

6

SUMMARY OF COMMON β-BLOCKERS USED FOR THE TREATMENT OF HYPERTENSION AND CARDIAC DISEASE

Generic Name	Trade Name(s)	Selectivity	Primary Indications*
Acebutolol	Sectral	β_1	Hypertension
Atenolol	Tenormin	β_1	Angina pectoris, hypertension, prevent reinfarction
Betaxolol	Kerlone	β_1	Hypertension
Bisoprolol	Zebeta	β_1	Hypertension
Carteolol	Cartrol	Nonselective	Hypertension
Esmolol	Emcyt	β_1	Dysrhythmias
Labetalol	Normodyne, Trandate	Nonselective	Hypertension
Metoprolol	Lopressor	β_1	Angina pectoris, hypertension, prevent reinfarction
Nadolol	Corgard	Nonselective	Angina pectoris, hypertension
Penbutolol	Levatol	Nonselective	Hypertension
Pindolol	Visken	Nonselective	Hypertension
Propranolol	Inderal	Nonselective	Angina pectoris, dysrhythmias, hypertension, prevent reinfarction, prevent vascular headache
Sotalol	Betapace	Nonselective	Dysrhythmias
Timolol	Blocardren	Nonselective	Hypertension, prevent reinfarction, prevent vascular headache

*Only indications listed in the United States product labeling are included in this table. All drugs are fairly similar pharmacologically, and some may be used for appropriate cardiovascular conditions not specifically listed in product labeling.

From Ciccone, CD: Pharmacology in Rehabilitation, ed 2. FA Davis, Philadelphia, 1996, p 282, with permission.

LYMPHATIC SYSTEM

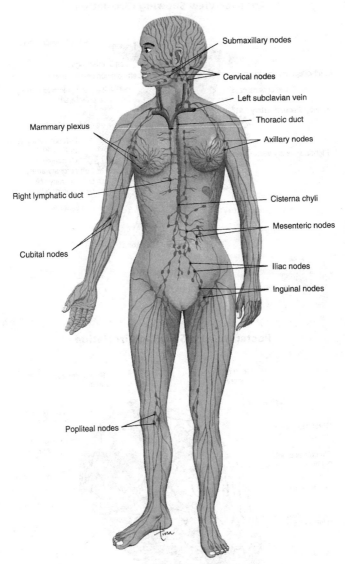

The lymphatic system, with major nodes illustrated.

THE HEART—EXTERNAL ANATOMY

Anterior View Showing Circulation

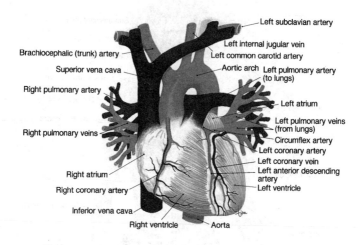

- Left subclavian artery
- Left internal jugular vein
- Left common carotid artery
- Aortic arch
- Left pulmonary artery (to lungs)
- Left atrium
- Left pulmonary veins (from lungs)
- Circumflex artery
- Left coronary artery
- Left coronary vein
- Left anterior descending artery
- Left ventricle
- Aorta

- Brachiocephalic (trunk) artery
- Superior vena cava
- Right pulmonary artery
- Right pulmonary veins
- Right atrium
- Right coronary artery
- Inferior vena cava
- Right ventricle

Posterior View Showing Circulation

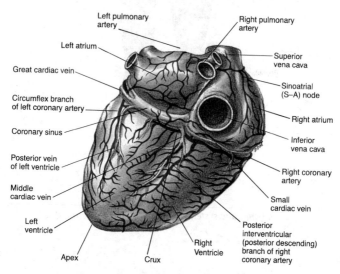

- Left pulmonary artery
- Right pulmonary artery
- Left atrium
- Superior vena cava
- Great cardiac vein
- Sinoatrial (S–A) node
- Circumflex branch of left coronary artery
- Right atrium
- Coronary sinus
- Inferior vena cava
- Posterior vein of left ventricle
- Right coronary artery
- Middle cardiac vein
- Small cardiac vein
- Left ventricle
- Posterior interventricular (posterior descending) branch of right coronary artery
- Apex
- Crux
- Right Ventricle

BLOOD SUPPLY TO THE HEART

Artery	Area Supplied
Circumflex artery	Inferior wall of left ventricle (when not supplied by right coronary artery)
	Left atrium
	Sinoatrial (SA) node (in approximately 40% of humans)

Coronary artery dominance is a term used to describe which artery descends posteriorly from the crux to the apex of the myocardium. The right coronary artery is dominant and branches into the *posterior descending branch* in approximately two thirds of humans; this is called *right dominance*. In these persons the right coronary artery supplies part of the left ventricle and ventricular septum. In the remaining third of humans, a branch of the circumflex is dominant, which is called *left dominance*, or dominance is from branches from both the right coronary artery and the circumflex artery, which is called a *balanced pattern*.

BLOOD SUPPLY TO THE CONDUCTION SYSTEM

There is considerable variation in the arterial venous branches to the myocardium. The table below lists the most common distributions.

Artery	Area Supplied
Right coronary artery (RCA)	Right atrium
	Right ventricle
	Inferior wall of left ventricle (in most humans)
	Atrioventricular (AV) node
	Bundle of His
	Sinoatrial (SA) node (in approximately 60% of humans)
Left anterior descending (LAD) artery	Left ventricle
	Interventricular septum
	Right ventricle
	Inferior areas of the apex
	Inferior areas of both ventricles

FOR MORE INFORMATION

Brannon, FJ, et al: Cardiac Rehabilitation: Basic Theory and Application, ed 2. FA Davis, Philadelphia, 1993.

Netter, FH: The CIBA Collection of Medical Illustrations, Vol 5, Heart. CIBA, Summit, NJ, 1978.

CONDUCTION SYSTEM OF THE HEART

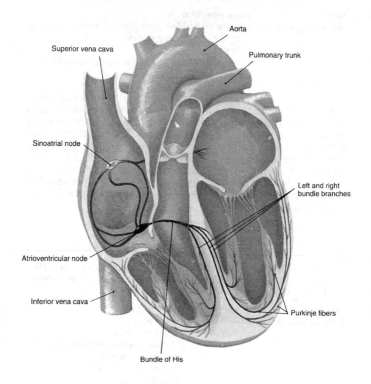

Aorta

Superior vena cava

Pulmonary trunk

Sinoatrial node

Left and right
bundle branches

Atrioventricular node

Inferior vena cava

Purkinje fibers

Bundle of His

ELECTROCARDIOGRAPHIC WAVES, SEGMENTS, AND INTERVALS

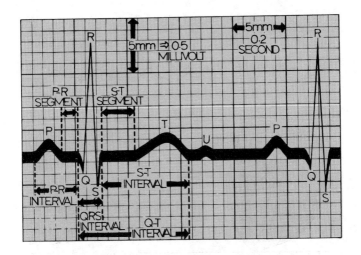

NORMAL RANGES OF ELECTROCARDIOGRAPHIC COMPONENTS		
	Duration	*Amplitude*
P wave	<.10 s	1–3 mm
PR interval	0.12–0.20 s	Isoelectric after the P-wave deflection
QRS	0.06–0.10 s	25–30 mm (maximum)
ST segment	0.12 s	−½–+1 mm
T wave	0.16 s	5–10 mm

ELECTROCARDIOGRAPHIC RECORDING OF MYOCARDIAL ACTIVITY

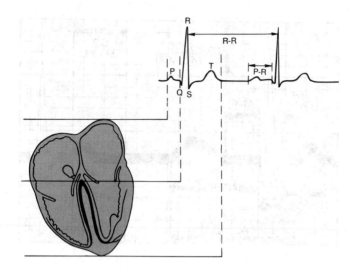

Electrocardiographic Component	Myocardial Event
P wave	Atrial depolarization
QRS complex	Ventricular depolarization
T wave	Ventricular repolarization

INTERPRETING THE ELECTROCARDIOGRAPH

Steps to Follow When Interpreting an Electrocardiogram Rhythm Strip

1. Calculate the rate.
2. Examine the rhythm and determine if regular or irregular.
3. Identify P waves.
4. Evaluate PR interval for duration and relationship of P wave to QRS complex.
5. Evaluate QRS complex for shape and duration.
6. Identify extra waves or complexes.
7. Determine clinical significance of a dysrhythmia.

Abbreviations Used
in Electrocardiographic Interpretations

APC (APB)	Atrial premature contraction (beat)
CHB	Complete heart block
JPC (JPB)	Junctional premature contraction (beat)
LAD	Left axis deviation
LAE	Left atrial enlargement
LAHB	Left anterior hemiblock
LBBB	Left bundle branch block
LVE	Left ventricular enlargement
LVH	Left ventricular hypertrophy
NPC (NPB)	Nodal premature contraction (beat)
NSR	Normal sinus rhythm
NSSTTW	Nonspecific ST- and T-wave changes
PAC (PAB)	Premature atrial contraction (beat)
PAT	Paroxysmal atrial tachycardia
PJC (PJB)	Premature junctional contraction (beat)
PNC (PNB)	Premature nodal contraction (beat)
PVC (PVB)	Premature ventricular contraction (beat)
RAE	Right atrial enlargement
RBBB	Right bundle branch block
RSR	Regular sinus rhythm
RVH	Right ventricular hypertrophy
SVT	Supraventricular tachycardia
VF	Ventricular fibrillation
VPC (VPB)	Ventricular premature contraction (beat)
VT	Ventricular tachycardia

FOR MORE INFORMATION

Brown, KR and Jacobson, S: Mastering Dysrhythmias: A Problem-Solving Guide. FA Davis, Philadelphia, 1988.

METHODS USED TO CALCULATE HEART RATES

Four methods can be used to calculate from an electrocardiogram rates with regular cardiac rhythms. When conduction is normal, both atrial and ventricular rates are identical.

Heart Rate Values

Normal	60 to 100 bpm
Bradycardia	less than 60 bpm
Tachycardia	greater than 100 bpm

When the rhythm is irregular, each beat in a 30 or 60 s rhythm strip should be counted to estimate the rate.

First Method for Calculating Rate

Multiply the number of QRS complexes in a 6-s strip (most electrocardiogram paper has markers every 1, 3, or 6 s) by 10 (chart speed = 25 mm/s). Estimate the portion of an RR interval when only a portion of one is contained at the end of 6 s.

Continued on following page

Second Method for Calculating Rate

Divide 300 by the number of whole or partial large boxes between two consecutive R waves.

Third Method for Calculating Rate

Find an R wave that falls on a large box line and count how many large boxes are in the interval before the next R wave. Memorize the values for each large box interval.

Heart Rate	Number of Large Boxes
300	1
150	2
100	3
75	4
60	5
50	6
43	7

Fourth Method for Calculating Rate

Divide 1500 by the number of small boxes between consecutive R waves.

Examples of Cardiac Rates

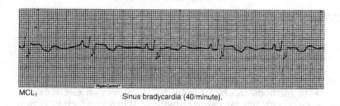

MCL₁   Sinus bradycardia (40/minute).

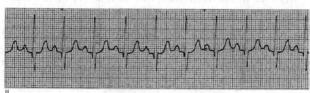

II   Regular or normal sinus rhythm (94/minute).

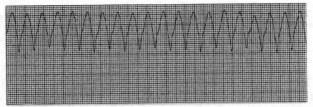

Ventricular tachycardia (180/minute).

ASSESSING THE REGULARITY OF AN ELECTROCARDIOGRAM RHYTHM STRIP

Examine the Rhythm and Determine if Regular or Irregular

Assess the regularity of the RR intervals. A regular rhythm has equally sized spaces between all intervals. An intermittently irregular rhythm is generally regular with occasional disruptions (extra beats, for example). A regularly irregular rhythm has a cyclical pattern of varying RR intervals. An irregularly irregular rhythm has no recurring pattern; RR intervals vary in an inconsistent manner.

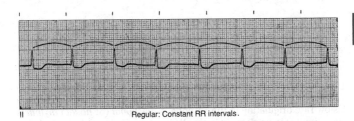

II   Regular: Constant RR intervals.

Examples of Irregular Rhythms

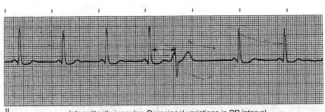

II   Intermittently irregular: Occasional variations in RR interval.

Continued on following page

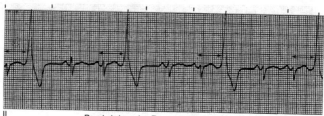

II

Regularly irregular: Every third RR interval varies.

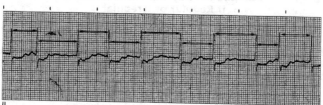

II

Irregularly irregular: Grossly irregular RR intervals.

Rhythm Names

Rhythms are generally named by the beat that initiates conduction to the ventricles and the rate. For example, *sinus bradycardia* is a slow rate originating in the SA node, a *junctional* (or *nodal*) *rhythm* is a normal rate originating in the AV junction, and *ventricular tachycardia* is a rapid rhythm orginating in the ventricles.

Examples of Named Rhythms

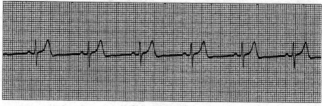

Sinus bradycardia.

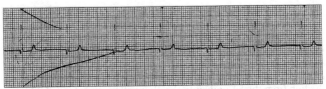

Sustained AV junctional rhythm.

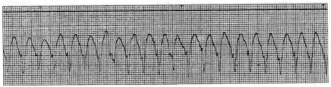

Ventricular tachycardia.

IDENTIFYING P WAVES

The presence of P waves indicates that myocardial conduction is initiated in the atria. A normal impulse initiated in the SA node has a P wave that is upright, rounded, and 1–3 mm tall. The P waves that are abnormally shaped include *flutter* (F) waves, which are also called *saw-toothed* and have a regular pattern; *fibrillation* (f), which are small, grossly irregular deflections on the baseline; and *premature* P waves, which look different and usually have a different PR interval than the regular P waves in a rhythm strip. (Premature beats are discussed under Identifying Extra Waves or Complexes.)

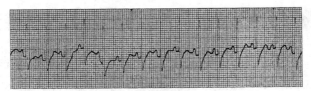

Normal P waves (sinus tachycardia).

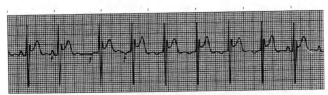

Alterations in P wave shapes.

Continued on following page

Evaluating the PR Interval for Duration and Relationship of P Wave to QRS Complex

The normal PR interval is between 0.12 and 0.20 s (3–5 small boxes). A shorter-than-normal PR interval indicates increased AV conduction or an atrial impulse that does not originate in the SA node. A longer-than-normal PR interval indicates a slowing of conduction from the SA node into the AV junction. A prolonged PR interval defines *atrioventricular heart block*. With normal conduction, a QRS complex should follow each P wave.

Type of Block	Characteristics
First degree	Prolonged PR interval; all P waves are followed by a QRS complex.
Second degree Mobitz type I (Wenckebach)	Progressive lengthening of the PR interval until one P wave is not conducted (no QRS follows a P wave). Occurs as a regular irregularity.
Mobitz type II	Atrial rate is regular, but some impulses are not conducted from the SA node through the AV junction. Ratio of conduction (e.g., 2:1 or 3:1) is regular. Occurs as a regular irregularity
Third degree (complete)	No conduction of impulse through the AV junction; no relationship between atrial and ventricular activity. Atrial and ventricular rhythms may be regular, but the ventricular rate is initiated below the AV node and is slow and independent of atrial activity.

TYPES OF ATRIOVENTRICULAR HEART BLOCKS

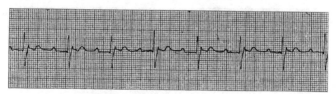

First degree AV block (PR interval is 0.32 sec).

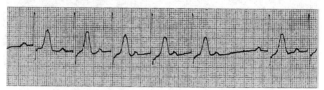

Second degree AV block; Mobitz type 1 (Wenckebach).

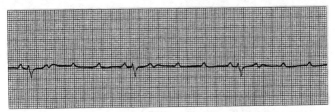

Second degree AV block; Mobitz type 2; 4:1 AV conduction ratio.

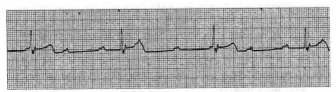

Third degree AV block (complete heart block).

EVALUATION OF QRS COMPLEX FOR SHAPE AND DURATION

All QRS complexes should be identical to one another. The normal duration of a QRS complex is 0.06–0.10 s (1.5–2.5 small boxes). Bundle branch blocks (BBBs) signify conduction interference down either the right or left bundle. Although both demonstrate a widened QRS complex, an RBBB has a notched and widened R component, and an LBBB has only a widened R. Bundle branch blocks are best diagnosed with a 12-lead ECG. Irregularities in ventricular conduction include flutter, fibrillation, and PVCs. Flutter and fibrillation usually develop following ventricular tachycardia and show a progressive degeneration of organized myocardial electrical activity (premature beats are discussed under Identifying Extra Waves and Complexes).

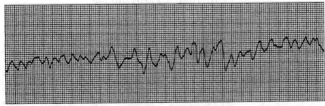

II   Coarse ventricular fibrillation.

Continued on following page

IDENTIFYING EXTRA WAVES OR COMPLEXES

Extra waves or complexes signify myocardial irritability. The problem may be atrial, junctional (nodal), and/or ventricular. The severity of a dysrhythmia is related to the location, frequency, and number of sites where extra beats are initiated.

Supraventricular Dysrhythmias

Premature atrial contractions (PACs) arise from an ectopic atrial focus. Their P waves look different from normal and also usually have a different PR interval. *Premature junctional (nodal) contractions* (PJCs) originate in the AV junction; the P wave may be inverted owing to retrograde conduction and may occur before, following, and buried within the QRS complex. Both PACs and PJCs have normally shaped QRS complexes and are generally not dangerous unless frequent or associated with signs and symptoms of altered hemodynamics.

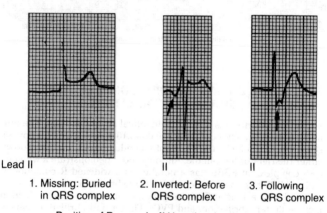

Lead II

1. Missing: Buried in QRS complex

2. Inverted: Before QRS complex

3. Following QRS complex

Position of P wave in AV junctional complexes.

Types of Premature Contractions

Ventricular Dysrhythmias

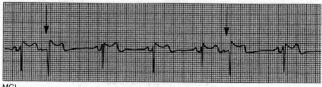

MCL₁   Premature atrial contractions (beats 2 and 6).

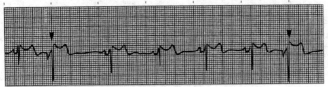

MCL₁   Premature junctional contractions (beats 2 and 7).

Premature ventricular contractions (PVCs) are the most dangerous and are classified by frequency and irritable foci. The PVCs are
not preceded by a P wave, are conducted abnormally through the
ventricles, and are characterized by wide, bizarre QRS complexes.
Unifocal PVCs arise from a single irritable focus and are identically
shaped; *multifocal PVCs* come from different sites and do not look
alike. Frequency of PVCs is described by the terms *single,
quadrigeminy* (one PVC every fourth beat), *trigeminy* (one every third
beat), and *bigeminy* (every other beat is a PVC). Paired PVCs are
called *couplets* and a run of PVCs is called a *salvo*. As PVCs signify
ventricular irritability, multiple sites and increasing frequency are
potentially lethal because the cardiac rhythm may disintegrate into
ventricular tachycardia, fibrillation, or asystole. More than six PVCs
per minute is considered dangerous. Particularly lethal is a PVC that
falls on a T wave (R on T phenomenon). It does not allow the ventricle to repolarize, and ventricular fibrillation is likely to ensue.

6

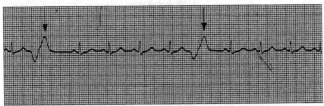

Two unifocal premature ventricular contractions (PVCs) (beats 2 and 7).

Types of Ventricular Dysrhythmias

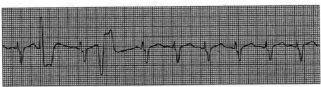

MCL₁   Multifocal PVCs (beats 2 and 4).

Continued on following page

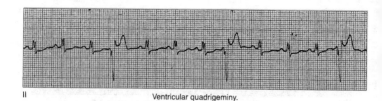

II   Ventricular quadrigeminy.

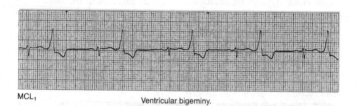

II   Ventricular trigeminy.

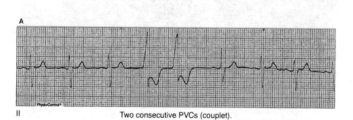

MCL₁   Ventricular bigeminy.

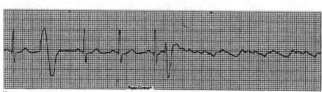

II   Two consecutive PVCs (couplet).

II   R on T phenomenon: a PVC during the vulnerable period (T wave) causes
                    ventricular fibrillation.

DETERMINING THE CLINICAL SIGNIFICANCE OF A DYSRHYTHMIA

Dysrhythmias result in varying degrees of abnormal hemodynamics. Cardiac output is decreased with very slow or very rapid rates.

Dysrhythmias Classified by Their Effect on Cardiac Output

Dysrhythmias Associated with Normal or Near Normal Hemodynamics (Generally Benign)

1. Sinus rhythm with premature atrial contractions
2. Sinus rhythm with premature junctional contractions
3. Artificial pacemaker rhythm with 1 : 1 capture
4. Atrial fibrillation with an average ventricular response between 60 and 100/min
5. Atrial flutter with an average ventricular response between 60 and 100/min
6. Sinus rhythm with first-degree AV block
7. Sinus rhythm with occasional premature ventricular contractions
8. Sinus bradycardia averaging 50–60/min
9. AV junctional rhythm averaging 50–60/min
10. Sinus rhythm with second-degree AV block Mobitz type 1
11. Isorhythmic AV dissociation

Dysrhythmias with Normal or Near Normal Hemodynamics but Which Are Potentially Dangerous

1. Sinus rhythm with short episodes of ventricular tachycardia
2. Sinus rhythm with short episodes of paroxysmal supraventricular tachycardia
3. Accelerated junctional rhythms
4. Artificial pacemaker rhythm with premature ventricular contractions that are new, multifocal, or couplets
5. Sinus rhythm with second-degree AV block Mobitz type 2
6. Atrial flutter or fibrillation with tachycardia ventricular rates
7. Sinus rhythm with sinus arrest
8. Sinus bradycardia with rates below 50/min

Dysrhythmias with Significantly Altered Hemodynamics

1. Ventricular tachycardia (with pulses)
2. Sinus rhythm or atrial fibrillation with complete heart block
3. Very slow (40/min or below) sinus, junctional, or idioventricular rhythms
4. Malfunctioning artificial pacemakers with idioventricular rhythms

Continued on following page

Dysrhythmias Associated with Absent Hemodynamics—Lethal Conditions

1. Ventricular fibrillation
2. Asystole
3. Pulseless ventricular tachycardia or flutter
4. Agonal idioventricular complexes
5. Electromechanical dissociation
6. Third-degree AV heart block with ventricular standstill

COMMON FORMS OF DYSRHYTHMIAS	
Classification	*Characteristic Rhythm*
Sinus Dysrhythmias	
Sinus tachycardia	>100 bpm
Sinus bradycardia	<60 bpm
Sick sinus syndrome	Severe bradycardia (<50 bpm); periods of sinus arrest
Supraventricular Dysrhythmias	
Atrial fibrillation and flutter	Atrial rate >30 bpm
Atrial tachycardia	Atrial rate >140–200 bpm
Premature atrial contractions	Variable
Atrioventricular Junctional Dysrhythmias	
Junctional rhythm	40–55 bpm
Junctional tachycardia	100–200 bpm
Conduction Disturbances	
Atrioventricular block	Variable
Bundle branch block	Variable
Fascicular block	Variable
Ventricular Dysrhythmias	
Premature ventricular contractions	Variable
Ventricular tachycardia	140–200 bpm
Ventricular fibrillation	Irregular, totally uncoordinated rhythm

From Ciccone, CD: Pharmacology in Rehabilitation, ed 2. FA Davis, Philadelphia, 1996, p 327, with permission.

Drug Treatment for Dysrhythmias

CLASSIFICATION OF DRUGS USED FOR DYSRHYTHMIAS	
Generic Names	*Trade Names*

Class I: Sodium Channel Blockers

Subclass A

Disopyramide	Norpace
Procainamide	Promine, Pronestyl
Quinidine	Cardioquin, Duraquin, others

Subclass B

Lidocaine	Xylocaine, Lidopen
Mexiletine	Mexitil
Moricizine*	Ethmozine
Phenytoin	Dilantin
Tocainide	Tonocard

Subclass C

Encainide	Enkaid
Flecainide	Tambocor
Propafenone	Rythmol

Class II: β-Blockers

Acebutolol	Sectral
Atenolol	Tenormin
Esmolol	Brevibloc
Metoprolol	Lopressor
Nadolol	Corgard
Oxprenolol	Trasicor
Propranolol	Inderal
Sotalol	Betapace
Timolol	Blocadren

Class III: Drugs That Prolong Repolarization

Amiodarone†	Cordarone
Bretylium	Bretylol

Class IV: Calcium Channel Blockers

Diltiazem	Cardizem
Verapamil	Calan, Isoptin

*Also has some class IC properties.

†Also has some class I properties.

From Ciccone, CD: Pharmacology in Rehabilitation, ed 2. FA Davis, Philadelphia, 1996, p 328, with permission.

CALCIUM CHANNEL BLOCKERS

Generic Name	Trade Name	Usual Oral Dose
Bepridil	Bepadin, Vascor	200–300 mg once a day
Diltiazem	Cardizem	60–90 mg 3 or 4 times a day
Felodipine	Plendil	5–10 mg once a day
Isradipine	DynaCirc	2.5–10 mg 2 times a day
Nicardipine	Cardene	20 mg 3 times a day
Nifedipine	Procardia	10–30 mg 3 or 4 times a day
Verapamil	Calan, Isoptin	80–160 mg 3 times a day

From Ciccone, CD: Pharmacology in Rehabilitation, ed 2. FA Davis, Philadelphia, 1996, p 315, with permission.

NORMAL VALUES FOR CARDIAC-RELATED BLOOD STUDIES

Test	Normal Values
Lipid Profile	
Cholesterol	100–200 mg/dl
Triglycerides	45–170 mg/dl
High-density lipoprotein	37–80 mg/dl
Low-density lipoprotein	95–185 mg/dl
Very-low-density lipoprotein	4–37 mg/dl
Apoprotein A	95–230 mg/dl
Apoprotein B	55–170 mg/dl

From University of Illinois at Chicago Medical Center, Department of Pathology.

CARDIAC EXAMINATION

auscultation: Listening to the intensity and quality of heart sounds as they vary over the surface of the chest. Four primary areas are identified over which to auscultate the cardiac valves.

AREAS TO AUSCULTATE FOR THE CARDIAC VALVES	
Valve	*Area to Auscultate*
Aortic	Second right intercostal space at right sternal border (base of heart)
Pulmonic	Second left intercostal space at left sternal border
Tricuspid	Fourth left intercostal space along lower left sternal border
Mitral	Fifth left intercostal space at midclavicular line (apical area)

FOR MORE INFORMATION

Seidel, HM, et al: Mosby's Guide to Physical Examination, ed 3. CV Mosby, St. Louis, 1995.

Sokolow, M, McIlroy, MB, Chietta, MD: Clinical Cardiology, ed 6. Lange Medical Publications, Los Altos, CA, 1993.

6

CARDIAC AUSCULTATION

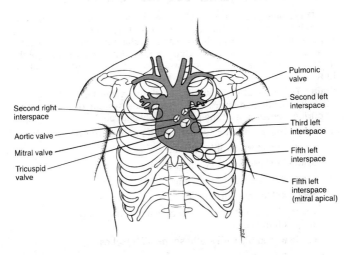

BASIC HEART SOUNDS

The four basic heart sounds are termed S_1, S_2, S_3, and S_4.

S_1 and S_2: Often referred to as "lub-dub," respectively, with S_1 being the first sound after the longest pause between pairs of beats.

S_1: Occurs at the onset of systole when the mitral and tricuspid valves close and should be loudest when auscultated over the apex of the heart (left lower sternal border).

S_2: Attributed to closure of the aortic and pulmonic valves and should be loudest over the base of heart (left upper sternal border). Systole is the period between S_1 and S_2, and diastole is the period between S_2 and the next S_1.

splitting of S_1 or S_2: Occurs when valves close asynchronously and may be a normal or pathologic finding.

> **A_2 and P_2:** When splitting is heard, S_2 is referred to as A_2 and P_2.
>
> **M_1 and T_1:** When splitting is heard, S_1 is referred to as M_1 and T_1.

S_3: Is difficult or impossible to hear without a stethoscope. It is associated with ventricular filling and occurs soon after S_2. A normal or physiologic S_3 is often found in young people. When S_3 is heard in older individuals with heart disease, it may indicate congestive failure and is called a *ventricular gallop*.

S_4: Is difficult or impossible to hear without a stethoscope. It is associated with ventricular filling as well as atrial contraction and occurs just before S_1. An audible S_4 is generally pathologic and may indicate hypertensive cardiovascular disease, coronary artery disease, postmyocardial infarction, aortic stenosis, or cardiomyopathy.

summation gallop: May be present with severe myocardial disease. It is a long heart sound that occurs when S_3 and S_4 blend together.

ventricular gallop: See S_3.

EXTRA HEART SOUNDS (MURMURS)

Described as *snaps*, *clicks*, *rubs*, and *murmurs*. Extra sounds are generally pathologic. Murmurs are caused by disturbances in the normal blood flow through the cardiac chambers and are usually classified based on their duration (timing), intensity, quality, pitch, location, and radiation. The following criteria are used for classification.

timing: During systole, diastole, or both. A murmur may be described as lasting an entire time period (holosystolic or pansystolic) or during a portion of a time period (early diastolic).

intensity: The system for evaluating the intensity of extra sounds is:

> **grade 1:** Softest audible murmur
>
> **grade 2:** Murmur of medium intensity
>
> **grade 3:** Loud murmur without thrill
>
> **grade 4:** Murmur with thrill
>
> **grade 5:** Loudest murmur that cannot be heard with stethoscope off the chest
>
> **grade 6:** Audible with stethoscope off the chest

quality: This describes the tone of the murmur, such as harsh, musical, blowing, rumbling. A crescendo murmur increases in intensity, a decrescendo murmur falls, and a crescendo-decrescendo murmur rises and then falls.

pitch: High, medium, or low pitched.

location: Area of the precordium in which the murmur is heard: aortic, pulmonic, tricuspid, mitral.

radiation: This describes when the sound of the murmur is transmitted to other regions of the body, such as across the chest, into the axilla or neck, or down the left sternal border.

THE CARDIAC CYCLE

The events of the cardiac cycle are depicted below, showing changes in left atrial pressure, left ventricular pressure, aortic pressure, ventricular volume, the ECG, and the phonocardiogram.

CARDIAC DYSFUNCTION

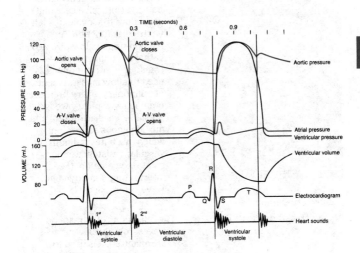

DIAGNOSTIC TESTS FOR CARDIAC DYSFUNCTION

Procedure	Description
Cardiac catheterization (for angiography)	The coronary arteries are injected with a contrast material, and the arterial system can be visualized with cinefluoroscopy: narrowing or occlusion of arteries can be evaluated.
Cardiac catheterization	Catheterization is used to measure intracardiac, transvalve, and pulmonary artery pressures and measure blood gas pressures to determine cardiac output and evaluate shunting.
Continuous hemodynamic monitoring	Pulmonary artery catheterization (Swan-Ganz) provides immediate cardiopulmonary pressure measurements. An invasive bedside (intensive care unit) procedure that evaluates left ventricular function. A balloon-tipped, flow-directed catheter, connected to a transducer and a monitor, is used to allow measurements of pulmonary artery pressure; pulmonary capillary wedge pressure; cardiac output; and mixed venous saturation, which evaluates pulmonary vascular resistance and tissue oxygenation. (See Interpreting Hemodynamic Waveforms, page 628.)
Echocardiography	
a. Transthoracic (TTE)	The reflections of ultrasound waves from cardiac surfaces are analyzed. It is used to evaluate left ventricular systolic function and the structure and function of cardiac walls, valves, and chambers; it can identify abnormal conditions such as tumors or pericardial effusion.
b. Transesophageal (TEE)	Transesophageal echocardiography is

Procedure	Description
	performed through the esophagus and stomach by a modified gastroscopy probe with one or two ultrasound transducers at its tip. TEE provides better image resolution and superior images of posterior cardiac structures. Continuous imaging is possible during operations or invasive procedures.
Electrocardiogram (ECG)	Surface electrodes record the electrical activity of the heart. A 12-lead ECG provides 12 views of the heart; it is used to assess cardiac rhythm, to diagnose the location, extent, and acuteness of myocardial ischemia and infarction; and to evaluate changes with activity.
Exercise stress tests	Numerous protocols for exercise tests have been used to assess responses to increased workloads with steps, treadmills, or bicycle ergometers. In conjunction with ECG and blood pressure recordings, patients are evaluated for exercise capacity, cardiac dysrhythmias, and diagnosis, prognosis, and management of coronary artery disease.
Hemodynamic monitoring	See continuous hemodynamic monitoring.
Holter monitoring	Continuous ambulatory ECG monitoring done by tape recording the cardiac rhythm for up to 24 h. It is used to evaluate cardiac rhythm, efficacy of medications, transient symptoms that may indicate cardiac disease, and *Continued on following page*

6

Procedure	Description
	pacemaker function; and to correlate symptoms with activity.
Pharmacologic stress tests	A noninvasive assessment for patients with coronary disease who are unable to achieve adequate cardiac stress with exercise.
Dipyridamole thallium	This potent vasodilator markedly enhances blood flow to normally perfused myocardium, whereas myocardium fed by stenotic coronary arteries demonstrates relative hypoperfusion and diminished thallium activity.
Dobutamine echocardiography	An incremental infusion is given causing an increase in the myocardial oxygen demand. Simultaneous evaluation of wall motion abnormalities, ECG, and BP are performed.
Phonocardiography	This test records cardiac sounds. It is used to time the events of the cardiac cycle and to confirm auscultatory findings.
Radionuclide angiography	Red blood cells tagged (marked) with a radionuclide are injected into blood. Ventricular wall motion can be evaluated and the ejection fraction determined; abnormal blood flow with valve and congenital defects can also be detected; techniques include gated-pool equilibrium studies and first-pass techniques.
Technetium-99m scanning (hot spot imaging)	Technetium-99m injected into blood is taken up by damaged myocardial tissue; this identifies and localizes acute myocardial infarctions

DIAGNOSTIC TESTS FOR CARDIAC DYSFUNCTION

Procedure	Description
Thallium-201 myocardial perfusion imaging (cold spot imaging)	Thallium-201 injected into blood at peak exercise; scanning identifies ischemic and infarcted myocardium, which does not take up thallium-201. It is used to diagnose coronary artery disease and perfusion, particularly when ECG is equivocal.

FOR MORE INFORMATION

Warren, JV and Lewis, RP: Diagnostic Procedures in Cardiology: A Clinician's Guide. Year Book Medical Publishers, Chicago, 1985.

ACSM's Resource Manual for Guidelines for Exercise Testing and Prescription, ed 2. Lea & Febiger, Philadelphia, 1993.

6

INTERPRETING HEMODYNAMIC WAVEFORMS

Right atrium

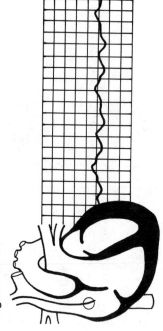

Normal Pressure

Mean: 1 to 6 mm Hg

Physiologic Significance

Right atrial (RA) pressures reflect mean RA diastolic (filling) pressure (equivalent to central venous pressure) and right ventricular (RV) end-diastolic pressure.

Clinical Implications

Increased RA pressure may signal RV failure, volume overload, tricuspid valve stenosis or regurgitation, constrictive pericarditis, or pulmonary hypertension.

Right ventricle

Normal Pressures
Systolic: 15 to 25 mm Hg
Diastolic: 0 to 8 mm Hg

Physiologic Significance
RV systolic pressure equals pulmonary artery systolic pressure; RV end-diastolic pressure reflects RV function and equals RA pressure.

Clinical Implications
RV pressures rise in mitral stenosis or insufficiency, pulmonary disease, hypoxemia, constrictive pericarditis, chronic congestive heart failure, atrial and ventricular septal defects, and patent ductus arteriosus.

Continued on following page

6

629

INTERPRETING HEMODYNAMIC WAVEFORMS (Continued)

Pulmonary artery

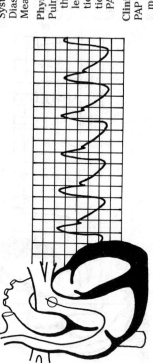

Normal Pressures

Systolic: 15 to 25 mm Hg
Diastolic: 8 to 15 mm Hg
Mean: 10 to 20 mm Hg

Physiologic Significance

Pulmonary artery pressure (PAP) reflects venous pressure in the lungs and mean filling pressure in the left atrium and left ventricle (if the mitral valve is normal), allowing detection of pulmonary congestion. PAP also reflects RV function since, in the absence of pulmonary stenosis, systolic PAP usually equals RV systolic pressure.

Clinical Implications

PAP rises in left ventricular (LV) failure, increased pulmonary blood flow (left or right shunting as in atrial or ventricular septal defects), and in any increase in pulmonary arteriolar resistance (as in pulmonary hypertension or mitral stenosis).

Pulmonary capillary wedge

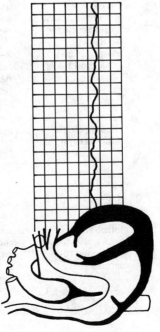

Normal Pressures

Mean: 5 to 12 mm Hg

Physiologic Significance

Pulmonary capillary wedge pressure (PCWP) accurately reflects both left atrial (LA) and LV pressures (if mitral stenosis is not present), because the heart momentarily relaxes during diastole as it fills with blood from pulmonary veins. At this instant, the pulmonary vasculature, left atrium, and left ventricle act as a single chamber with identical pressures. Thus, changes in PAP and PCWP reflect changes in LV filling pressure.

Clinical Implications

PCWP rises in LV failure, mitral stenosis or insufficiency, and pericardial tamponade. It decreases in hypovolemia.

FROM

Nurse's Clinical Library: Cardiovascular Disorders. Springhouse Corporation, Springhouse, Pa, 1984, pp. 43–46. Used with permission from Cardiovascular Disorders/Nurse's Clinical Library. © 1984 Springhouse Corporation. All rights reserved.

6

DIAGNOSIS OF ACUTE MYOCARDIAL INFARCTION

Signs and Symptoms

Signs and symptoms of acute myocardial infarction (AMI) include pain similar to that for angina pectoris. There is a heaviness, squeezing, or tight feeling in the chest; nausea and vomiting; lightheadedness; dyspnea and hypotension; sweating; weakness; and apprehension. There may be fever, shock, and cardiac failure.

Myocardial Enzymes

Tissue necrosis causes enzymes to be released into the blood. Enzymes released by myocardial damage demonstrate a characteristic pattern and duration of pressure in the blood.

MYOCARDIAL ENZYMES		
Abbreviation for Enzyme	Enzyme (Normal Value)	Description
AST (formerly called SGOT)	Aspartate aminotransferase (serum glutamic-oxaloacetic transaminase) (<45 U/mL)	Enzyme appears in serum within hours, peaks at 12–24 h, falls to normal within 2–7 d. AST is also released due to damage to muscle, brain tissue, and other internal organs.
CPK (CK)	Creatine phosphokinase (20–232 U/mL)	Enzyme appears in serum within hours, peaks within 24 h, falls to normal within 3–5 d. CPK is also released due to damage to brain tissue and skeletal muscle.
CK-MB	Creatine kinase myocardial band isoenzyme (0–8 ng/mL)	Isoenzyme of CPK more specific for myocardial damage; appears in serum at 4–6 h, peaks at 12–24 h, falls to normal within 48 h.

Abbreviation for Enzyme	Enzyme (Normal Value)	Description
REL INDEX	Relative index (0–2.5%)	Relative index calculations are only of value if CK-MB is >8 ng/mL and CPK exceeds upper limit. An index >2.5% is highly suggestive of myocardial damage.
LDH (LD)	Lactate dehydrogenase (<600 U/mL)	Enzyme begins to rise 12–24 h, peaks by day 3, and returns to normal within 8–12 d. LDH is also released due to damage to brain, red blood cell tissue, kidney, lung, and spleen.

Elevation of Enzymes after Acute Myocardial Infarctions

6

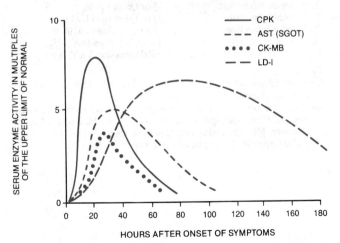

Stylized depiction (assembled from multiple sources) of the time-activity curves of CPK, CK-MB, LD-1, and AST (SGOT), following onset of acute myocardial infarction (defined on the basis of sentinel-persistent chest pain).

Electrocardiographic Changes After Myocardial Infarctions

Serial 12-lead ECG recordings are used to diagnose the presence and evolution of AMI. Injury is localized by the presence of abnormal waves on specific ECG leads.*

A. *Sequential phases in infarction*

1. Acute	ST elevation (earliest change). Tall, hyperacute T waves. New Q or QS wave.
2. Evolving	Deep T-wave inversions may persist; usually returns to normal (months). ST elevation returns to baseline (days). Q or QS waves may decrease in size, rarely disappear.

B. *Infarction type*

1. Subendocardial intramural	ST-T changes: ST depression or T-wave inversion. Without QRS changes.
2. Transmural	Abnormal Q or QS waves in leads overlying the infarct. ST-T changes.

C. *Infarction site*

1. Anterior infarction:	Q or QS in V_1–V_4.
2. Lateral infarction:	Q or QS in lead I, aVl.
3. Inferior infarction:	Q or QS in leads II, III, aVF.
4. Posterior infarction:	Large R waves in V_1–V_3. ST depression V_1, V_2, or V_3.

---

*Standard 12-lead electrocardiogram: leads I to III, aVR, aVl, and aVF are limb leads; V_1 to V_6 are chest leads.

Based on Goldberger, A and Goldberger, E: Clinical Electrocardiography—A Simplified Approach, ed 2. CV Mosby, St. Louis, 1985; and Conover, MB: Understanding Electrocardiography—Physiological and Interpretive Concepts, ed 3. CV Mosby, St. Louis, 1980.

GUIDELINES FOR HELPING PATIENTS RESUME WALKING SOON AFTER MYOCARDIAL INFARCTIONS

Before Exercise

Ask about chest discomfort, dyspnea, and faintness (if present, check with physician before proceeding).

Measure blood pressure and heart rate (if >160/100 or <90/60 mm Hg or if heart rate is >110 or <60 bpm, check with physician before starting).

Check orthostatic blood pressure before beginning standing range-of-motion exercise or walking. If blood pressure falls more than 20 mm Hg or if fall is associated with symptoms of faintness, have patient lie down and notify physician.

During Exercise

Ask patient to report symptoms, particularly chest discomfort, dyspnea, or faintness. If symptoms occur, discontinue exercise until checking with physician.

Ask for rating of perceived exertion.

Immediately After Exercise

Ask patient about symptoms.

Measure heart rate, blood pressure, and rating of perceived exertion. If symptoms occur, blood pressure falls more than 20 mm Hg, or heart rate rises more than 20 bpm over resting rate, check with physician before continuing.

From Fletcher, GF, et al: Exercise Standards: A Statement for Healthcare Professionals from the American Heart Association. American Heart Association, Dallas, 1995 p. 608.

TYPES OF ANGINA PECTORIS

Classification	Description	ECG	Treatment
Stable angina	Myocardial oxygen demand exceeds oxygen supply. Pain is brought on by physical exertion or stress, often occurs after eating. Discomfort is most often substernal, precordial, or in the epigastric region with radiation to the left arm, jaw, or neck.	ST-segment depression (horizontal or down sloping) occurs during ischemia episodes.	Usually treated with either a β-blocker or long-acting nitrate; relieved by rest
Variant (Prinzmetal's) angina	Myocardial oxygen supply decreases due to coronary vasospasm. It may occur at rest and in a circadian manner at a similar time of day (often in the early morning hours); more common in women (younger than 50).	ST-segment elevation, occurs sometimes unaccompanied by pain. Less frequent is ST-segment depression.	Treated primarily with calcium channel blockers
Unstable (preinfarction, crescendo)	Myocardial oxygen supply decreases at the same time that oxygen demand increases. It may occur at any time (with rest or activity). Pain distribution is similar to that which occurs with typical stable angina, but it may be more intense and last for several hours.	ST-segment depression or elevation occurs	May require a combination of drugs (a calcium channel blocker and a β-blocker)
Syndrome X	Chest pain that is seemingly ischemic in origin but with a normal arteriogram and normal ECG; it may be referred pain.	Normal ECG	

FOR MORE INFORMATION

Ciccone, CD: Pharmacology in Rehabilitation, ed 2. FA Davis. Philadelphia, 1996. Irwin, S and Tecklin, JS: Cardiopulmonary Physical Therapy, ed 3. CV Mosby. St. Louis, 1995.

Levels of Angina

1+   Light or barely noticeable.
2+   Moderate, bothersome.
3+   Severe and very uncomfortable.
4+   Most severe pain ever experienced.

Causes of Chest Pain

acute cholecystitis
coronary artery disease
esophagitis
herpes zoster
musculoskeletal disorders: axillary muscle pain, referred pain,
   rib fractures, osteoarthritis, osteochondritis, arthritis
peptic ulcer
pericarditis
pneumothorax
pulmonary embolism
thoracic aortic dissection

BASED ON

Abrams, WB, et al (eds): The Merck Manual of Geriatrics, ed 2. Merck
Research Laboratories, Whitehouse Station, NJ, 1995, pp 632–634.

6

ORGANIC NITRATES USED FOR THE TREATMENT OF ANGINA PECTORIS

Dosage Form	Onset of Action	Duration of Action
Nitroglycerin		
Oral	20–45 min	4–6 h
Buccal (extended release)	2–3 min	3–5 h
Sublingual	1–3 min	30–60 min
Ointment	30 min	4–8 h
Transdermal patches	Within 30 min	8–24 h
Isosorbide dinitrate		
Oral	15–40 min	4–6 h
Oral (extended release)	30 min	12 h
Chewable	2–5 min	1–2 h
Sublingual	2–5 min	1–2 h
Erythrityl tetranitrate		
Oral	30 min	Up to 6 h
Chewable	Within 5 min	2 h
Buccal	Within 5 min	2 h
Sublingual	Within 5 min	2–3 h
Pentaerythritol tetranitrate		
Oral	20–60 min	4–5 h
Amyl nitrate		
Inhaled	30 s	3–5 min

From Ciccone, CD: Pharmacology in Rehabilitation, ed 2. FA Davis, Philadelphia, 1996, p 311, with permission.

β-BLOCKERS USED TO TREAT ANGINA PECTORIS

Generic Name	Trade Name	Usual Oral Dose
Acebutolol	Sectral	200–600 mg 2 times a day
Atenolol	Tenormin	50–100 mg once a day
Carteolol	Cartrol	2.5–10.0 mg once a day
Labetalol	Normodyne, Trandate	200–400 mg 2 times a day
Metoprolol	Lopressor	50–200 mg 2 times a day
Nadolol	Corgard	40–240 mg once a day
Penbutolol	Levatol	20 mg once a day
Pindolol	Visken	5–20 mg 2 times a day
Propranolol	Inderal	10–120 mg 2–4 times a day
Sotalol	Betapace	80–160 mg 2 times a day
Timolol	Blocadren	10–30 mg 2 times a day

From Ciccone, CD: Pharmacology in Rehabilitation, ed 2. FA Davis, Philadelphia, 1996, p 314, with permission.

FUNCTIONAL AND THERAPEUTIC CLASSIFICATIONS OF PATIENTS WITH DISEASES OF THE HEART

Classification	Permissible Workloads Continuous–Intermittent	Maximal
Functional		
Class I	4.0–6.0 cal/min	6.5 METs
	Patients with cardiac disease but without resulting limitations of physical activity. Ordinary physical activity does not cause undue fatigue, palpitation, dyspnea, or anginal pain.	
Class II	3.0–4.0 cal/min	4.5 METs
	Patients with cardiac disease resulting in slight limitation of physical activity. Patients are comfortable at rest. Ordinary physical activity results in fatigue, palpitation, dyspnea, or anginal pain.	
Class III	2.0–3.0 cal/min	3.0 METs
	Patients with cardiac disease resulting in marked limitation of physical activity. Patients are comfortable at rest. Less than ordinary physical activity causes fatigue, palpitation, dyspnea, or anginal pain.	
Class IV	1.0–2.0 cal/min	1.5 METs
	Patients with cardiac disease resulting in inability to carry on any physical activity without discomfort. Symptoms of cardiac insufficiency or of the anginal syndrome may be present even at rest. If any physical activity is undertaken, discomfort is increased.	
Therapeutic		
Class A	Patients with cardiac disease whose physical activity need not be restricted in any way.	
Class B	Patients with cardiac disease whose ordinary physical activity need not be restricted but who should be advised against severe or competitive efforts.	

Continued on following page

Classification	Permissible Workloads Continuous–Intermittent	Maximal
Class C	Patients with cardiac disease whose ordinary physical activity should be moderately restricted and whose more strenuous efforts should be discontinued.	
Class D	Patients with cardiac disease whose ordinary physical activity should be markedly restricted.	
Class E	Patients with cardiac disease who should be at complete rest or confined to bed or chair.	

METs = metabolic equivalents.
Reprinted by permission of the American Heart Association, New York.

TREATMENT OF CORONARY ARTERY DISEASE

Coronary Artery Bypass Grafts

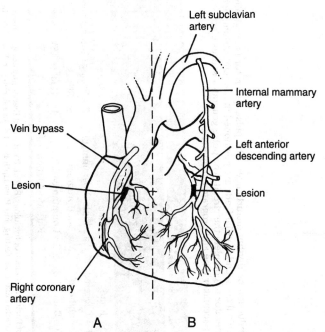

Coronary artery bypass graft procedures. (A) Saphenous vein bypass graft. Leg vein is sutured to ascending aorta and to right coronary artery beyond critical stenosis, creating vascular conduit to shunt blood around blockage to ischemic myocardium. (B) Mammary artery graft procedure. Mammary artery is anastomosed to anterior descending branch of left coronary artery distal to blockage so blood flow is re-established.

Pacemakers

Pacemakers are implanted to help manage conduction or rhythm disturbances. The pulse generator is surgically implanted into a subcutaneous pouch in the pectoral or abdominal area. Endocardial leads are positioned in the right atrium, right ventricle, or both. The lead wire is connected to the pulse generator to complete the circuit. The pulse generator senses electrical activity in the heart and stimulates the heart according to the pacemaker type and program parameters.

			NBG PACEMAKER CODE		
Position	I	II	III	IV	V
Category	Chamber(s) Paced	Chambers Sensed	Response to Sensing	Programmability/ Modulation	Antitachyarrhythmia Functioning
	O = None	O = None	O = None	O = None	O = None
	A = Atrium	A = Atrium	T = Triggered	P = Simple Programmable	P = Pacing (Antitachyarrhythmia)
	V = Ventricle	V = Ventricle	I = Inhibited	M = Multiprogram	S = Shock
	D = Dual (A&V)	D = Dual (A&V)	D = Dual (T&I)	C = Communicating	D = Dual (P&S)
				R = Rate Modulation	

NBG = NASPE/BPEG generic code (North American Society of Pacing and Electrophysiology/British Pacing and Electrophysiology Group.
From American College of Sports Medicine: Guidelines for Graded Exercise Testing and Prescription, ed 4. Lea & Febiger, Philadelphia, 1991, p 143, with permission.

Percutaneous Transluminal Coronary Angioplasty

Percutaneous transluminal coronary angioplasty (PTCA) is a nonsurgical technique using a balloon-tipped catheter to achieve coronary reperfusion. Under fluoroscopic guidance the PTCA catheter is advanced across the middle of the coronary lesion. The balloon is inflated and reduces the constriction by physically splitting the atheromatous plaque and stretching the arterial wall.

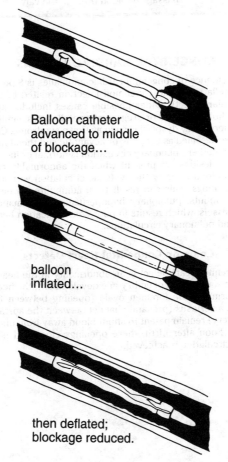

Balloon catheter advanced to middle of blockage...

balloon inflated...

then deflated; blockage reduced.

Events leading to successful percutaneous transluminal coronary angioplasty (PTCA).

VALVULAR DYSFUNCTION

Type	Description
Atresia	Congenital absence or closure.
Prolapse	Typically of the mitral valve; valve cusp falls back into atrium during systole.
Regurgitation	Incompetent valve closure allows blood to flow backwards; this is also called *insufficiency*.
Stenosis	Valve becomes stiff and fibrotic, obstructing the passage of blood through the valve.

CONGENITAL CARDIAC LESIONS

The incidence of congenital cardiac anomalies is 8 per 1000 live births. Rubella is the most common infection related to congenital cardiovascular defects. Other possible causes include exposure to x-rays, alcohol, infections or drugs, maternal diabetes, family history, and some hereditary dysplasias such as Down syndrome. Cardiac defects can be classified as cyanotic or acyanotic and then further categorized by whether pulmonary circulation is normal or increased.

Cyanotic lesions are present when the abnormality causes deoxygenated blood to enter the systemic circulation without passing through the lungs. This can result from admixture, as occurs with right-to-left shunts; pulmonary hypoperfusion; or transposition of the great vessels, which results in poor communication between the systemic and pulmonary circulations.

Common Congenital Heart Defects

A congenital heart defect is an abnormality in the heart's structure. By the eighth week of embryonic development, the heart is well formed. Normally, the foramen ovale (opening between the atria) and ductus arteriosus (prenatal channel between the aorta and pulmonary artery) remain patent to shunt blood away from unexpanded fetal lungs. Soon after birth, these openings close and normal extrauterine circulation is achieved.

With normal cardiovascular development, the heart's low pressure right side receives unoxygenated blood from the body and delivers it to the lungs for reoxygenation; in turn, the heart's high pressure left side receives oxygenated blood from the lungs and delivers it to all body parts. But improper development can obstruct or alter this blood-flow pattern. The result? A congenital defect—either acyanotic or cyanotic. Acyanotic defects shunt oxygenated blood from the left to the right heart, but do not mix unoxygenated blood in the systemic circulation. Cyanotic defects shunt blood from the right to the left heart and permit unoxygenated blood to flow from the left ventricle to all parts of the body, resulting in cyanosis.

To identify a congenital heart defect, take a careful history and make a thorough assessment. Always be alert for signs of inadequate oxygenation, such as cyanosis, nail-bed clubbing, and labored breathing. Also, watch for inadequate cardiac output and CHF, murmurs, and easy fatigability. If a congenital heart defect has been diagnosed, help parents to understand and accept the condition and teach them to prevent complications.

FROM

Nurse's Clinical Library: Cardiovascular Disorders. Springhouse Corporation, 1984, pp 180–181.

6

CONGENITAL HEART DEFECTS

Congenital Defect	Assessment Findings
Ventricular septal defect (VSD) Abnormal opening in the ventricular septum allows shunting of oxygenated blood from left ventricle to mix with unoxygenated blood in right ventricle. Results from inadequate development of septal tissue during fetal life. Defect varies from size of pinhole to absence of entire septum. Most defects are small and close spontaneously by ages 4 to 6. May cause pulmonary artery hypertension in sizable left-to-right shunts.	**History:** In small VSD, unremarkable. In medium-size VSD, increased susceptibility to respiratory infection and easy fatigability. In large VSD, feeding difficulty, poor weight gain, frequent respiratory infections, and markedly increased fatigability. **Inspection:** In large VSD, child is thin, small, and tachypneic, with prominent anterior chest wall and active precordium. **Palpation:** In small VSD, cardiac thrill at left sternal border. In medium-size to large VSD, possible liver enlargement from CHF; PMI displaced to left, with significant cardiomegaly. **Auscultation:** In small VSD, loud, harsh systolic murmur at left sternal border. In medium to large VSD, rumbling systolic murmur heard best at lower left sternal border; loud, widely split S_2. With pulmonary artery hypertension, quieter murmur but loud, booming pulmonic S_2.
Atrial septal defect (ASD) One or more openings between the atria (includes ostium secundum, ostium primum, and sinus venosus) allow blood to shunt from left to right. Condition caused by delayed or incomplete closure of foramen ovale or atrial septum. Results in right heart volume overload. Depending on size of the defect, it often goes undetected in preschoolers and may lead to CHF and pulmonary vascular disease in adults.	**History:** In child, usually good health and growth; at times, frequent respiratory tract infections and fatigability after extreme exertion. In child with ostium primum, feeding difficulty, dyspnea, frequent respiratory infections. In adult, pronounced fatigability and dyspnea on exertion (after age 40); syncope and hemoptysis in severe pulmonary vascular disease. **Inspection:** In child with ostium primum, growth retardation. In adult, cyanosis and clubbing of fingers.

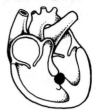

Diagnostic tests

Chest X-ray: In small VSD, normal. In medium-size to large VSD, enlarged left atrium and left ventricle, prominent pulmonary vascular markings. With pulmonary artery hypertension, enlarged right atrium and ventricle and pulmonary artery.

ECG: In small VSD, normal. In medium-size to large VSD, left ventricular hypertrophy. With pulmonary artery hypertension, right ventricular hypertrophy.

Echocardiography: May detect VSD and its location, determine size of left-to-right shunt, and suggest pulmonary hypertension; more useful in identifying associated lesions and complications.

Cardiac catheterization: Confirms size of VSD; calculates degree of shunting; determines extent of pulmonary hypertension; detects associated defects.

Treatment

Medical: In small VSD, conservative management. In medium-size to large VSD, bed rest, oxygen, digoxin, diuretics, and fluid restrictions for acute CHF; prophylactic antibiotics to prevent infective endocarditis; monitoring to detect pulmonary artery hypertension.

Surgical: In medium-size to large VSD, closure or patch graft, using cardiopulmonary bypass and deep hypothermia, during preschool years.

6

Chest X-ray: Enlarged right atrium and right ventricle and prominent pulmonary artery, increased pulmonary vasculature, small aorta.

ECG: May be normal, but prolonged PR interval, right axis deviation, varying degrees of right bundle branch block, right ventricular

Medical: Not usually necessary, except in ostium primum with accompanying CHF.

Surgical: Direct closure or patch graft recommended during preschool or early school-age years.

Continued on following page

Congenital Defect

Assessment Findings

Palpation: Possible thrill accompanies murmur.

Auscultation: In a child, soft early to mid-systolic murmur, heard at second or third left intercostal space; fixed and widely split S_2. In large shunts, low-pitched diastolic murmur heard at lower left sternal border. In older patients with large ASD and obstructive pulmonary vascular disease, right ventricular hypertrophy with accentuated S_2, and fixed wide splitting; possible pulmonary ejection click and audible S_4.

Patent ductus arteriosus (PDA)

Patent duct between the descending aorta and pulmonary artery bifurcation allows left-to-right shunting of blood from aorta to pulmonary artery. Caused by failure of the ductus to close after birth. Results in recirculation of arterial blood through lungs and increased left-heart work load. In time, can precipitate pulmonary vascular disease and infective endocarditis.

History: In premature infant, frank CHF. In child, mild symptoms of heart disease, such as frequent respiratory tract infections, slow motor development, and fatigability. In adult, fatigability and dyspnea on exertion (by age 40).

Inspection: In premature infant, signs of CHF.

Palpation: In infant or child with large PDA, possible thrill at left sternal border and a prominent left ventricular impulse.

Auscultation: Loud, continuous machinery murmur heard at left upper sternal border and under left clavicle that may obscure S_1; S_3 in CHF; widened pulse pressure.

Coarctation of aorta

Constriction of the aorta near the site of the ligamentum arteriosum (remnant of the fetal ductus arteriosus). May be classified as preductal or postductal. It may result from spasm and constriction of smooth muscle in ductus

History: In infant with preductal coarctation: signs of CHF. In some infants with postductal coarctation: possible CHF in first few months of life. In others: normal growth and health. In some children: headaches, epistaxis, fatigue, or cold feet. In adult: dyspnea, syncope,

Diagnostic tests	Treatment

hypertrophy, and, in ostium primum, left axis deviation. In adult, possible atrial fibrillation.

Echocardiography: Measures extent of right ventricular enlargement and may locate ASD.

Cardiac catheterization: Confirms ASD, determines volume of shunting, and detects pulmonary vascular disease.

Chest X-ray: Increased pulmonary vascular markings and prominent pulmonary arteries. If shunt is large, enlarged left atrium, left ventricle and aorta.

ECG: May be normal or show left ventricular hypertrophy.

Echocardiography: Detects PDA and reveals enlarged left atrium and left ventricle.

Cardiac catheterization: Shows PDA. Increased PA pressure indicates large shunt, or, if PA pressure exceeds systemic arterial pressure, severe pulmonary vascular disease. Allows calculation of blood volume crossing ductus.

Medical: CHF regimen; cardiac catheterization deposits a plug in ductus to stop shunting; administration of indomethacin (a prostaglandin inhibitor) induces ductus spasm and closure.

Surgical: In infant with CHF who fails to respond to treatment, ductal ligation. After age 1, ligation and division of ductus.

Patent ductus arteriosus

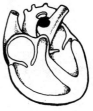

6

Coarctation of aorta

Chest X-ray: In preductal coarctation, shows cardiomegaly. In postductal coarctation, shows enlarged left atrium and ventricle and

Medical: In infant with preductal coarctation, CHF regimen. Balloon angioplasty shows promise in relieving this anomaly in infants. A balloon- *Continued on following page*

649

Congenital Defect

Assessment Findings

arteriosus as it closes, or from abnormal development of aortic arch.

claudication, headaches, and leg cramps.

Inspection: Infant often displays signs of CHF; peripheral cyanosis in end stages of severe untreated coarctation. In adolescents, visible aortic pulsations in suprasternal notch due to collateral circulation.

Palpation: Hepatomegaly in infant with CHF. Increased amplitude of peripheral pulses in arms; weak, absent, or delayed pulses in legs.

Auscultation: In preductal coarctation, normal heart sounds and absence of murmurs. In CHF, S_3 or S_4. In postductal coarctation, continuous systolic murmur over back if collateral circulation is extensive. In severe coarctation, loud S_2.

Tetralogy of Fallot

Four defects: ventricular septal defect (VSD), overriding aorta, pulmonary stenosis, right ventricular hypertrophy. Results from incomplete development of ventricular septum and pulmonic outflow tract. Coexisting VSD and obstructed blood flow from right ventricle cause unoxygenated blood to shunt right to left, and to mix with oxygenated blood, resulting in cyanosis.

History: After 3 to 6 months, cyanosis. In some infants: intense cyanotic "blue" spells (dyspnea, deep sighing respirations, bradycardia, fainting, seizures, loss of consciousness), precipitated by awakening, crying, straining, infection, or fever. In older child: decreased exercise tolerance, increased dyspnea on exertion, growth retardation, eating difficulties, squatting when short of breath.

Inspection: Remarkable cyanosis, even during rest. Older child displays clubbing of fingers and toes.

Palpation: Thrill along left sternal border. Prominent right ventricular impulse or heave at inferior septum.

Auscultation: Loud systolic murmur along entire left sternal border, which may diminish or obscure pulmonic component of S_2. Possible continuous murmur over back if

Diagnostic tests	Treatment
dilated ascending aorta.	tipped catheter is advanced through the femoral artery up the aorta to the area of coarctation. The balloon is rapidly inflated and deflated many times, forcing open the area of coarctation.
ECG: In preductal coarctation, shows right ventricular hypertrophy. In postductal coarctation, shows left ventricular hypertrophy.	
Echocardiography: May show increased left ventricular muscle thickness, aortic valve abnormalities, site of defect, and associated defects.	**Surgical:** Resection with anastomosis of aorta or insertion of prosthetic graft usually recommended between ages 4 and 8, unless unmanageable CHF develops in infant with preductal coarctation.
Cardiac catheterization: Locates site of defect, evaluates collateral circulation, measures pressure in the left and right ventricles and in ascending and descending aortas, and detects associated defects.	
Aortography: Locates site of defect.	

Tetralogy of Fallot

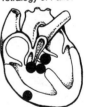

Chest X-ray: Normal cardiac size, decreased pulmonary vascular markings, and a boot-shaped cardiac silhouette. ventricular hypertrophy, right

ECG: Shows right axis deviation, and, occasionally, right atrial hypertrophy.

Echocardiography: Identifies VSD and pulmonary stenosis. Detects enlarged right ventricle and displaced aorta.

Cardiac catheterization: Confirms diagnosis by detecting pulmonary stenosis and VSD, visualizing overriding aorta, and

Medical: Avoidance of cyanosis is key objective. If it occurs, knee-chest position and administration of oxygen and oxygenation. Administration of morphine improve propranolol may relieve spasm of right ventricular outflow tract and improve oxygen saturation. Prophylactic antibiotics aim to prevent infective endocarditis. Continuous assessment aims to detect other serious bacterial infections and polycythemia.

Surgical: Palliative *Continued on following page*

Congenital Defect   Assessment Findings

extensive pulmonary collateral circulation develops.

Transposition of the great arteries

Great arteries are reversed: aorta leaves right ventricle and pulmonary artery leaves left ventricle, producing two noncommunicating circulatory systems. Unoxygenated blood flows through right atrium and ventricle and out the aorta to systemic circulation; oxygenated blood flows from lungs to left atrium and ventricle and out the pulmonary artery to lungs.

History: In infant, cyanosis. In older child, cyanosis, frequent respiratory infections, diminished exercise tolerance, fatigability.

Inspection: In infant, cyanosis, tachypnea, dyspnea (worsens with crying); poor feeding. In older child, dyspnea and clubbing of fingers.

Palpation: Hepatomegaly due to CHF.

Auscultation: S_2 louder than normal, but no murmur during first days of life. Murmurs may later be associated with ASD, VSD, PDA, or pulmonary stenosis. Gallop rhythm possible with CHF.

Diagnostic tests	Treatment
ruling out other cyanotic heart defects.	surgery, such as Blalock-Taussig, Potts-Smith-Gibson, or Waterston procedures, enhances blood flow to lungs to reduce hypoxia. Corrective surgery relieves pulmonary stenosis and closes VSD. Administration of prophylactic antibiotics continues after surgery.

Chest X-ray: Often normal in first days of life. Within days or weeks, enlarged right atrium and right ventricle (oblong shape). Also shows increased pulmonary vascular markings.

ECG: May be normal in first days of life. Later, reveals right axis deviation, right ventricle hypertrophy, and possibly right atrial hypertrophy.

Echocardiography: Demonstrates reversed aorta and pulmonary artery, and records echoes from both semilunar valves simultaneously, because of aortic valve displacement.

Medical: Balloon septostomy enlarges foramen ovale and improves oxygenation; CHF regimen; administration of alprostadil maintains open ductus arteriosus in newborns.

Surgical: Recommended during first years of life. Mustard or Senny procedure redirects venous return to appropriate ventricle.

Transposition of great arteries

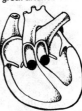

6

FROM

Nurse's Clinical Library: Cardiovascular Disorders. Springhouse Corporation, 1984, pp 180–181.

HEART FAILURE

Heart failure results when the myocardium is unable to maintain adequate circulation of the blood for respiration and metabolism. There may be failure of the right or left ventricle or both.

TYPES OF HEART FAILURE	
Type	**Description**
Backward	Venous return to the heart is reduced, with resulting venous stasis and congestion.
Congestive	Systemic congestion (edema, enlarged liver, elevated venous pressure) due to right heart failure and/or pulmonary congestion due to left heart failure.
Forward	Cardiac output is greatly reduced due to left ventricular failure, as after myocardial infarction when the ventricle has lost contractility.
High output	Cardiac failure that results from conditions that increase the amount of circulation, as with a large arteriovenous fistula or anemia.
Low output	Failure of the heart to maintain adequate cardiac output due to insufficient venous return, as with hemorrhage.

COMPARISONS OF RIGHT- AND LEFT-SIDED HEART FAILURE	
Right	**Left**
Elevated end-diastolic right ventricular pressure	Elevated end-diastolic left ventricular pressure
Systemic congestion: Enlarged liver Ascites Jugular venous distention Dependent (pitting) edema	Pulmonary congestion: Pulmonary edema Dyspnea, orthopnea Paroxysmal nocturnal dyspnea Cough Bronchospasm (Cardiac asthma)
Fatigue Anorexia and bloating	Fatigue
Oliguria, nocturia	Oliguria

COMPARISONS OF RIGHT- AND LEFT-SIDED HEART FAILURE
(Continued)

Right	Left
Cyanosis (capillary stasis)	Cyanosis (central)
Pleural effusion (R > L)	Tachycardia
Unexplained weight gain	
Etiology:	Etiology:
Mitral stenosis	Hypertension
Pulmonary parenchymal or vascular disease	Coronary artery disease
	Aortic valve disease
Pulmonic or tricuspid valvular disease	Cardiomyopathies
	Congenital heart defects
Infective endocarditis	Infective endocarditis
	High-output conditions
	Various connective tissue disorders

FOR MORE INFORMATION

Merck Manual, ed 16. Merck, & Co., Rahway, NJ, 1992.

DRUGS USED IN CONGESTIVE HEART FAILURE

Drug Group	Primary Effect
Digitalis glycosides Deslanoside Digitoxin Digoxin	Increase cardiac pumping ability.
Diuretics Thiazides, loop diuretics, and so on	Decrease vascular fluid volume.
Angiotensin-converting enzyme inhibitors Benazepril Captopril Enalapril Lisinopril Quinapril Ramipril	Prevent angiotensin-induced vasoconstriction; limit aldosterone secretion.
Others Amrinone, milrinone Dopamine, dobutamine Vasodilators	Increase myocardial contractility. Increase myocardial contractility. Decrease peripheral vascular resistance.

From Ciccone, CD: Pharmacology in Rehabilitation, ed 2. FA Davis, Philadelphia, 1996, p 339, with permission.

SAMPLE PHASE I CARDIAC REHABILITATION PROGRAM

		CARDIAC PATIENT PROGRESSION		
Level	Suggested Day	Supervised Exercise	CCU/Ward Activity	Educational Topics
1	1–2 (CCU)	Passive ROM, ankle pumps, breathing exercise (1.0–1.5 METs)	Bedrest, bedside commode, feed self, partial self-care	Orientation to CCU
2	2–3 (CCU)	Active ROM of upper extremities (supine)	Sit in chair 15 min, partial self-bath	Anatomy and physiology of coronary disease, cholesterol/lipids
3	3–4 (ward)	Active ROM (sitting), calisthenics and walking (50–75 ft)	Sit in chair 15–30 min bid-tid, feed self in chair	Pulse monitoring, activity diary, carbohydrates/protein
4	4–6	Calisthenics (2–3 METs), walk 2–3 min	Bathroom privilege, simulated shower, dress in clothes	Energy costs of various activities, sodium and blood pressure

5	5–8	Calisthenics (2.0–3.5 METs), walk 3–5 min, walk up 3–5 steps	In chair most of day, shower with help	Home exercise program, nutrition labeling, food fads and myths, work simplification
6	6–9	Calisthenics (2.5–4.0 METs), walk 5–7 min, walk down flight of stairs	Previous activity, light crafts, shower by self	Aerobic vs anaerobic, vitamins and minerals, eating out
7	7–10	Calisthenics (2.5–4.0 METs), walk up flight of stairs	Previous activity, exercise testing	Exercise prescription; long-term management of exercise, stress, and nutrition; outpatient rehab program

CCU = coronary care unit; METs = metabolic equivalents; ROM = range of motion.
Reprinted from Physical Therapy, Davidson, DM and Maloney, CA: Recovery after cardiac events. 1985, vol 65, p 1821, with the permission of the APTA.

EFFECTS OF MEDICATIONS ON HEART RATE, BLOOD PRESSURE, ELECTROCARDIOGRAPHIC FINDINGS (ECG), AND EXERCISE CAPACITY

Medications	Heart Rate		Blood Pressure Rest (R) and Exercise (E)	ECG		Exercise Capacity
	Rest	Exercise		Rest	Exercise	
Beta blockers (including labetalol)	↓*	↓	↓	↓ HR*	↓ ischemia†	↑ in patients with angina; ↓ or ↔ in patients without angina
Nitrates	↑	↑ or ↔	↓ (R) or ↔ (E)	↑ HR	↑ or ↔ HR ↓ ischemia†	↑ in patients with angina; ↔ in patients without angina; ↑ or ↔ in patients with congestive heart failure (CHF)
Calcium channel blockers						
Nifedipine	↑	↑	↓	↑ HR	↑ HR ↓ ischemia†	↑ in patients with angina; ↔ in patients without angina
Diltiazem	↓	↓	↓	↓ HR	↓ HR ↓ ischemia†	↑ in patients with angina; ↔ in patients without angina
Verapamil	↓	↓	↓	↓ HR	↓ HR ↓ ischemia†	↑ in patients with angina; ↔ in patients without angina

		May produce nonspecific ST-T wave changes	May produce ST segment depression	Improved only in patients with fibrillation or in patients with CHF
Digitalis	↓ in patients with atrial fibrillation and possibly CHF; not significantly altered in patients with sinus rhythm	↔	↔		↔, except possibly in patients with CHF (see text)
Diuretics	↔	↔ or ↓	↔	May cause PVCs and "false-positive" test results if hypokalemia occurs	↔
Vasodilators					
Nonadrenergic vasodilators	↑ or ↔	↓	↑ or ↔ HR	↑ or ↔ HR	↔, except ↑ or ↔ in patients with CHF
α-Adrenergic blockers	↔	↓	↔	↔	↔
Antiadrenergic agents without selective blockade of peripheral receptors	↓ or ↔	↓	↓ or ↔ HR	↓ or ↔ HR	↔

Continued on next page

6

EFFECTS OF MEDICATIONS ON HEART RATE, BLOOD PRESSURE, ELECTROCARDIOGRAPHIC FINDINGS (ECG), AND EXERCISE CAPACITY (Continued)

| Medications | Heart Rate | | Blood Pressure Rest (R) and | ECG | | Exercise Capacity |
	Rest	Exercise	Exercise (E)	Rest	Exercise	
Antiarrhythmic agents						
Class I						
Quinidine	↑ or ↔	↑ or ↔	↑ or ↔ (R)	May prolong QRS and QT inter-vals	Quinidine may cause "false-negative" test results	↕
Disopyramide			↔ (E)			
Procainamide	↕	↕	↕	May prolong QRS and QT inter-vals	Procainamide may cause "false-positive" test results	↕
Phenytoin						
Tocainide						
Mexiletine						
Encainide						
Flecainide						
Class II						
Beta blockers	(see previous entry)					
Class III						
Amiodarone	↓	→	↕	↕	↕	↕
Class IV						
Calcium channel blockers	(see previous entry)					

660

Medication					
Bronchodilators Methylxanthines	↑ or ↔	↑ or ↔	↑	↑ or ↔ HR; may produce PVCs	↑ or ↔ HR; may produce PVCs	Bronchodilators ↑ exercise capacity in patients limited by bronchospasm
Sympathomimetic agents	↑ or ↔	↑ or ↔	↑, ↔, or ↓	↑ or ↔ HR	↑ or ↔ HR
Cromolyn sodium	↔	↔	↔	↔	↔
Corticosteriods	↔	↔	↔	↔	↔
Hyperlipidemic agents	Clofibrate may provoke arrhythmias, angina in patients with prior myocardial infarction				
	Dextrothyroxine may ↑ HR and BP at rest and during exercise, provoke arrhythmias, and worsen myocardial ischemia and angina				
	Nicotinic acid may ↓ BP				
	Probucol may cause QT interval prolongation				
	All other hyperlipidemic agents have no effect on HR, BP, and ECG				
Psychotropic medications:					
Minor tranquilizers	May ↓ HR and BP by controlling anxiety; no other effects				
	↑ or ↔	↑ or ↔	↓ or ↔	(see text)	(see text)
Antidepressants	↑ or ↔	↑ or ↔	↓ or ↔	(see text)	May cause "false-positive" test results
Major tranquilizers	↑ or ↔	↑ or ↔	↓ or ↔	↑ or ↔	May cause "false-positive" or

Continued on next page

6

EFFECTS OF MEDICATIONS ON HEART RATE, BLOOD PRESSURE, ELECTROCARDIOGRAPHIC FINDINGS (ECG), AND EXERCISE CAPACITY (Continued)

Medications	Heart Rate		Blood Pressure Rest (R) and Exercise (E)	ECG		Exercise Capacity
	Rest	Exercise	Exercise (E)	Rest	Exercise	
Lithium	↔	↔	↔	May cause T-wave changes and arrhythmias	"false-negative" test results May cause T-wave changes and arrhythmias	
Nicotine	↑ or ↔	↑ or ↔	↑	↑ or ↔ HR; may provoke ischemia, arrhythmias	↑ or ↔ HR; may provoke ischemia, arrhythmias	↔, except ↓ or ↔ in patients with angina
Antihistamines	↔	↔	↔	↔	↔	↔
Cold medications with sympathomimetic agents	Effects similar to those described in *Sympathomimetic agents*, although magnitude of effects is usually diminished					↔

Medication	Heart Rate	Blood Pressure	ECG	Exercise Capacity
Thyroid medications Only levothyroxine	↑	↑	↑ HR; provoke arrhythmias; ↑ ischemia	↔, unless angina worsened
Alcohol	↔	Chronic use may have role in ↑ BP	May provoke arrhythmias	↔
Hypoglycemic agents Insulin and oral agents	↔	↔	↔	↔
Dipyridamole	↑ ↔	↔ →	↔	↔
Anticoagulants	↔	↔	↔	↔
Antigout medications	↔ ↔	↔ ↔	↔ ↔	↔
Antiplatelet medications	↔	↔	↔	↔
Pentoxifylline	↔	↓	↔	↑ or ↔ in patients limited by intermittent claudication

*Beta blockers with ISA lower resting HR only slightly. ↑, increase; ↔, no effect; ↓, decrease.
†May prevent or delay myocardial ischemia.
From American College of Sports Medicine: Resource Manual for Guidelines for Exercise Testing and Prescription. Philadelphia: Lea & Febiger, 1988, pp 276—279, with permission.

6

ENERGY CONSUMPTION

Metabolic Equivalents

Metabolic equivalents (METs) are used to compare the energy cost of various activities to the resting state. Oxygen consumption in a resting state is estimated to be approximately 3.5 ml O_2/kg per minute, which is 1 MET. The oxygen consumption of an individual for a given activity is usually expressed in liters per minute or milliliters per kilogram per minute. Energy expenditure in calories depends on the weight of the individual. When the individual's weight and oxygen consumption are known, the energy expenditure in calories can be estimated.

Conversions

$$1 \text{ MET} = 3.5 \text{ ml } O_2/\text{ml per minute}$$
$$1 \text{ MET} = 1 \text{ kcal/kg per minute}$$
$$1 \text{ L } O_2/\text{min} = 5 \text{ kcal}$$

Example: A 110-pound person performs a 5-MET activity for 20 minutes.

$$110 \text{ lb} = 50 \text{ kg } (2.2 \text{ lb} = 1 \text{ kg})$$

Oxygen consumption =

$$5 \times 3.5 \text{ ml } O_2/\text{kg/min} = 17.5 \text{ ml } O_2/\text{kg per minute}$$

Expressed in liters per minute = 5×3.5 ml O_2/kg per minute $\times 50$ kg
$$= 875 \text{ ml } O_2/\text{min}$$

divided by 1000 (to convert milliliters to liters) = 0.875 L O_2/min

Calories consumed = 0.875×5 kcal/min = 4.375 kcal/min

Total caloric consumption = 4.375 kcal/min $\times 20$ min = 87.5 cal

NORMAL VALUES FOR MAXIMAL OXYGEN UPTAKE AT DIFFERENT AGES

Age, y	Men	Women
20–29	43 ± 7.2 12 METs	36 ± 6.9 10 METs
30–39	42 ± 7.0 12 METs	34 ± 6.2 10 METs
40–49	40 ± 7.2 11 METs	32 ± 6.2 9 METs
50–59	36 ± 7.1 10 METs	29 ± 5.4 8 METs
60–69	33 ± 7.3 9 METs	27 ± 4.7 8 METs
70–79	29 ± 7.3 8 METs	27 ± 5.8 8 METs

MET indicates metabolic equivalent; 1 MET = 3.5 mL · kg^{-1} · min^{-1} oxygen uptake. Values are expressed as milliliters per kilogram per minute.

From Fletcher, GF, et al: Exercise Standards: A Statement for Healthcare Professionals from the American Heart Association. American Heart Association, Dallas, 1995.

6

SUMMARY OF METABOLIC CALCULATIONS

$\dot{V}O_2$ Mode (units)	=	Horizontal Component	+	Vertical or Resistive Component	+	Resting Component	Comments
Walking $(ml \cdot kg^{-1} \cdot min^{-1})$	=	$m \cdot min^{-1} \times \left(0.1 \dfrac{ml \cdot kg^{-1} \cdot min^{-1}}{m \cdot min^{-1}} \right)$	+	grade (frac) $\times$ $m \cdot min^{-1}$ $\times 1.8 \dfrac{ml \cdot kg^{-1} \cdot min^{-1}}{m \cdot min^{-1}}$	+	$3.5\ ml \cdot kg^{-1} \cdot min^{-1}$	1. For speeds of 50–100 $m \cdot min^{-1}$ (1.9–3.7 $mi \cdot h^{-1}$) 2. $1.8 \dfrac{ml}{kg \cdot m} \times \dfrac{m \cdot min^{-1}}{1.8 \dfrac{ml \cdot kg \cdot min^{-1}}{m \cdot min^{-1}}}$ 3. $1\ mi \cdot h^{-1} = 26.8\ m \cdot min^{-1}$
Running $(ml \cdot kg^{-1} \cdot min^{-1})$	=	$m \cdot min^{-1} \times \left(0.2 \dfrac{ml \cdot kg^{-1} \cdot min^{-1}}{m \cdot min^{-1}} \right)$ ▲	+	grade (frac) $\times$ $m \cdot min^{-1}$ $\times$ $1.8 \dfrac{ml \cdot kg^{-1} \cdot min^{-1}}{m \cdot min^{-1}} \times 0.5$ ▲	+	$3.5\ ml \cdot kg^{-1} \cdot min^{-1}$	1. For speeds > 134 $m \cdot min^{-1}$ (>5.0 $mi \cdot h^{-1}$) 2. If truly jogging (not walking), this equation can also be used for speeds between 80 and 134 $m \cdot min^{-1}$ (3–5 $mi \cdot h^{-1}$) 3. Formula applies to level running off the treadmill, but not to grade running off the treadmill

▨▨▨ Leg Ergometer ($ml \cdot min^{-1}$)	= None	+ $\dfrac{kg \cdot m}{min} \times \dfrac{2\ ml}{kg \cdot m}$ ▲	+ $3.5\ ml \cdot kg^{-1} \cdot min^{-1} \times kg\ (BW)$ ▲	1. For work rates between 300–1200 $kg \cdot m \cdot min^{-1}$ $\dfrac{kg \cdot m}{min} = kg \times \dfrac{m}{rev} \times \dfrac{rev}{min}$ 2. Multiply resting component by body weight (kg) to convert to $ml \cdot min^{-1}$ 3. Monarch = 6 $m \cdot rev^{-1}$ Tunturi = 3 $m \cdot rev^{-1}$
▨▨▨ Arm Ergometer ($ml \cdot min^{-1}$)	= None	+ $\dfrac{kg \cdot m}{min} \times 3\ \dfrac{ml}{kg \cdot m}$ ▲	+ $3.5\ ml \cdot kg^{-1} \cdot min^{-1} \times kg\ (BW)$ ▲	1. For work rates between 150–750 $kg \cdot m \cdot min^{-1}$ $\dfrac{kg \cdot m}{min} = kg \times \dfrac{m}{rev} \times \dfrac{rev}{min}$ 2. ▲ 3. Multiply resting component by body weight (kg) to convert to $ml \cdot min^{-1}$

Continued on next page

6

SUMMARY OF METABOLIC CALCULATIONS (Continued)

$\dot{V}O_2$ Mode (units)	= Horizontal Component	+ Vertical or Resistive Component	+ Resting Component	Comments
Stepping ($ml \cdot kg^{-1} \cdot min^{-1}$)	$= \dfrac{\text{▨ steps}}{min} \times 0.35 \dfrac{ml \cdot kg^{-1} \cdot min^{-1}}{steps \cdot min^{-1}}$ ▲	$+ \left(\dfrac{\text{▨ m}}{\text{▨ steps}} \times \dfrac{\text{▨ steps}}{min} \times 1.33\right) \times 1.8 \dfrac{ml \cdot kg^{-1} \cdot min^{-1}}{m \cdot min^{-1}}$	+ Included in horizontal and vertical components	1. 1.33 includes both positive component of going up (1.0) + negative component of going down (0.33) = 1.33 ▲ 2. Stepping height in meters

Key: ▨ indicates values to be obtained from the patient to be used in calculations.

▲ note change in constant.

From American College of Sports Medicine: Guidelines for Exercise Testing and Prescription, ed 4. Lea & Febiger, Philadelphia, 1991, pp 296–297, with permission.

668

APPROXIMATE ENERGY REQUIREMENTS IN METABOLIC EQUIVALENTS FOR HORIZONTAL AND GRADE WALKING

Percent Grade	1.7	2.0	2.5	3.0	3.4	3.75
mi · h⁻¹ / m · min⁻¹	45.6	53.7	67.0	80.5	91.2	100.5
0	2.3	2.5	2.9	3.3	3.6	3.9
2.5	2.9	3.2	3.8	4.3	4.8	5.2
5.0	3.5	3.9	4.6	5.4	5.9	6.5
7.5	4.1	4.6	5.5	6.4	7.1	7.8
10.0	4.6	5.3	6.3	7.4	8.3	9.1
12.5	5.2	6.0	7.2	8.5	9.5	10.4
15.0	5.8	6.6	8.1	9.5	10.6	11.7
17.5	6.4	7.3	8.9	10.5	11.8	12.9
20.0	7.0	8.0	9.8	11.6	13.0	14.2
22.5	7.6	8.7	10.6	12.6	14.2	15.5
25.0	8.2	9.4	11.5	13.6	15.3	16.8

From American College of Sports Medicine: Guidelines for Exercise Testing and Prescription, ed 4. Lea & Febiger, Philadelphia, 1991, p 298, with permission.

669

6

APPROXIMATE ENERGY REQUIREMENTS IN METABOLIC EQUIVALENTS FOR HORIZONTAL AND UPHILL JOGGING/RUNNING

Percent Grade	mi · h⁻¹						
	5	6	7	7.5	8	9	10
	m · min⁻¹						
	134	161	188	201	215	241	268
Outdoors on a Solid Surface							
0	8.6	10.2	11.7	12.5	13.3	14.8	16.3
2.5	10.3	12.3	14.1	15.1	16.1	17.9	19.7
5.0	12.0	14.3	16.5	17.7	18.8		
7.5	13.8	16.4	18.9				
10.0	15.5	18.5					
On a Treadmill							
0	8.6	10.2	11.7	12.5	13.3	14.8	16.3
2.5	9.5	11.2	12.9	13.8	14.7	16.3	18.0
5.0	10.3	12.3	14.1	15.1	16.1	17.9	19.7
7.5	11.2	13.3	15.3	16.4	17.4	19.4	
10.0	12.0	14.3	16.5	17.7	18.8		
12.5	12.9	15.4	17.7	19.0			
15.0	13.8	16.4	18.9				

From American College of Sports Medicine: Guidelines for Exercise Testing and Prescription, ed 4. Lea & Febiger, Philadelphia, 1991, p 299, with permission.

APPROXIMATE ENERGY EXPENDITURE IN METABOLIC EQUIVALENTS DURING BICYCLE ERGOMETRY*

Body (kg)	Weight (lb)	Exercise Rate (kg · m · min⁻¹ and Watts)						
		300 / 50	450 / 75	600 / 100	750 / 125	900 / 150	1050 / 175	1200 / 200
50	110	5.1	6.9	8.6	10.3	12.0	13.7	15.4
60	132	4.3	5.7	7.1	8.6	10.0	11.4	12.9
70	154	3.7	4.9	6.1	7.3	8.6	9.8	11.0
80	176	3.2	4.3	5.4	6.4	7.5	8.6	9.6
90	198	2.9	3.8	4.8	5.7	6.7	7.6	8.6
100	220	2.6	3.4	4.3	5.1	6.0	6.9	7.7

*VO_2 for zero load pedaling is approximately 550 ml · min⁻¹ for 70- to 80-kg subjects.
From American College of Sports Medicine: Guidelines for Exercise Testing and Prescription, ed 4. Lea & Febiger, Philadelphia, 1991, p 299, with permission.

6

671

APPROXIMATE METABOLIC EQUIVALENT VALUES FOR VARIOUS ACTIVITIES

These values should be used as guidelines only. There is much individual variation in energy expenditure depending on how an activity is performed (e.g., speed, technique). One MET equals 3.5 ml O_2/kg per minute.

Activity	METs
Ambulation, braces and crutches	6.5
Archery	3–4
Auto, radio, TV repair	2–3
Backpacking	5–11
Badminton	4–9+
Basketball (game)	7–12+
Basketball (nongame)	3–9
Beating carpets	4
Bedside commode	3
Billiards	2.5
Bowling	2–4
Boxing (sparring)	8.3
Boxing (in ring)	13.3
Bricklaying	3.5
Canoeing, rowing, kayaking	3–8
Carpentry	2–7
Carrying 80-lb load	7–8
Cleaning windows	3
Climbing hills	5–10+
Cricket	4.6–7.4
Cycling (pleasure)	3–8+
Cycling, 5.5 mph	3.5
Cycling, 10 mph	7
Cycling, 11 mph	6–7
Cycling, 12 mph	7–8
Cycling, 13 mph	9
Dancing (aerobic)	6–9
Dancing (social, square, tap)	3.7–7.4
Desk work	1.5–2
Digging ditches	7–8
Dressing, undressing	2–2.3
Driving car	2
Fencing	6–10+
Field hockey	8
Fishing (stream wading)	5–6
Fishing (from bank)	2–4
Gardening (wheelbarrow)	4–10
Gardening (weeding)	3–5
Gardening (raking)	3–6
Gardening (hoeing, digging)	4–8
Golf (power cart)	2–3
Golf (walk, carry bag)	4–7
Hand sewing	1
Handball	8–12+

Activity	METs
Hiking (cross-country)	3–7
Horse ploughing	5
Horseback riding (galloping)	8.2
Horseback riding (trotting)	6.6
Horseback riding (walking)	2.4
Horseshoe pitching	2–3
Housework (heavy: scrubbing, making beds)	3–6
Housework (light: sweeping, ironing, polishing)	2–4
Hunting (big game, dragging)	3–14
Hunting (bow or gun, small game)	3–7
Ironing, standing	3.5
Jogging, 5 mph	7–8
Judo	13.5
Kneading dough	2.5
Maching sewing	1.5
Mopping	3.5
Mountain climbing	5–10+
Mowing lawn, on cart	2
Mowing lawn, power mower	4–5
Mowing lawn, hand mower	4–6
Music playing	2–3
Paddleball, racquetball	8–12
Painting, plumbing (home)	3–8
Painting (recreational)	1.5
Paperhanging	4–5
Peeling potatoes	2.5
Plastering	3.5
Playing piano	2
Radio assembly	2.5
Rope jumping (120–140 skips/min)	11–12
Rope jumping (60–80 skips/min)	9
Running, 6 min/mi	16.3
Running, 7 min/mi	14.1
Running, 8 min/mi	12.5
Running, 9 min/mi	11.2
Running, 10 min/mi	10.2
Running, 11 min/mi	9.4
Running, 12 min/mi	8.7
Sailing	2–5
Sawing hardwood	7–8
Scrubbing, standing	2.5
Scuba diving	5–10
Sexual intercourse	5–5.5+
Shoveling	6–10+
Showering	3.5–4.2
Shuffleboard	2–3

Continued on following page

6

Activity	METs
Skating, ice and roller	5–8
Skiing, cross-country	6–12+
Skiing, downhill	5–8
Sledding, tobogganing	4–8
Snow shoveling (wet snow)	8–15
Snow shoveling (powder snow)	6–9
Snowshoeing	7–14
Soccer	5–12+
Splitting/sawing wood, cutting trees (hand saw)	5–10
trees (power saw)	2–4
Squash	8–12+
Stair climbing	4–8
Stairs, carrying 24 lb, up 8 steps	10
Stairs, up 8 steps	5–5.5
Stairs, down flight	4.5–5.2
Swimming	4–8+
Table tennis	3–5
Tending furnace	8.5
Tennis	4–9+
Touch football	6–10
Tractor ploughing	3.5
Using bedpan	4
Volleyball	3–6
Walking, 1.7 mph	2.3
Walking, 2 mph	2.5
Walking, 2.5 mph	2.9
Walking, 3 mph	3.3
Walking, 3.4 mph	3.6
Walking, 3.75 mph	3.9
Walking, 4 mph	4.6
Walking, 4.5 mph	5.4
Walking, 5 mph	6.9
Walking, 5.5 mph	8.6
Walking upstairs	4–8
Walking downstairs	4–5
Washing face, hands	2
Washing/hanging clothes	2.5–3.5
Watch repairing	1.5
Water skiing	5–7
Wheelchair propulsion	2
Woodworking (light)	2–3

EXERCISE PRESCRIPTION

INTENSITY. For healthy individuals, 65%–90% of age-adjusted maximum heart rate or 50%–85% of maximum oxygen consumption. Cardiac patients should have a stress test or exercise at lower intensities initially.

DURATION. Fifteen to 60 minutes per exercise session should be scheduled.

FREQUENCY. Three to 5 days per week should be scheduled. No more than 2 days off should occur between exercise sessions.

Exercise Prescription by Heart Rate

The age-adjusted maximum heart rate (AAMHR) for an individual can be estimated by subtracting age from 220. The training heart rate (THR) can then be calculated.

$$\text{THR range} = 0.65\ (220 - \text{age}) \text{ to } 0.90\ (220 - \text{age})$$

The Karvonen equation uses the individual's resting heart rate to establish a THR range:

$$\text{THR range} = 0.65 \text{ to } 0.9\ (\text{AAMHR} - \text{resting HR}) + \text{resting HR}$$

BASED ON

American College of Sports Medicine: Guidelines for Exercise Testing and Prescription, ed 3. Lea & Febiger, Philadelphia, 1986, pp 31–42, 67, with permission.

6

Exercise Prescription by Metabolic Equivalents

Activities of appropriate intensity can be selected if an individual's functional capacity in METs is known. An intensity of 60%–70% of the functional capacity is considered an appropriate training range. If 60% of maximum MET is used, add the maximum MET level to 60, divide this by 100, and multiply this value by maximum METs.

Example for an individual with a 5-MET maximum:

$$\frac{(60 + 5)}{100} = 0.65$$

$0.65 \times 5 \text{ METs} = 3.25 \text{ METs (average training intensity)}$

Exercise Prescription by Relative Exertion

BORG SCALE FOR RATING PERCEIVED EXERTION	
Fifteen-Grade Scale	*Ten-Grade Scale*
6	0 Nothing
7 Very, very light	0.5 Very, very weak (just noticeable)
8	1 Very weak
9 Very light	2 Weak (light)
10	3 Moderate
11 Fairly light	4 Somewhat strong
12	5 Strong (heavy)
13 Somewhat hard	6
14	7 Very strong
15 Hard	8
16	9
17 Very hard	10 Very, very strong (almost maximum)
18	
19 Very, very hard	* Maximum
20	

*The rating of perceived exertion scales. The original scale (6–20) on the left and the newer 10-point category scale with ratio properties on the right.

From Borg, GAV: Psychophysical bases of perceived exertion. Med Sci Sports Exerc 14:377, 1982, with permission.

GUIDELINES FOR EXERCISE TRAINING USED IN CARDIAC REHABILITATION

GUIDELINES FOR ELECTROCARDIOGRAPHIC MONITORING IN EXERCISE TRAINING	
Activity Classification	*ECG Monitoring*
A Apparently healthy	Not required
B Known stable CAD, low risk for vigorous exercise	Monitored and supervised for activity instruction (usually 6–12 sessions)
C Moderate to high risk for cardiac complications during exercise and/or unable to self-regulate or to understand recommended activity levels	Monitored and supervised (usually 6–12 sessions or more)

CAD = coronary artery disease.

From Fletcher, GF, et al: Exercise Standards: A Statement for Healthcare Professionals from the American Heart Association. American Heart Association, Dallas, 1995.

CONTRAINDICATIONS FOR ENTRY INTO INPATIENT AND OUTPATIENT EXERCISE PROGRAMS

The following criteria may be used as contraindications for program entry:
1. Unstable angina
2. Resting systolic blood pressure over 200 mm Hg or resting diastolic blood pressure over 100 mm Hg
3. Significant drop (20 mm Hg or more) in resting systolic blood pressure from the patient's average level that cannot be explained by medications
4. Moderate to severe aortic stenosis
5. Acute systemic illness or fever
6. Uncontrolled atrial or ventricular dysrhythmias
7. Uncontrolled tachycardia (>100 bpm)
8. Symptomatic congestive heart failure
9. Third-degree heart block
10. Active pericarditis or myocarditis
11. Recent embolism
12. Thrombophlebitis
13. Resting ST displacement (>3 mm)
14. Uncontrolled diabetes
15. Orthopedic problems that would prohibit exercise

From American College of Sports Medicine: Guidelines for Exercise Testing and Prescription, ed 4. Lea & Febiger, Philadelphia, 1991, p 126, with permission.

6

CRITERIA FOR TERMINATION OF AN INPATIENT EXERCISE SESSION

The following guidelines may be used to terminate the exercise session for cardiac inpatients:
1. Fatigue
2. Failure of monitoring equipment
3. Light-headedness, confusion, ataxia, pallor, cyanosis, dyspnea, nausea, or any peripheral circulatory insufficiency
4. Onset of angina with exercise
5. Symptomatic supraventricular tachycardia
6. ST displacement (3 mm) horizontal or downsloping from rest
7. Ventricular tachycardia (3 or more consecutive PVCs)
8. Exercise-induced left bundle branch block
9. Onset of 2° and/or 3° AV block
10. R on T PVCs (one)
11. Frequent multifocal PVCs (30% of the complexes)
12. Exercise hypotension (>20 mm Hg drop in systolic blood pressure during exercise)
13. Excessive blood pressure rise: systolic ≥220 or diastolic ≥110 mm Hg
14. Inappropriate brachycardia (drop in heart rate >10 beats · min^{-1}) with increase or no change in workload

From American College of Sports Medicine: Guidelines for Exercise Testing and Prescription, ed 4. Lea & Febiger, Philadelphia, 1991, p 127, with permission.

GUIDELINES FOR EXERCISE TESTING USED IN CARDIAC REHABILITATION

CRITERIA FOR STOPPING AN EXERCISE TEST

1. Progressive angina (stop at 3+ level or earlier on a scale of 1+ to 4+)
2. Ventricular tachycardia
3. Any significant drop (20 mm Hg) of systolic blood pressure or a failure of the systolic blood pressure to rise with an increase in exercise load
4. Light-headedness, confusion, ataxia, pallor, cyanosis, nausea, or signs of severe peripheral circulatory insufficiency
5. Greater than 4 mm horizontal or downsloping ST depression or elevation (in the absence of other indicators of ischemia)
6. Onset of second- or third-degree AV block
7. Increasing ventricular ectopy, multiform PVCs, or R on T PVCs
8. Excessive rise in blood pressure: systolic pressure >250 mm Hg; diastolic pressure >120 mm Hg
9. Chronotropic impairment
10. Sustained supraventricular tachycardia
11. Exercise-induced left bundle branch block
12. Subject requests to stop
13. Failure of the monitoring system

From American College of Sports Medicine: Guidelines for Exercise Testing and Prescription, ed 4. Lea & Febiger, Philadelphia, 1991, p 72, with permission.

CRITERIA FOR AN ABNORMAL EXERCISE TEST

1. One millimeter or more of exercise-induced ST-segment depression or elevation relative to the Q-Q line, lasting 0.08 seconds or more from the J-point
2. Chest discomfort typical of angina induced or increased by exercise
3. Ventricular tachycardia or frequent (>30%) premature ventricular contractions, or multifocal premature ventricular contractions
4. Exercise-induced left or right bundle branch block
5. Significant drop (>10 mm Hg) in systolic blood pressure during exercise, or failure of the systolic blood pressure to rise with an increase in exercise intensity after the initial adjustment period
6. Sustained supraventricular tachycardia
7. R on T premature ventricular contractions
8. Exercise-induced second- or third-degree heart block
9. Postexercise U-wave inversion
10. Inappropriate bradycardia

From American College of Sports Medicine: Guidelines for Graded Exercise Testing and Exercise Prescription, ed 3. Lea & Febiger, Philadelphia, 1986, p 22, with permission.

COMMONLY USED TREADMILL PROTOCOLS SHOWING SPEED, GRADE, AND MINUTES OF TESTING

BRUCE PROTOCOL

Stage	mph	Grade %	Minutes	MET Requirement*		
				Men	Women	Cardiac
I	1.7	10	1	3.2	3.1	3.6
			2	4.0	3.9	4.3
			3	4.9	4.7	4.9
II	2.5	12	4	5.7	5.4	5.6
			5	6.6	6.2	6.2
			6	7.4	7.0	7.0
III	3.4	14	7	8.3	8.0	7.6
			8	9.1	8.6	8.3
			9	10.0	9.4	9.0
IV	4.2	16	10	10.7	10.1	9.7
			11	11.6	10.9	10.4
			12	12.5	11.7	11.0
V	5.0	18	13	13.3	12.5	11.7
			14	14.1	13.2	12.3
			15	15.0	14.1	13.0

Continued on following page

COMMONLY USED TREADMILL PROTOCOLS SHOWING SPEED, GRADE, AND MINUTES OF TESTING
(Contiued)

NAUGHTON-BALKE PROTOCOL

mph	Grade (%)	Minutes	METs
3.0	2.5	2	4.3
(Constant)	5.0	2	5.4
	7.5	2	6.4
	10.0	2	7.4
	12.5	2	8.4
	15.0	2	9.5
	17.5	2	10.5
	20.0	2	11.6
	22.5	2	12.6

MODIFIED BALKE PROTOCOL

mph	Grade (%)	Minutes	METs
2.0	0	3	2.5
2.0	3.5	3	3.5
2.0	7.0	3	4.5
2.0	10.5	3	5.4
2.0	14.0	3	6.4
2.0	17.5	3	7.4
3.0	12.5	3	8.5
3.0	15.0	3	9.5
3.0	17.5	3	10.5
3.0	20.0	3	11.6
3.0	22.5	3	12.6

*MET values are indicated for each stage or minute *completed*. Note that women and cardiac patients achieve *lower* $\dot{V}O_2$ for equivalent workload. Holding on to front rail will *increase* the apparent MET capacity.

From American College of Sports Medicine: Guidelines for Exercise Testing and Prescription, ed 4. Lea & Febiger, Philadelphia, 1991, p 61, with permission.

BRANCHING TREADMILL PROTOCOL

Exercise Intensity (METs)	Treadmill Speed (mph)* at Percent Grade						
	2.0	1	2.5	2.75	3.0	3.25	3.5
2	0	0					
3	1.5	1	0	0	0	0	0
4	5	4	3	2	1.5	1	0.5
5	9	7	6	5	4	3	2.5
6	12.5	10	9	7.5	6.5	5.5	5
7	16	13.5	12	10	9	7.5	7
8	20	17.5	15	13	11	10	9
9		20	17.5	15	13.5	12	11
10			20	18	16	14	13
11				21	18	16.5	15
12					21	19	17

*Treadmill speed is initially selected at 0% grade to produce a brisk walking pace (2–3 mph) compatible with each patient's gait. Treadmill speed may be subsequently increased or decreased in branching increments of 0.25 mph (within the range of 2.0–3.5 mph) to maintain optimum walking speed. The percent of grade in the corresponding speed column is increased every 2 min to produce 1-MET increments in work intensity.

From American College of Sports Medicine: Guidelines for Exercise Testing and Prescription, ed 4. Lea & Febiger, Philadelphia, 1991, p 62.

6

EXERCISE PROTOCOLS: OXYGEN AND MET VALUES

Functional Class	Clinical Status	O₂ Cost ml/kg/min	METS	Bicycle Ergometer (1 WATT = 6.1 Kpm/min) FOR 70kg BODY WEIGHT Kpm/min	Bruce 3min Stages mph/%gr	Balke-Ware % Grade at 3.3mph 1min Stages	USAFSAM MPH/%GR	"Slow" USAFSAM MPH/%GR	McHenry MPH/%GR	Stanford %Grade at 3mph / at 2mph	ACIP MPH/%GR	CHF MPH/%GR	METS
Normal and I	Healthy, Dependent on Age, Activity	56.0	16		5.5/20		3.3/25						16
		52.5	15		5.0/18	26					3.4/24.0		15
		49.0	14		4.2/16	25 / 24	3.3/20		3.3/21				14
		45.5	13	1500		23 / 22			3.3/18		3.1/24.0		13
		42.0	12	1350		21 / 20	3.3/15				3.0/21.0		12
	Sedentary Healthy	38.5	11	1200	3.4/14	19 / 18			3.3/15	22.5	3.0/17.5	3.4/14.0	11
		35.0	10	1050		17 / 16	3.3/10	2/25	3.3/12	20.0	3.0/14.0	3.0/15.0	10
		31.5	9	900		15 / 14		2/20	3.3/9	17.5	3.0/10.5	3.0/12.5	9
		28.0	8	750		13 / 12	3.3/5	2/15	3.3/6	15.0	3.0/7.0	3.0/10.0	8
		24.5	7	600	2.5/12	11 / 10		2/10		12.5		3.0/7.5	7
II		21.0	6	450		9 / 8	3.3/0	2/5		10.0 / 17.5	3.0/3.0	2.0/10.5	6
	Limited	17.5	5	300	1.7/10	7 / 6		2/0	2.0/3	7.5 / 14.0		2.0/7.0	5
III		14.0	4	150	1.7/5	5 / 4	2.0/0	2/0		5.0 / 10.5	2.5/2.0	2.0/3.5	4
	Symptomatic	10.5	3		1.7/0	3 / 2				2.5 / 7.0	2.0/0.0	1.5/0.0	3
IV		7.0	2			1				0 / 3.5		1.0/0.0	2
		3.5	1										1

USAFSAM = U.S. Air Force School of Aerospace Medicine; ACIP = asymptomatic cardiac ischemia pilot; CHF = congestive heart failure (Modified Naughton); Kpm/min = kilopond meters per minute; and %GR = percent grade. From Froelicher, VF, et al: Exercise and the Heart: Clinical Concepts, ed 3. Mosby–Year Book, Inc., St. Louis, 1993, p 17, with permission.

Pediatrics

7

VITAL SIGNS AND BLOOD GAS VALUES FOR CHILDREN

	Newborn	Older Infant and Child
Respiratory rate	40–60	20–30 ($\leq$6 y)
		15–20 (>6 y)
Heart rate	120–200	100–180 ($\leq$3 y)
		70–150 (>3 y)
Po_2 (mm Hg)	60–90	80–100
Pco_2 (mm Hg)	30–35	30–35 ($\leq$2 y)
		20–24 (>2 y)
Blood pressure (mm Hg)		
Systolic	60–90	75–130 ($\leq$3 y)
		90–140 (>3 y)
Diastolic	30–60	45–90 ($\leq$3 y)
		50–80 (>3 y)
Arterial oxygen saturation (%)	87–89 (low)	95–100
	94–95 (high)	
	90–95 (preterm infant)	

Data from Comer, DM. Pulse oximetry: Implications for practice. Journal of Obstetrics, Gynecology, and Neonatal Nursing 21:35, 1992; and Pagtakhan, RD and Chernick, V: Intensive Care for Respiratory Disorders. In Kendig, EL and Chernick, V (eds): Disorders of the Respiratory Tract in Children, ed 4. WB Saunders, Philadelphia, 1983, pp 145–168.

Adapted from Kelly, MK: Children with Ventilator Dependence. In Campbell, SK: Physical Therapy for Children. WB Saunders, Philadelphia, 1994, p 675, adapted with permission.

PHYSICAL DEVELOPMENT FROM BIRTH TO ONE YEAR

| Age | Physical Development | |
	Length Range	Weight Range
Birth		
Boys	18¼–21½ in.	5½–9¼ lb
	46.4–54.4 cm	2.54–4.15 kg
Girls	17¾–20¾ in.	5¼–8½ lb
	45.4–52.9 cm	2.36–3.81 kg
1 mo		
Boys	19¾–23 in.	7–11¾ lb
	50.4–58.6 cm	3.16–5.38 kg
Girls	19¼–22½ in.	6½–10¾ lb
	49.2–56.9 cm	2.97–4.92 kg
3 mo		
Boys	22¼–25¾ in.	9¾–16¼ lb
	56.7–65.4 cm	4.43–7.37 kg
Girls	21¾–25 in.	9¼–14¾ lb
	55.4–63.4 cm	4.18–6.74 kg
6 mo		
Boys	25–28½ in.	13¾–20¾ lb
	63.4–72.3 cm	6.20–9.46 kg
Girls	24¼–27¾ in.	12¾–19¼ lb
	61.8–70.2 cm	5.79–8.73 kg
9 mo		
Boys	26¾–30¼ in.	16½–24 lb
	68.0–77.1 cm	7.52–10.93 kg
Girls	26–29½ in.	15½–22½ lb
	66.1–75.0 cm	7.0–10.17 kg
12 mo		
Boys	28¼–32 in.	18½–26½ lb
	71.7–81.2 cm	8.43–11.99 kg
Girls	27½–31¼ in.	17¼–24¾ lb
	69.8–79.1 cm	7.84–11.24 kg

Adapted from Thomas, CL (ed): Taber's Cyclopedic Medical Dictionary, ed 18. FA Davis, Philadelphia, 1997, p 1592, with permission.

7

FONTANELS

The fontanels of the infant are shown in the figure. The posterior fontanel closes between 2 and 3 months of age; the anterior fontanel closes between 16 and 18 months of age.

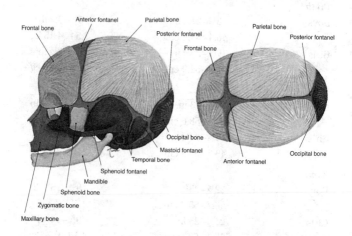

VARIATIONS IN FEMORAL NECK SHAFT ANGLE WITH AGE

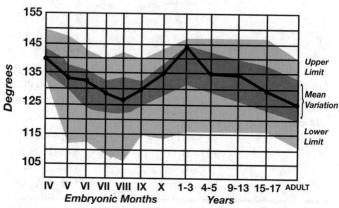

Redrawn from Von Lanz, T and Mayet, A: Die gelenkorper des menschlichen hufgelenkes in der progredienten phase iherer umwegigen ausformung. Z Anat 117:317, 1953. As in appearing in Hensinger, RN: Standards in Pediatric Orthopedics: Tables, Charts, and Graphs Illustrating Growth. Raven Press, New York, 1986, p 49.

VARIATIONS IN FEMORAL ANTEVERSION ANGLES WITH AGE

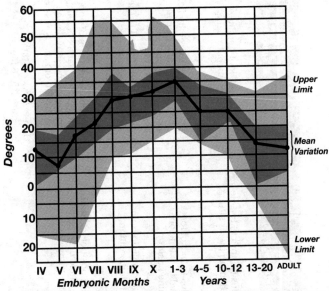

Redrawn from Von Lanz, T and Mayet, A: Die gelenkorper des menschlichen hufgelenkes in der progredienten phase iherer umwegigen ausformung. Z Anat 117:317, 1953. As in appearing in Hensinger, RN: Standards in Pediatric Orthopedics: Tables, Charts, and Graphs Illustrating Growth. Raven Press, New York, 1986, p 53.

DEVELOPMENTAL ASSESSMENT

REFLEX TESTING

Reflexes	Stimulus	Response
Primitive/Spinal		
Flexor withdrawal	Noxious stimulus (pinprick) to sole of foot; tested in supine or sitting position	Toes extend, foot dorsiflexes, entire leg flexes uncontrollably. Onset: 28 wk Integrated: 1–2 mo
Crossed extension	Noxious stimulus to ball of foot of extremity fixed in extension; tested in supine position	Opposite lower extremity flexes, then adducts and extends. Onset: 28 wk gestation Integrated: 1–2 mo
Traction	Grasp forearm and pull up from supine into sitting position	Grasp and total flexion of the upper extremity occur. Onset: 28 wk gestation Integrated: 2–5 mo
Moro	Sudden change in position of head in relation to trunk: drop patient backward from sitting position	Extension, abduction of upper extremities, hand opening, and crying followed by flexion, adduction of arms across chest occur. Onset: 28 wk gestation Integrated: 5–6 mo

Startle	Sudden loud or harsh noise	Sudden extension or abduction of arms, crying occur. Onset: birth Integrated: persists
Grasp	Maintained pressure to palm of hand (palmer grasp) or to ball of foot under toes (plantar grasp)	Flexion of fingers or toes is maintained. Onset: palmar: birth; plantar: 28 wk Integrated: palmar: 4–6 mo; plantar: 9 mo
Tonic/Brain Stem		
Asymmetrical tonic neck (ATNR)	Rotation of the head to one side	Flexion of skull limbs, extension of the jaw limbs, "bow and arrow" or "fencing" posture occur. Onset: birth Integrated: 4–6 mo
Symmetrical tonic neck (STNR)	Flexion or extension of the head	With head flexion: flexion of arms, extension of legs occur; with head extension: extension of arms, flexion of legs occur. Onset: 4–6 mo Integrated: 8–12 mo

Continued on following page

REFLEX TESTING (Continued)

Reflexes	Stimulus	Response
Symmetrical tonic labyrinthine (TLR or STLR)	Prone or supine position	With prone position: increased flexor tone/flexion of all limbs occur; with supine: increased extensor tone/extension of all limbs occur. Onset: birth Integrated: 6 mo
Positive supporting	Contact to the ball of the foot in upright standing position	Rigid extension (cocontraction) of the lower extremities occurs. Onset: birth Integrated: 6 mo
Associated reactions	Resisted voluntary movement in any part of the body	Involuntary movement in a resting extremity occurs. Onset: birth–3 mo Integrated: 8–9 y
Neck righting action on the body (NOB)	Passively turn head to one side; tested in supine	Body rotates as a whole (log rolls) to align the body with the head. Onset: 4–6 mo Integrated: 5 y

Body righting acting on the body (BOB)	Passively rotate upper or lower trunk segment: tested in supine	Body segment not rotated follows to align the body segments. Onset: 4–6 mo Integrated: 5 y
Labyrinthine head righting (LR)	Occlude vision; alter body position by tipping body in all directions	Head orients to vertical position with mouth horizontal. Onset: birth–2 mo Integrated: persists
Optical righting (OR)	Alter body position by tipping body in all directions	Head orients to vertical position with mouth horizontal. Onset: birth–2 mo Integrated: persists
Body righting acting on head (BOH)	Place in prone or supine position	Head orients to vertical position with mouth horizontal. Onset: birth–2 mo Integrated: 5 y
Protective extension (PE)	Displace center of gravity outside the base of support	Arms or legs extend and abduct to support and to protect the body against falling. Onset: arms: 4–6 mo; legs: 6–9 mo Integrated: persists

Continued on following page

7

REFLEX TESTING (Continued)

Reflexes	Stimulus	Response
Equilibrium reactions—tilting (ER)	Displace the center of gravity by tilting or moving the support surface (e.g., with a movable object such as an equilibrium board or ball)	Curvature of the trunk toward the upward side along with extension and abduction of the extremities on that side occurs; protective extension on the opposite (downward) side occurs. Onset: prone 6 months; supine 7–8 mo; sitting 7–8 mo; quadruped 9–12 months; standing 12–21 mo. Integrated: persists
Equilibrium reactions—postural fixation	Apply a displacing force to the body, altering the center of gravity in its relation to the base of support; can also be observed during voluntary activity	Curvature of the trunk toward the external force with extension and abduction of the extremities on the side to which the force was applied occurs. Onset: prone 6 months; supine 7–8 mo: sitting 7–8 mo; quadruped 9–12 months; standing 12–21 mo Integrated: persists

NORMAL DEVELOPMENT

Postural Control

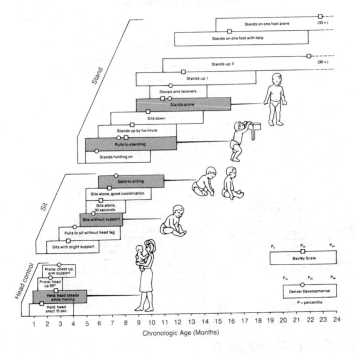

Continued on following page

7

NORMAL DEVELOPMENT (Continued)

Manual Skills
(control of prehension)

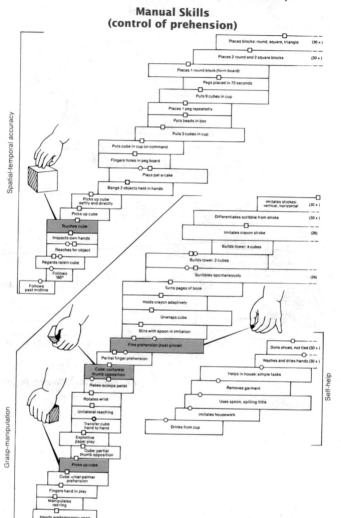

From Keogh, J and Sugden, D: Movement Skill Development. Macmillan, New York, 1985, with permission.

Locomotor Skills

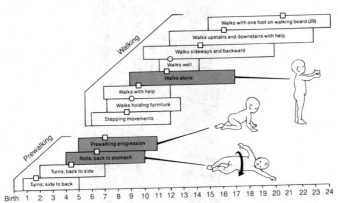

From Keogh, J and Sugden, D: Movement Skill Development. Macmillan, New York, 1985, with permission.

APGAR SCORES

Sign	Score (for each item)		
	0	1	2
Heart rate	Absent	Slow (<100)	>100
Respiratory effort	Absent	Slow, irregular	Good; crying
Muscle tone	Limp	Some flexion of extremities	Active motion
Reflex irritability	No response	Grimace	Cough or sneeze
Color	Blue, pale	Body pink; extremities blue	Completely pink

CLASSIFICATION OF BIRTH INJURIES

Cerebral Birth Injury

Damage to the nervous system by complications during pregnancy, labor, delivery, or the immediate neonatal period. It is associated with a number of predisposing factors related to maternal health, maternal age, social status, labor and delivery, birth weight, gestation, and parity. The most common mechanisms are asphyxia (which may be chronic or acute) and trauma.

intraventricular hemorrhage—not related to trauma: More common in premature infants and with respiratory distress syndrome.

compression head injury—compression of the head: Most likely in full-term or postmature infants, many of whom are large for their gestational age. May present as subarachnoid, subdural, or (infrequently) cerebellar hemorrhage.

Fractures

Most of these lesions heal without treatment; however, the infant may be more comfortable when the fracture is immobilized.

skull fractures: Fissure fractures are not uncommon but are usually of little significance. Depressed fractures (a "pond" fracture) may result from pressure on the sacral promontory. The majority resolve spontaneously.

clavicle fractures: This fracture may occur during breech delivery if the baby's arms become displaced or may be the result of a difficult vertex delivery. Recovery is likely without treatment; however, it is usual to immobilize the upper arm against the chest. The baby should always be examined for a concurrent brachial plexus injury.

humeral fractures: This fracture may occur when a displaced arm is pulled down during a breech delivery. The baby should always be examined for nerve damage.

femoral fractures: This fracture may occur when a leg is pulled down during delivery of a breech presentation with extended legs. The fracture may be immobilized by bandaging the affected limb to the abdomen.

Nerve Lesions

abducens palsy: Transient abducens palsy occurs in a significant proportion of children born after prolonged labor and those who are delivered by forceps. Usually there is full recovery after a few days or weeks.

facial palsy: Pressure from a forceps blade may injure the extracranial part of the facial nerve. Facial palsy occasionally occurs following a spontaneous vaginal delivery. Recovery may be expected within 2–3 wk.

Erb's palsy: Trauma to the C5 and C6 spinal roots due to excessive traction on the neck during a delivery, such as a difficult breech extraction or vertex delivery, where there has been difficulty with delivery of the shoulders. The affected arm lies limply at the infant's

Continued on following page

7

side, with the hand pronated and wrist slightly flexed. Recovery is usually complete within 2 wk.

other brachial plexus injuries: The C4 root may be implicated in addition to Erb's palsy, thereby affecting function of the diaphragm with possible resultant acute respiratory distress. Much less common are damage to the lower roots (C7–T1).

radial palsy: Involvement of the radial nerve usually by subcutaneous fat necrosis or spontaneously due to pressure as a result of malposition in utero. Complete recovery is expected.

spinal cord injuries: These lesions are rare; however, they may occur following a breech delivery or with spinal fractures or subluxations. They occur most commonly in the cervical and thoracic region and are produced by traction on the vertebral column during delivery. There may also be an additional lesion to the brachial plexus due to tearing of the cervical roots from the spinal cord.

FOR MORE INFORMATION

Campbell, AGM and McIntosh, N (eds): Forfar and Arneil's Textbook of Pediatrics, ed 4. Churchill Livingstone, New York, 1992.

CLASSIFICATION OF CEREBRAL PALSY

There are many different classifications of cerebral palsy. Confusion and incompatability between terminology can result. The most widely used system of classification, adopted by the American Academy for Cerebral Palsy (now the American Academy of Cerebral Palsy and Developmental Medicine), is based on clinical presentation. The system is based on the topographic distribution of muscle tone (reflex disorders) and movement disorders. This particular classification system is useful clinically because it describes cerebral palsy in terms of the motor deficit and distribution. An important limitation of this classification system is that it does not take into consideration developmental changes that commonly occur in the child with cerebral palsy.

The following classification begins with a description of the physiological (motor) disorder followed by specific subtypes of cerebral palsy that include topology.

spasticity: It is characterized by increased muscle tone (hyperreflexia), stereotyped and limited movements, pathologic stretch reflexes with clonus, persistence of primitive and tonic reflexes, and poor development of postural reflex mechanisms.

spastic hemiplegia: One side of the entire body is affected, the upper extremity more than the lower extremity. It is often associated with strabismus, oral motor dysfunction, somatosensory dysfunction, and perceptual learning disorders. Seizures often develop with maturity.

spastic triplegia: The extremities, usually both legs and one arm, are invovled. It may represent incomplete quadriplegia.

spastic quadriplegia (tetraplegia): It is often related to birth asphyxia in term infants or grade 3 and 4 intraventricular bleeds in immature infants. There is involvement of all four extremities as well as head, neck, and trunk. It often presents first with hypotonia. In severe disorders, the child's posture and movement are dominated by either flexion or extension tone. Ability to move against gravity is very slight. It is associated with problems with vision, hearing, seizures, mental retardation, and oral-motor abilities.

spastic diplegia: Terminology is seldom used. It is most frequently related to problems of prematurity. The total body is affected (bilateral paralysis); there is greater involvement in trunk and lower extremities than upper extremities and face. One side often is more involved than the other (double hemiplegia). Associated problems occur with speech, oral-motor function, and esotropia (crossed eyes).

athetosis (dyskinetic syndrome): It is characterized by an abnormal amount and type of involuntary motion with varying amounts of tension, normal reflexes, and asymmetric involvement. Abnormal movements are exaggerated by voluntary movement, postural adjustments, and changes in emotion or speech. Often it is associated with impaired speech and poor respiratory and oral-motor control; it is related to erythroblastosis and birth asphyxia. (Note: not all of the following classification of athetosis have been adopted by the American Academy of Cerebral Palsy; they are included for completeness.)

rotary athetoid: Common type that involves muscles that function as rotators; rotary motion usually slow. Feet describe circular motion, hands pronate and supinate, and shoulders internally and externally rotate. There are varying degrees of muscle tension.

tremor (tremorlike) athetoid: Common type that involves irregular and uneven involuntary contraction and relaxation involving flexors and extensors, abductors and adductors. Rotary motion is not seen.

dystonic athetoid: Extremities, head, neck, and trunk assume distorted positions. There is increased muscle tone. Different abnormal positions may be assumed over time.

choreoathetoid: Involuntary, unpredictable, small movements of the distal parts of the extremities.

tension athetoid: A state of increased muscle tension blocking involuntary athetoid movements. Tension is not constant. Tension must be the dominant characteristic for this classification to be applicable; it is normally a temporary classification.

nontension athetoid: Involuntary movements without increased muscle tone. It is a temporary classification identifying a treatment phenomena and is frequently seen as an initial symptom of cerebral palsy in small babies.

flailing athetoid: A rare type of athetosis. Arms and legs are thrown violently from shoulder and hip, but there is little involvement of hands, wrists, fingers, or knees.

ataxia (ataxic cerebral palsy): It is associated with developmental deficits of the cerebellum, it is characterized by disturbance in the
Continued on following page

sense of balance and equilibrium, dyssynergias, and low postural tone. There is bilateral distribution affecting trunk and legs more than arms and hands, as well as a widespread stance and gait. Spastic diplegia and athetosis are often concomitant. Ataxia often follows initial stage of hypotonia. Associated problems include nystagmus, poor eye tracking, delayed and poorly articulated speech, astereognosis, and poor depth perception.

hypotonia (flaccid cerebral palsy): Often a transient stage in the evolution of athetosis or spasticity, it is characterized by decreased muscle tone, real or apparent weakness, and increased range of movement. A child typically assumes "froglike" position when placed supine and uses hands to support trunk during sitting.

mixed types: Any child with cerebral palsy that does not fit characterizations described. This label is used most commonly to indicate spastic diplegia mixed with athetosis.

FOR MORE INFORMATION

Campbell, SK: Pediatric Neurologic Physical Therapy. Churchill Livingstone, New York, 1984.

Campbell, SK: Physical Therapy for Children. WB Saunders, Philadelphia, 1994.

Thompson, GH, Rubin, IL, and Bilenker, RM: Comprehensive Management of Cerebral Palsy. Grune & Stratton, New York, 1982.

CLASSIFICATION OF MUSCULAR DYSTROPHY

Type	Onset	Inheritance	Course
Duchenne's	1–4 y	X-linked	Rapidly progressive; loss of walking by 9–10 y; death in late teens
Becker's	5–10 y	X-linked	Slowly progressive; maintain walking past early teens; life span into third decade
Congenital	Birth	Recessive	Typically slow but variable; shortened life span
Congenital myotonic	Birth	Dominant	Typically slow with significant intellectual impairment
Childhood-onset facioscapulohumeral	First decade	Dominant/recessive	Slowly progressive loss of walking in later life; variable life expectancy
Emery-Dreifus	Childhood to early teens	X-linked	Slowly progressive with cardiac abnormality and normal life span

From Stuberg, WA: Muscular Dystrophy and Spinal Muscular Atrophy. In Campbell, SK: Physical Therapy for Children. WB Saunders, Philadelphia, 1994, p 297, with permission.

7

VIGNOS FUNCTIONAL RATING SCALE FOR DUCHENNE'S MUSCULAR DYSTROPHY

1. Walks and climbs stairs without assistance
2. Walks and climbs stairs with aid of railing
3. Walks and climbs stairs slowly with aid of railing (over 25 s for eight standard steps)
4. Walks, but cannot climb stairs
5. Walks assisted, but cannot climb stairs or get out of chair
6. Walks only with assistance or with braces
7. In wheelchair: sits erect and can roll chair and perform bed and wheelchair ADL
8. In wheelchair: sits erect and is unable to perform bed and wheelchair ADL without assistance
9. In wheelchair: sits erect only with support and is able to do only minimal ADL
10. In bed: can do no ADL without assistance

ADL = activities of daily living.
From Stuberg, WA: Muscular Dystrophy and Spinal Muscular Atrophy. In Campbell, SK: Physical Therapy for Children. WB Saunders, Philadelphia, 1994, p 300, with permission.

CLASSIFICATION OF SPINAL MUSCULAR ATROPHY

Type	Onset	Inheritance	Course
Acute child-onset, type I, Werdnig-Hoffmann (acute)	0–3 mo	Recessive	Rapidly progressive; severe hypotonia; death within first year
Chronic childhood-onset, type II, Werdnig-Hoffmann (chronic)	3 mo–4 y	Recessive	Rapid progress that stabilizes; moderate to severe hypotonia; shortened life span
Juvenile-onset, type III, Kugelberg-Welander	5–10 y	Recessive	Slowly progressive; mild impairment

From Stuberg, WA: Muscular Dystrophy and Spinal Muscular Atrophy. In Campbell, SK: Physical Therapy for Children. WB Saunders, Philadelphia, 1994, p 312, with permission.

7

TYPES OF SPINA BIFIDA

A normal spine with an intact spinal cord is seen on the left. Illustrations of types of spina bifida (midline closure defects) are to the right. Although defects may occur anywhere along the vertebral column, they are most common in the lumbar and lumbosacral regions.

Spina bifida occulta is a failure of the vertebral lamina to develop and is usually asymptomatic; however, it may be associated with other birth defects. Spina bifida with meningocele is a midline defect with herniation of the meninges. Depending on the severity of the herniation and associated problems, there may or may not be any neural defect. Spina bifida with meningomyelocele is a midline defect with herniation of neural tissue. In addition to neural deficits, this condition may be life-threatening due to complications such as infection (meningitis) and hydrocephalus.

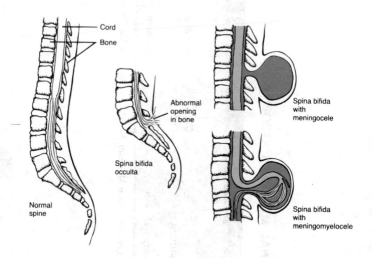

Cord

Bone

Abnormal opening in bone

Spina bifida occulta

Normal spine

Spina bifida with meningocele

Spina bifida with meningomyelocele

RECOMMENDATIONS FOR PARTICIPATION IN COMPETITIVE SPORTS FOR CHILDREN WITH DISORDERS OR MEDICAL CONDITIONS

Disorder/Condition	Contact/ Collison	Limited Contact/ Impact	Strenuous	Moderately Strenuous	Nonstrenuous
				Noncontact	
Atlantoaxial Instability	No	No	Yes[1]	Yes	Yes
Acute Illnesses	2	2	2	2	2
Cardiovascular					
Carditis	No	No	No	No	No
Hypertension					
Mild	Yes	Yes	Yes	Yes	Yes
Moderate	3	3	3	3	3
Severe	3	3	3	3	3
Congenital heart disease	4	4	4	4	4

Continued on following page

7

RECOMMENDATIONS FOR PARTICIPATION IN COMPETITIVE SPORTS FOR CHILDREN WITH DISORDERS OR MEDICAL CONDITIONS (Continued)

Disorder/Condition	Contact/ Collison	Limited Contact/ Impact	Noncontact		
			Strenuous	Moderately Strenuous	Nonstrenuous
Eyes					
Absence or loss of function of one eye	5	5	5	5	5
Detached retina	6	6	6	6	6
Inguinal Hernia	Yes	Yes	Yes	Yes	Yes
Kidney: Absence of one	No	Yes	Yes	Yes	Yes
Liver: Enlarged	No	No	Yes	Yes	Yes
Musculoskeletal Disorders	7	7	7	7	7
Neurologic					
History of serious head or spine trauma, repeated concussions, or craniotomy	7	7	Yes	Yes	Yes
Convulsive disorder					
Well controlled	Yes	Yes	Yes	Yes	Yes
Poorly controlled	No	No	Yes[8]	Yes	Yes[9]
Ovary: Absence of One	Yes	Yes	Yes	Yes	Yes

Respiratory					
Pulmonary insufficiency					
Asthma	Yes[10]	Yes[10]	Yes[10]	Yes[10]	Yes[10]
Sickle Cell Trait	Yes	Yes	Yes	Yes	Yes
Skin: Boils, Herpes, Impetigo, Scabies	Yes[11]	Yes[11]	Yes	Yes	Yes
Spleen: Enlarged	No	No	No	Yes	Yes
Testicle: Absence or Undescended	Yes[12]	Yes[12]	Yes	Yes	Yes

[1] Swimming: no butterfly, breast stroke, or diving starts.
[2] Needs individual assessment, e.g., contagiousness to others, risk of worsening illness.
[3] Needs individual assessment.
[4] Patients with mild forms can be allowed a full range of physical activities; patients with moderate to severe forms, or who are postoperative, should be evaluated by a cardiologist before athletic participation.
[5] Availability of American Society for Testing and Materials (ASTM)-approved eye guards may allow competitor to participate in most sports, but this must be judged on an individual basis.
[6] Consult ophthalmologist.
[7] Needs individual assessment.
[8] No swimming or weight lifting.
[9] No archery or riflery.
[10] May be allowed to compete if oxygenation remains satisfactory during a graded stress test.
[11] No gymnastics with mats, martial arts, wrestling, or contact sports until not contagious.
[12] Certain sports may require a protective cup.

From American Academy of Pediatrics, Committee on Sports Medicine and Fitness: Recommendations for participation in competitive sports. Pediatrics 81:737, 1994, with permission.

MEASUREMENT INSTRUMENTS USED IN PEDIATRICS

Name	Type of Test	Age
Alberta Infant Motor Scale (AIMS)	Motor performance: assesses postural control in supine, prone, sitting, and standing	0–18 mo
Assessment, Evaluation and Programming System for Infants and Children	Behavioral, motor performance; social skills: assesses fine motor, gross motor, adaptive, cognitive, social-communication, social	1 mo–3 y
Assessment of Movement Activity in Infants	Motor performance: assesses antigravity movement and posture	Infants
Battelle Developmental Inventory (BDI)	Behavioral: determines level of development to determine eligibility for educational intervention; areas tested are personal-social, adaptive, motor, communication, cognition	1 mo–9 y
Bayley Scales of Infant Development II (Bayley II)	Developmental: assesses cognitive, motor, behavioral	0–42 mo
Brigance Inventory of Early Development	Developmental: represents a comprehensive profile of developmental status examining gross motor, fine motor, self-help, prespeech, speech and language, general knowledge and comprehension, early academic skills	Birth–7 y
Bruininks-Oseretsky Test of Motor Proficiency	Developmental: assesses gross motor, fine motor, upper limb coordination	4½–14½ y

The Carolina Curriculum for Infants and Toddlers with Special Needs (2nd ed)	Behavioral: assesses cognition, communication, gross motor, fine motor, self-help	0–36 mo
Chandler Movement Assessment of Infants: Screening Test (CMAI-ST)	Neurologic: screens for movement disorders; tone, primitive reflexes, automatic reactions, volitional movement	Infants below 12-mo developmental level
DeGangi-Berk Test of Sensory Integration (TSI)	Sensory: assesses underlying sensory motor mechanisms; postural control, bilateral motor integration, reflex integration	3–5 y
Denver Development Screening Test II (DDST-II), (Denver II)	Developmental: detects potential developmental problems in the areas of gross motor, fine motor, language, personal-social	2 wk–6 y
Developmental Test of Visual-Motor Integration (VMI)	Developmental: assesses visual-motor skills	2–15 y
Early Learning Accomplishment Profile (ELAP)	Developmental: determines skill levels through task analyses; gross motor, fine motor, cognitive, language, self-help, social-emotional	Birth–36 mo
Erhardt Developmental Prehension Assessment (EDPA)	Developmental: used to describe the components of prehension; involuntary arm/hand patterns, primary voluntary movements, prewriting skills	Birth–15 mo
Functional Independence Measure for Children (Wee-FIM)	Functional: measures severity of disability; self-care, sphincter control, mobility, locomotion, communication, social, cognition, gross motor, fine motor, language, personal-social, adaptive	6 mo–7 y

Continued on following page

7

MEASUREMENT INSTRUMENTS USED IN PEDIATRICS (Continued)

Name	Type of Test	Age
Revised Gesell and Amatruda Developmental Neurological Exam	Developmental: assesses gross motor, fine motor, language, personal-social, adaptive	4 wk–5 y
Gross Motor Function Measure (GMFM)	Evaluates change in motor function of children with cerebral palsy; lying and rolling, sitting, crawling, and kneeling, standing, walking, and running and jumping	Best suited for children 2–5 y with cerebral palsy
Hawaii Early Learning Profile (HELP)	Behavioral: determines developmental level; cognition, language, gross motor, fine motor, social, self-help	0–36 mo
Harris Infant Neuromotor Test (HINT)	Developmental: screening tool designed to detect early signs of cognitive or neuromotor delays	Infants 3–12 mo
Home Observation for Measurement of the Environment (HOME)	Determines the impact of home environment on the child; emotional and verbal responsiveness of parents, acceptance of child, organization of environment, provision of appropriate play materials, parental involvement, opportunities for stimulation	Birth–36 mo
Infant Monitoring Questionnaires (IMQ)	Developmental: determines developmental level through parent report; communication, gross motor, fine motor, adaptive, personal-social	4–36 mo
The Infant Motor Screen (IMS)	Neurologic: tone, primitive reflexes, automatic responses	Preterm infants at corrected ages 4–16 mo
Infant Neurological International Battery (INFANIB)	Neurologic: tone, reflexes, automatic responses, head and trunk control	Neonates–9 mo

Infant Toddler Scale for Every Baby (ITSE)	Developmental: cognitive, communication, physical, social-emotional, adaptive	3–42 mo
Milani-Comparetti Motor Development Screening (M-C) Test	Determines neuromotor maturation of infants; reflexes, motor milestones	1–16 mo
Miller Assessment of Preschoolers (MAP)	Developmental: identifies children with mild to moderate delays; sensorimotor, cognitive	33–68 mo
Movement Assessment Battery for Children (Movement ABC)	Developmental: identifies and describes motor impairments; manual dexterity, balance, ball handling, visual-motor	4–12 y
Movement Assessment of Infants (MAI)	Neurologic: tone, reflexes, automatic reactions, volitional movement	0–12 mo
Naturalistic Observation of Newborn Behavior (NONB)	Behavioral: used to develop a profile of infants' physiologic and behavioral responses to environmental demands and care giving; behavioral state, autonomic responses, motor	Neonates–4 wk post-term
Neonatal Behavioral Assessment Scale (NBAS)	Determines interactive behavior and neuromotor status; state, tone, reflexes, interactive behavior	Birth–1 mo
Neonatal Oral-Motor Assessment Scale (NOMAS)	Identifies oral motor dysfunction; jaw and tongue patterns during nutritive and non-nutritive sucking	Neonate
Neurobehavioral Assessment of Preterm Infant (NAPI)	Adaptive-transactive, neurologic: determines neurobehavioral status and effects of intervention; state, behavior, reflexes, motor patterns, tone	32–42 wk gestation

Continued on following page

7

MEASUREMENT INSTRUMENTS USED IN PEDIATRICS (Continued)

Name	Type of Test	Age
The Neurological Assessment of the Preterm and Full-term Newborn Infant	Neurologic: Evaluates functional neurologic status; tone, posture, spontaneous movement, primitive reflexes, tendon reflexes	Infants 38–42 wk gestation
Nursing Child Assessment Satellite Training Teaching and Feeding Scales (NCAST)	Adaptive-transactive: assesses parental responsiveness to infant and infant-caregiver interaction; sensitivity to cues, response to distress, social-emotional growth, cognitive growth, clarity of cues, responsiveness to parent	Teaching 0–3 y, feeding 0–1 y
Peabody Developmental Motor Scales	Developmental: reflexes, gross motor, fine motor	0–83 mo
Pediatric Evaluation of Disability Inventory (PEDI)	Functional: self-care, mobility, and social function	6 mo–7½ y
Quick Neurological Screening Test (QNST)	Neuromotor: determines risk for learning disabilities; motor maturity, fine and gross motor control, motor planning, spatial organization, visual and auditory perception, balance	6–17 y
Scales of Independent Behavior (SIB)	Developmental, functional: motor, social and communication, personal and community living, behavior problems	Birth to adulthood
Screening Test for Evaluating Preschoolers (First Step)	Developmental: identifies children in need of comprehensive evaluation; cognition, communication, motor, social-emotional, adaptive	33–74 mo

Sensory Integration and Praxis Test (SIPT)	Sensory: assesses vestibular, proprioception, kinesthesia, tactile, visual	4–8 y, 11 mo
Test of Infant Motor Performance (TIMP)	Motor performance: identifies deficits in postural control; ability to orient and stabilize head in space and in response to stimulation, selective control of distal movements, antigravity control of trunk and extremities	32 wk gestation to 4 mo post-term
Test of Sensory Functions in Infants (TSFI)	Sensory: assesses tactile, deep pressure, visual-tactile integration, adaptive motor, ocular-motor, reactivity to vestibular stimulation	4–18 mo
Toddler and Infant Motor Evaluation (TIME)	Motor performance: assesses repertoires of movements through observations; neurologic foundations, stability, mobility, motor organization	Birth–42 mo
Transdisciplinary Play Based Assessment	Adaptive-transactive, developmental: determines developmental skill levels, learning style, and interaction through structured play; cognition, communication and language; sensorimotor, social-emotional	6 mo–6 y

Based on Long, TM and Cintas, HL: Handbook of Pediatric Physical Therapy. Williams & Wilkins, Baltimore, 1995, pp 56–79.

7

Geriatrics

8

PROPORTION OF PERSONS ≥65 AND ≥85 IN THE POPULATION: INCLUDING PROJECTIONS THROUGH 2040 (numbers in thousands)

Year	Total Population (all ages)	≥65 y		≥85 y	
		Number	Percentage of Total	Number	Percentage of 65+
1960	179,323	16,560	9.2	929	5.6
1980	226,546	25,550	11.3	2,240	8.8
1990	248,710	31,079	12.5	3,021	9.7
2000	274,815	34,886	12.7	4,289	12.3
2020	322,602	53,627	16.6	6,480	12.1
2040	364,349	75,588	20.7	13,221	17.5

From Abrams, WB, et al (eds): Merck Manual of Geriatrics, ed 2. Merck Research Laboratories, Whitehouse Station, NJ, 1995, p 1352, with permission. Sources: U.S. Bureau of the Census. Current Population Reports, Special Studies, 823-178, Sixty-Five Plus in America. Washington, DC, U.S. Government Printing Office, 1992; and U.S. Bureau of the Census, Current Population Reports, P25-1092, Population Projection of the United States, by Age, Sex, Race, and Hispanic Origin: 1992 to 2050. Washington, DC, U.S. Government Printing Office, 1992.

LEADING CAUSES OF DEATH AMONG PERSONS 65 AND OLDER (1990 data)

Cause of Death	Number of Deaths	Death Rate (per 100,000 population)	Percentage of All Deaths in Those ≥ 65 Years Old
All causes	1,542,493	4,963.2	100.0
Heart disease	594,858	1,914.0	38.6
Malignant neoplasms, including neoplasms of lymphatic and hematopoietic tissues	345,387	1,111.3	22.4
Cerebrovascular diseases	125,409	403.5	8.1
Chronic obstructive pulmonary disease and associated conditions	72,755	234.1	4.7
Pneumonia and influenza	70,485	226.8	4.6
Diabetes mellitus	35,523	114.3	2.3
Accidents and adverse effects	26,213	84.3	1.7
Motor vehicle accidents	7,210	23.2	0.5
All other accidents and adverse effects	19,003	61.1	1.2
Nephritis, nephrotic syndrome, and nephrosis	17,306	55.7	1.1
Atherosclerosis	17,158	55.2	1.1
Septicemia	15,351	49.4	1.0
All other causes, residual	222,048	2,045.9	14.4

From Abrams, WB, et al (eds): Merck Manual of Geriatrics, ed 2. Merck Research Laboratories, Whitehouse Station, NJ, 1995, p 1356, with permission. Source: National Center for Health Statistics. Advanced report of final mortality statistics, 1990. Monthly Vital Statistics Report, vol 41, no. 7, Suppl. Public Health Service, Hyattsville, MD, 1993.

8

VARIATIONS IN VITAL SIGNS BY AGE

Age	Average Temperature	Pulse Rate at Rest/Min		Respiratory Rate/Min	Mean Blood Pressure (mm Hg)
		Average	Range		
Newborn	36.1–37.7 C 97.0–100.0 F (axilla)	125	70–190	30–80	78 Systolic 42 Diastolic By flush technique: 30–60
1 y	37.7 C 99.7 F	120	80–160	20–40	96 Systolic 65 Diastolic
2 y	37.2 C 98.9 F	110	80–130	20–30	100 Systolic 63 Diastolic
4 y		100	80–120	20–30	97 Systolic 64 Diastolic
6 y	37.0 C 98.6 F (oral)	100	75–115	20–25	98 Systolic 65 Diastolic
8 y		90	70–110		106 Systolic 70 Diastolic

Age				
10 y	90	70–110	17–22	110 Systolic 72 Diastolic
12 y	Male: 85 Female: 90	65–105 70–110	17–22	116 Systolic 74 Diastolic
14 y	Male: 80 Female: 85	60–100 65–105		120 Systolic 76 Diastolic
16 y	Male: 75 Female: 80	55–95 60–100	15–20	123 Systolic 76 Diastolic
18 y	Male: 70 Female: 75	50–90 55–95	15–20	126 Systolic 79 Diastolic
Adult	Same as 18 years		15–20	120 Systolic 80 Diastolic
Elderly (over 70 y)	36.0 C 96.8 F	Same as 18 years	15–20	Diastolic pressure may increase

From Kozier, B, et al: Techniques of Clinical Nursing, ed 4. Addison-Wesley, Redwood City, CA, 1993, p 161, with permission.

TARGET HEART RATES FOR TRAINING OF OLDER PERSONS IN BEATS PER MINUTE (BPM)

Maximum Heart Rate (bpm) = 220 − Age in Years

Heart Rate Reserve (bpm) =
Maximum Heart Rate (bpm) − Heart Rate at Rest (bpm)

Target Heart Rate Range =
30% and 45% of Heart Rate Reserve (bpm) +
Heart Rate at Rest (bpm)

Example: 75-year-old man with resting heart rate of 86 bpm

220 − 75 = 145 bpm (Maximum Heart Rate)
145 − 86 = 59 bpm (Heart Rate Reserve)
18 (30% of Heart Rate Reserve) + 86 (Heart Rate at Rest) =
104 bpm (Lower Limit of Target)
27 (45% of Heart Rate Reserve) + 86 (Heart Rate at Rest) =
113 bpm (Upper Limit of Target)

Target Heart Rate Range = 104–113 bpm

BASED ON

Abrams, WB, et al (eds): Merck Manual of Geriatrics, ed 2. Merck Research Laboratories, Whitehouse Station, NJ, 1995, pp 434–440.

CHANGES IN LABORATORY VALUES WITH AGING

Increased	Unchanged	Decreased
Prostate-specific antigen (PSA)	Blood urea nitrogen (BUN)	Creatinine clearance
Serum cholesterol	Erythrocyte sedimentation rate	Dihydroepiandrosterone
Serum copper	Hemoglobin	Plasma gammatocopherol (vitamin E)
Serum ferritin	Leukocyte zinc	Plasma vitamin C
Serum fibrinogen	RBC count	Serum 1,25-dihydroxycholecalciferol
Serum glucose	Serum alkaline phosphatase	Serum calcium
Serum norepinephrine	Serum carotene	Serum iron
Serum triglycerides	Serum creatinine	Serum phosphorus
Serum uric acid	Serum IgM, IgG, IgA	Serum selenium
	Serum pantothenate	Serum testosterone
	Serum riboflavin	Serum thiamine
	Serum vitamin A	Serum vitamin B_{12}
	WBC count	Serum vitamin B_6
		Serum zinc
		Triiodithyronine

RBC = red blood cell; WBC = white blood cell.
From Abrams, WB, et al (eds): Merck Manual of Geriatrics, ed 2. Merck Research Laboratories, Whitehouse Station, NJ, 1995, p 1433, with permission.

OVERVIEW OF INSTRUMENTS COMMONLY USED FOR GERIATRIC PATIENTS

Instrument	Administered by	Answered by	Score Range* (poor–good)	Test Time (min)
Katz ADL	Interviewer	Proxy†	0–6	2–4
Lawton IADL	Interviewer, self-administered	Proxy† or subject	9–27	3–5
Folstein Mini Mental State	Interviewer	Subject	0–30	5–15
Yesavage Geriatric Depression Scale	Interviewer, self-administered	Subject	15–30	3–6
Tinetti Balance & Gait Evaluation	Interviewer, self-administered	Subject	0–28	5–15

*Scores are those suggested by test designers.
†Proxy is a person designated to answer questions for the patient as specified by the test designer. Poor score indicates limitations in function.
ADL = activities of daily living; IADL = instrumental activities of daily living.
Based on Abrams, WB, et al (eds): Merck Manual of Geriatrics, ed 2. Merck Research Laboratories, Whitehouse Station, NJ, 1995, pp 227–231.

	OFFICE OF TECHNOLOGY ASSESSMENT'S ESTIMATE OF THE PROPORTION OF HIP FRACTURE PATIENTS AGE 50 AND OVER WHO DIE OF ANY CAUSE BY 1-YEAR POST-FRACTURE		
Age	All Hip Fracture Patients	Male Hip Fracture Patients	Female Hip Fracture Patients
50–64	*	*	7%
65–74	14%	22%	10
75–84	21	34	17
85+	31	48	28
Totals	**24**	**36**	**21**

*Data not available to determine these proportions.
Data from Office of Technology Assessment, 1993.
From U.S. Congress, Office of Technology Assessment: Hip Fracture Outcomes in People Age 50 and Over—Background Paper, OTA-BP-H-120. U.S. Government Printing Office, Washington, DC, July 1994.

	ONE-YEAR MORTALITY FOR HIP FRACTURE PATIENTS, BY TYPE OF FRACTURE, TYPE OF TREATMENT, AGE, AND GENDER, 1986		
Age	Trochanteric Hip Fracture with Reduction and Internal Fixation	Cervical Hip Fracture with Reduction and Internal Fixation	Partial Hip Replacement
65–74	13%	10%	12%
75–85	20	18	19
85+	29	29	29
Males			
65–74	19	16	21
75–85	30	31	33
85+	43	44	46
Females			
65–74	10	8	10
75–85	17	14	16
85+	27	26	26

Data from U.S. Department of Health and Human Services, Health Care Financing Administration, Special Report, Vol 3, June 1990.
From U.S. Congress, Office of Technology Assessment: Hip Fracture Outcomes in People Age 50 and Over—Background Paper, OTA-BP-H-120. U.S. Government Printing Office, Washington, DC, July 1994.

FALLS AMONG PEOPLE 65 YEARS OF AGE AND OLDER

Epidemiology of Falls

Falls are the leading cause of accidental deaths in persons after 65 years of age.

Falls are the seventh leading cause of death among people older than 65 years.

In the United States 75% of deaths from falls occur in the 12% of the population that is older than 65 years.

From 75 years of age the rate of death from falls rises nonlinearly for both genders and all racial groups.

Until age 75 years falls occur more frequently in women. The frequency is the same for both genders between ages 75 and 85 years, and after 85 years, white men have the highest death rate from falls.

Thirty-three percent of healthy community-dwelling elders (older than 65 years) fall annually.

Sixty-seven percent of nursing home residents fall annually.

Between 33% and 67% of older patients in hospital-like environments fall annually.

Although most falls occur indoors, there is no seasonal, location, or hourly correlation with when falls occur.

Sequelae from falls or prolonged floor contact after falls include fear of falling, dehydration, pressure sores, hypothermia, pneumonia, and rhabdomyolysis.

Forty percent of older individuals have a fear of falling, with half avoiding activities behind essential ADLs because of this fear.

Falls contribute to 40% of admissions to nursing homes.

Whites who fall have twice the hip fracture rate as persons from other racial groups.

Five percent of falls among older people will result in fractures.

Ten to twenty percent of falls among older people will result in soft-tissue injuries, with 50% of these requiring medical care.

Seventy percent of emergency room visits by people older than 75 years are due to falls.

Only 50% of individuals older than 85 years who are hospitalized after a fall live for 1 year.

The most common fractures as a result of falls among the elderly are humeral, wrist, pelvis, and hip, with the presence of osteoporosis making fractures more likely.

Hip Fractures Due to Falls

The most serious fracture (i.e., with the greatest likelihood of morbidity and mortality) after falls in the elderly are hip fractures (greater than 250,000 per year in people older than 65 years).

Twenty percent of women reaching age 80 will have sustained a hip fracture during their lifetime.

The risk of hip fracture from falls doubles with use of certain antipsychotic and long-acting benzodiazepine drugs.

Five percent of hip fractures result in death during hospitalization.

Overall mortality from hip fractures in the elderly 1 year after hip fracture is 12%–67%.

Fifty percent of the elderly who are able to walk before a hip fracture cannot do so after the fracture, and 50% are unable to live independently after hip fracture.

FOR MORE INFORMATION

National Center for Health Statistics: Data from the National Interview Survey, 1984, Supplement on Aging, and the 1980 Longitudinal Studies on Aging, Washington, DC.

Age-Related Physiologic Changes Contributing to Falls Among Older Persons

Reduced vision: diminished accommodation, acuity, loss of peripheral vision, reduced tolerance of glare, diminished contrast sensitivity and darkness adaptation, and impaired contextual processing of visual inputs

Hearing and balance: impaired speech comprehension, compromised tonal discrimination, reduced hair cells in cochlea, and reduced endolymph

Other central nervous system factors: reduced reaction time, dyskinesia in lower limbs, heightened sway, and poor gait

BASED ON

Horak, FH, Shupert, CL, and Myrka, A: Components of postural dyscontrol: A review. Neurobiology of Aging 10:727, 1989. Abrams, WB, et al (eds): Merck Manual of Geriatrics, ed 2. Merck & Co., Whitehouse Station, NJ, 1995, p 67.

8

Continued on following page

Medical Conditions That Predispose Older Persons to Falls

System	Disorders
Neurologic	Stroke, transient ischemic attacks, Parkinson's disease, delirium, seizures, myelopathy, cerebellar disorders, carotid sinus supersensitivity, peripheral neuropathy
Cardiovascular	Myocardial infarction, orthostatic hypotension, cardiac arrhythmias
Gastrointestinal	Bleeding, diarrhea, defecation syncope, postprandial syncope
Metabolic	Hypothyroidism, hypoglycemia, anemia, hypokalemia, dehydration, hyponatremia
Genitourinary	Incontinence, nocturia, micturition syncope
Musculoskeletal	Deconditioning, arthritis, proximal limb myopathy
Psychologic	Depression, anxiety

Based on Abrams, WB, et al (eds): Merck Manual of Geriatrics, ed 2. Merck Research Laboratories, Whitehouse Station, NJ, 1995, p 68.

Types of Medications Associated with Falls in Older Persons

Benzodiazepines
Diuretics
Narcotics
Phenothiazines
Select antihypertensives
Tricyclic antidepressants

BASED ON

Abrams, WB, et al (eds): Merck Manual of Geriatrics, ed 2. Merck Research Laboratories, Whitehouse Station, NJ, 1995, p 68.

Injury Prevention in Older Persons: Factors to Evaluate and Recommended Actions to Follow

Factor	Recommendations
Screening	Periodic review of existing or potential problem areas.
Health	Periodic check of height, weight, activity levels, sudden changes in life habits, changes in footwear or leg circumference/pain.
Accident check	Review home environment for obstacles and preventive additions in lighting, fixtures, appliance placement, etc.
Lifestyle	Regular checks for changes in exercise, overt behavior, medication intake, alcohol or tobacco intake.
Exercise	Weight-bearing and aerobic exercise 20–30 min, at least 3 times/wk. Daily stretching, group activity.
Nutrition	Protein: 0.6–1.0 g/kg per day; low fat (<30% calories); low-cholesterol intake; minimal daily allowances of vitamins and minerals in foods and supplements; 1.0–1.5 g calcium in daily diet, with additional supplements for older women; adequate fiber and complex sugars (starchy foods); moderate salt intake; weight reduction, as appropriate.

Environmental Modifications to Reduce the Likelihood of Falls Among Older Persons

Bathroom

Bath tub: eliminate slippery surfaces by installing materials with a high coefficient of friction, install grab bars, eliminate unstable towel racks near the tub and shower

Toilet seat: raise seat if too low

Cabinets: check for adequate room lighting and safe distances required to reach objects

Medications: assure that there is correct and legible labeling of adequate size to be read

Continued on following page

8

Stairs

Step heights: reduce to 6 in. or less if possible

Handrails: install rails if they are not present, and extend the rail beyond the top and bottom steps

Inclines: assure that all inclined surfaces are not too long to be managed by the person using them, and make certain there are places where someone can rest

Surfaces: install nonskid material on all steps

Lighting: assure proper lighting, including night lights and the use of color contrast materials at step edges

Kitchen

Cabinets: make cabinets at heights where persons do not have to reach excessively to access them

Floor: eliminate slippery surfaces including waxed surfaces that are slippery

Appliances: assure that there is correct and legible labeling of adequate size to be read for all controls

Tables: check the stability of table legs; assure that curved legs do not impede walking paths

Chairs: check for sturdiness and eliminate friction-free legs (rollers, etc.) height

General Considerations

Rugs: eliminate frayed edges, curves, or materials that do not contrast with under surface

Appliances: arrange electrical cords that could impede walk ways

Chairs: provide chairs with arms for body support or assistance from sit-to-stand position; eliminate unstable furniture (tables and chairs)

Positioning: arrange furniture to minimize obstacles in major thoroughfares

Temperature: check temperature controls to assure a comfortable environment

BASED ON

Tideiksaar, R: Preventing falls: Home hazard checklist to help older patients protect themselves. Geriatrics 41:26, 1986.

Abrams, WB, et al (eds): Merck Manual of Geriatrics, ed 2. Merck Research Laboratories, Whitehouse Station, NJ, 1995, pp 74–77.

Factors to Evaluate Regarding Falls in Older Persons

From history:
    Activity at time of fall
    Concurrent events (at the time of the fall): light headedness, palpitations, apnea, chest pain, disorientation, vertigo, loss of consciousness, incontinence
    Location of fall
    Accounts by witnesses to fall
    History of previous falls
    Medication use

Examination:
    Visual fields and acuity
    Look for bruises, edema, indications of arthritis, podiatric limitations
    Examine for axial-spinal discomfort or the sudden onset of pain
    Mental status: orientation, memory
    Balance and gait: examine sit-to-stand maneuver, walking, Romberg or modified Romberg, stair climbing, examine how patient bends
    Variability in blood pressure, heart rate and rhythm and the presence of heart murmurs

BASED ON

Abrams, WB, et al (eds): Merck Manual of Geriatrics, ed 2. Merck Research Laboratories, Whitehouse Station, NJ, 1995, pp 71–73.

AGE OF ONSET OF MOVEMENT DISORDERS IN OLDER PERSONS

Disorder	Typical Age of Onset
Essential (senile) tremor	after 60 years
Parkinson's disease	50–79 years
Progressive supranuclear palsy	after 60 years
Senile chorea	after 60 years
Shy-Drager syndrome	after 55 years in men (the disease occurs predominantly in males)
Spasmodic torticollis	20–50 years

8

ASSESSMENT TOOLS USED FOR GERIATRIC PATIENTS
Measurement of Mental Function for Geriatric Patients

COGNITION

Elements Tested	Types of Items Tested	Instruments Used
Attention span/concentration	Block designs	Evaluation Scale
Intelligence	Correct observed behaviors	Extended Dementia Scale
Learning ability	Math problems	Face-Hand Test
Memory: distant	Puzzles or word problems	Geriatric Interpersonal Dementia Rating Scale
Memory: recent	Recall of distant news events	Memory and Information Test
Orientation	Recall of birth date	Mental Status Questionnaire
Perceptual ability	Recall of old personal events	Mini-Mental State Exam
Problem solving/judgment	Recall of messages	Misplaced Objects Test
Psychomotor ability	Recall of time	PGC Mental Status
Social intactness	Recall of place	Quick Test
	Recall of recent events	Set Test
	Recall of own name	Short Portable MSQ

Types of Items Tested	Instruments Used
Simulated situations	VIRO Orientation Scale
Vocabulary tests	Visual Counting Test
	WAIS (complete or abridged)
	Wechsler Memory Scale

AFFECTIVE FUNCTIONING

Elements Tested	Types of Items Tested	Instruments Used
Demoralization	Appetite disturbances	Affect Balance Scale
Depression, endogenous	Psychophysiological apathy	Beck Depression Inventory
Depression, reactive	Sadness	Hopkins Symptom Checklist
Suicidal risk	Sense of failure	Zung Self-Rating Depression Scale
	Sleep disturbances	
	Suicidal thoughts	
	Symptoms	
	Tearfulness	
	Withdrawal	

Continued on following page

ASSESSMENT TOOLS USED FOR GERIATRIC PATIENTS (Continued)

GENERAL MENTAL HEALTH

Elements Tested	Types of Items Tested	Instruments Used
Affective impairment	Numerous items gathered through clinical observation, questionnaire, or projective testing	Emotional Problems Questionnaire
Cognitive mental health		Gerontological Apperception Test
Paranoia		London Psychogeriatric Rating Scale
Presence of psychopathology		Nurses Observation for Inpatient Evaluation
		OARS Mental Health Section
Substance abuse		Psychological Well-Being Interview
		Savage-Britton Index
		Screening Score of Psychiatric Symptoms
		Senior Apperception Test

Based on Kane, RA and Kane, RL: Assessing the Elderly: A Practical Guide to Measurement. Lexington Books, Lexington, MA, 1981, pp 81–94.

TESTS OF HIGHER COGNITIVE FUNCTIONS
(by region of brain affected)

Lobe	Test (patient required tasks)
Frontal	Points finger each time examiner makes fist and makes fist each time examiner points
Temporal	Dominant hemisphere: standard aphasia testing (spontaneous speech, repetition, comprehension, writing and naming)
	Nondominant hemisphere: interprets affect of others (identifies behavior represented in photos of faces or interprets affect based on examiner's voice)
Parietal	Dominant hemisphere: names fingers, knows left from right, performs calculations using paper, reading
	Nondominant hemisphere: reproduces match stick figure made by examiner
Occipital	Matches color and objects if unable to name them

Based on Gallo, JJ, Reichel, W, and Andersen, LM: Handbook of Geriatric Assessment, ed 2. Aspen, Gaithersburg, MD, 1995.

MENTAL STATUS ASSESSMENT INSTRUMENTS USED FOR GERIATRIC PATIENTS

Category Fluency: This test requires respondents to identify as many items as possible in each of four categories. The test is not timed, and the maximum items in each category is 10 for a total score of 40. Scores of less than 15 are abnormal, with 80% of demented elderly people scoring at this level.

Cognitive Capacity Screen: This test is designed to detect cognitive impairments in patients with medical illness. There are 30 questions with 1 point given per correct answer. A score less than 20 is usually associated with dementia or may be due to a low level of education. The test contains some unique questions designed to test abstraction.

Folstein Mini–Mental State Examination: This test of cognitive function has two parts. The first part assesses orientation, memory, and attention. The second part evaluates the patient's ability to name objects, follow verbal or written commands, and write a sentence. Maximum score is 30 points. Normal scores approximate 28. Individuals who score 9.7, 19, and 25 are patients with dementia, patients with depression with cognitive impairment, and patients with affective disorders, respectively.

Kokmen Short Test of Mental Status: This test examines intellectual tasks including abstract thinking. There are eight categories and a maximum score of 38 points. A score of 29 or less indicates that a patient is demented with a sensitivity of 95.5% and a specificity of 91.4% (Kokmen, E, Naessens, JM, and Offest, KA: A short test of men-

Continued on following page

tal status: Description and preliminary results. Mayo Clin Proc 62:281, 1987).

Mattis Dementia Rating Scale: This test has 144 tasks and is based on the presumption that if a respondent can answer the first question in a given section correctly, then subsequent questions in that section will also be answered correctly. Scores range from 0–144. Most individuals who do not have dementia will score greater than 85. Patients with dementia take 30–45 minutes to complete the test while older individuals who are not demented can complete it in 10–15 minutes.

Orientation-Memory-Concentration Test: Individuals are asked six questions. Each question is given a score based on the number of errors and a weighted factor. When the weighted score is 10 or more, the patient is mentally impaired. Normally older persons score 6 or less. The memory phase and counting backward questions are answered incorrectly by respondents who are developing dementia. (Katzman, R, Braun, T, and Fuld, P: Validation of a short orientation-memory-concentration test of cognitive impairment. Am J Psychiat 140:734, 1983.)

Short Portable Mental Status Questionnaire: This test has 10 questions addressing personal history, calculation, remote memory, and orientation. More than three errors suggest mental impairment. Accuracy of answers and education of the respondent must be considered. For example, verification of mother's maiden name must be ascertained.

FOR MORE INFORMATION

Gallo, JJ, Reichel, W, and Andersen, LM: Handbook of Geriatric Assessment, ed 2. Aspen, Gaithersburg, MD, 1995, pp 37–68.
National Center for Cost Containment: Geropsychological Assessment Resource Guide. United States Department of Commerce, National Technical Information Service, Milwaukee, WI, 1993.

DEPRESSION SCALES USED FOR GERIATRIC PATIENTS

Beck Depression Inventory: This test addresses 21 characteristics associated with depression, and each item is scored from 0–3. A score greater than 21 suggests depression.

Center of Epidemiologic Studies Depression Scale (CES-D): This test contains 20 items. For each item, respondents are asked to report the number of days that they have experienced symptoms during the previous week. Scores above 27 indicate the likelihood of depression.

General Health Questionnaire: This 60-item test is self-administered and is designed to detect mental distress. The scaled version contains 28 items that test four categories: somatic symptoms, anxiety and insomnia, social dysfunction, and depression. Scores of 4 or 5 are often seen as a cutoff, with higher scores indicating depression.

Geriatric Depression Scale: This questionnaire consists of 30 "yes" or "no" items. The test is scored by assigning a point for each answer matching the "yes" or "no" response assigned to it. Scores above 10 or 11 indicate depression.

Zung Self-Rating Depression Scale: This scale contains 20 statements rated by four possible levels of applicability to self, and each is scored on a 1 to 4 basis. The scale uses a Likert scale, with a total raw score of 80 possible. An index is generated by dividing the raw score by 80; therefore, a score of 1 is the maximum score. Eighty-eight percent of patients diagnosed as depressed from a psychiatric examination had a score of .50 or higher, and the same percentage of patients who were not depressed had scores of less than .50.

FOR MORE INFORMATION

Kane, RA and Kane, RL: Assessing the Elderly: A Practical Guide to Measurement. Lexington Books, Lexington, MA, 1981.

Spreen, O and Strauss, E: A Compendium of Neuropsychological Tests. Oxford, New York, 1991.

ACUTE CONFUSIONAL (DELIRIUM) STATES IN OLDER PERSONS

Signs and Symptoms of Confusional (Delirium) States in Older Persons

Anxiety, agitation
Clouded consciousness
Delusions
Diffuse electroencephalogram slowing
Disorientation to time or space
Disrupted thinking
Enhanced symptoms at night
Impaired attention or concentration
Impaired memory
Increased restlessness
Perceptual disturbances (illusions or hallucinations)
Rapid onset
Reduced wakefulness
Speech abnormalities

Extracranial Causes of Confusional (Delirium) States in Older Persons

Alcohol withdrawal
Anesthetic use
Drug withdrawal after prolonged use
Environmental alterations
Giant cell arteritis
Hip fracture
Hypercapnia
Hypoxia
Infections
Intoxication
Metabolic disturbances
Myocardial infarction

Continued on following page

Intracranial Causes of Confusional (Delirium) States in Older Individuals

Infections (e.g., meningitis)
Seizures
Stroke
Subdural hematoma
Tumors

BASED ON

Abrams, WB, et al (eds): Merck Manual of Geriatrics, ed 2. Merck Research Laboratories, Whitehouse Station, NJ, 1995, pp 1141–1146.

DEFINITIONS OF SLEEP PATTERNS IN OLDER PERSONS

transient insomnia: poor sleep over a few nights; may be caused by stress, work, or time zone changes

short-term insomnia: poor sleep over less than 1 month; may be related to acute medical or psychological conditions

long-term insomnia:

problems falling asleep of over 1-month duration that may be related to anxiety, poor sleep habits, medical problems, medication-related sleep disorders, or changes in activity levels, or **frequent awakening** that may be related to depression, medication-related sleep disorders, sleep apnea, medical problems, or changes in activity levels

BASED ON

Abrams, WB, et al (eds): Merck Manual of Geriatrics, ed 2. Merck Research Laboratories, Whitehouse Station, NJ, 1995, pp 110–115.

MALNUTRITION IN OLDER PERSONS

Systemic Changes Contributing to Malnutrition (Protein Deficiency) in Older Persons

Circulatory: pedal edema, orthostatic hypotension, pressure sores
Musculoskeletal: fatigue, reduced muscle strength, hip fracture, lack of energy
Immunologic: reduced natural killer cell activity, decreased serum antibody response to antigens, infections, increased interactions between drugs
Other: altered thyroid function, weight changes

Factors Contributing to Malnutrition (Protein Deficiency) in Older Persons

Alcoholism
Cancer
Chronic infection
Chronic obstructive pulmonary disease
Dental/facial pathology
Depression
Dysphagia
Excessive low-fat diet
Hypercalcemia
Hyperthyroidism
Impaired senses (taste, smell)
Inability to gather or prepare food
Loneliness
Medication intake (e.g., theophylline)
Medication withdrawal
Pheochromocytoma
Poverty
Rapid satiation

BASED ON

Abrams, WB, et al (eds): Merck Manual of Geriatrics, ed 2. Merck Research Laboratories, Whitehouse Station, NJ, 1995, pp 8–11.

PHYSIOLOGICAL CHANGES WITH AGING THAT PREDISPOSE OLDER PERSONS TO HYPOTHERMIA

Compromised cutaneous sensation: altered perception of cold
Compromised proprioception: altered awareness of joint position
Changes in autonomic nervous system function: reduced shivering response, compromised peripheral circulation, poor vasoconstrictor response to cold, orthostatic hypotension
Changes in central nervous system: dementia, poor judgment

BASED ON

8

Abrams, WB, et al (eds): Merck Manual of Geriatrics, ed 2. Merck Research Laboratories, Whitehouse Station, NJ, 1995, pp 51–57.

Measurement, Assessment, and Outcomes

9

DISABLEMENT MODELS

NAGI SCHEME

ACTIVE PATHOLOGY		IMPAIRMENT		FUNCTIONAL LIMITATION		DISABILITY
(interruption or interference with normal processes, and efforts of the organism to regain normal state)	→	(anatomic, physiologic, mental, or emotional abnormalities or loss)	→	(limitation in performance at the level of the whole organism or person)	→	(limitation is performance of socially defined roles and tasks within a sociocultural and physical environment)

INTERNATIONAL CLASSIFICATION OF IMPAIRMENTS, DISABILITIES, AND HANDICAPS (ICIDH)

"DISEASE"		IMPAIRMENT		DISABILITY		HANDICAP
(the intrinsic pathology or disorder)	→	(loss or abnormality of psychological, physiologic, or anatomic structure or function at organ level)	→	(restriction or lack of ability to perform an activity in normal manner)	→	(disadvantage due to impairment or disability that limits or prevents fulfillment of a normal role [depends on age, sex, sociocultural factors] for the person)

NATIONAL CENTER FOR MEDICAL REHABILITATION RESEARCH				
PATHOPHYSIOLOGY →	IMPAIRMENT →	FUNCTIONAL LIMITATION →	DISABILITY →	SOCIETAL LIMITATION
(interruption with normal physiologic developmental processes or structures)	(loss or abnormality of cognitive, emotional, physiologic, or anatomic structure or function)	(restriction or lack of ability to perform an action in the manner or range consistent with the purpose of an organ or organ system)	(limitation or inability in performing tasks, activities, and roles to levels expected within physical and social contexts)	(restriction attributable to social policy or barriers that limit fulfillment of roles)

Rprinted from Physical Therapy, Jette, AM: Physical disablement concepts for physical therapy research and practice. 1994, vol 74, p 380, with the permission of the APTA.

9

TERMS USED IN MEASUREMENT

The following terms are from the American Physical Therapy Association's (APTA's) Standards for Tests and Measurements in Physical Therapy Practice. Phys Ther. 71:589–622, 1991. For more information, see Rothstein, JM, and Echternach, JL: Primer on Measurement: An Introductory Guide to Measurement Issues. APTA, Alexandria, Virginia, 1993.

Alternate-forms (parallel-forms) reliability: see *reliability*

Assessment: Measurement, quantification, or placing a value or label on something; assessment is often confused with evaluation; an assessment results from the act of assessing (see *evaluation* and *examination*)

Attribute: A variable; a characteristic or quality that is measured

Classification (categorization): Assignment of an individual or an entity to a group; assignment is based on rules; groups are defined so that they allow all pertinent entities or individuals to belong to the defined groups (classes or categories are exhaustive) and so that they allow entities or individuals to belong to only one possible group (classes or categories are mutually exclusive)

Clinical decision: a determination that relates to direct patient care, indirect patient care, acceptance of patients for treatment, and whether patients should be referred to other practitioners (this definition is modified from that presented by Charles Magistro at a conference on Clinical Decision Making held under APTA auspices in October 1988 in Lake of the Ozarks, Missouri); a diagnosis that leads therapist to take an action is a form of a clinical decision: clinical decisions result in actions; when direct supporting evidence for clinical decisions is lacking, such decisions are based on clinical opinions

Clinical opinion: a belief or idea that a physical therapist holds regarding a patient; this opinion may be based on the use of tests and measurements, but is not directly supported by evidence relating to those tests and measurements; clinical opinions are based on the therapist's evaluation of available information; clinical decisions (i.e., determinations that cause the therapist to take an action) that are based on the therapist's synthesis of information are based on the clinical opinions of that therapist.

Concurrent validity: see *validity*

Construct: a concept developed for the purpose of measurement; support for the construct is through logical argumentation based on the theoretical and research evidence (see *construct validity* listed under *validity*)

Construct validity: see *validity*

Content validity: see *validity*

Criterion-based (criterion-related) validity: see *validity*

Data: synonymous with measurements (see *measurement*)

Derived measurement: a measurement of an attribute that is obtained as the result of a mathematical operation applied to an existing measurement of some other attribute; an example is the measurement of leg-length difference, which is derived by subtracting one leg-length measurement from another

Evaluation: a judgment based on a measurement; often confused with assessment and examination (see *assessment* and *examination*); evaluations are judgments of the value or worth of something

Examination: a test or a group of tests used for the purpose of obtaining measurements or data (see *assessment* and *evaluation*).

False-negatives: persons who test negatively for some attribute but who, in fact, have that attribute (see *true-negatives*)

False-positives: persons who test positively for some attribute but who, in fact, do not have that attribute (see *true-positives*)

Instrument: a machine, a questionnaire, or any device that is used as part of, or as a test to obtain, measurements

Internal consistency: see *reliability*

Intertester reliability: see *reliability*

Intratester reliability: see *reliability*

Measure: the act of obtaining a measurement (datum)

Measurement: the numeral assigned to an object, event, or person or the class (category) to which an object, event, or person is assigned according to rules

Normalization: a process that yields a new or transformed measurement that is mathematically derived to change the distribution of measurements; normalization procedures are often used to change the distribution of data to make the distribution more congruent with a bell-shaped (or normal) curve

Objective measurement: a measurement that is not affected by some aspect of the person obtaining the measurement; the opposite of a subjective measurement (see *subjective measurement*); measurements cannot be totally objective, because the term *objective* relates to the reliability of measurements, especially in the intertester reliability; objectivity and reliability are measured along a continuum

Operational definition: a set of procedures that guides the process of obtaining a measurement; includes descriptions of the attribute that is to be measured, the conditions under which the measurement is to be taken, and the actions that are to be taken in order to obtain the measurement

Parallel-forms (alternate-forms) reliability: see *reliability*

Practicality of a test: the usefulness of a test based on issues relating to personnel, time, equipment, cost of administration, and impact on the person taking a test

Predictive validity: see *validity*

Predictive value of a measurement: the degree of certainty that can be associated with a positive or negative finding (measurement) obtained on a diagnostic test; the predictive value of a positive measurement is the ratio formed by dividing the number of true-positives by the number of all positive findings; the predictive value of a negative measurement is the ratio formed by dividing the number of true-negatives by the number of all negative findings

Continued on following page

Prescriptive validity: see *validity*

Primary purveyor: see *purveyor*

Purveyor: any person (or organization) who develops a test or any person (or organization) who offers, promotes, or requires the use of a test; a purveyor is also a person who advocates use of specific tests through the publication of research or scholarly articles or through teaching

> **Primary purveyor:** a person who develops, promotes, or requires the use of tests; this definition includes persons within clinical institutions who require the use of specific tests; persons who conduct continuing education courses in which a major component involves the advocacy of the use of specific testing procedures are primary purveyors; any person (or organization) who promotes (advocates) the use of tests by selling testing equipment, manuals, books, or similar materials is a primary purveyor; in the case of books or articles that serve as test manuals, the primary purveyor is the author; persons who sell instruments that may be used for testing, but who do not describe or advocate specific testing procedures, are not purveyors (see purveyor, *secondary purveyor*, and *tertiary purveyor*).

> **Second purveyor:** any researcher or other person who publishes a scholarly work that examines aspects of tests and who, in that scholarly work, suggests (advocates) that a test be used; a secondary purveyor is not the initial source of information on a test (i.e., did not supply the manual or the original information on the test) (see *purveyor, primary purveyor*, and *tertiary purveyor*)

> **Tertiary purveyor:** any person who teaches or prepares instructional material that describes specific tests or specific uses of measurements; this definition includes, but is not limited to, persons teaching in academic institutions, clinical educators, and continuing educators who are not acting in the role of primary or secondary purveyors (see purveyor, *primary purveyor*, and *secondary purveyor*)

Reactivity: the degree to which the process of taking a test affects a measurement or other measurements taken on the same person in the future; examples are learning and physiologic effects of taking tests

Reliability: the consistency or repeatability of measurements; the degree to which measurements are error-free and the degree to which repeated measurements will agree

> **Internal consistency:** the extent to which items or elements that contribute to a measurement reflect one basic phenomenon or dimension

> **Intertester reliability:** the consistency or equivalence of measurements when more than one person takes the measurements; indicates agreement of measurements taken by different examiners

> **Intratester reliability:** the consistency or equivalence of measurements when one person takes repeated measurements separated in time; indicates agreement in measurements over time

Parallel-forms (alternate-forms) reliability: the consistency or agreement of measurements obtained with different (alternative) forms of a test; indicates whether measurements obtained with different forms of a test can be used interchangeably

Test-retest reliability: the consistency or repeated measurements separated in time; indicates stability (reliability) over time

Score (grade): the numeric (quantitative) or verbal (qualitative) descriptor used to characterize the result of a test; a score is a measurement (see measurement)

Secondary purveyor: see purveyor

Sensitivity of a test: an indication of how well a diagnostic test identifies people who should have a positive finding; the numeric representation of sensitivity is a ratio formed by dividing the number of persons with a true-positive response on a test by the number of persons who should have had a positive response (i.e., the number of persons who are known to have properties that would indicate that they should test positive)

Specificity of a test: an indication of how well a diagnostic test identifies people who should have a negative finding; the numeric representation of specificity is a ratio formed by dividing the number of persons with a true-negative response on a test by the number of persons who should have had a negative response (i.e., the number of persons who are known to have properties that would indicate that they should test negative)

Standardization: a process by which a score is converted (transformed) into a relative score by using indices of central tendency and variability; a commonly used standardized score is the z score; the term *standardization* is also used to describe the process of standardization, however, does not ensure reliability, because reliability can only be determined through the collection of data (see *reliability*)

Subjective measurement: a measurement that is affected by some aspect of the person obtaining the measurement (contrasts with objective measurement); subjectivity relates to the reliability of measurements, especially the intertester reliability; the more subjective the measurement, the less reliable the measurement; subjectivity, like reliability, is measured along a continuum

Tertiary purveyor: see *purveyor*

Test: a procedure or set of procedures that is used to obtain measurements (data); the procedures may require the use of instruments

Test manual: a booklet or book prepared by a primary test purveyor to guide the process of obtaining a measurement and to provide documentation and justification for the test

Test setting: the environment in which a test is given, including the physical setting and the characteristics of that setting

Test user: one who chooses tests, interprets test scores, or makes decisions based on test scores (this definition is from *Standards for Educational and Psychological Tests.* American Psychological Association, Washington, DC, 1974, p 1)

Continued on following page

Test-retest reliability: see *reliability*

Transformation of measurements: the application of a mathematical operation for the purpose of changing the value or distribution of measurements, such as is done in the process of standardization or normalization

True-negatives: persons who test negatively for some attribute and who, in fact, do not have that attribute (see *false-negatives*)

True-positives: persons who test positively for some attribute and who, in fact, have that attribute (see *false-positives*)

Validity: the degree to which a useful (meaningful) interpretation can be inferred from a measurement

> **Concurrent validity:** a form of criterion-based validity in which an inferred interpretation is justified by comparing a measurement with supporting evidence that was obtained at approximately the same time as the measurement being validated
>
> **Construct validity:** the conceptual (theoretical) basis for using a measurement to make an inferred interpretation; evidence for construct validity is through logical argumentation based on theoretical and research evidence (see *construct*)
>
> **Content validity:** a form of validity that deals with the extent to which a measurement is judged to reflect the meaningful elements of a construct and not any extraneous elements
>
> **Criterion-based (criterion-related) validity:** three forms of criterion-based validity exist: concurrent validity, predictive validity, and prescriptive validity; the common element is that, with each of these forms of validity, the correctness of an inferred interpretation can be tested by comparing a measurement with either a different measurement or data obtained by other forms of testing
>
> **Predictive validity:** a form of criterion-based validity in which an inferred interpretation is justified by comparing a measurement with supporting evidence that is obtained at a later point in time; examines the justification of using a measurement to say something about future events or conditions
>
> **Prescriptive validity:** a form of criterion-based validity in which the inferred interpretation of a measurement is the determination of the form of treatment a person is to receive; prescriptive validity is justified based on the successful outcome of the chosen treatment

$$\text{Sensitivity} = \frac{TP}{TP + FN} \times 100$$

$$\text{Relative Risk} = \frac{\dfrac{TP}{TP + FP}}{\dfrac{FN}{TN + FN}}$$

$$\text{Specificity} = \frac{TN}{FP + TN} \times 100$$

$$\begin{array}{l}\text{Predictive Value of} = \dfrac{TP}{TP + FP} \times 100 \\ \text{Abnormal Test}\end{array}$$

TP = true-positives or those with abnormal test and disease; FN = false-negatives or those with normal test and disease; TN = true-negatives or those with normal test and no disease; FP = false-positives or those with abnormal test and no disease. Predictive value of an abnormal response is the percentage of individuals with an abnormal test who are sick. Relative risk, or risk ratio, is the relative occurrence of a disease in the group with an abnormal test compared with those with a normal test.

From Froelicher, VF and Marcondes, GD. Manual of Exercise Testing. Mosby-Yearbook, St Louis, MO; 1989:97, with permission.

STANDARDS FOR TESTS
AND MEASUREMENTS IN PHYSICAL
THERAPY PRACTICE

Standards for Test Users (Indicated with a U)

The following terms are from the American Physical Therapy Association's (APTA's) Standards for Tests and Measurements in Physical Therapy Practice. Phys Ther. 71:589–622, 1991. For more information, see Rothstein, JM and Echternach, JL: Primer on Measurement: An Introductory Guide to Measurement Issues. APTA, Alexandria, Virginia, 1993.

The Standards in this section describe requirements for test users. The following is the definition of a test user.

Test user: one who chooses tests, interprets test scores, or makes decisions based on test scores (this definition is from *Standards for Educational and Psychological Tests.* American Psychological Association, Washington, DC, 1974, p 1)

Organization of the Standards for Test Users: Four basic types of Standards are found in the Standards for Test Users. The Standards listed first detail the general knowledge that a test user must have. The majority of the Standards in this section deal with specific requirements that a user should consider when performing specific tests. These Standards include issues relating to the choice of tests, the performance of testing, observing the rights of test takers, and the use of obtained measurements. The last two Standards, U44 and U45, describe the requirements test users should observe in interpreting and reporting test results.

9

Continued on following page

U1. Persons should not become test users unless they are prepared to adhere to the Standards and understand the requirements for test purveyors.

U2. Test users must have a basic understanding of local, state, and federal laws governing the use of tests in their practice settings.

U34. Test users must have a basic knowledge of the theory and principles of tests and measurements.

U3.1. Test users must understand what constitutes a measurement, what constitutes a test, and the role of instruments in obtaining measurements.

U3.2. Test users must understand the differences between clinical opinions (impressions) that are not based on valid measurements and inferences that are based on the use of valid measurements.

U3.3. Test users must understand what constitutes an operational definition and the importance of using operational definitions.

U3.4. Test users must understand the different levels of measurement (i.e., nominal, ordinal, interval, and ratio) and the mathematical operations that are appropriate for each level.

U3.5. Test users must understand types of validity and how these types of validity relate to the use of measurements.

U3.6. Test users must understand types of reliability and validity and how these qualities relate to clinical decisions and other uses of measurements.

U3.7. Test users must have a basic understanding of the methods used to assess reliability and validity (e.g., statistics and research designs).

U3.8. Test users must understand the relationship between reliability and validity and the differences between the two qualities.

U3.9. Test users must understand what constitutes meaningful normative data and how such data can be used.

U3.10. Test users must understand the differences between objective measurements and subjective measurements and the implications of using each type of measurement.

U3.11. Test users must understand the meaning and use of the terms *false-negatives, false-positives, true-negatives, true-positives, predictive value of a measurement, specificity of a test,* and *sensitivity of a test.*

U3.12. Test users must understand the importance of knowing the technical specifications of instruments.

U3.13. Test users must understand the importance of calibrating instruments.

U3.14. Test users must have a basic understanding of the methods and effects of normalizing or standardizing measurements.

U3.15. Test users must understand the meaning and implications of reactivity to tests.

U4. Test users must have background knowledge in basic, applied, and clinical sciences related to the selection, administration, and interpretation of each test they use.

U5. Test users must understand the theoretical bases (construct and content validity) for the tests they use, and they must have knowledge about the attribute (characteristic) being measured.

U6. Test users must be familiar with the development of tests that they use and the test settings in which those tests have been developed and used.

U7. Test users must understand how a test they are using relates to similar tests or previous versions of the same test.

U8. Test users must be able to justify the selection of tests they use. Test users must also be prepared to supply logical arguments to justify the rejection of tests they choose not to use.

> **U8.1.** Test users must consider the safety of subjects in selecting tests and should consider the benefits to be obtained from a test in view of potential risks to the subject.

> **U8.2.** Test users should consider the practicality of the test (e.g., personnel, time, equipment, cost of administration, and impact on the person taking the test) in selecting tests and in planning examination procedures.

U9. Test users must be able to identify their sources of information regarding tests they use. Test users must be able to specify where they obtained information (e.g., rationale and directions) for selecting and conducting a test.

> **U9.1.** Test users should not cite a test manual as a source of information unless they have personally examined a complete copy of the test manual. Test users should not conduct tests unless they have examined all relevant sections of a complete copy of the test manual.

U10. Test users must understand all operational definitions related to tests they use.

> **U10.1.** Test users must understand the operational definitions for attributes that the test measures.

> **U10.2.** Test users must understand the operational definitions for terms used to describe the population for whom the test is intended.

> **U10.3.** Test users must understand the operational definitions for terms to describe potential test users.

> **U10.4.** Test users must understand the operational definitions for terms used to describe components of the test or test instruments.

> **U10.5.** Test users must understand the operational definitions for any terms created by purveyors of the test.

Continued on following page

U10.6. Test users must be able to identify and understand the operational definitions for any terms used in a noncustomary matter.

U11. Test users must be able to describe the population for whom the test was designed. Test users must be able to relate this description to the persons they are testing.

U12. Test users must be able to determine before they use a test whether they have the ability to administer that test. The determination should be based on an understanding of the test user's own skills and knowledge (competency) as compared with the competencies described by the test purveyor.

U12.1. Test users must be able to describe the potential consequences of administering a test that they do not have the skills or knowledge to administer.

U12.2. Test users who have doubts about their ability to administer a test should report this information when they report test results (e.g., their reservations about the quality of their measurements should be discussed).

U13. Test users must follow instructions provided by purveyors for all tests they administer.

U13.1. Test users must understand instructions for administering all tests that they use. Test users must be able to describe all of the equipment and activities needed for obtaining, recording, and interpreting the measurements. Test users must be able to identify the source of the instructions.

U13.2. Test users who deviate from accepted directions for obtaining a measurement should not use published data or documentation relative to reliability and validity to justify their use of the measurement.

U14. Test users must know what information and instructions are to be given to the person being tested. Test users should be able to answer questions about the test and related subjects.

U14.1. Test users who do not give the purveyor's specified instructions to persons being tested, or test users who are unable to give these instructions, should not use published data or documentation relative to reliability and validity to justify their use of the measurements.

U15. Test users must know the physical settings in which the test should be given and the possible effects of conducting the test in other settings.

U16. Test users must be able to identify any conditions or behaviors in the person being tested that may compromise the reliability or validity of their measurements (e.g., if modified position must be used in manual muscle testing because of a deformity). Test users who observe such conditions or behaviors should note these observations in their reports of any resultant measurements. Test users who believe that the effect on their measurements could be significant should include a discussion of the implications of these observations in their reports.

U17. Test users must have a basic understanding of the instruments they use as part of a test.

U17.1. Test users must know relevant technical information regarding performance characteristics of any machines, recording devices, transducers, computer interfaces, and similar instruments they use. Test users should be able to identify the source of this information. If this information is not available, the test user must be able to discuss the implications and limitations of using such instruments.

U17.2. Test users must be able to describe how instruments they use to manipulate or process information in order to obtain measurements. Test users should identify the source of this information. If this information is not available, the test user must be able to discuss the implications and limitations of using such instruments.

U18. Test users must know how to use any instruments required to obtain the desired measurements. This Standard includes, where appropriate, the test user knowing how to choose machine settings and other user-selected options. Test users must be able to discuss the effects of all options on their measurements and the consequences of selecting the incorrect options.

U19. Test users must be able to describe how instruments they use for a test are calibrated, including the means of testing calibration. Tests users must know the course of action to be taken when calibration is needed.

U20. Test users, for all the tests they use, should be able to describe variations in the test procedures that are available. Test users must be able to describe variations that are known not to impair the quality of the measurements and those variations that are known to lead to measurements of questionable validity.

U21. Test users who deviate from accepted directions for obtaining a measurement should not use published data or documentation relative to reliability and validity to justify their use of the measurement.

U21.1. Test users who administer tests in settings other than those recommended by the purveyor should not use published data or documentation relative to reliability and validity to justify their use of the measurement.

U22. Test users have a responsibility to suggest further testing when they have serious concerns about the quality of the measurements they obtain or when they believe that other tests or other personnel can be used to obtain better measurements.

U23. Test users who are required to derive or transform measurements must have sufficient training and knowledge to derive or transform those measurements. Test users must have the background information and skills needed to derive measure-

Continued on following page

ments or make categorizations necessary for interpretation of their measurements (e.g., how to normalize or standardize a score or how to classify a measurement).

U24. Test users must be aware of any normative data for the measurements they are obtaining (see Standard U44.3 for guidelines on using normative data to interpret measurements; see Standard U45.10 for guidelines on reporting measurements related to normative data). Test users should be able to evaluate critically normative data and use the data for clinical decision making.

U25. Test users must make every effort to control the environment (test setting) in which they test in order to maintain consistent conditions between tests. These efforts are needed to ensure that the validity and reliability of a measurement are not compromised.

U26. Test users must make every effort when personal information is being obtained to control the environment (test setting) in which they administer tests in order to preserve the privacy of the person taking the test.

U27. Test users must be able to discuss common errors in the interpretation of the measurements they use.

U28. Test users must make every effort to minimize the effects of reactivity associated with the tests they use.

U29. Test users should report to the purveyor of the test any problems regarding a test or any associated instruments.

U30. Test users should communicate with other test users and purveyors regarding their experiences with tests.

U31. Test users must avoid getting persons prior knowledge about the nature of a test when such knowledge is known to compromise the validity of the measurements.

U32. Test users are responsible for maintaining confidentiality of test results. Confidentiality of results should be in accordance with standard practices in the institution or community in which the test user obtains the measurements. Results should not be shared with any persons (or organizations) who are known to be unwilling to report the right of confidentiality of the person who was tested.

U33. Test users should not share results of tests with persons (or organizations) who are likely to misuse that information.

U34. Test users must respect the rights of persons whom they test.

    U34.1. Test users must respect the right of persons to refuse to be tested. Test users must allow persons to discontinue participation in any test at any time without recrimination or prejudice against that person.

    U34.2. Test users must inform persons whom they test of potential risk and benefits that persons may experience as a result of taking the test.

    U34.3. Test users must respect the right of persons being tested to know the results of tests, the interpretations of those test results, and with whom the test results will be shared. The right of the person to know the results of tests does not imply that all test users must personally supply this information. In some cases, test results may be supplied by the professional who originated a referral or who is coordinating treatment.

U34.4. Test users who fail to adhere to the Standards and who use tests inappropriately, especially in terms of drawing unwarranted conclusions from results, violate the rights of persons being tested.

U34.4.1. Test users who misrepresent their clinical opinions as being based on test results when evidence for such opinions is not found in the research literature violate the rights of persons taking tests. (For example: A test user may use a battery of tests to determine the ability of a patient with low back pain to function in an industrial environment. In this hypothetical example, the test battery yields a measurement that is supposed to predict the type of work that the patient may do safely. There is, in this example, evidence for the validity of this inference. However, based on this test user's observations, the test user concludes that the patient is malingering. This is the test user's clinical opinion; it is not based on the validated use of the measurement. The test user does not violate the rights of the person taking the test by having or presenting clinical opinions, but would violate the person's rights by contending that the measurement could be used to infer malingering.)

U35. Test users must maintain records in such a manner that information about tests and measurements is accurate and is not likely to be distorted or lost. Abbreviations used in communications should be limited to those that appear in established references.

U36. Test users have a responsibility to report inappropriate test use to proper authorities.

U36.1. Test users who know that a person's rights are not being observed during testing must make every effort to change that situation.

U37. Test users should select tests based on what is best for the person being tested. Test selection based on considerations of personal benefit to the test user, test purveyor, or the referring practitioner is inappropriate.

U38. Test users, in clinical practice, should avoid the use of tests that were designed solely for research purposes. Such tests, when they are used in the clinical setting, should be identified
Continued on following page

in all reports as research tests that have not necessarily been shown to be reliable or valid in clinical use.

U39. Test users should not assign persons to conduct tests unless they know that such persons are qualified to conduct the tests.

U40. Test users should not make promotional claims for their testing procedures that are not supported by research literature.

> **U40.1.** Test users are responsible for the critical evaluation of all claims of test purveyors and should not merely repeat the claims of purveyors without critical evaluation of these claims.

U41. Test users should assist in the development and refinement of testing procedures by sharing their knowledge of tests and assisting in the collection of data where appropriate.

U42. Test users have a responsibility to periodically review the test procedures they and their colleagues use in their institutions (practice settings) to ensure that appropriate use of measurements is being made and that the rights of persons tested are being observed.

> **U42.1.** Test users, as part of their periodic review of test procedures, should examine whether the normative data they are using appear to relate to their clinical setting.

> **U42.2.** Test users, as part of their periodic review of test procedures, should attempt to estimate the reliability of measurements in their practice settings. All forms of reliability relevant to the practice settings should be assessed.

U43. Test users who use tests that do not meet the Standards should be aware that these tests do not meet the Standards. Test users, therefore, should interpret results of these tests with caution and share these reservations with all persons who receive test results.

U44. Test users must follow the basic rules and principles of measurement when they interpret results of tests they use. (The following Standards provide guidelines for interpreting measurements. These Standards are not meant to supersede or in any way modify the requirements specified elsewhere in the Standards for Test Users.)

> **U44.1.** Test users must limit their interpretations of measurements to the inferences for which those measurements have been shown to be valid.

> **U44.2.** Test users must consider the error associated with their measurements when they interpret their test results. Reliability and validity estimates should be considered when the test user makes interpretations of measurements. (For example: Reliability studies have indicated that a measurement varies as much as 10% between repeated tests. Therefore, a change of less than 10% on that measurement may be due, at least in part, to measurement error. Test users who note changes the second time they take measurements should consider, before they make in-

terpretations, that the change may not reflect real change, but may be due solely to measurement error.)

U44.3. Test users must consider whether normative data are available for the measurements they interpret. Test users must consider the sources of the normative data and how applicable these data are to the measurements they are interpreting.

U44.3.1. Test users should use all available information when using normative data for interpretations of measurements.

U44.3.1.1. Test users using normative data should interpret any measurement that is interval or ratio scaled in terms of how that measurement relates to measures of central tendency, measures of variability, and percentiles.

U44.3.1.2. Test users using normative data should interpret any measurement that is nominal or ordinal scaled in terms of the proportion of persons in the population that can be expected to belong to the same classification.

U44.4. Test users must consider the limitations of their measurements when they classify persons into diagnostic groups based on the presence or absence of a finding (e.g., use of cut scores or tests to determine a positive or negative finding). Test users should use all available data in making their interpretations.

U44.4.1. Test users must consider the percentages of false-positives and false-negatives for a diagnostic test when interpreting measurements. If this information is not available, test users should understand the limitations of making interpretations based on their measurements.

U44.4.2. Test users must consider the sensitivity of the diagnostic test they are using when they interpret their measurements. If this information is not available, test users should understand the limitations of making interpretations based on their measurements.

U44.4.3. Test users must consider the specificity of the diagnostic test they are using when they interpret their measurements. If this information is not available, test users should understand the limitations of making interpretations based on their measurements.

U44.4.4. Test users consider the predictive values of positive and negative findings when they inter-

Continued on following page

pret their measurements obtained with a diagnostic test. If this information is not available, test users should understand the limitations of making interpretations based on their measurements.

U44.5. Test users must avoid overinterpreting the results of their tests. Test users are responsible for understanding both the certainty and the uncertainty with which they can make judgments based on their measurements.

U44.6. Test users must consider whether changes (e.g., attributable to development or learning) in the person being tested may alter performance on subsequent tests. Test users, when appropriate, should discuss in their reports of test results the possibility of change in the future. Test users should not imply that a test result represents an immutable state when there is a reason to believe that the test result may differ if the test is repeated at some future time.

U44.7. Test users must consider the conditions under which they conduct tests and the extent to which results are generalizable to other test situations (e.g., testing in other places or at other times).

U44.8. Test users must identify whether their interpretations are based on the results of multiple measurements obtained with the same test or on the results of a single measurement.

U44.9. Test users must identify whether any of their interpretations are not supported by research evidence of validity. Such interpretations must be clearly identified as being based on the test user's personal opinion.

U45. Test users reporting the results of tests must supply adequate information so that these results can be understood. (The following Standards provide guidelines for reporting about measurements. These Standards are not meant to supersede or in any way modify the requirements specified elsewhere in the Standards for Test Users.)

U45.1. Test users should specify, when more than one form of a test exists, the specific form of the test used when they report their results.

U45.2. Test users should report measurements in the form specified by the purveyor's instructions. Test users should justify any deviations from standard methods of reporting.

U45.3. Test users should use only the terms that are defined in test manuals or in other supporting literature when they discuss tests or measurements. Descriptive terms that are not defined should be avoided, because such terms may encourage inappropriate interpretation of results.

U45.4. Test users, in reporting test results, should use terms in a customary manner or describe how terms are being used differently. Test users should justify deviations from commonly accepted uses of terms in their reports.

U45.5. Test users must consider estimates of reliability and validity when reporting test results. Test users should report estimates of the errors associated with a measurement when they report test results. (For example: Reliability studies have indicated that a measurement varies as much as 10% between repeated measurements. Therefore, a change of less than 10% may be due, at least in part, to measurement error. Test users who note changes the second time they take measurements, in reporting such measurements, should also report that the change in the measurement may not reflect real change. The change may be solely due to measurement error. A report of the reliability estimate or standard error, in this case, would be useful in the test user's report.)

U45.6. Test users should include warnings about common misinterpretations of their measurements in reports of their measurements.

U45.7. Test users should report any significant effects of reactivity when they report the results of their tests.

U45.8. Test users who use a variation of a test must indicate, when they report test results, that a variation was used. The test users must note whether they believe that the variation may have affected the quality of their measurements. Test users who believe the variation had a significant effect on the measurements should discuss this belief in all reports of test results.

U45.9. Test users should report any aspect of the test that may cast doubt on test results (e.g., ways in which the person tested differed from the population for which the test was designed or any observation the test user made during testing).

U45.10. Test users, in reports of test results, should relate their measurements to normative data, if available. Test users should report the source of the normative data they use and, if necessary, discuss how applicable the data are to the measurements they are reporting (see Standard U44.3 for guidelines on using normative data to interpret measurements).

U45.10.1. Test users using normative data, when they report test results, should report all information necessary to understand the test user's interpretation of the measurements.

U45.10.1.1. Test users using normative data for measurements that are interval or ratio scaled should report

Continued on following page

9

their test results in terms of how the measurements relate to measures of central tendency, measures of validity, and percentiles.

U45.10.1.2. Test users who report classifications in their test results should also report the proportion of persons in the population who can be expected to belong to that classification. The test user, if requested, should be able to cite the source of the data used to determine the proportions.

U45.11. Test users reporting the results of their tests should indicate whether any data were transformed (normalized or standardized). Test users, in their reports, should justify the use of transformations, if this is not customary practice.

U45.12. Test users who base their interpretations of test results on the mean of multiple measurements should note this fact in their reports of test results. Test users should justify the use of the mean of multiple measurements in clinical reports, if this is not customary practice.

U45.13. Test users who base their interpretations on a single measurement chosen from a group of measurements (e.g., the best of three trials) should note this fact when they report test results. Test users, in their reports, should justify the use of the single measurement and the criteria used to select the measurement, if this is not customary practice.

U45.14. Test users who base their interpretations on the results of a variety of tests should note this fact when they discuss their measurements. Test users should justify their selection of the tests in reporting test results.

U45.15. Test users should note in their reports of test results the specific criteria they use for clinical decisions. When a specific measurement (e.g., cut score) is used for a clinical decision, the test user, in all reports, should justify the use of that specific measurement.

OUTCOME INSTRUMENTS: LISTED ALPHABETICALLY
(Including Those That Measure Impairments and Disabilities)

Test	Description	For More Information	Examines
Action Research Arm Test	Used to determine level of functional recover of the upper extremity after a CVA. Four subscales examine the ability to grasp, grip, pinch, and perform gross motor tasks.	Caroll, D, et al: A quantitative test of upper extremity function. Journal of Chron Disease 18:479–491, 1965.	Upper extremity function after a CVA
Alberta Infant Motor Scale (AIMS)	Used to examine delays in the development of motor performance. The scale consists of 58 items examining motor performance in four positions: prone, supine, sitting, and standing.	Piper MC, et al: Construction and validation of the Alberta Infant Motor Scale (AIMS). Can J Public Health 83:46–50, 1992.	Impairments
Barthel Index	Used to measure functional independence and is derived from scoring the following activities: feeding, wheelchair transfer, self-bathing, dressing, sphincter control, stairway navigation, toileting, personal hygiene, ambulation, and wheelchair propulsion.	Mahoney, FI, and Barthel, DW: Functional evaluation: The Barthel Index. Maryland State Medical Journal 14:62–65, 1965.	Disability

Continued on following page

9

OUTCOME INSTRUMENTS: LISTED ALPHABETICALLY (Continued)

Test	Description	For More Information	Examines
Bayley Scales of Infant Development	Used to examine motor and mental development in children from birth to 30 months of age. (Bayley II has been expanded to permit assessment of children up to 42 months). There is a mental scale and a psychomotor scale.	(For the Bayley II: Bayley, N: Bayley II. Psychological Corporation, San Antonio, TX, 1993.) Palisano, RJ: Concurrent and predictive validities of the Bayley Motor Scale and the Peabody Developmental Motor Scales. Phys Ther 66:1714–1719, 1986.	Impairments
Berg Balance Scale	Used to examine a person's ability to maintain posture or to control movement during 14 conditions that represent successively smaller bases of support. Conditions include sitting, standing, and single-leg stance.	Berg, KO, et al: Measuring balance with the elderly: Validation of an instrument. Can J Public Health 1992, (suppl) 83:7–11.	Balance
Bruininks-Oseretsky Test of Motor Proficiency (BOTMP)	Used to examine gross and fine motor skills in children 4.5 to 14.5 years of age. There are 46 items in eight subtests. The subtests for gross motor performance examine running speed, balance, bilateral coordination, and strength. The subtests for fine motor performance examine response speed, visual-motor control, upper limb speed and	Krus, PH, and Bruininks, RH: Structure of motor abilities in children. Percept Mot Skills 52:119–129, 1981. Spiegel, AN, et al: The early motor profile: Correlation with the Bruininks-Oseretsky Test of Motor Performance. Percept Mot Skills 1990;71:645–646.	Impairments

	dexterity, and upper limb coordination.		
Canadian Neurological Scale (CNS)	Used to determine neurologic status during the acute phase after a CVA. Subscales examine mentation, motor function, and motor response.	Cote, R, et al: The Canadian Neurological Scale: Validation and reliability assessment. Neurology 39:638–643, 1989.	Post CVA Neurological Status
Chedoke-McMaster Stroke Assessment	Used to examine both impairments and disabilities in persons who have had CVAs. The impairment inventory has six subscales to measure recovery of postural control; control of the arm, hand, leg, and foot; and shoulder pain. There are two disability subscales one examines gross motor function and the other walking. Classification of recovery is based primarily on the stages described by Brunnstrom, and the system was designed to be used with the Uniform Data System for Medical Rehabilitation (UDS).	Gowland, C, et al: Measuring physical impairment and disability with the Chedoke-McMaster Assessment. Stroke 24:58–63, 1993.	Impairments and disabilities

Continued on following page

9

OUTCOME INSTRUMENTS: LISTED ALPHABETICALLY (Continued)

Test	Description	For More Information	Examines
Chronic Respiratory Disease Questionnaire (CRQ)	Used to examine the quality of life in persons with chronic lung disease via a self-administered questionnaire dealing with dyspnea, fatigue, and emotional function, and how well individuals cope with their illnesses.	Guyatt, G, et al: A measure of quality of life for clinical trials in chronic lung disease. Thorax 42:773–778, 1987.	Quality of life
Clinical Outcome Variable Scale (COVS)	Used to examine physical mobility by using measures from the Patient Evaluation Conference System (PECS). Four items were added from the Canadian Physiotherapy Association's Health Status Rating Scale.	Seaby, L, et al: Reliability of a physiotherapy functional assessment used in a rehabilitation setting. Physiotherapy Canada 41:264–271, 1989.	Mobility
Dual Inclinometer Method of Measuring Spinal Mobility	Two inclinometers are used to measure motion of the lower back while hip motion is eliminated from the measurement. Motion can be measured in flexion and in extension.	Mayer, TG, et al: Use of noninvasive techniques for quantification of spinal range of motion in normal subjects and chronic low back dysfunction. Spine 9:588–595, 1984.	Spinal mobility
Emory Motor Test	Used to examine speed of movement using 21 timed upper extremity movements that progress from single-joint motions to complete limb motions for functional tasks. Applicable to patients with traumatic brain injury and CVAs.	Taub, E, et al: Technique to improve chronic motor deficit after stroke. Arch Phys Med Rehabil 74:347–354, 1993.	Recovery after cerebral injury

Fugl-Meyer Assessment of Sensorimotor Recovery After Stroke	Used to evaluate upper and lower extremity motor function, balance, pain, and range of motion in patients after CVAs. The test requires judgment on quality of movements and is based on the degree of independence.	Fugl-Meyer, AR. Post-stroke hemiplegia assessment of physical properties. Scand J Rehabil Med 7:85–93, 1980.	Recovery after CVA
Functional Independence Measure (FIM)	Used to determine outcomes for persons undergoing rehabilitation. Part of the UDS, the FIM is used to examine the degree of dependence in performing 23 items in the following areas: mobility, locomotion, communication, self-care, cognition, social adjustment, and sphincter control.	Hamilton, B, et al: A uniform national data system for medical rehabilitation. In Fuhrer, MJ (ed): Rehabilitation Outcomes: Analysis and Measurement. Paul H. Brooks, Baltimore, MD, 1987, pp 137–147. Keith, RA, et al: The Functional Independence Measure. Advances in Clinical Rehabilitation 1:6–18, 1987.	Functional independence
Functional Reach Test	Used to assess the ability to reach forward along a sagitally placed ruler without the subject's feet moving. The test is used to characterize balance abilities.	Duncan, PW, et al: Functional Reach: a new clinical measure of balance. J Gerontology 45:M192–M197, 1990.	Balance

Continued on following page

9

OUTCOME INSTRUMENTS: LISTED ALPHABETICALLY (Continued)

Test	Description	For More Information	Examines
Gross Motor Function Measure (GMFM)	Used to examine change over time in gross motor function in children with cerebral palsy who perform at a level up to that expected of a 5 year old. The test consists of 88 items tested with the child lying and rolling to supine, crawling, and kneeling, sitting, standing, walking, running, and jumping.	Russell, D, et al: The Gross Motor Function Measure: A means to evaluate the effects of physical therapy. Dev Med Child Neurol 31:341–351, 1989.	Impairments
Gross Motor Performance Measure (GMPM)	Used to examine the quality of movement in children with cerebral palsy and was designed to be used with GMFM. The test consists of 20 items that evaluate alignment of the body in space, coordination, ability to isolate movements (dissociated movements), ability to maintain postures (stability), and weight shifting.	Boyce, W, et al. Gross Motor Performance Measure for children with cerebral palsy: Study design and preliminary findings. Can J Public Health 1992, (suppl) 83: S34–S40.	
Harris Infant Neuromotor Test (HINT)	The HINT is a 20-minute screening tool designed to detect early signs of cognitive or neuromotor delays in at-risk infants, ranging in age from	Harris, SR: Content validity of the Harris Infant Neuromotor Test. Phys Ther 76:727–737, 1996. Harris, SR: Parents' and care givers'	Developmental status

	perception of their children's development. Dev Med Child Neurol 36:918–923, 1994.	
Inclinometer Method of Measuring Spinal Mobility	3–12 months. Intended for use by physical therapists, occupational therapists, family physicians, pediatricians, or community health nurses, the HINT manual is in the development stages and available for use as of 1997. Used to measure spinal motion through the placement of an inclinometer on the segment of the spine being measured.	Loebl, WY: Measurement of spinal posture and spinal movement. Annals of Physical Medicine 9:104–110, 1967.	Spinal mobility
Katz ADL Index	Used to characterize the degree of dependence on an 8-point ordinal scale for each of six areas: bathing, dressing, toileting, transfers, feeding, and continence. Different members of an interdisciplinary contribute scores. It has been applied primarily to the elderly, but it has also been used to assess children. The index is not disease specific and has been used on patients with a variety of diagnoses.	Katz, S, et al: Progress in the development of the Index of ADL. Gerontologist 10:20–30, 1970. Staff of the Benjamin Rose Hospital: Multi disciplinary studies of illness in aged persons. II. A new classification of functional status in activities of daily living. Journal of Chronic Disease 9:55–62, 1959.	ADL

Continued on following page

9

OUTCOME INSTRUMENTS: LISTED ALPHABETICALLY (Continued)

Test	Description	For More Information	Examines
Kenny Self-Care Evaluation	Use to measure ADL for the purposes of setting goals and monitoring a patient's overall progress in improving ADL skills. The following categories are examined by scoring 85 tasks: bed activities, transfers, locomotion, dressing, personal hygiene, bowel and bladder function, and feeding.	Donaldson, SW, et al: A unified ADL evaluation form. Arch Phys Med Rehabil 54:175–179, 1973. Kerner, JF, et al: Activities of daily living: Reliability and validity of gross vs specific ratings. Arch Phys Med Rehabil 62:161–166, 1981.	ADL
Klein-Bell Activities of Daily Living Scale	Used to assess ADL of adults with disability due to any cause. Six subscales consisting of 170 items examine dressing, mobility, elimination, bathing/hygiene, eating and emergency communication.	Klein, RM, and Bell, B. Self-care skills: Behavioral measurement with Klein-Bell ADL Scale. Arch Phys Med Rehabil 63:335–338, 1982.	ADL
Level of Rehabilitation Scale (LORS-II)	Used by interdisciplinary teams to assess ADL, mobility, and communication. Developed to meet criteria set forth by the Commission on Accreditation of Rehabilitation Facilities. Nurses, physical therapists, occupational therapists, and speech therapists contribute to	Carey, RG, and Posovac, EJ: Rehabilitation program evaluation using a revised level of rehabilitation scale (LORS-II). Arch Phys Med Rehabil 63:367–370, 1982. Velozo, CA, et al: Functional scale discrimination at admission and	ADL

	the scoring. The scoring criteria are based on degree of independence; the higher the score the more independent the person.	discharge: Rasch analysis of the Level of Rehabilitation Scale-III. Arch Phys Med Rehabil 76:705–712, 1995.	
Modified Schöber Method for Measuring Spinal Mobility	See Schöber Method for Measuring Spinal Mobility (Modified)		
Motor Assessment Scale (MAS)	Used to determine level of motor recovery after CVAs. The scale evaluates eight types of movement and includes an additional test for muscle tone.	Carr, JH, et al: Investigation of a new motor assessment scale for stroke patients. Phys Ther 65:175–178, 1985.	Motor recovery
Movement Assessment of Infants (MAI)	Used to screen and evaluate the motor status of high risk infants from birth to 12 months of age (adjusted to date of conception). The test examines 65 items dealing with muscle tone, primitive reflexes, automatic reactions, and volitional movements.	Piper, MC, et al: Early developmental screening: Sensitivity and specificity of chronological and adjusted scores. Dev Behavioral Pediatrics 13:95–101, 1992.\nWashington, K, and Dietz, J: Performance of full-term six months old infants on the Movement Assessment of Infants. Pediatric Physical Therapy 7:65–74, 1995.	Impairments

Continued on following page

9

OUTCOME INSTRUMENTS: LISTED ALPHABETICALLY (Continued)

Test	Description	For More Information	Examines
Oswestry Low Back Pain Disability Questionnaire	Used to measure a patient's perceived disability due to low back pain based on 10 areas of limitation in performance. These include pain, personal care, lifting, walking, sitting, standing, sleeping, sex life, social life, and traveling.	Fairbank, JCT, et al: The Oswestry Low Back Pain Disability Questionnaire. Physiotherapy 66:271–273, 1980.	Low back disability
Patient Evaluation Conference System (PECS)	Used to detect small changes in function in persons undergoing rehabilitation. This 79-item test is divided into 14 subscales reflecting various components of the rehabilitation process. Each subscale is scored by the rehabilitation professional responsible for that area of care.	Harvey, RF, et al: Functional performance assessment: A program approach. Arch Phys Med Rehabil 62:456–461, 1981. Korner-Bitensky, N, et al: Motor and functional recovery after stroke: Accuracy of physical therapists' predictions. Arch Phys Med Rehabil 70:95–99, 1989.	Changes in function
Peabody Developmental Motor Scale	Used to examine gross motor (including reflexes) and fine motor skills in children from birth to 83 months of age.	Palisano, RJ: Concurrent and predictive validities of the Bayley Motor Scale and the Peabody Developmental Motor Scales. Phys Ther 66:1714–1719, 1986. Stokes, NA, et al: The Peabody developmental fine motor scale: An interrater reliability study. Am J Occup Ther 44:334–340, 2990.	Impairments

Pediatric Evaluation of Disability Inventory (PEDI)	Used to examine the functional performance of children between the ages of 6 months and 7 years, as well as the level of caregiver assistance needed by the child.	Feldman, AB, et al: Concurrent and construct validity of the Pediatric Evaluation of Disability Inventory. Phys Ther 70:602–610, 1990.	Disability and functional limitations
PULSES Profile	Used to determine the level of function in chronically ill institutionalized persons. Six subscales assess physical condition, upper limb functions, lower limb functions, sensory components (sight and communication), excretory functions, and support factors (including those based on patient performance and family and financial support).	Granger, CV, et al: Functional status measurement and medical rehabilitation outcomes. Arch Phys Med Rehabil 57:103–109, 1976. Granger, CV, et al: Outcome of comprehensive medical rehabilitation: Measurement by PULSES profile and Barthel Index. Arch Phys Med Rehabil 60:145–154, 1979.	Function in institutionalized persons
Rivermead Mobility Index	Used to examine mobility in a functional context for patients with neurologic conditions.	Collen, FM, et al: The Rivermead Mobility Index: A Further Development of the Rivermead Motor Assessment. International Disabilities Studies 13:50–54, 1991.	Functional mobility

Continued on following page

9

OUTCOME INSTRUMENTS: LISTED ALPHABETICALLY (Continued)

Test	Description	For More Information	Examines
Roland and Morris Disability Questionnaire	Used as a "disability index" for low back pain by adding the with the phrase Sickness Impact Profile "because of my back" to statements from the SIP	Roland, M, and Morris R: A study of the natural history of back pain. Development of a reliable and sensitive measure of disability in low-back pain. Spine 8:141–144, 1983.	Low back disability
Schöber Method for Measuring Spinal Mobility (Modified)	Used to assess spinal mobility by measuring the increase between the two marks on the low back (to assess flexion).	Macrae, IF, and Wright, V: Measurement of back movement. Ann Rheum Diseases 28:584–589, 1969.	Spinal mobility
Self-Paced Walking Test	Used to estimate maximal oxygen uptake by having patients walk 128 M at three self-selected paces (slow, normal, and fast). Measures of speed and heart rate are then used to estimate maximal oxygen uptake.	Bassey, EJ, et al: Self-paced walking as a method of exercise testing in elderly and young men. Clinical Science and Molecular Medicine 51:609–612, 1976.	Impairment

Short-form Health Survey (SF-36)	Used to examine a person's perceptions of health status. The survey is designed for use in a variety of settings as a non–disease-specific instrument. It contains 36 items that assess eight health concepts, including perceived limitations in physical, social, and usual role activities; pain; mental health; and well-being.	Brazier, JE, et al: Validating the SF-36 health survey questionnaire: New outcome measure for primary care. BMJ 305:160–164, 1992. Ware, JE, and Sherbourne, CD: The MOS 36-item short-form health survey (SF-36). I. Conceptual framework and item selection. Med Care 30:473–481, 1992.	Perceived health status
Sickness Inventory Profile (SIP)	Used to examine a person's perceived health-related behaviors, providing a non–disease-specific measure of disease-related dysfunction. The SIP assesses 12 categories of activities: sleep and rest, eating, work, home management, recreation, ambulatory mobility, body care and movement, social interaction, alertness, emotional behavior, and communication.	Bergner, M, et al: The sickness impact profile: Development and final revision of a health status measure. Med Care 19:787–805, 1981.	Perceived health status

Continued on following page

9

OUTCOME INSTRUMENTS: LISTED ALPHABETICALLY (Continued)

Test	Description	For More Information	Examines
Six-Minute Walking Test	Derived from the 12-minute walking test, this instrument is used to estimate maximal oxygen uptake for persons with disabilities. The measure is also widely thought to reflect other variables, such as psychological status and other factors that can influence walking speed and distance.	Butland, RJA, et al: Two-, six-, and 12-minute walking tests in respiratory disease. BMJ 284:1607–1608, 1982. Guyatt GH, et al: How should we measure function in patients with chronic heart and lung disease. Journal of Chron Disease 38:517–524, 1985. Guyatt GH, et al. The 6-minute walk: A new measure of exercise capacity in patients with chronic heart failure. Can Med Assoc J 132:919–923, 1985.	Impairment
Sorensen Test for Endurance of Back Muscles	Used to examine a prone subject's ability to maintain the trunk in a horizontal position when the trunk is not supported.	Biering-Sorensen F: Physical measurements as risk indicators for low-back trouble over a one-year period. Spine 9:106–119, 1984.	Back muscle function
Timed "Up and Go" Test	Used to assess the mobility of frail elderly persons with a variety of diagnoses by timing them as they rise from a chair, stand, walk for 3 M, return and sit.	Mathias, S, et al: Balance in elderly patients: the "get-up and go" test. Arch Phys Med Rehabil 67:387–389, 1986. Podsiadlo, D, et al: The timed "up and go": A test of basic functional	Basic mobility in the frail elderly

			Impairment
Visual Analogue Scale for Dyspnea	Used to examine patients perceptions of how difficult it is to breath by use of either a 100-mm or 30-cm line. Anchoring the low end of the scale are the expressions "minimum shortness of breath" or "not at all breathless." At the high end, the anchors are "maximum breathlessness" or "worst possible breathlessness."	mobility for frail elderly persons. J Am Geriatr Soc 39:142–148, 1991. Muza, SR: Comparison of scales used to quantitate the sense of effort to breath in patients with chronic obstructive pulmonary disease. Am Rev Respir Dis 141:909–913, 1990.	
Visual Analogue Scale for Pain (VAS)	Used to examine patients' perceptions of pain along a 100-mm horizontal line. Anchoring the low end of the scale is the expression "no pain." At the high end of the scale, the anchor is "pain as bad as it could be."	Dixon, JS, and Bird, HA. Reproducibility along a 10 cm. Vertical visual analogue scale. Ann Rheum Dis 40:87–89, 1981.	Pain

ADL = Activities of daily living; CVA = cerebrovascular accident.

9

HYPOTHESIS-ORIENTED ALGORITHM FOR CLINICIANS

In 1986, Rothstein and Echternach published an algorithm for clinical decision making called the hypothesis-oriented algorithm for clinicians (HOAC). The purpose of the algorithm was to provide rehabilitation practitioners with a framework for clinical decision making, self-evaluation, and documentation. A central feature of the algorithm is the idea that all treatments must be based on a conceptual theme, that is, hypotheses as to why patients have problems or may anticipate developing problems. Problems and goals are usually at the level of disability or functional loss, whereas hypothesized causes of problems or disabilities are usually due to impairments or a pathological processes. Another important feature is that it forces clinicians to make explicit assumptions and to describe expectations for change with temporal predictions (e.g., the re-evaluation schedule indicates when the clinician expects changes to occur at levels of impairment and disability).

A unique aspect of the algorithm is the use of criterion measures to test the correctness of all hypotheses (which are usually related to the level of impairments) generated by the clinician. One criterion measure is used for each hypothesis. For example, if a person's inability to walk is hypothesized to be solely due to weakness of the quadriceps muscles, then the criterion measure would be a given level of force that the clinician believes the patient would need. If the patient achieves the criterion and is still unable to walk, then the hypothesis would, at best, have been incomplete or possibly totally incorrect.

The algorithm has two parts. Part One leads clinicians through the process of evaluation, hypothesis generation, and the development of treatment strategies (overall purposes) and tactics (specific treatments). In addition, it provides logical junctures where clinicians may seek and document the need for consultations or referrals. Part Two takes the clinician through the processes of re-evaluation, with concrete items being considered (i.e., implementation of tactics and formulation of strategies) before theoretical issues (i.e., is the hypothesis correct?).

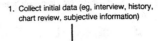

HYPOTHESIS-ORIENTED ALGORITHM FOR CLINICIANS
PART ONE

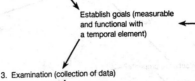

1. Collect initial data (eg, interview, history, chart review, subjective information)

2. Generate a problem statement

Establish goals (measurable and functional with a temporal element)

3. Examination (collection of data)

Referral to other practitioner (if no hypotheses can be generated)

4. Generate working hypotheses about why goals are or cannot be met at the present time (establish testing criteria for each hypothesis)

Ask whether goals are viable
- if no, modify
- if yes, proceed

5. Plan reevaluation methodology (schedule dates for reevaluations)

Consultation, if needed

6. Plan treatment strategy based on hypotheses (overall treatment approach)

7. Plan tactics to implement strategy (specifics of treatment plan)

8. Implement tactics (treatment)

Continued on following page

9

HYPOTHESIS-ORIENTED ALGORITHM FOR CLINICIANS

PART TWO

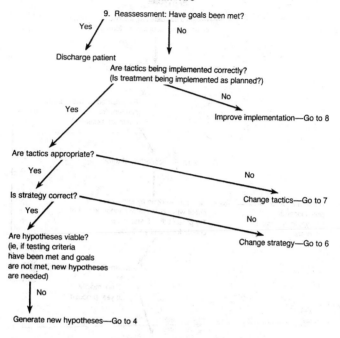

9. Reassessment: Have goals been met?

Yes → Discharge patient

No → Are tactics being implemented correctly? (Is treatment being implemented as planned?)

No → Improve implementation—Go to 8

Yes → Are tactics appropriate?

No → Change tactics—Go to 7

Yes → Is strategy correct?

No → Change strategy—Go to 6

Yes → Are hypotheses viable? (ie, if testing criteria have been met and goals are not met, new hypotheses are needed)

No → Generate new hypotheses—Go to 4

FOR MORE INFORMATION

Echternach JL, and Rothstein JM: Hypothesis-oriented algorithms. Phys Ther 69:559–564, 1989.

Rothstein, JM, and Echternach, JL: Hypothesis-oriented algorithm for clinicians: A method for evaluation and treatment planning. Phys Ther 66:1388–1394, 1986. Reprinted from Physical Therapy with the permission of the APTA.

TYPES OF MUSCLE CONTRACTIONS

When excitation-contraction coupling occurs in skeletal muscle, actinomyosin is formed. The formation of the cross-bridges between the two contractile proteins results in a contraction, that is, the actin filaments being pulled toward the middle of the sarcomere. This is what occurs with all muscle contractions. However, depending on the relationship of the external load (resistance) to the tension generated, there may or may not be sliding of the actin filaments with a resultant decrease in the distance between z lines. Therefore, there is only one type of muscle contraction. However, it has become customary to refer to contraction types based on whether there is shortening of the whole muscle.

Concentric contractions occur when the external load (resistance) is such that when excitation-contraction coupling occurs there is shortening of the sarcomere leading to a decrease in the length of the whole muscle. In practice this means that a limb segment will be moved in the direction of the muscle tension vector.

Isometric contractions occur when the external load (resistance) is such that when excitation-contraction coupling occurs there is shortening of the sarcomere in order to take up any slack in the muscle or connective tissue, but there will be no observable change in the length of the whole muscle. In practice this means that a limb segment will not move.

Eccentric contractions occur when the external load (resistance) is such that when excitation-contraction coupling occurs there is lengthening of the sarcomere leading to an increase in the length of the whole muscle. In practice this means that a limb segment will be moved in the direction opposite the muscle tension vector.

Type of Contraction	Forces	Function	Mechanical Work
Concentric	$M_m > M_r$	Acceleration	Positive ($W = F [+ D]$)
Isometric	$M_m = M_r$	Fixation	Zero (no change in length)
Eccentric	$M_m < M_r$	Deceleration	Negative ($W = F [- D]$)

Force Relationships in Different Types of Muscular Contractions

M_r: Resistance moment. This is due to the weight of the limb segment and any load applied to that segment.

M_m: Rotary moment of the muscular force. This is the rotary component that is resolved from the tensile force created when a muscle contracts.

W = work.
F = force.
D = distance.

Based on forces and using the above notation, the three types of muscle contractions can be described. This table is based in part on Komi, PV: The stretch-shortening cycle and human power output. In Jones, NL, et al (eds): Human Muscle Power. Human Kinetics, Champaign, IL, 1986, pp 27–39.

FOR MORE INFORMATION

Rodgers, MM and Cavanagh, PR: Glossary of biomechanical terms, concepts and units. Phys Ther 64:1886, 1984.

Soderberg, GL: Kinesiology: Application to Pathological Motion. Williams & Wilkins, Baltimore, 1986.

BIOMECHANICAL, KINESIOLOGICAL, KINETIC, AND KINEMATIC TERMS (in alphabetical order)

acceleration: Rate of change in velocity; for translatory motion expressed in distance per second squared, for angular motion expressed in degrees per second squared.

action line: See *force*.

active insufficiency: See *muscle insufficiency*.

agonist muscle: A muscle or group of muscles whose contractions may be considered primarily responsible for causing a movement (see *antagonist muscle*).

antagonist muscle: A muscle that can oppose the action of an agonist (see *agonist muscle*); therefore, for a muscle to be an antagonist, it must be referenced to an agonist.

bending: The result of a load applied to a structure such that movement occurs about an axis, with tension and compression occurring on opposite sides of the material bending.

Blix's curve: See *length-tension curve*.

center of gravity: The center of mass, which is also the point where the resultant force of gravity is said to be acting.

center of mass: Same as center of gravity; see *center of gravity*.

composition of forces: Adding two or more forces to show the single resultant force that is formed.

compression: A load in which collinear forces act in opposite directions so as to push a material together.

concentric contraction: See *muscle contractions*.

concurrent force system: See *force systems*.

creep: Progressive deformation over time of a material, even though the load is constant.

density: Mass per unit volume.

derivatives: The process of deriving one quantity from another by analysis of a curve or a function.

Continued on following page

differentiation: A calculus technique used in kinematics to determine the rate of change of a quantity.

direction of forces: See *force.*

dynamics: The study of bodies in motion and the forces acting on them.

eccentric contraction: See *muscle contractions.*

energy: A fundamental quantity that represents the capacity to do work, expressed in ergs, joules, foot-pounds, or calories.

fatigue: In material science it is the failure of a material due to repetitive loading.

force: The vector quantity that reflects how one body acts on another, that is, attracts, repels, pulls, or pushes. In newtonian terms, force equals mass times acceleration. Units of force are dynes, newtons, or pounds. Force is a vector and is described like any other vector by the following four characteristics:

> **action line:** The path on which the force is acting.
>
> **direction:** Whether the force is attracting or repelling (pushing or pulling).
>
> **magnitude:** Strength of the force.
>
> **point of application:** Where the force acts on a body.

force couple: Two equal and opposite forces acting from different directions so as to turn an object about a fixed point.

force systems: Ways in which forces may be combined.

> **concurrent:** All the forces meet at one point.
>
> **general:** A collection of forces in a plane that cannot be defined by one of the other systems.
>
> **linear:** All the forces are acting along one line.
>
> **parallel:** All the forces are acting in the same plane but not along the same line.

force-velocity relationship: The relationship between the force a muscle can generate at a given length and the rate at which the muscle shortens. This relationship is present at constant rates of stimulation (i.e., in vitro electrical stimulation) and is inverse for concentric muscle contractions and direct for eccentric contractions up to a point where a plateau is reached.

free body diagram: A graphic representation of all the forces acting upon a body.

friction: A force that is in opposition to movement of two contacting bodies, with the force being parallel to the contacting surfaces.

general force system: See *force systems.*

gravity: The attractive force between two masses as defined by Newton's Law of Universal Gravitation. Force is equal to the gravitational constant (g).

$$g = \frac{mass_1 \times mass_2}{(\text{distance between masses})^2}$$

ground reaction forces: Forces that act on the body as a result of the body interacting with the supporting surface.

hysteresis: The property of a material such that the stress-strain relationship is different during loading and unloading; because of internal friction a material exhibiting hysteresis uses energy during loading or unloading.

impulse: The time a force acts on a body, expressed in units of $kg \times m/s$ or $lb \times ft/s$.

inertia: The quality that maintains a body at rest or in a constant state of motion (i.e., equilibrium) unless acted on by an external force (as defined by Newton's First Law).

integration: The technique in calculus that determines the area under a curve (in reference to the x axis).

inversion of muscle action: A term used to describe the event where a secondary action of a muscle changes owing to joint position; for example, the hip adductors can normally also cause flexion at the hip joint. However, if the femur is fully flexed at the hip, then the adductors can extend the hip because they have undergone inversion of their function.

isokinetic movement: Constant velocity movement.

isometric contraction: See *muscle contractions.*

isotonic contraction: See *muscle contractions.*

joint forces: Forces that act on articular surfaces and are due to muscular action, gravity, and inertia.

kinematics: The branch of dynamics that deals with motion (velocity and acceleration) but excludes consideration of mass and force.

kinetic energy (KE): The mechanical energy in a system that comes from its motion (during translatory motions, $KE = \frac{1}{2} m \times v^2$, where m = mass and v = velocity).

kinetics: A branch of dynamics that deals with forces.

length-tension curve: The plotted relationship of a muscle's length and the isometric tension that muscle can generate; because tension is measured directly, length-tension relationships can be measured only in vivo.

lengthening contraction: A term originated by physiologists who used it to describe an eccentric contraction; the term is actually an oxymoron (see *muscle contractions*).

levers: A system consisting of two forces and a fulcrum that alters a mechanical advantage.

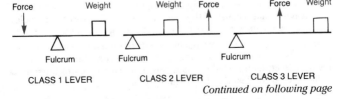

10

Continued on following page

linear force system: See *force systems.*

mass: As defined by Newton's Second Law, equal to the force on an object divided by the acceleration of the object. On earth, weight is a mass divided by the acceleration due to the earth's gravity.

mechanical advantage: A measure of efficiency equal to the ratio formed by dividing the output of a system by the input to the system. Its maximum value is 1 (i.e., 100% efficiency).

mechanics: A branch of physics that deals with energy and forces and their relationship to movement, equilibrium, and deformation.

modulus of elasticity: The ratio of stress to strain.

moment arm: The perpendicular distance from the action of a force to the axis of rotation.

moment of force: The product of a force times the perpendicular distance (moment arm) from the axis of rotation.

momentum: Mass times velocity.

motion types: Motion in space may be divided into two types: rotary movement, where movement occurs in an arc around a fixed point, and translatory movement, where a body moves in space from one point to another.

muscle contractions: Muscles contract in one set manner; that is, muscles create tension due to the formation of actinomyosin cross-bridges. However, depending on the load applied to the muscle, different types of events may occur (see table of muscle contractions).

    concentric contraction: A contraction in which the origins and insertions of the contracting muscle are brought closer together owing to the action of the muscle.

    eccentric contraction: A contraction in which the origins and insertions of a contracting muscle are moved away from each other by an external force, even though the muscle is contracting.

    isokinetic contraction: This is not really a type of contraction and is a term often used incorrectly. There can be an isokinetic movement (i.e., constant velocity movement), but there is no unique contractile event.

    isometric contraction: A contraction in which no noticeable shortening of the muscle takes place.

    isotonic contraction: This is not really a type of contraction, but rather a term that has been used widely to describe many different things. Originally the term was applied to in vivo experiments where a muscle worked against a constant load; therefore, the term cannot be directly applied to moving loads in an intact body. However, the term has been used to describe contractions where the body lifts a given weight, even though the gravitational vector of the weight changes, as does the muscle's moment arm, and as a result the load is not constant.

muscle insufficiency: This occurs when the tension produced by a muscle is reduced because the muscle is contracting from an extremely lengthened or shortened position. Two types of muscle insufficiency were described by Brunnstrom.

active insufficiency: This type is thought to occur when a two-joint muscle contracts across two joints at the same time. As a result, tension development can be severely compromised because the muscle is at the extreme left (shortened) side of its length-tension curve.

passive insufficiency: This type is thought to occur when a two-joint muscle is stretched across two joints at the same time. As a result, tension development can be severely compromised because the muscle is at the extreme right (lengthened) side of its length-tension curve.

negative work: A term coined by A. V. Hill to describe the work done by a muscle during an eccentric contraction when the muscle is actually working in opposition to the work being done on a limb segment. Mechanical work is not being performed by the muscle, although physiologic work is taking place.

Newton's Laws:

First Law (Law of Inertia): A body remains at rest or continues to move uniformly unless that body is acted on by a force.

Second Law (Law of Momentum): A change in momentum of a body is proportional to the magnitude and duration of the force acting on it (proportional to the impulse).

Third Law (Law of Reaction): Action and reaction are equal; therefore, any force acting on one body will be counteracted by an equal and opposite force.

parallel force systems: See *force systems*.

passive insufficiency: See *muscle insufficiency*.

point of application: See *force*.

potential energy: The mechanical energy of a body that is a result of the body's position in space (potential energy = mass × gravitational constant × distance).

power: The rate of doing work (work per unit time).

pressure: Force divided by the area over which it is applied (force per unit area).

prime mover: A term similar to *agonist* but preferred by some because it does not imply that a muscle is working against an antagonist. See *agonist muscle* and *antagonist muscle*.

resolution of forces: Computing the elements of a force; determining the constituent forces from a single force.

resting length: The length at which the muscle can generate the maximum amount of active tension. Because tension cannot be measured in intact human muscles, we do not know the resting length of any human muscle. Therefore, resting length is not the same as the anatomical position.

rotary motion: See *motion types*.

scalar quantity: A quantity having only magnitude. Scalars can be added arithmetically (e.g., quantified such as speed, time, and temperature).

Continued on following page

10

shear: A force acting tangentially to a surface.

shortening contraction: A term originated by physiologists to describe a concentric contraction as opposed to an eccentric contraction. The term is actually redundant (see *muscle contractions*).

shunt muscles: According to MacConnail and Basmajian, muscles that cause stabilization (or joint compression), or a shunt component is the part of muscle action that causes joint stabilization (see *spurt muscles*).

speed: The magnitude of velocity, expressed as distance per unit time.

spurt muscles: According to MacConnail and Basmajian, muscles that cause rotation, or a spurt component is the part of a muscle action that causes rotation (see *shunt muscles*).

statics: The study of bodies at rest and forces in equilibrium, as contrasted to dynamics, which deals with bodies in motion.

strain: Deformation (lengthening or shortening) of an object due to external loading.

stress: Internal forces developed within a body due to externally applied loads.

stress relaxation: A property of a material such that when that material is suddenly strained and maintained at that strain level it exhibits decreasing stress.

synergist: A muscle that contracts along with an agonist to assist that muscle in performing an action or to stabilize body parts to allow the agonist to cause movement (see *agonist muscle*).

tension: A load in which collinear forces attempt to pull something apart.

torque: Moment of a rotary force; same as *moment*.

translatory motion: See *motion types*.

vector quantity: A quantity having magnitude, direction, and a point and line of application.

velocity: A vector that describes displacement. The term is often confused with *speed* (a scalar); however, speed represents only the magnitude of velocity.

viscoelasticity: The property of a material that exhibits hysteresis, stress relaxation, and creep.

volume: Space occupied by an object as measured in cubic units.

weight: The force with which a body is attracted to the earth; mass $\times$ g (the gravitational constant), expressed in units of dynes, newtons, and pounds.

work: Force times distance (see *negative work*).

FOR MORE INFORMATION

Rogers, MM and Cavanagh, PR: Glossary of biomechanical terms, concepts and units. Phys Ther 64:1886, 1984.

Smith, LK, Weiss, EL, and Lehmkuhl, LD: Brunnstrom's Clinical Kinesiology, ed 5. FA Davis, Philadelphia, 1996.

Soderberg, GL: Kinesiology: Application to Pathological Motion. Williams & Wilkins, Baltimore, 1986.

Temporal Processing of the Electromyographic Signal

Illustration of Several Common Methods of Signal Processing

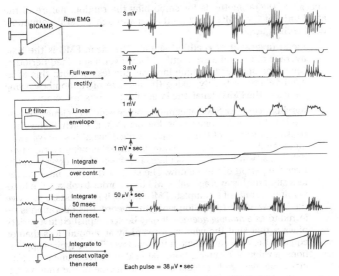

Several common methods of signal processing (definitions on pages 786 and 787).

raw electromyography (EMG): Visual inspection of the raw EMG is the most common way of examining muscle activity as it changes with time. The raw signal allows for visual inspection of the size and shape of individual muscle potentials. The amplitude of the raw EMG when reported should be that seen at the electrodes and should not reflect the gain of any amplifiers in the recording system.

full-wave rectification: The rectifier generates the absolute value of the EMG, usually with a positive polarity.

half-wave rectification: This is accomplished by eliminating negative values of the signal. Full-wave rectification is preferred because it retains all of the energy of the signal. Because simple averaging of the signal does not provide useful information, rectification of the signal is commonly used before further signal conditioning (such as moving averages or integration) is conducted. A visual examination of the full-wave rectified signal indicates the changing contraction level of the muscle.

Continued on following page

linear envelope: Low-pass filtering of the full-wave rectified signal produces a linear envelope of the signal. It is a type of moving average that follows the trend of the EMG and closely resembles the shape of the muscle tension curve. To represent muscle tension without body movement artifact, the low-pass filter should cut off at about 6 Hz (3 dB) and be at least a second-order type. This form of signal conditioning is often incorrectly confused with integration.

averages: Digital methods for smoothing the random nature of the amplitude of the EMG can be attained through several commonly used techniques.

mean (average) of rectified signal: The mean EMG is the time average of the full-wave rectified EMG over a specified period of time. The shorter this time interval, the less smooth this averaged value will be. By taking the average of randomly varying values of the EMG signal, the larger fluctuations are removed.

moving averages: Several common processing techniques are employed; the most common is low-pass filter, which follows the peaks and valleys of the full-wave rectified signal (see *linear envelope*). Another common procedure is a digital moving-average type defining a "window" that calculates the mean of the detected EMG over the period of the window. The shorter this time interval, the less smooth this average value will be. In order to obtain the time-varying average of a complete EMG record, it is necessary to move the time window T duration along the record; this operation is referred to as a *moving average*. It may be accomplished in a variety of ways that shift the window forward by an amount less than or equal to the time equivalent of the window *(T)*. For typical applications, a value of T ranging from 100–200 ms is recommended. Normally the average is calculated for the middle of the window because it does not introduce a lag in its output; special forms of weighting (exponential, triangular, etc.) can also be applied and should be specified along with the window width, T.

ensemble average: An ensemble average is accomplished digitally for those applications in which the average pattern of the EMG is required for repetitive or evoked responses (e.g., electrically elicited contractions). The time-averaged waveform has an amplitude in mV, and the number of averages is important to report, as well as the standard error at each point in time.

integrated EMG (iEMG or IEMG): A widely used procedure in electromyography that is frequently confused with signal averaging techniques or linear envelope detection. The correct interpretation of integration is purely mathematical and means "area under the curve"; the correct units are millivolts $\times$ seconds (mV·s) or microvolts $\times$ seconds (µV·s). There are many methods of integrating the EMG; three common procedures are illustrated and described.

integrate over contraction: The simplest form of integration starts at some preset time and continues during the total time of muscle activity. Over any desired period of time, the IEMG can be seen in millivolts.

resetting of the integrated signal: The integrated signal is reset to 0 at regular intervals of time, usually from 50–200 ms (the time should be specified); such a scheme yields a series of peaks that represents the trend of the EMG amplitude with time (similar to a moving average). The sum of all the peaks in any given contraction should equal the IEMG over that contraction.

integration with voltage level reset: The integration begins before the contraction. If the muscle activity is high, the integrator rapidly charges up to the reset level; if low activity occurs, the integrator takes longer to reach reset. Thus the activity level is reflected in the frequency of resets. High frequency of resets (sometimes called *pips*) means high muscle activity; low frequency means low level activity, as seen by the low trace in the illustration above. Each reset represents a value of IEMG and should be specified; the product of the number of resets times this calibration yields the total IEMG over any given time period.

root-mean-square (RMS) value: A method that is not as commonly used as other methods but gaining in popularity with the availability of analog chips that perform the RMS procedure. The RMS is an electronic average representing the square root of the average of the squares of the current or voltage; RMS provides a nearly instantaneous output of the power of the EMG signal.

FOR MORE INFORMATION

Basmajian, JV and De Luca, CJ: Muscles Alive: Their Functions Revealed by Electromyography, ed 5. Williams & Wilkins, Baltimore, 1985.

Winter, DA: Biomechanics of Human Movement. John Wiley & Sons, New York, 1979.

Winter, DA (Chairman): Units, Terms and Standards in the Reporting of EMG Research. Report of the Ad Hoc Committee of the International Society of Electrophysiological Kinesiology (ISEK), 1980.

Continued on following page

10

TERMS USED IN ELECTROMYOGRAPHY

Terminology	Units	Comments/ Recommendations
Amplifier gain	Ratio or dB	Must be sufficient to produce an output of $+/-1$ V; input bias and offset currents $<$ 50 pA (picoamperes); input equivalent noise < 2 μV RMS.
Input resistance or impedance	Ω	Must be $100–1000$ mΩ; minimum of 100 times skin impedance.
Common mode rejection ratio (CMMR)	Ratio or dB	90 dB or better.
Filter cutoff or bandwidth	Hz	Specify type and order of filter; minimum of $5–500$ Hz (3 dB) is required.
EMG (raw signal)	mV	
EMG (average)	mV	Specify averaging period.
EMG (full-wave rectified)	mV	
EMG (nonlinear detector)	mV	Specify nonlinearity (i.e., square law).
EMG (linear envelope)	mV	Specify cutoff frequency and type of low-pass filter.
Integrated EMG (IEMG or iEMG)	mV·s	Specify integration period.
Integrated EMG with reset every T seconds	mV·s or μV·s	Specify T (ms).
Integrated EMG to threshold and reset	mV·s or μV·s	Specify threshold (mV·s).

NORMAL GAIT
Divisions of the Gait Cycle

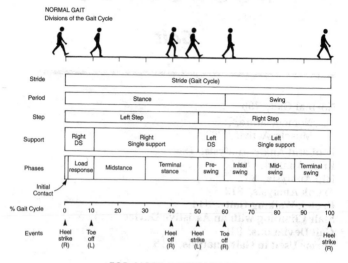

NORMAL GAIT
Divisions of the Gait Cycle

Stride	Stride (Gait Cycle)							
Period	Stance				Swing			
Step	Left Step				Right Step			
Support	Right DS	Right Single support		Left DS	Left Single support			
Phases	Load response	Midstance	Terminal stance	Pre-swing	Initial swing	Mid-swing	Terminal swing	

Initial Contact

% Gait Cycle	0	10	20	30	40	50	60	70	80	90	100
Events	Heel strike (R)	Toe off (L)			Heel off (R)	Heel strike (L)	Toe off (R)				Heel strike (R)

FOR MORE INFORMATION

Craik, RL and Otis, CA: Gait Analysis: Theory and Application. Mosby Year Book, St. Louis, 1995.

Nomenclature used to describe the divisions of the gait cycle has expanded over the years to include the terminology based on functional significance, as well as the traditional terminology based on events occurring between the first foot movement and ground contact. The preceding figure shows these divisions for a normal subject in terms of percentages of the gait cycle. The *stride* is depicted as the interval in the gait cycle between two sequential initial contacts with the same foot. A *step* is the interval between initial contact with one foot and then the other foot (e.g., right to left). Support times are divided into phases of *double (limb) support* (weight bearing is shared by both lower extremities) and *single (limb) support* (weight bearing is on one lower extremity). Each of the functional phases and events depicted in the figure are defined in greater detail for traditional and Rancho Los Amigos nomenclature.

traditional nomenclature: The events taking place during the phase are named, for the most part, according to the events that take place at the foot, for example, heel strike.

Ranchos Los Amigos nomenclature: The events taking place during the phases are named, for the most part, according to the purpose of the phase, for example, initial contact.

TERMS USED TO DESCRIBE GAIT
FOR OBSERVATIONAL ANALYSIS

Traditional	*Rancho Los Amigos*

STANCE PHASE

Heel strike: The beginning of the stance phase when the heel contacts the ground.

Foot flat: The portion of the stance phase that occurs immediately after heel strike, when the sole of the foot contacts the floor.

Midstance: The point at which the body passes directly over the reference extremity.

Heel-off: The point following midstance at which time the heel of the reference extremity leaves the ground.

Toe-off: The point after heel-off when only the toe of the reference extremity is in contact with the ground.

Initial contact: The beginning of the stance phase when the heel or another part of the foot contacts the ground.

Loading response: The portion of the stance phase from immediately after initial contact until the contralateral extremity leaves the ground.

Midstance: The portion of the stance phase that begins when the contralateral extremity leaves the ground and ends when the body is directly over the supporting limb.

Terminal stance: The portion of the stance phase from midstance to a point just prior to initial contact of the contralateral extremity.

Preswing: The portion of stance from the initial contact of the contralateral extremity to just prior to the liftoff of the reference extremity. This portion includes toe-off.

SWING PHASE

Acceleration: The portion of beginning swing from the moment the toe of the reference extremity leaves the ground to the point when the reference extremity is directly under the body.

Midswing: Portion of the swing pause when the reference extremity passes directly below the body. Midswing extends from the end of

Initial swing: The portion of swing from the point when the reference extremity leaves the ground to maximum knee flexion of the same extremity.

Midswing: Portion of the swing phase from maximum knee flexion of the reference extremity to a vertical tibial position.

Continued on following page

11

Traditional	*Rancho Los Amigos*
acceleration to the beginning of deceleration.	
Deceleration: The swing portion of the swing phase when the reference extremity is decelerating in preparation for heel strike.	Terminal swing: The portion of the swing phase from a vertical position of the tibia of the reference extremity to just prior to initial contact.

From O'Sullivan, SB and Schmitz, TJ: Physical Rehabilitation: Assessment and Treatment, ed 3. FA Davis, Philadelphia, 1994, p 169, with permission.

FOR MORE INFORMATION

Craik, RL and Otis, CA: Gait Analysis: Theory and Application. Mosby Year Book, St. Louis, 1995.

Muscles Controlling Gait
Muscle Sequence Controlling the Foot During Stance

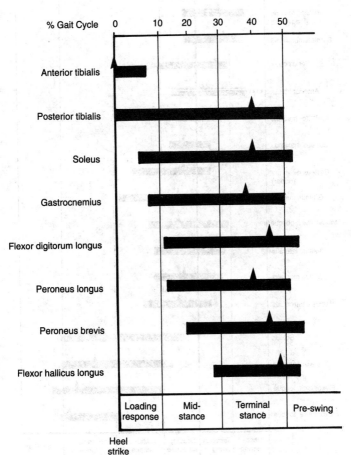

Continued on following page

Lower Extremity Muscle Sequence for Stance

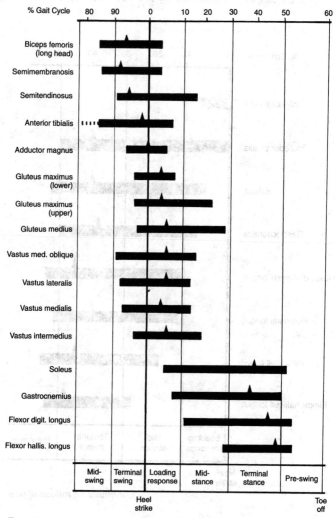

From Perry, J: Gait Analysis: Normal and Pathologic Function. Slack, Thorofare, NJ, 1992, p 163, with permission.

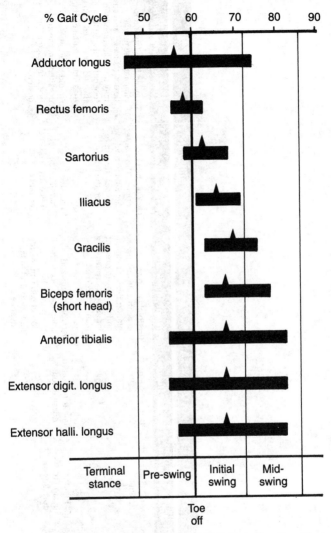

Lower Extremity Muscle Sequence for Swing

% Gait Cycle   50   60   70   80   90

Adductor longus

Rectus femoris

Sartorius

Iliacus

Gracilis

Biceps femoris
(short head)

Anterior tibialis

Extensor digit. longus

Extensor halli. longus

| Terminal stance | Pre-swing | Initial swing | Mid-swing |

Toe
off

From Perry, J: Gait Analysis: Normal and Pathologic Function. Slack, Thorofare, NJ, 1992, p 163, with permission.

NORMAL GAIT: FOOT AND ANKLE: STANCE PHASE (as seen from a lateral view)

Portion of Phase	Angular Motion	Normal Moment	Normal Muscle Activity	Result of Weakness	Possible Compensation
Heel strike to foot flat	0 – 15° Plantar flexion	Plantar flexion	Pretibial group acts eccentrically to oppose plantar flexion moment and thereby to prevent foot slap by controlling plantar flexion.	Lack of ability to oppose the plantar flexion moment causes the foot to slap the floor.	To avoid foot slap and to eliminate the plantar flexion moment, heel strike may be avoided and the foot either placed flat on the floor or placed with the toes first at initial contact.
Foot flat through midstance	15° Plantar flexion to 10° dorsiflexion	Plantar flexion to dorsiflexion	Gastrocnemius and soleus act eccentrically to oppose the dorsiflexion moment and to control tibial advance.	Excessive dorsiflexion and uncontrolled tibial advance.	To avoid excessive dorsiflexion, the ankle may be maintained in plantar flexion.

Midstance to heel-off	10° – 15° Dorsiflexion	Dorsiflexion	Gastrocnemius and soleus contract eccentrically to oppose the dorsiflexion moment and control tibial advance.	Excessive dorsiflexion and uncontrolled forward motion of tibia.	The ankle may be maintained in plantar flexion; if the foot is flat on the floor, the dorsiflexion moment is eliminated and a step-to gait is produced.
Heel-off to toe-off	15° Dorsiflexion to 20° plantar flexion	Dorsiflexion	Gastrocnemius, soleus, peroneus brevis, peroneus longus, flexor hallicus longus contract to plantar flex the foot.	No roll-off.	Whole foot is lifted off the ground.

From O'Sullivan, SB and Schmitz, TJ: Physical Rehabilitation: Assessment and Treatment, ed 3. FA Davis, Philadelphia, 1994, p 169.

11

GAIT DEVIATIONS: FOOT AND ANKLE: STANCE PHASE (as seen from a lateral view)			
Portion of Phase	**Deviation**	**Description**	**Possible Causes**	**Analysis**
Initial contact	Foot slap	At heel strike, forefoot slaps the ground.	Weak dorsiflexors or atrophy of dorsiflexors	Look for muscle weakness at ankle. Look for steppage gait (excessive hip and knee flexion) in swing phase.
	Toes first	Toes contact ground instead of heel. A tiptoe posture may be maintained throughout the phase, or the heel may contact the ground.	Leg length discrepancy; contracted heel cord; plantar flexion contraction; hyper-reflexive plantar flexors; flaccidity of dorsiflexors; painful heel	Compare leg lengths and look for hip and/or knee flexion contractures. Analyze reflex activity and timing of activity in plantar flexors. Check for pain in heel.
	Foot flat	Entire foot contacts the ground at heel strike.	Excessive fixed dorsiflexion; flaccid or weak dorsiflexors	Check range of motion at ankle. Check for hyperextension at the knee and persistence of immature gait pattern.
Midstance	Excessive positional plantar flexion	Tibia does not advance to neutral from 10° plantar flexion.	No eccentric contraction of plantar flexors; could be due to flaccidity/ weakness in plantar	Check for hyper-reflexive or weak quadriceps; hyperextension at the knee; hip hyperextension;

Gait deviation	Description	Possible causes	Assessment
		flexors; surgical overrelease, rupture, or contracture of Achilles tendon	backward- or forward-leaning trunk. Check for weakness in plantar flexors or rupture of Achilles tendon.
Heel lift in midstance	Heel does not contact ground in midstance.	Hyper-reflexive plantar flexors	Check reflexes of plantar flexors, quadriceps, hip flexors, and adductors.
Excessive positional dorsiflexion	Tibia advances too rapidly over the foot, creating a greater than normal amount of dorsiflexion.	Inability of plantar flexors to control tibial advance; knee flexion or hip flexion contractures	Look at ankle muscles, knee and hip flexors, range of motion, and position of trunk.
Toe clawing	Toes flex and "grab" floor	Plantar grasp reflex that is only partially integrated; positive supporting reflex; hyper-reflexive toe flexors	Check plantar grasp reflex, positive supporting reflexes, and range of motion of toes.
Push-off (heel-off to toe-off) — No roll-off	Insufficient transfer of weight from lateral heel to medial forefoot	Mechanical fixation of ankle and foot; flaccidity or inhibition of plantar flexors, inverters, and toe flexors; rigidity/cocontraction of plantar flexors and dorsiflexors; pain in forefoot	Check range of motion at ankle and foot. Check muscle function and reflexes at ankle. Look at dissociation between posterior foot and forefoot.

From O'Sullivan, SB and Schmitz, TJ: Physical Rehabilitation: Assessment and Treatment, ed 3. FA Davis, Philadelphia, 1994, p 176.

11

NORMAL GAIT: FOOT AND ANKLE: SWING PHASE (as seen from a lateral view)

Portion of Phase	Angular Motion	Normal Moment	Normal Muscle Activity	Result of Weakness	Possible Compensation
Acceleration to midswing	Dorsiflexion to neutral	Plantar flexion	Dorsiflexors contract to bring the ankle into neutral and to prevent the toes from dragging on the floor.	Footdrop and/or toe dragging	Hip and knee flexion may be increased to prevent toe drag, or the hip may be hiked or circumducted. Sometimes vaulting on the contralateral limb may occur.
Midswing to deceleration	Neutral	Plantar flexion	Dorsiflexion	Footdrop and/or toe dragging	Hip and knee flexion may be increased to prevent toe drag. The swing leg may be circumducted, or vaulting may occur on the contralateral side.

From O'Sullivan, SB and Schmitz, TJ: Physical Rehabilitation: Assessment and Treatment, ed 3. FA Davis, Philadelphia, 1994, p 170.

GAIT DEVIATIONS: FOOT AND ANKLE: SWING PHASE (as seen from a lateral view)			
Portion of Phase	Deviation	Description	Possible Causes	Analysis
Swing	Toe drag	Insufficient dorsiflexion (and toe extension) so that forefoot and toes do not clear floor	Flaccidity or weakness of dorsiflexors and toe extensors; hyper-reflexiveness of plantar flexors; inadequate knee or hip flexion	Check for ankle, hip, and knee range of motion. Check for strength and reflexes at hip, knee, and ankle.
	Varus	Foot excessively inverted	Hyper-reflexive invertors; flaccidity or weakness of dorsiflexors and evertors; extensor pattern	Check for muscle reflexes of invertors and plantar flexors. Check force of dorsiflexors and evertors. Check for extensor pattern of the lower extremity.

From O'Sullivan, SB and Schmitz, TJ: Physical Rehabilitation: Assessment and Treatment, ed 3. FA Davis, Philadelphia, 1994, p 176.

11

NORMAL GAIT: KNEE: STANCE PHASE (as seen from a lateral view)

Portion of Phase	Angular Motion	Normal Moment	Normal Muscle Activity	Result of Weakness	Possible Compensation
Heel strike to foot flat	Flexion 0°–15°	Flexion	Quadriceps contracts initially to hold the knee in extension and then eccentrically to oppose the flexion moment and to control the amount of flexion.	Excessive knee flexion because the quadriceps cannot oppose the flexion moment	Plantar flexion at ankle so that foot flat instead of heel strike occurs. Plantar flexion eliminates the flexion moment. Trunk leans forward to eliminate the flexion moment at the knee and therefore may be used to compensate for quadriceps weakness.
Foot flat through midstance	Extension 15°–5°	Flexion to extension	Quadriceps contracts in early part, and then no activity is required.	Excessive knee flexion initially	Same as above in early part of midstance. No compensation required in later part of phase.
Midstance to heel-off	5° Flexion to 0° (neutral)	Flexion to extension	No activity is required.		None is required.
Heel-off to toe-off	0°–10° Flexion	Extension to flexion	Quadriceps is required to control amount of knee flexion.		

From O'Sullivan, SB and Schmitz, TJ: Physical Rehabilitation: Assessment and Treatment, ed 3. FA Davis, Philadelphia, 1994, p 170.

GAIT DEVIATIONS: KNEE: STANCE PHASE (as seen from a lateral view)			
Portion of Phase	**Deviation**	**Description**	**Possible Causes**	**Analysis**
Initial contact (heel strike)	Excessive knee flexion	Knee flexes or buckles rather than extends as foot contacts ground.	Painful knee; hyper-reflexive knee flexors or weak or flaccid quadriceps; short leg on contralateral side.	Check for pain at knee, reflexes of knee flexors, strength of knee extensors, and leg lengths; anterior pelvic tilt.
Foot flat	Knee hyper-extension (genu recurvatum)	There is a greater-than-normal extension at the knee.	Flaccid/weak quadriceps and soleus compensated for by pull of gluteus maximus; spasticity of quadriceps; accommodation to a fixed ankle plantar flexion deformity.	Check force and reflexes of knee and ankle flexors, and range of motion at ankle.
Midstance	Knee hyper-extension (genu recurvatum)	During single limb support, tibia remains in back of ankle mortice as body weight moves over foot; ankle is plantar flexed.	Same as above.	Same as above.

Continued on following page

11

	GAIT DEVIATIONS: KNEE: STANCE PHASE (as seen from a lateral view) (Continued)		
Portion of Phase	**Deviation**	**Description**	**Possible Causes**	**Analysis**
Push-off (heel-off to toe-off)	Excessive knee flexion	Knee flexes to more than 40° during push-off	Center of gravity is unusually forward of pelvis; this could be due to rigid trunk, knee/hip flexion contractures; flexion-withdrawal reflex; dominance of flexion synergy in middle of recovery from CVA.	Look at trunk posture, knee and hip range of motion, and flexor synergy.
	Limited knee flexion	The normal amount of knee flexion (40°) does not occur.	Overactive quadriceps and/or plantar flexors.	Look at reflexes of hip, knee, and ankle muscles.

CVA = cerebrovascular accident.
From O'Sullivan, SB and Schmitz, TJ: Physical Rehabilitation: Assessment and Treatment, ed 3. FA Davis, Philadelphia, 1994, p 177.

NORMAL GAIT: KNEE: SWING PHASE (as seen from a lateral view)				
Portion of Phase	Angular Motion	Normal Muscle Activity	Result of Weakness	Possible Compensation
Acceleration to midswing	40°–60° Flexion	There is little or no activity in quadriceps; biceps femoris (short head), gracilis, and sartorius contract concentrically.	Inadequate knee flexion	Increased hip flexion, circumduction, or hiking
Midswing	60°–30° Extension			
Deceleration	30°–0° Extension	Quadriceps contracts concentrically to stabilize knee in extension in preparation for heel strike.	Inadequate knee extension	

From O'Sullivan, SB and Schmitz, TJ: Physical Rehabilitation: Assessment and Treatment, ed 3. FA Davis, Philadelphia, 1994, p 170.

11

GAIT DEVIATIONS: KNEE: SWING PHASE (as seen from a lateral view)

Portion of Phase	Deviation	Description	Possible Causes	Analysis
Acceleration to midswing	Excessive knee flexion	Knee flexes more than 65°.	Diminished preswing knee flexion, flexor-withdrawal reflex, dysmetria	Look at reflexes of hip, knee, and ankle muscles; test for reflexes and dysmetria.
	Limited knee flexion	Knee does not flex to 65°.	Pain in knee, diminished range of knee motion, extensor spasticity; circumduction at the hip	Assess for pain in knee and knee range of motion; test reflexes at knee and hip.

From O'Sullivan, SB and Schmitz, TJ: Physical Rehabilitation: Assessment and Treatment, ed 3. FA Davis, Philadelphia, 1994, p 177.

NORMAL GAIT: HIP: STANCE PHASE (as seen from a lateral view)

Portion of Phase	Angular Motion	Normal Moment	Normal Muscle Activity	Result of Weakness	Possible Compensation
Heel strike to foot flat	30° Flexion	Flexion	Erector spinae, gluteus maximus, hamstrings	Excessive hip flexion and anterior pelvic tilt owing to inability to counteract flexion moment	Trunk leans backward to prevent excessive hip flexion and to eliminate the hip flexion moment.
Foot flat through midstance	30° Flexion to 5° (neutral)	Flexion to extension	Gluteus maximus at beginning of period to oppose flexion moment; then activity ceases as moment changes from flexion to extension	At the beginning of the period, excessive hip flexion and anterior pelvic tilt owing to inability to counteract flexion moment	At beginning of the period, subject may lean trunk backward to prevent excessive hip flexion; however, once the flexion moment changes to an extension moment, the subject no longer needs to incline the trunk backward.
Midstance to heel-off	Extension	Extension	No activity	None	None required.
Heel-off to toe-off	10° Extension to neutral	Extension	Iliopsoas, adductor, magnus, and adductor longus	Undetermined	Undetermined.

From O'Sullivan, SB and Schmitz, TJ: Physical Rehabilitation: Assessment and Treatment, ed 3. FA Davis, Philadelphia, 1994, p 171.

807

11

GAIT DEVIATIONS: HIP: STANCE PHASE (as seen from a lateral view)				
Portion of Phase	**Deviation**	**Description**	**Possible Causes**	**Analysis**
Heel strike to foot flat	Excessive flexion	Flexion exceeds 30°.	Hip and/or knee flexion contractures; knee flexion caused by weak soleus and quadriceps, hyper-reflexive of hip flexors.	Check hip and knee range of motion and force of soleus and quadriceps. Check reflexes of hip flexors.
Heel strike to foot flat	Limited hip flexion	Hip flexion does not attain 30°.	Weakness of hip flexors; limited range of hip flexion; gluteus maximus weakness	Check force of hip flexors and extensors. Analyze range of hip motion.
Foot flat to midstance	Limited hip extension	The hip does not attain a neutral position.	Hip flexion contracture, hyper-reflexive hip flexors	Check hip range of motion and reflexes of hip muscles.

Internal rotation	An internally rotated position of the extremity.	Hyper-reflexive internal rotators; weakness of external rotators; excessive forward rotation of opposite pelvis	Check reflexes of internal rotators and force of external rotators. Measure range of motion of both hip joints.
External rotation	An externally rotated position of the extremity.	Excessive backward rotation of opposite pelvis	Assess range of motion at both hip joints.
Abduction	An abducted position of the extremity.	Contracture of the gluteus medius; trunk lateral lean over the ipsilateral hip	Check for abduction pattern.
Adduction	An adducted position of the lower extremity.	Hyper-reflexive hip flexors and adductors such as seen in spastic diplegia; pelvic drop to contralateral side	Assess reflexes of hip flexors and adductors. Test force of hip abductors.

From O'Sullivan, SB and Schmitz, TJ: Physical Rehabilitation: Assessment and Treatment, ed 3. FA Davis, Philadelphia, 1994, p 178.

NORMAL GAIT: HIP: SWING PHASE (as seen from a lateral view)

Portion of Phase	Angular Motion	Normal Moment	Normal Muscle Activity	Result of Weakness	Possible Compensation
Acceleration to midswing	20° – 30° Flexion	None	Hip flexor activity to initiate swing: iliopsoas, rectus femoris, gracilis, sartorius, tensor fascia lata	Diminished hip flexion, causing an inability to initiate the normal forward movement of the extremity and to raise the foot off the floor	Circumduction and/or hip hiking may be used to bring the leg forward and to raise the foot high enough to clear the floor.
Midswing to deceleration	30° Flexion to neutral	None	Hamstrings	A lack of control of the swinging leg; inability to place limb in position for heel strike	

From O'Sullivan, SB and Schmitz, TJ: Physical Rehabilitation: Assessment and Treatment, ed 3. FA Davis, Philadelphia, 1994, p 175.

		GAIT DEVIATIONS: HIP: SWING PHASE (as seen from a lateral view)		
Portion of Phase	**Deviation**	**Description**	**Possible Causes**	**Analysis**
Swing	Circumduction	A lateral circular movement of the entire lower extremity consisting of abduction, external rotation, adduction, and internal rotation	A compensation for weak hip flexors or a compensation for the inability to shorten the leg so that it can clear the floor	Check force of hip flexors, knee flexors, and ankle dorsiflexors. Check range of motion in hip flexion, knee flexion, and ankle dorsiflexion. Check for extensor pattern.
	Hip hiking	Shortening of the swing leg by action of the quadratus lumborum	A compensation for lack of knee flexion and/or ankle dorsiflexion; also may be a compensation for extensor spasticity of swing leg	Check force and range of motion at knee, hip, and ankle. Also check reflexes at knee and ankle.
	Excessive hip flexion	Flexion >20°–30°	Attempt to shorten extremity in presence of footdrop; flexor pattern	Check force and range of motion at ankle and foot. Check for flexor pattern.

From O'Sullivan, SB and Schmitz, TJ: Physical Rehabilitation: Assessment and Treatment, ed 3. FA Davis, Philadelphia, 1994, p 178.

11

GAIT DEVIATIONS: TRUNK: STANCE PHASE

Portion of Phase	Deviation	Description	Possible Causes	Analysis
Stance	Lateral trunk lean	A lean of the trunk over the stance extremity (gluteus medius gait/trendelenburg gait)	A weak or paralyzed gluteus medius on the stance side cannot prevent a drop of pelvis on the swing side, so a trunk lean over the stance leg helps compensate for the weak muscle. A lateral trunk lean also may be used to reduce force on hip if a patient has a painful hip.	Check force of gluteus medius and assess for pain in the hip.
	Backward trunk lean	A backward leaning of the trunk; resulting in hyperextension at the hip (gluteus maximus gait)	Weakness or paralysis of the gluteus maximus on the stance leg; anteriorly rotated pelvis.	Check for force of hip extensors. Check pelvic position.

Forward trunk lean	A forward leaning of the trunk, resulting in hip flexion	Compensation for quadriceps weakness; the forward lean eliminates the flexion moment at the knee; hip and knee flexion contractures.	Check force of quadriceps.
	A forward flexion of the upper trunk	Posteriorly rotated pelvis.	Check pelvic position.

From O'Sullivan, SB and Schmitz, TJ: Physical Rehabilitation: Assessment and Treatment, ed 3. FA Davis, Philadelphia, 1994, p 179.

CRUTCH-WALKING GAITS

three-point gait: Both crutches are moved forward with the affected limb. This non-weight-bearing gait can be used if the patient has one normal lower limb that can tolerate full weight bearing. For example, this mode of crutch walking is used after hip or knee operations. A modified three-point gait is the partial-weight-bearing gait during which the affected extremity is allowed to bear some weight when both crutches are on the ground.

four-point gait: One crutch is advanced in this gait pattern, followed by advancement of the opposite lower extremity. Only one leg or crutch is off the floor at a time, leaving three points for support, making this a very stable and safe gait. This gait can be used for the patient who is able to move his legs alternately but who has poor balance or is not able to bear full weight bilaterally without the support of crutches.

partial-weight-bearing gait: See *three-point gait.*

two-point gait: A modification of the four-point gait. The right crutch and left leg move together, and the left crutch and right leg move together. It is close to the natural rhythm of walking.

swing-to gait: Both crutches are moved forward together, and the lower extremities are then swung forward to a position between the crutches. This gait is often used by paraplegic patients who are unable to move their legs alternately.

swing-through gait: Both crutches are moved forward together, and the lower extremities are then swung forward to a position beyond the crutches. This gait is often used by paraplegic patients who are unable to move their legs alternately.

BASED ON

O'Sullivan, SB and Schmitz, TJ: Physical Rehabilitation: Assessment and Treatment, ed 3. FA Davis, Philadelphia, 1994, pp 268–269, with permission.

TECHNIQUES USED TO CLIMB STAIRS WHILE USING ASSISTIVE DEVICES

The sequences presented here describe stair-climbing techniques without the use of a railing. When a secure railing is available, the patient should be instructed to use it always.

I. Cane
   A. Ascending
      1. The unaffected lower extremity leads up.
      2. The cane and affected lower extremity follow.
   B. Descending
      1. The affected lower extremity and cane lead down.
      2. The unaffected lower extremity follows.
II. Crutches: three-point gait (non-weight-bearing gait)
   A. Ascending
      1. The patient is positioned close to the foot of the stairs. The involved lower extremity is held back to prevent "catching" on the lip of the stairs.

2. The patient pushes down firmly on both handpieces of the crutches and leads up with the unaffected lower extremity.
3. The crutches are brought up to the stair that the unaffected lower extremity is now on.

   B. Descending
1. The patient stands close to the edge of the stair such that the toes protrude slightly over the top. The involved lower extremity is held forward over the lower stair.
2. Both crutches are moved down *together* to the *front* half of the next step.
3. The patient pushes down firmly on both handpieces and lowers the unaffected lower extremity to the step that the crutches are now on.

III. Crutches: partial-weight-bearing gait
   A. Ascending
1. The patient is positioned close to the foot of the stairs.
2. The patient pushes down on both handpieces of the crutches and distributes weight partially on the crutches and partially on the affected lower extremity while the unaffected lower extremity leads up.
3. The involved lower extremity and crutches are then brought up together.

   B. Descending
1. The patient stands close to the edge of the stair such that the toes protrude slightly over top of the stair.
2. Both crutches are moved down *together* to the *front* half of the next step. The affected lower extremity is then lowered (depending on patient skill, these may be combined). *Note:* When crutches are not in floor contact, greater weight must be shifted to the uninvolved lower extremity to maintain a partial-weight-bearing status.
3. The uninvolved lower extremity is lowered to the step the crutches are now on.

IV. Crutches: two- and four-point gait
   A. Ascending
1. The patient is positioned close to the foot of the stairs.
2. The right lower extremity is moved up and then the left lower extremity.
3. The right crutch is moved up and then the left crutch is moved up (patients with adequate balance may find it easier to move the crutches up together).

   B. Descending
1. The patient stands close to the edge of the stair.
2. The right crutch is moved down and then the left (may be combined).
3. The right lower extremity is moved down and then the left.

From O'Sullivan, SB and Schmitz, TJ: Physical Rehabilitation: Assessment and Treatment, ed 3. FA Davis, Philadelphia, 1994, p 273, with permission.

TERMS USED TO DESCRIBE COMMON
GAIT DEVIATIONS (in alphabetical order)

Gait deviations (limps) take on many forms, and their etiologies may be complex. The list below is not meant to be all-inclusive. Only the most common patterns are listed, and only the most common etiologies for those patterns are noted.

antalgic gait (painful gait): Avoidance of weight bearing on the affected side, shortening of the stance phase, and an attempt to unload the limb as much as possible. In addition, the painful region is often supported by one hand, while the other arm is outstretched. This pattern is often the result of pain caused by injury to the hip, knee, ankle, or foot.

arthrogenic gait: Elevation of the pelvis and circumduction of the leg on the involved side with exaggerated plantar flexion of the opposite ankle. This pattern is often due to stiffness, laxity, or deformity of the hip or knee and is often seen with fusion of these joints or after the recent removal of a cylinder cast.

ataxic gait: This gait may take two forms, depending on the pathology.

> **spinal ataxia:** A gait deviation that is characterized by the patient walking with a broad base and throwing out the feet, which come down first on the heel and then on the toes with a slapping sound or "double tap." It is characteristic for patients to watch their feet while walking. In milder cases, the gait may appear near normal with the eyes open, but when the patient is asked to walk with eyes closed, the patient staggers, becomes unsteady, and may be unable to walk. This gait is thought to result from the disruption of sensory pathways in the central nervous system, as occurs with tabes dorsalis or multiple sclerosis.

> **cerebellar ataxia:** A gait deviation that is equally severe when the patient walks with eyes open or closed. The gait is wide based, unsteady, and irregular. The patient staggers and is unable to walk tandem or to follow a straight line. This form of ataxia occurs with cerebellar lesions. If the disease is localized to one hemisphere, there is persistent deviation or swaying toward the affected side.

calcaneous gait: See *gastrocnemius-soleus gait.*

crouch gait: Bilateral impairment typified by excessive hip and knee flexion, excessive plantar flexion, and anterior pelvic tilt. A characteristic gait of children with diplegia, quadriplegia, or paraplegia.

digitigrade: Walking on toes (see *equinus gait*).

dorsiflexor gait: See *footdrop gait.*

dystrophic (penguin) gait: There is a pronounced waddling element to this gait. The patient rolls the hips from side to side during the stance phase of every forward step in order to shift the weight of the body. There is an exaggerated lumbar lordosis while walking or standing. It usually presents as a difficulty in running or climbing stairs. This gait is encountered in various myopathies and is most typical of muscular dystrophy.

equinus gait: Excessive plantar flexion usually associated with fixed ankle deformity, contracture, or extensor hyperactivity (see *digitigrade*).

flaccid gait: See *hemiplegic gait.*

footdrop (dorsiflexor or steppage) gait: The patient lifts the knee high and slaps the foot to the ground on advancing to the involved side. This gait is typical of patients with weak or paralyzed dorsiflexor muscles.

gastrocnemius-soleus (calcaneus) gait: This deviation is demonstrated best when the patient walks up an incline. At push-off, the heel does not come off the ground, and the affected side lags compared to the other side. This gait results from weakness to the gastrocnemius and/or the soleus muscles.

genu recurvatum gait: Excessive knee extension (hyperextension) during the stance phase of gait.

gluteus maximus (hip extensor) gait: A lurching gait characterized by a posterior thrust of the thorax at heel strike to maintain hip extension of the stance leg. The knee is tightly extended in midstance, which slightly elevates the hip on that side. This gait usually results from weakness to the gluteus maximus muscle.

gluteus medius (trendelenburg) gait: In the uncompensated gluteus medius limp, the pelvis dips more when the unaffected limb is in swing phase and there is an apparent lateral protrusion of the stance hip; if necessary, the patient may use a steppage gait to clear the swing leg. The gluteus medius gait commonly occurs owing to weakness of the gluteus medius muscle or with congenital dislocations of the hip or with coxa vara. If the gluteus medius is absent or extremely weak, a compensated gait appears where the patient shifts the trunk to the affected side during the stance phase.

hemiplegic or hemiparetic (flaccid) gait: The patient swings the paretic leg outward and ahead in a circle (circumduction) or pushes it ahead. Heel strike is often missing, and the patient strikes with the forefoot. This gait is present when one leg is shorter than the other or with a deformity in one of the bones of the leg.

hip extensor gait: See *gluteus maximus gait.*

painful gait: See *antalgic gait.*

Parkinsonian gait: This is a highly stereotypical gait in which the patient has impoverished movement of the lower limb. There is generalized lack of extension at the ankle, knee, hip, and trunk. Diminished step length and a loss of reciprocal arm swing are noted. Patients have trouble initiating movement, and this results in a slow and shuffling gait characterized by small steps. Because patients with parkinsonism often exhibit flexed postures, their centers of gravity project forward, causing a festinating gait. The patients, in an attempt to regain their balance, take many small steps rapidly. The rapid stepping causes the patients to increase their walking speed. In some cases patients will break into a run and can only stop their forward progression when they run into an object. Less common than the forward propulsive gait pattern is a retropulsive pattern that occurs when patients lose their balance in a backward direction (retropulsion is more common in patients with cerebellar lesions).

Continued on following page

penguin gait: See *dystrophic gait.*

plantigrade: Simultaneous floor contact by the forefoot and heel.

scissors gait: Excessive hip adduction during swing causing the swing limb to cross the stance limb.

steppage gait: See *footdrop gait.*

stiff-knee gait: Failure of the knee to flex during stance and swing phase of gait.

Trendelenburg gait: See *gluteus medius gait.*

unguligrade: Tip-toe walking.

FOR MORE INFORMATION

Craik, RA and Otis, CA: Gait Analysis: Theory and Application. Mosby Year Book, St. Louis, 1995.

Perry, J: Gait Analysis: Normal and Pathologic Function. Slack, Thorofare, NJ, 1992.

TERMS AND MEASUREMENTS USED IN KINETIC AND KINEMATIC ANALYSIS OF GAIT

acceleration: Rate of change in velocity per unit time, for translatory motion expressed in distance per second squared, for angular motion expressed in radians per second squared or degrees per second squared.

accelerometer: An instrument that measures acceleration.

angular acceleration: See *acceleration.*

automated motion analysis: A system that senses and quantifies limb motion without operator intervention.

base of support: The distance between left and right foot contacts as measured in a plane transverse to the line of progression during gait.

body weight vector: A force vector indicating the orientation and magnitude of body weight relative to one or more joints of interest.

cadence: Number of steps per unit time.

center of (foot) pressure (COP): The location of the mean weight-bearing force relative to the plane of foot support; often used to quantify postural sway.

cycle time: See *stride time.*

degree of toe out or toe in: See *foot angle.*

double support time: The amount of time during the gait cycle when both lower extremities are in contact with the ground; for example, when the right leg is in stance phase and the left heel comes in contact with the ground, the period of left double support begins and continues until the right foot comes off the ground.

electrogoniometer: A potentiometer device attached to a limb to record angular joint position.

foot angle: The angle of foot placement with respect to the line of progression.

footswitch: A device that measures the time of floor contact with respect to a designated area of the foot.

force plate (platform): A platform set on or into the floor that is instrumented to measure ground reaction forces and/or moments imposed on it.

ground reaction forces: Forces created as a result of foot contact with supporting surface. These are equal in magnitude and opposite in direction to those applied by the limb to the supporting surface.

joint forces: Forces present at articular surfaces resulting from muscle activity, gravity, and inertia.

light-emitting diode (LED): An active kinematic marker, usually of infrared light, that is placed singularly or in clusters on limb or joint segments to record time-histories of movement as recorded by infrared-sensitive cameras.

moment: See *torque*.

speed: Distance divided by time, the rate of displacement of an object; a scalar quantity.

> **free speed:** Normal walking speed; also called *preferred speed*.

stabilogram: A plot of COP displacement in the plane of support during quiet standing; used to quantify postural sway.

step length: The distance between heel strike of one leg and heel strike of the contralateral leg. Left and right step lengths are usually measured because they may differ.

step time: The time between heel strike of one leg and heel strike of the contralateral leg. Left and right step times are usually measured because they may differ.

step width: See *base of support*.

stride time: The time between successive occurrences of the same phase of gait, usually measured in seconds from heel strike of one leg to heel strike of the same leg. Left and right stride times are usually measured because they may differ.

swing time: The time that a foot is off the ground during one gait cycle. Left and right swing times are usually measured because they may differ.

torque: The product of a force times the perpendicular distance (moment arm) from the axis of rotation to the line of action of the force.

velocity: A vector that describes displacement. The term is often confused with speed (a scalar); however, speed represents only the magnitude of velocity.

> **angular velocity:** A vector that describes displacement around an axis; units are radians per seconds or degrees per second.

> **linear velocity:** A vector that describes translation of a body in space; moment in a straight line; in gait, usually expressed in meters per second.

Continued on following page

width of walking base: See *base of support.*

work: Force times distance.

FOR MORE INFORMATION

Craik, RA and Otis, CA: Gait Analysis: Theory and Application. Mosby Year Book, St. Louis, 1995.

Perry, J: Gait Analysis: Normal and Pathologic Function. Slack, Thorofare, NJ, 1992.

$\text{S}\ \text{E}\ \text{C}\ \text{T}\ \text{I}\ \text{O}\ \text{N}\ \mathbf{1}\ \mathbf{2}$

Prosthetics and Orthotics

CLASSIFICATION OF LONGITUDINAL AND TRANSVERSE DEFECTS IN LIMB BUD DEVELOPMENT

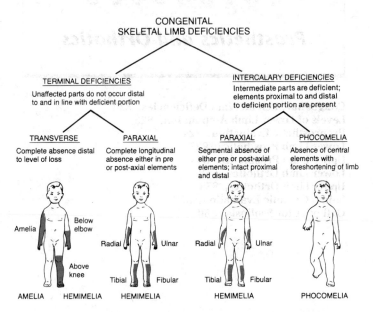

From Hall, CB, Brooks, MD, and Dennis, JF: Congenital skeletal deficiencies of the extremities: Classification and fundamentals of treatment. JAMA 181:591, 1962, with permission.

LEVELS OF AMPUTATION—
LOWER EXTREMITY

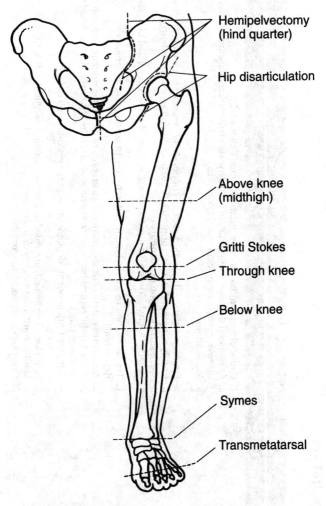

Hemipelvectomy
(hind quarter)

Hip disarticulation

Above knee
(midthigh)

Gritti Stokes

Through knee

Below knee

Symes

Transmetatarsal

From Thomson, A, Skinner, A, and Piercy, J: Tidy's Physiotherapy, ed 12. Butterworth-Heineman, Boston, p 261, with permission.

GUIDE FOR PREPROSTHETIC EVALUATION

Item to Be Evaluated	Observe for:
Medical status	1. Cause of amputation (disease, tumor, trauma, congenital)
	2. Associated diseases/symptoms (neuropathy, visual disturbances, cardiopulmonary disease, renal disease, congenital anomalies)
	3. Medications
Psychological	1. Emotional status (depression, denial, cooperativeness, enthusiasm, motivation)
	2. Family situation (interest, support, level of understanding, ability to help)
	3. Work situation (job opportunity)
	4. Prosthetic goals (desire for a prosthesis, anticipated activity level and lifestyle)
Activities of daily living	1. Transfers (bed to wheelchair, to toilet, to tub, to automobile; independent, dependent)
	2. Ambulatory status (with crutches, walker; type of gait; independent, dependent)
	3. Home (architectural barriers, safety rails; stairs; other hazards, such as small rugs, unsturdy rails)
	4. Self-care (independent, dependent; includes residual limb care)
Skin	1. Scar (location; healed, unhealed; adherent, mobile; invaginated, flat, thickened, keloid; from other surgery or a burn)
	2. Open lesions (size, shape, exudate)

Residuum	
Length	Bone length; soft-tissue, redundant-tissue length; the length of the below-knee limb is usually measured from the medial tibial plateau, and the above-knee limb from the ischial tuberosity or the greater trochanter
Shape	Cylindrical, conical, hourglass, "dog-ears," bulbous, above-knee adductor roll

3. Moisture (moist, dry, crusting)
4. Sensation (absent, diminished, hypersensitive to touch or pressure)
5. Grafts (location, type, degree of healing)
6. Dermatologic lesions (psoriasis, eczema, acne vulgaris, dermatitis, boils, epidermold cysts)

Vascularity (both limbs if cause of amputation is vascular disease)

1. Pulses (femoral, popliteal, dorsalis pedis, posterior tibial)
2. Color (cyanotic, redness)
3. Temperature (cool, warm)
4. Edema (circumference measurements)
5. Pain (in dependent position, throbbing, claudication)
6. Trophic changes (shininess, dryness, loss of hair)

Neurologic

1. Sensation (light touch, pressure, joint proprioception; both limbs)
2. Neuroma (location, tenderness)
3. Phantom (sensation; pain; description; throbbing, burning, electrical; duration)
4. Mental status (alert, senile; intelligent, limited ability to understand)

Range of motion

1. Hips (flexion, abduction, or external rotation contracture)
2. Knee (flexion contracture)
3. Ankle (plantar flexion contracture)

Continued on following page

825

GUIDE FOR PREPROSTHETIC EVALUATION (Continued)

Item to Be Evaluated	Observe for:
Strength	Major muscle groups; adaptation must be made for shortened lever arm
Prior prosthesis	Type, components, problems, gait deviations
Compression device	Type, applied independently, remains secure, provides adequate compression without excessive pressure on bony prominences
Footwear	Accommodates deformities on contralateral foot. Has accommodative insert if pressure sensation is impaired

From Sanders, GT: Lower Limb Amputations: A Guide to Rehabilitation. FA Davis, Philadelphia, 1986, p. 373, with permission.

Below-Knee Prosthetic Evaluation

The following table lists the various elements that should be checked as part of the evaluation of a below-knee prosthesis. Elements to be checked (standards) are in the left column and possible causes of a failure to meet the standards are in the right column.

Standard	Possible Deficiencies
Dons prosthesis easily	1. Socket too small; residual limb edematous 2. Technique improper 3. Medial wedge contour unsatisfactory (supracondylar suspension)
Stands comfortably 1. Anterior heel and sole flat on floor	1. Socket too far anterior, causing knee to flex and weight to be borne primarily on sole 2. Socket too far posterior, causing knee to feel forced backward and weight to be borne primarily on heel
2. Medial and lateral borders of sole flat on floor	1. Socket too abducted, causing excessive loading laterally 2. Socket too adducted, causing excessive loading medially
Stands with pelvis level, both knees extended	Pelvis may tilt toward prosthetic side and/or contralateral hip and knee may flex if: 1. Heel cushion or prosthetic foot bumper too soft 2. Prosthetic foot dorsiflexed 3. Socket too flexed 4. Socket too loose, causing residual limb to lodge too deeply 5. Shank too short

Continued on following page

Below-Knee Prosthetic Evaluation (Continued)

Standard	Possible Deficiencies
Minimal (<0.5 cm) slippage when prosthesis is lifted during standing	1. Suspension inadequate 2. Socket too large
Stands with thigh corset, if present, well fitted 1. Uprights conform to thigh contour 2. Mechanical knee joints close to the thigh, in line with the epicondyles 3. Corset flat on thigh, without gapping or pinching 4. Corset edges not touching each other	1. Uprights improperly contoured 2. Joints set too far or too close to the thigh 3. Joints set too far proximal or distal to the epicondyles, interfering with sitting comfort 4. Corset improperly set on uprights 5. Corset shape unsuitable for wearer's thigh 6. Corset too large
Appearance satisfactory	1. Shank does not match contour or color of contralateral limb

Sits comfortably with knees flexed 90°	1. Posterior socket brim inadequate:
	  a. Too sharp
	  b. Too high
	  c. Insufficient provision for hamstring tendons
	2. Cuff suspension attached to the socket too far anterior or distal (cuff suspension)

3. Mechanical knee joints attached to the socket too far anterior or distal (thigh corset suspension)
4. Medial wedge contour unsatisfactory (supracondylar suspension)

Kneels comfortably

1. Because kneeling requires acute knee flexion, the same deficiencies that interfere with sitting hamper kneeling

Walks comfortably with minimal deviation

1. See Below-Knee Prostheses: Gait Deviations and Their Causes

Walks with adequate suspension

1. Cuff attached to the socket too far anteriorly (cuff suspension)
2. Socket loose (supracondylar suspension)

Walks quietly

1. Prosthetic foot improperly fitted to shoe
2. Prosthetic foot joints loose (articulated assembly)
3. Mechanical knee joints loose (thigh corset suspension)

With prosthesis removed, construction satisfactory

1. Plastic lamination not uniform
2. Edges rough
3. Foot not joined to shank with smooth transition
4. Stitching inadequate
5. Rivets not flush with surface
6. Cosmetic cover inadequate

Continued on following page

Below-Knee Prosthetic Evaluation (Continued)

Standard	Possible Deficiencies
Skin unblemished by prosthesis 10 min after removal	1. Socket too tight 2. Socket too loose, sliding during walking and/or causing residual limb to bear too much load distally 3. Corset too tight (thigh corset suspension) 4. Medial wedge contour unsatisfactory (supracondylar suspension)
Wearer satisfied	1. Any deficiency noted above 2. Discomfort within residual limb or proximal joints 3. Psychosocial dysfunction 4. At final evaluation, insufficient training

Based on Prosthetics and Orthotics Staff: Lower Limb Prosthetics, rev ed. New York University, New York, 1981; and American Academy of Orthopedic Surgeons: Atlas of Limb Prosthetics: Surgical and Prosthetic Principles, ed 2. CV Mosby, St. Louis, 1992.

Below-Knee Prostheses: Gait Deviations and Their Causes

Deviation	Prosthetic Causes	Biological Causes
Excessive knee flexion in early stance	Insufficient plantar flexion Stiff heel cushion or plantar bumper Excessive socket flexion Socket malaligned too far anteriorly Excessive posterior placement of cuff tabs	Knee flexion contracture Weak quadriceps
Insufficient knee flexion in early stance	Excessive plantar flexion Soft heel cushion or plantar bumper Insufficient socket flexion Socket malaligned too far posteriorly	Pain at anterodistal aspect of residual limb Weak quadriceps Extensor hyper-reflexia Arthritis of the knee
Excessive lateral thrust	Excessive inset of foot Excessive socket adduction	
Medial thrust	Outset of foot Insufficient socket adduction	

Continued on following page

12

Below-Knee Prostheses: Gait Deviations and Their Causes (Continued)

Deviation	Prosthetic Causes	Biological Causes
Early knee flexion in late stance "drop-off"	Insufficient plantar flexion Distal end of keel or toe break misplaced posteriorly Soft dorsiflexion stop Excessive socket flexion Socket malaligned too far anteriorly Excessive posterior placement of cuff tabs	Knee flexion contracture
Delayed knee flexion in late stance "walking uphill"	Excessive plantar flexion Distal end of keel or toe break misplaced anteriorly Stiff dorsiflexion stop Insufficient socket flexion Socket malaligned too far posteriorly	Extensor hyper-reflexia Knee arthritis

Based on Prosthetics and Orthotics Staff: Lower Limb Prosthetics, rev ed. New York University, New York. 1981; and American Academy of Orthopedic Surgeons: Atlas of Limb Prosthetics: Surgical and Prosthetic Principles, ed 2. CV Mosby, St. Louis, 1992.

Above-Knee Prosthetic Evaluation

The following table lists the various elements that should be checked as part of the evaluation of an above-knee prosthesis. Elements to be checked (standards) are in the left column and possible causes of a failure to meet the standards are in the right column.

Standard	Possible Deficiencies
Dons prosthesis easily	1. Socket too small; residual limb edematous
	2. Suction valve not located below residual limb or at bottom of anterior surface of socket
	3. Technique improper
Stands comfortably	1. Proximal flesh roll caused by improper donning or too small a socket
	2. Greater trochanter and/or distal femoral socket concavities inadequate
	3. Quadrilateral socket:
	a. Adductor longus tendon not in channel
	Socket too large, causing anteromedial discomfort
	Socket too small
	b. Medial brim sharp
	c. Ischial tuberosity not on posterior brim
	Socket too large, causing residual limb to lodge too deeply and impinge anteromedially
	Socket too small, causing posterior discomfort
	d. Posterior brim not parallel to floor
	4. Ischial containment socket:
	a. Socket too small; posteromedial corner does not cover ischial tuberosity
	b. Socket too large; posterior wall gaps
	c. Socket impinges on coccyx and/or pubis

Continued on following page

Above-Knee Prosthetic Evaluation (Continued)

Standard	Possible Deficiencies
Stands with pelvis level, both knees extended (*Note:* If prosthesis has a manually locked knee unit, shank should be 1 cm short to provide for clearance during swing phase.)	Pelvis may tilt toward prosthetic side and/or contralateral hip and knee may flex if: 1. Heel cushion or prosthetic foot bumper too soft 2. Prosthetic foot dorsiflexed 3. Socket too loose, causing residual limb to lodge too deeply 4. Shank too short
Stands relaxed with prosthetic knee extended	1. Unlocked prosthetic knee unit: knee bolt too far anterior to line from hip to anterior border of heel, or ankle bolt of articulated foot-ankle assembly 2. Locked prosthetic knee unit: defective lock
Appearance satisfactory	Shank and/or thigh section do not match contour or color of contralateral limb
Sits comfortably with knees flexed 90°; should be able to lean forward to touch shoe	1. Anterior wall too high, impinging on abdomen 2. Posterior wall too thick or not parallel with chair seat 3. Insufficient posteromedial socket concavity (quadrilateral socket) 4. Mechanical hip joint not superior and anterior to greater trochanter (pelvic band suspension) 5. Pelvic band not contoured to torso (pelvic band suspension)

Walks comfortably with minimal deviation	See Above-Knee Prostheses: Gait Deviations and Their Causes

Walks with adequate suspension	1. Suction suspension:
	  a. Socket too large
	  b. Lateral socket wall not contacting thigh
	  c. Lateral socket wall too short
	  d. Greater trochanter concavity inadequate
	  e. Suction valve clogged with glue, powder, or perspiration
	2. Silesian bandage auxiliary suspension:
	  a. Lateral attachment not superior and posterior to greater trochanter
	  b. Anterior attachment (single attachment or midpoint between double anterior attachment) too high
	3. Pelvic band suspension:
	  a. Band not between iliac crest and greater trochanter
	  b. Mechanical hip joint not superior and anterior to greater trochanter

Walks quietly	1. Prosthetic foot improperly fitted to shoe 2. Prosthetic foot joints loose (articulated assembly) 3. Extension stop in the knee unit insufficiently padded 4. Loose mechanism in knee unit 5. Fluid-controlled knee unit leaking

Continued on following page

835

Above-Knee Prosthetic Evaluation (Continued)

Standard	Possible Deficiencies
With prosthesis removed, construction satisfactory	1. Socket interior rough
	2. Knee and ankle clearance excessive or insufficient
	3. Posterior thigh and shank not contoured to permit acute knee flexion
	4. Posterior thigh and shank not congruent when prosthetic knee is flexed fully
	5. Rigid socket lacks resilient back pad to absorb noise when sitting and to reduce clothing abrasion
	6. Knee lock, if present, malfunctions
	7. Plastic lamination or molding not uniform
	8. Foot not joined to shank with smooth transition
	9. Stitching inadequate
	10. Rivets not flush with surface
	11. Cosmetic cover is inadequate
Skin unblemished by prosthesis 10 min after removal	1. Socket too tight
	2. Socket too loose, sliding during walking and/or causing residual limb to bear too much load distally
	3. Socket does not cover proximal medial thigh, permitting fleshy bulge
	4. Socket edges too sharp
	5. Inappropriate number of stump socks
Wearer satisfied	1. Any deficiency noted above
	2. Discomfort felt within the residuum limb or proximal joints
	3. Psychosocial dysfunction
	4. At final evaluation, insufficient training

Above-Knee Prostheses: Gait Deviations and Their Causes

Deviation	Prosthetic Causes	Biological Causes
Lateral trunk bending	Short prosthesis Inadequate lateral wall adduction Sharp or excessively high medial wall Malalignment in abduction	Weak abductors Abduction contracture Hip pain Very short residual limb Instability
Wide walking base (abducted gait)	Long prosthesis Excessive abduction of hip joint Inadequate lateral wall adduction Sharp or excessively high medial wall Malalignment in abduction	Abduction contracture Adductor tissue roll Instability
Circumduction	Long prosthesis Excessive stiffness of knee unit Inadequate suspension Small socket Excessive plantar flexion	Abduction contracture Poor knee control
Medial (lateral) whip	Faulty socket contour Malrotation of knee unit	

Continued on following page

Above-Knee Prostheses: Gait Deviations and Their Causes (Continued)

Deviation	Prosthetic Causes	Biological Causes
Rotation of foot on heel strike	Stiff heel cushion or plantar bumper Malrotation of foot	
Uneven heel rise	Inadequate knee friction Lax or taut extension aid	Excessively forceful hip flexion
Terminal swing impact	Insufficient knee friction Taut extension aid	
Foot slap	Soft heel cushion or plantar bumper	
Uneven step length	Faulty socket contour Inadequate knee friction Lax or taut extension aid	Weak hip musculature Hip flexion contracture Instability
Lordosis	Inadequate support from posterior brim Inadequate socket flexion	Hip flexion contracture Weak hip extensors
Vaulting	Long prosthesis Inadequate suspension Inadequate knee friction Excessive plantarflexion Small socket	Walking speed exceeding that for which friction in a sliding friction knee unit was adjusted

Based on Prosthetics and Orthotics Staff: Lower Limb Prosthetics, rev ed. New York University, New York, 1981; and American Academy of Orthopedic Surgeons: Atlas of Limb Prosthetics: Surgical and Prosthetic Principles, ed 2. CV Mosby, St. Louis, 1992.

Hip-Disarticulation Prosthetic Evaluation

The following table lists the various elements that should be checked as part of the evaluation of a hip-disarticulation prosthesis. Elements to be checked (standards) are in the left column and possible causes of a failure to meet the standards are in the right column.

Standard	Possible Deficiencies
Dons prosthesis easily	1. Socket too small; residual limb edematous 2. Technique improper
Stands comfortably	1. Socket improperly contoured over the iliac crests 2. Residual limb not sufficiently lateral in socket 3. Ischial tuberosity not covered by socket 4. Perineal flesh roll below socket
Stands with pelvis almost level Pelvis should tilt slightly toward prosthetic side; a 1-cm lift under the prosthesis should restore level pelvic alignment. Slight shortness aids clearance during swing phase	1. Heel cushion or prosthetic foot bumper too soft 2. Prosthetic foot dorsiflexed 3. Shank or thigh section too short
Stands relaxed, with prosthetic hip and knee extended	1. A straight line joining the mechanical hip and knee joint fails to pass at least 3.5 cm posterior to the heel 2. Hip extension stop too thick *Continued on following page*

Continued on following page

Hip-Disarticulation Prosthetic Evaluation (Continued)

Standard	Possible Deficiencies
Minimal (< 0.5 cm) slippage when prosthesis is lifted during standing	1. Socket too large 2. Residual limb not sufficiently lateral in socket 3. Socket depressions over the iliac crests too shallow or too high
Appearance satisfactory	1. Shank and/or thigh section do not match contour or color of contralateral limb
Sits comfortably with knees flexed 90°	1. Hip extension stop too thick 2. Mechanical hip joint displaced too far posteriorly or too far distally 3. Posterior wall of thigh section not parallel with chair seat 4. Socket too large 5. Socket improperly contoured over the ischium 6. Residual limb not sufficiently lateral in socket 7. Waistband inadequately flared or too low 8. Proximal socket brim inadequately flared or too low 9. Knee extension aid fails to swivel to permit full knee flexion
Walks comfortably with minimal deviation	1. Because prosthesis is intentionally short, wearer may bend laterally 2. Hip instability, caused by failure of hip extension stop to contact socket in early stance, because

either the stop is too thin or the mechanical hip joint is too posterior

3. Knee instability, caused by failure of knee extension in early stance, because either the hip extension stop is too thick or the mechanical hip joint is displaced anteriorly

Walks with adequate suspension

1. Socket too large
2. Socket depressions over the iliac crests too shallow or too high
3. Contralateral side of socket provides insufficient support
4. Lateral waistband too loose

Walks quietly

1. Prosthetic foot improperly fitted to shoe
2. Prosthetic foot joints loose (articulated assembly)
3. Extension stop in knee unit insufficiently padded
4. Loose mechanism in knee or hip unit
5. Fluid-controlled knee unit leaking

With prosthesis removed, construction satisfactory

1. Socket interior rough
2. Knee and ankle clearance excessive or insufficient
3. Posterior thigh and shank not contoured to permit acute knee flexion

Continued on following page

Hip-Disarticulation Prosthetic Evaluation (Continued)

Standard	Possible Deficiencies
	4. Posterior thigh and shank not congruent when prosthetic knee flexed fully
	5. Plastic lamination not uniform
	6. Foot not joined to shank with smooth transition
	7. Stitching inadequate
	8. Rivets not flush with surface
	9. Cosmetic cover inadequate
Skin unblemished by prosthesis 10 min after removal	1. Socket too tight
	2. Socket too loose, sliding during walking
	3. Socket edges too sharp
Wearer satisfied	1. Any deficiency noted above
	2. Discomfort within amputated limb or proximal joints
	3. Psychosocial dysfunction
	4. At final evaluation, insufficient training

Based on Prosthetics and Orthotics Staff: Lower Limb Prosthetics, rev ed. New York University, New York, 1981; and American Academy of Orthopedic Surgeons: Atlas of Limb Prosthetics: Surgical and Prosthetic Principles, ed 2. CV Mosby, St. Louis, 1992.

Upper Limb Prosthetic Evaluation

The following table lists the various elements that should be checked as part of the evaluation of an upper limb prosthesis. Elements to be checked (standards) are in the left column and possible causes of a failure to meet the standards are in the right column.

Standard	Possible Deficiencies
Dons prosthesis easily	1. Socket too tight 2. Harness too complex 3. Technique improper

Wearing prosthesis, moves upper limb through satisfactory excursion comfortably.	Below-elbow, above-elbow, and shoulder prosthesis:
	    Chest strap too tight (chest strap suspension)
	
	Below-elbow and above-elbow prostheses:
	1. Axilla loop too small and/or unpadded
	2. Front support strap not in deltopectoral groove
	    (figure-of-eight suspension)
	
	Below-elbow prosthesis:
	1. Socket anterior brim restricts elbow flexion
	2. Socket posterior brim restricts elbow extension
	3. Socket too loose, reducing transmission of
	    forearm pronation and supination to the socket
	4. Elbow hinge pinches flesh
	5. Triceps pad or cuff improperly aligned
	    Continued on following page

Continued on following page

Upper Limb Prosthetic Evaluation (Continued)

Standard	Possible Deficiencies

Terminal device opens and closes satisfactorily. Active opening and closing should equal passive excursion when forearm is perpendicular to torso. Below-elbow prosthesis: full excursion should be obtained also with terminal device at waist and at mouth. Above-elbow and shoulder prostheses: active excursion at waist and at mouth should be at least half of the mechanical range.	Above-elbow prosthesis:
	 1. Socket anterior brim restricts shoulder flexion to $< 90°$
	 2. Socket lateral brim restricts shoulder abduction to $< 90°$
	 3. Socket posterior brim restricts shoulder hyperextension to $< 30°$
	
	 1. Cable-controlled terminal device:
	   a. Cable malaligned
	   b. Cable too long or too short
	   c. Cable path has sharp bends
	   d. Cable housing too long
	   e. Cross of figure-of-eight harness too far toward residual side
	   f. Control attachment strap on or above scapular spine
	   g. Chest strap too loose (chest strap suspension)
	   h. Leather lift loop too large or too distal
	   i. Terminal device adjustments, e.g., two-position thumb, malfunctioning
	 2. Myoelectrically controlled terminal device:
	   a. Electrodes improperly located

Prosthesis operates efficiently. Below-elbow prosthesis: force at terminal device should equal at least 80% of force measured at control attachment strap of harness. Above-elbow and shoulder prostheses: terminal device force should be at least 70% of force measured at control attachment strap.	b. Socket too loose, preventing electrode contact with skin c. Battery inadequately charged 1. Cable malaligned 2. Cable too long 3. Cable path has sharp bends
Minimal slippage when 23-kg (50-lb) axial stress is applied to prosthesis. Below-elbow supracondylar socket should not slip more than 1 cm. All other sockets should not slip more than 2.5 cm.	1. Socket too loose 2. Harness attachments insecure 3. Shoulder saddle too small (chest strap suspension) 4. Inappropriate number of stump socks

Limbs equal in length when elbows are extended.
1. Prosthetic hand should be at same level as sound hand
2. Hook should be at same level as thumb of sound hand
	1. Below-elbow, above-elbow, and shoulder prostheses:
	  a. Forearm too short or too long
	  b. Terminal device too small or too large
	2. Above-elbow and shoulder prostheses: Humeral section too short or too long

Wrist unit rotates and, if lock is present, locks satisfactorily	1. Friction adjustment too tight or too loose 2. Locking mechanism malfunctions

Continued on following page

845

Upper Limb Prosthetic Evaluation (Continued)

Standard	Possible Deficiencies
Above-elbow and shoulder prostheses: Elbow unit moves and locks satisfactorily. Maximum of 45° shoulder flexion needed to flex elbow fully	1. Cable malaligned 2. Cable too long 3. Cable housing too long 4. Cable housing ends abut before full elbow flexion is achieved 5. Cross of figure-of-eight harness too far toward residual side 6. Control attachment strap on or above scapular spine 7. Chest strap too loose (chest strap suspension) 8. Leather lift loop too large, too short, or improperly located 9. Leather lift loop folds or does not pivot 10. Elastic suspensor strap too loose or too taut 11. Locking mechanism malfunctions 12. Turntable too loose or too tight

Appearance satisfactory	1. Terminal device too large or too small
	2. Prosthetic hand:
	  a. Glove improperly installed
	  b. Glove stained or torn
	  c. Glove color does not match contralateral limb

	3. Forearm and humeral section, if present, does not match contour or color of contralateral limb
With prosthesis removed, construction is satisfactory	1. Plastic lamination not uniform 2. Edges of socket or housing rough 3. Stitching inadequate 4. Rivets not flush with surface 5. Cosmetic cover inadequate
Skin appears unblemished by prosthesis 10 min after removal	1. Socket or harness too tight 2. Socket edges rough 3. Axilla loop too small or unpadded
Wearer is satisfied	1. Any deficiency noted above 2. Discomfort within residual limb or proximal joints 3. Psychosocial dysfunction 4. At final evaluation, insufficient training

Based on Prosthetics and Orthotics Staff: Upper-Limb Prosthetics. New York University, New York, 1986; and Atkins, DJ and Meier, RH III (eds): Comprehensive Management of the Upper-Limb Amputee. Springer-Verlag, New York, 1989.

ORTHOTIC EVALUATION

Lower Limb Orthotic Evaluation

The following table lists the various elements that should be checked as part of the evaluation of a lower limb orthosis. Elements to be checked (standards) are in the left column and possible causes of a failure to meet the standards are in the right column.

Standard	Possible Deficiencies
Dons orthosis easily	1. Shoe or proximal components too small 2. Fastenings unsuitable 3. Shoe does not open sufficiently. Blucher design, in which anterior borders of lace stays are not attached, provides maximum opening 4. Shoe does not detach from proximal components. Shoe insert, split stirrup, and caliper are easier to don than solid stirrup 5. Insufficient trimline of plastic ankle-foot orthosis
Stands comfortably	1. Shoe too tight, especially at metatarsophalangeal joints 2. Shoe too short, contacting toetips 3. Shoe insert or foot valgus/varus correction strap contour unsatisfactory 4. Knee valgus/varus correction strap contour unsatisfactory 5. Shells, bands, and uprights too tight 6. Calf band presses on fibular head

Stands with pelvis level, both knees extended (*Note*: If orthosis has a locked knee joint, 1-cm shortening provides for clearance during swing phase)

7. Medial and lateral uprights not at midline of leg: If too posterior, reduces areas of calf shell or band; if too anterior, may permit unstable knee to hyperextend
8. Posterior upright not at posterior midline of leg
9. Mechanical ankle and knee joint stops set improperly
10. Medial upright impinges into perineum
11. Lateral upright contacts greater trochanter
12. Trimline of plastic orthotic impinges on bony prominence

Shoe elevation inadequate to compensate for limb shortness

Stands relaxed.

1. Knee and hip locks not engaged securely
2. Ankle or knee joint in inappropriate amount of flexion

Patellar-tendon bearing or proximal thigh brim, if included, reduces weight bearing at the heel

Brim contour inadequate to support weight proximally

Appearance satisfactory

Orthosis design or construction excessively bulky

Continued on following page

Lower Limb Orthotic Evaluation (Continued)

Standard	Possible Deficiencies
Sits comfortably with knees flexed 105° (*Note:* Orthosis limiting dorsiflexion will restrict acute knee flexion)	1. Proximal border of calf shell or band too sharp or too high 2. Mechanical ankle joints not level with distal tip of medial malleolus 3. Mechanical knee joints not level with medial femoral epicondyle 4. Mechanical hip joints not superior and anterior to greater trochanter 5. Pelvic band not contoured to torso
Walks comfortably with minimal deviation	See Lower Limb Orthoses: Gait Deviations and Their Causes
With orthosis removed, construction satisfactory	1. Edges rough 2. Metal nicked 3. Stitching inadequate 4. Rivets not flush with surface 5. Shoe heel and sole not level, including shoes with wedges 6. Insert does not fit snugly in shoe 7. Mechanical ankle, knee, or hip joints bind when moved

8. Mechanical ankle or knee joints do not contact simultaneously at full flexion and at full extension
9. Lengthening provision inadequate (child's orthosis)
10. Sharp edge on trimline of plastic orthotic

1. Orthosis too tight
2. Mechanical ankle joints not level with distal tip of medial malleolus, causing calf band to abrade leg (if orthosis permits dorsiflexion)
3. Evidence of inadequate pressure relief over bony prominences

1. Any deficiency noted above
2. Discomfort within the lower limb or back
3. Psychosocial dysfunction
4. At final evaluation, insufficient training

Skin unblemished by orthosis 10 min after removal

Wearer satisfied

Based on Prosthetics and Orthotics Staff: Lower-Limb Prosthetics, rev ed. New York, New York University, 1981; American Academy of Orthopedic Surgeons: Atlas of Orthotics, ed 2. CV Mosby, St. Louis, 1981; Redford, JB (ed): Orthotics Etcetera, ed 3. Williams & Wilkins, Baltimore, 1986.

Lower Limb Orthoses: Gait Deviations and Their Causes

Deviation	Orthotic Causes	Biological Causes
Lateral trunk bending	Excecesive height of medial upright of KAFO Excessive abduction of hip joint Insufficient shoe lift to compensate for leg shortening	Weak abductors Abduction contracture Dislocated hip Hip pain Instability
Hip hiking	Hip or knee lock uncompensated by contralateral shoe lift Pes equinus uncompensated by contralateral shoe lift Inadequate plantar flexion stop or dorsiflexion spring	Weak hip flexors Hip extensor hyper-reflexia Decreased hip or knee flexion ROM Decreased dorsiflexion ROM
Internal (external) hip rotation	Transverse plane malalignment	Weak lateral (medial) hip musculature
Circumduction	Hip or knee lock uncompensated by contralateral shoe lift Pes equinus uncompensated by contralateral shoe lift Inadequate plantar-flexion stop or dorsiflexion spring	Weak hip flexors Abduction contracture Decreased hip or knee flexion ROM Decreased dorsiflexion ROM

Deviation		
Wide walking base	Excessive height of medial upright of KAFO	Weak abductors
	Excessive abduction of hip joint	Abduction contracture
	Knee lock uncompensated by contralateral shoe lift	Instability
		Genu valgum
Excessive medial (lateral) foot contact	Transverse plane malalignment	Weak invertors (evertors)
		Pes valgus (varus)
		Genu valgum (varum)
Anterior trunk bending	Inadequate knee lock	Weak quadriceps
Posterior trunk bending		Weak hip extensors
Lordosis		Hip flexion contracture
		Weak hip extensors
Hyperextended knee	Inadequate support from the brim of a weight-relieving KAFO	Weak quadriceps
	Genu recurvatum inadequately controlled by plantar stop and excessively concave calf band	Lax knee ligaments
		Extensor hyper-reflexia
Knee instability	Inadequate knee lock	Knee flexion contracture
	Inadequate dorsiflexion stop	Weak quadriceps

Continued on following page

Lower Limb Orthoses: Gait Deviations and Their Causes (Continued)

Deviation	Orthotic Causes	Biological Causes
Inadequate dorsiflexion control	Inadequate plantar flexion stop or dorsiflexion spring	Weak dorsiflexors Extensor hyper-reflexia
Vaulting	Hip or knee lock uncompensated by contralateral shoe lift Pes equinus uncompensated by contralateral shoe lift Inadequate plantar flexion stop or dorsiflexion spring	Weak hip flexors Abduction contracture Decreased hip or knee flexion ROM Decreased dorsiflexion ROM

KAFO = Knee-ankle-foot orthosis, ROM = range of motion.
Based on Prosthetics and Orthotics Staff: Lower-Limb Prosthetics, rev ed. New York University, New York, 1981; American Academy of Orthopedic Surgeons: Atlas of Orthotics, ed 2. CV Mosby, St. Louis, 1981; Redford, JB (ed): Orthotics Etcetera, ed 3. Williams & Wilkins, Baltimore, 1986.

Upper Limb Orthotic Evaluation

The following table lists the various elements that should be checked as part of the evaluation of an upper limb orthosis. Elements to be checked (standards) are in the left column and possible causes of a failure to meet the standards are in the right column.

Standard	Possible Deficiencies
Dons orthosis easily	1. Orthosis too tight 2. Orthosis too complex 3. Technique improper 4. Fastenings unsuitable
Wearing orthosis, moves fingers comfortably	1. Mechanical joints not congruent with anatomic joints. 2. Components press on bony prominences 3. Wrist strap does not lie between metacarpal bases and wrist crease
Orthosis promotes maximum function (except for orthosis intended to promote rest)	1. Palmar surface of finger tips obstructed 2. Opponens bar does not provide adequate ulnar-directed force on thumb metacarpal 3. Opponens bar does not extend to palmar edge of thumb metacarpal 4. Thumb abduction bar does not maintain adequate abduction

Continued on following page

12

Upper Limb Orthotic Evaluation (Continued)

Standard	Possible Deficiencies
Orthosis promotes maximum function (except for orthosis intended to promote rest)	5. Thumb abduction bar restricts thumb interphalangeal or index metacarpophalangeal joint motion
	6. Palmar or dorsal bars do not conform to contour of distal transverse arch
	7. Metacarpophalangeal extension stop ineffective
	8. Thumb and index and middle fingers not aligned to provide desired grasp, either three-jaw chuck or lateral grasp
	9. Forearm bar too long or too short
	10. Forearm bar does not maintain wrist in desired position
	11. Electric microswitch actuator unsatisfactory
	12. Battery inadequately charged
	13. Utensil holder too large or too small

Appearance satisfactory.	1. Orthosis excessively bulky or complex.
With orthosis removed, construction satisfactory.	1. Edges rough 2. Plastic molding not uniform 3. Rivets not flush with surface 4. Mechanical joints bind when moved
Skin unblemished by orthosis 10 min after removal.	1. Orthosis too tight 2. Orthosis too loose, permitting slippage during function 3. Edges rough
Wearer is satisfied.	1. Any deficiency noted above 2. Discomfort within the upper limb 3. Psychosocial dysfunction 4. At final evaluation, insufficient training.

Based on American Academy of Orthopedic Surgeons: Atlas of Orthotics, ed 2. CV Mosby, St. Louis, 1981; and Redford, JB (ed): Orthotics Etcetera, ed 3. Williams & Wilkins, Baltimore, 1986.

Spinal Orthotic Evaluation

The following table lists the various elements that should be checked as part of the evaluation of a spinal orthosis. Elements to be checked (standards) are in the left column and possible causes of a failure to meet the standards are in the right column.

Standard	Possible Deficiencies
Dons orthosis easily	1. Orthosis too tight 2. Thoracic band too long 3. Technique improper
Stands comfortably	1. Pelvic or thoracic band too narrow or not conforming to torso 2. Pelvic band at or above posterior superior iliac spines 3. Pelvic band terminates posterior to lateral midline of torso 4. Thoracic band above inferior angles of scapulae 5. Thoracic band not horizontal 6. Posterior uprights press on vertebrae 7. Interscapular band too short, too long, or too high 8. Subclavicular extensions of the thoracic band, if present, too high or too low 9. Abdominal support too small 10. Suprapubic pad, if present, impinges on pelvis 11. Sternal plate, if present, too high 12. Occipital plate, if present, too low
Appearance satisfactory	1. Orthosis design or construction excessively bulky

Sits comfortably	1. Pelvic band below greater trochanters or contacting chair
	2. Thoracic band too high
	3. Interscapular band too low
	4. Abdominal support too large or inferior border too low or too high
	5. Posterior uprights press on vertebrae
	6. Pads impinge on clavicles
With orthosis removed, construction satisfactory	1. Edges rough
	2. Metal nicked
	3. Stitching inadequate
	4. Rivets not flush with surface
	5. Plastic molding not uniform
Skin unblemished by orthosis 10 min after removal	1. Orthosis too tight
	2. Pelvic or thoracic band improperly contoured
Wearer satisfied	1. Any deficiency noted above
	2. Discomfort within the trunk or neck
	3. Psychosocial dysfunction

Based on American Academy of Orthopedic Surgeons: Atlas of Orthotics, ed 2. CV Mosby, St. Louis, 1981; Redford, JB (ed): Orthotics Etcetera, ed 3. Williams & Wilkins, Baltimore, 1986; Prosthetics and Orthotics Staff: Spinal Orthotics. New York University, New York, 1987.

Evaluation of Orthotics for Scoliosis

The following table lists the various elements that should be checked as part of the evaluation of orthoses used to treat scoliosis. Elements to be checked (standards) are in the left column and possible causes of a failure to meet the standards are in the right column.

Standard	Possible Deficiencies
Dons orthosis easily	1. Orthosis too tight 2. Technique improper 3. Pelvic girdle straps too short 4. Pelvic girdle opening insufficient
Stands comfortably	1. Pads too snug or too small 2. Pelvic girdle too tight 3. Pelvic girdle anteroinferior border contacts pubis 4. Pelvic girdle anterosuperior border too low or too high 5. Pelvic girdle superolateral border contacts ribs 6. Pelvic girdle does not accommodate iliac spines 7. Thoracic pad strap not centered on pad 8. Thoracic pad spans fewer than three ribs 9. Lumbar pad impinges on pelvis or vertebrae 10. Shoulder ring or sling improperly contoured 11. Sternal pad too high 12. Pads or frame interfere with deep breathing or arm motion

Appearance satisfactory	1. Pelvic girdle superolateral border gaps
	2. Uprights not contoured to the torso
	3. Shoulder ring or sling improperly contoured
Sits comfortably	1. Pelvic girdle anteroinferior border too low, contacting chair
	2. Pelvic girdle anteroinferior border too low, impinging on thighs
	3. Pelvic girdle lateral border impinges on greater trochanters
With orthosis removed, construction satisfactory	1. Uprights not covered with plastic or leather
	2. Edges rough
	3. Metal nicked
	4. Stitching inadequate
	5. Rivets not flush with surface
	6. Plastic molding not uniform
Skin unblemished by orthosis 10 min after removal Painless reddening is satisfactory just above the ilium and beneath pads.	1. Pads impinge on bony prominences
	2. Pelvic girdle too tight or too loose
Wearer satisfied	1. Any deficiency noted above
	2. Discomfort within the trunk or neck
	3. Psychosocial dysfunction

Based on American Academy of Orthopedic Surgeons: Atlas of Orthotics, ed 2. CV Mosby, St. Louis, 1981; Redford, JB (ed): Orthotics Etcetera, ed 3. Williams & Wilkins, Baltimore, 1986; Prosthetics and Orthotics Staff: Spinal Orthotics. New York University, New York, 1987.

12

Psychology and Psychiatry

NEUROPSYCHOLOGICAL TESTS LISTED ALPHABETICALLY

Name of Test	Description
Aphasia Screening Test	A test that screens for aphasia and associated disorders. Items assess speech comprehension, oral expression, speech repetition, naming, oral reading, reading comprehension, writing, written and oral calculation, and constructional (drawing) ability. The test is not timed but takes under 15 min.
Autobiographical Memory Interview (AMI)	A standardized test of retrograde amnesia using information and events from a patient's own life. The test is not timed but takes under 30 min.
Beck Depression Inventory	A self-report, multiple-choice instrument for measuring the presence and severity of depression-related symptoms. The test is not timed but takes under 15 min.
Beery Development Test of Visual-Motor Integration (BDI)	An assessment of drawing ability by requiring patients to copy increasingly difficult geometric figures from models. The test is not timed but takes under 15 min.
Behavioral Inattention Test (BIT)	A comprehensive assessment of neglect syndromes using items that require line crossing, letter cancellation, star cancellation, figure copying, line bisection, drawing, picture scanning, telephone dialing, reading, telling and setting time on a clock, coin sorting, writing, map navigation, and card sorting. The test is not timed but takes under 1 h.
Benton Facial Recognition Test	An assessment of ability to match and discriminate faces. The test is not timed but takes under 30 min.
Benton Judgment of Line Orientation Test	An assessment of ability to judge the orientation of lines in space. The test is not timed but takes under 30 min.

Benton Motor Impersistence Test	An assessment of ability to maintain various movements or positions involving the eyes, tongue, mouth, and head. The test is sensitive to presence of motor disinhibition. The test takes under 15 min.
Benton Right-Left Orientation Test	An assessment of ability to distinguish right vs left from one's own perspective and from the perspective of a person facing the opposite direction. The test is not timed but takes under 10 min.
Benton Visual Form Discrimination Test	An assessment of ability to match and discriminate visual forms. The test is not timed but takes under 15 min.
Benton Visual Retention Test (BVRT)	An assessment of ability to learn and retain visual and spatial information using sets of designs. Available in five alternate forms and administration formats. The test takes under 15 min.
Boston Diagnostic Aphasia Examination (BDAE)	This examination provides a thorough and comprehensive assessment of oral and written language disorder. It includes subtests measuring fluency, comprehension, naming, repetition, oral reading, reading comprehension, and written and oral spelling. It also includes supplementary tests in many areas permitting for a more refined assessment. The test may take over 1 hr.
Boston Naming Test (BNT)	A test of confrontation naming using pictures of objects. Names vary from high frequency to low frequency words, and phonemic and semantic cues are provided. The test is not timed but takes under 15 min.
California Verbal Learning Test (CVLT)	An assessment of ability to learn and retain verbal information using mock shopping lists. It permits a sophisticated process-oriented analysis of memory performance that delineates factors responsible for a given level of impairment. The test takes under 1 hour, including a 20-min delayed recall interval.

Continued on following page

NEUROPSYCHOLOGICAL TESTS LISTED ALPHABETICALLY (Continued)

Name of Test	Description
Category Test (CT)	A measure of abstract reasoning, problem solving, and executive functioning. Patients must compare stimuli for similarities and differences to discover an abstract rule governing success or failure. The test also incorporates a memory trial. The test is not timed but takes under 45 min.
Controlled Oral Word Association Test (COWAT)	An assessment of word fluency using three trials in which words beginning with a target letter are named within a defined period. The test takes 3 min.
Dementia Rating Scale (DRS)	A brief measure of attention, initiation, perseveration, constructional ability, abstract conceptualization, and memory. The test is suitable for patients with severe impairment who might be untestable by other means. Useful in the diagnosis of dementia. The test is not timed but takes under 1 h.
Finger Tapping Test (FTT)	Patients tap a key with their index finger as rapidly as possible while a counter records the number of taps. The test is administered to each hand separately to assess motor speed and coordination. The test takes under 10 min.
Grooved Pegboard Test	Patients attempt to rapidly insert ridged pegs into variously oriented slots. The test is administered to each hand separately to assess fine motor coordination and speed. The test takes under 10 min.
Halstead-Reitan Battery (HRB)	A battery comprised of the Sensory Perceptual Examination, use of a hand dynamometer, Category Test, Tactual Performance Test, Seashore Rhythm Test, Speech Sounds Perception Test, Finger Tapping Test, Grooved Pegboard Test, Aphasia Screening Test, and several additional tests. The battery is designed to detect, lateralize, localize, and measure the severity

of brain damage. It is often supplemented with additional tests of memory, intellectual functioning, and personality. Depending on the tests included, it takes from 3–8 h (could be longer).

Ishihara Test for Color Blindness
A test that detects the most common forms of congenital and acquired color blindness. The test is not timed but takes under 10 min.

Line Bisection Test (LB)
A test that detects the presence of a neglect syndrome using lines of various lengths and in various positions on a page, which patients attempt to bisect. The test is not timed but takes under 10 min.

Luria-Nebraska Neuropsychological Battery (LNNB)
A battery that attempts to represent a standardized and normed version of Luria's Neuropsychological Investigation (see next listing). The battery includes scales to measure motor functions, rhythm and pitch perception and production, tactile and visual perception, language, writing, reading, arithmetic, memory, and intellectual ability. It also includes supplemental scales consisting of right and left sensorimotor items and items considered pathognomic of brain damage. The validity and reliability of the battery continues to be investigated. The test is not timed but takes under 3 h.

Luria's Neuropsychological Investigation
A compilation of examination techniques and procedures derived from the work of the neuropsychologist Aleksandr Luria. Items cover the same areas as the Luria-Nebraska (see previous listing). The test is not timed but takes under 3 h.

Memory Assessment Scales (MAS)
A comprehensive battery of tests assessing ability to learn and retain lists, prose, names and faces, and designs. The test also includes subtests measuring various aspects of attention. The test takes under 1 h.

Minnesota Multiphasic Personality Inventory 2 (MMPI 2)
The most widely used standardized and normed measure of personality and emotional disorders. It uses a true-false response format. It includes several validity scales useful for determining patients' response biases, scales covering the major psychiatric disorders, and a broad range of personality variables. The test is not timed but takes between 90 min and 2 h.

Continued on following page

13

NEUROPSYCHOLOGICAL TESTS LISTED ALPHABETICALLY (Continued)

Name of Test	Description
Paced Auditory Serial Addition Test (PASAT)	An assessment of sustained attention and speed of information processing using a serial addition task presented on audiotape. The test takes under 20 min.
Peabody Individual Achievement Test (PIAT)	A standardized test of academic achievement measuring general knowledge, spelling, arithmetic, and reading ability. The test is not timed but takes under 45 min.
Rivermead Behavioural Memory Test (RBMT)	An assessment of ability to learn and retain new information using everyday memory content, including names, faces, an appointment, prose, and a route. Incorporating everyday content, the test potentially gives greater ecologic validity than other instruments. It is available in four parallel forms. The test takes under 30 min.
Seashore Rhythm Test	An assessment of auditory perception using pairs of rhythmic beats, presented by audiotape, which patients must judge as the same or different. The test takes from 15–20 min.
Sensory-Perceptual Examination	A standardization of procedures from neurologic examinations. The test includes confrontation testing of visual fields, unilateral and bilateral simultaneous stimulation perception, detection of fingers touched, detection of numbers traced on fingers, discrimination of coins, and visual recognition of tactually presented shapes. The test is not timed but takes under 20 min.
Speech Sounds Perception Test	An assessment of ability to identify nonsense syllables that match those presented via an audiotape. The test is used for detecting brain damage and subtle language deficits. The test takes from 15–20 min.
Tactual Performance Test (TPT)	An assessment of tactile perception and memory using variously shaped blocks that blindfolded patients attempt to fit into slots on a board. Each hand is tested separately and then together. Patients then attempt to draw shapes from memory in their correct spatial position. The test takes approximately 40 min.

Test of Visual Neglect	A test that detects neglect syndromes by requiring patients to make hatch marks through lines placed in what appear to be random positions on a page. The test is not timed but takes under 10 min.
Three-Dimensional Block Construction	Patients attempt to construct three-dimensional models (presented as actual three-dimensional models or in photographs) using blocks of various sizes and shapes. The test is not timed, but takes under 30 min.
Token Test	An assessment of language comprehension using increasingly long and complex commands relating to manipulation of tokens of varying colors, sizes, and shapes. The test is not timed but takes under 30 min.
Vigil	A computerized continuous performance test measuring vigilance or the ability to sustain attention over time. The test takes 16 min.
Vineland Adaptive Behavior Scales	A standardized and normed instrument assessing personal and social skills. Separate forms can be administered as an interview or questionnaire or can be completed by an observer (e.g., a teacher). Administration time varies with the form used, but the test takes under 90 min.
Visual Object and Space Perception Battery (VOSP)	A battery that includes tests that assess various aspects of visual and spatial perception including discrimination of forms, identification of incomplete letters, identification of objects depicted as rotated silhouettes, dot counting, determination of the position of points in space, and estimation of quantity. The test is not timed but takes under 30 min.
Visual Search and Attention Test (VSAT)	An assessment of neglect syndrome using four letter and shape cancellation tasks. The test takes under 15 min.

Continued on following page

NEUROPSYCHOLOGICAL TESTS LISTED ALPHABETICALLY (Continued)

Name of Test	Description
Wechsler Adult Intelligence Scale–Revised (WAIS-R, as a Neuropsychological Instrument)	A test that applies the process-oriented approach to the traditional WAIS-R subtests to obtain qualitatively richer data for neuropsychological interpretation of intellectual deficits. It modifies the traditional WAIS-R subtests and adds several test variations, allowing the examiner to determine factors responsible for a given level of impairment. The test is not timed but takes under 3 h.
WAIS-R	The most widely used standardized and normed measure of intellectual functioning, incorporating verbal and performance subscales. Subscales examine attention, general information, vocabulary, numerical reasoning, verbal abstracting, pictorial reasoning, puzzle construction, and other intelligence-related abilities. The arithmetic and several performance subscales are excluded. This test takes under 90 min.
Wechsler Memory Scale–Revised	A widely used comprehensive battery of tests assessing the ability to learn and retain new information. The battery includes list, paired associate, prose, and design learning tasks. It also incorporates measures of attention. The test takes under 1 h.
Western Aphasia Battery	A comprehensive assessment of oral and written language disorders, with items measuring fluency, naming, repetition, comprehension, reading, writing, and spelling. The test also includes items that assess praxis, calculations, and constructional abilities. The test is not timed but takes under 30 min.
Wide Range Achievement Test Revised (WRAT-R)	A standardized test of academic achievement measuring spelling, arithmetic, and reading (word pronunciation) ability. The test takes under 30 min.
Wisconsin Card Sorting Test	A measure of abstract reasoning, problem solving, and executive functioning using a sorting task. A highly sensitive measure of frontal lobe functioning and of the presence of brain damage. The test is not timed but takes under 1 h.

FOR MORE INFORMATION

Lezak, MD: Neuropsychological Assessment, ed 3. Oxford University Press, New York, 1994.

Spreen, O and Strauss, E: A Compendium of Neuropsychological Tests: Administration, Norms, and Commentary. Oxford University Press, New York, 1991.

Stringer, AY: A Guide to Adult Neuropsychological Diagnosis. FA Davis, Philadelphia, 1996.

NEUROPSYCHOLOGICAL TESTS LISTED BY FUNCTION TESTED

For descriptions of the tests, see Neuropsychological Tests Listed Alphabetically, pages 864–870.

Abstraction and Cognitive Functioning

Category Test
Wisconsin Card Sorting Test

Affective State

Beck Depression Inventory
Minnesota Multiphasic Personality Inventory (MMPI)
Vineland Adaptive Behavior Scales

Attention

Paced Auditory Serial Addition Test
Vigil

Composite Batteries

Dementia Rating Scale
Halstead-Reitan Battery
Luria-Nebraska Neuropsychological Battery
Luria's Neuropsychological Investigation

Intellectual

Peabody Individual Achievement Test
Wechsler Adult Intelligence Scale Revised (WAIS-R)
Wide Range Achievement Test 3

Language

Aphasia Screening Test
Boston Diagnostic Aphasia Examination
Boston Naming Test
Controlled Oral Word Association Test
Speech Sounds Perception Test
Token Test
Western Aphasia Battery

Memory

Autobiographical Memory Interview
Benton Visual Retention Test
California Verbal Learning Test
Memory Assessment Scales
Rivermead Behavioural Memory Test
Wechsler Memory Scale—Revised

Motor

Beery Development Test of Visual-Motor Integration
Benton Motor Impersistence Test
Finger Tapping Test
Grooved Pegboard Test
Three-Dimensional Block Construction

13

Perception

Behavioral Inattention Test
Benton Facial Recognition Test
Benton Judgment of Line Orientation Test
Benton Right-Left Orientation Test
Benton Visual Form Discrimination Test
Ishihara Test for Color Blindness
Line Bisection Test
Seashore Rhythm Test
Sensory-Perceptual Examination
Tactual Performance Test
Test of Visual Neglect
Visual Object and Space Perception Test
Visual Search and Attention Test

FOR MORE INFORMATION

Lezak, MD: Neuropsychological Assessment, ed 3. Oxford University Press, New York, 1994.

Spreen, O and Strauss, E: A Compendium of Neuropsychological Tests: Administration, Norms, and Commentary. Oxford University Press, New York, 1991.

Stringer, AY: A Guide to Adult Neuropsychological Diagnosis. FA Davis, Philadelphia, 1996.

PSYCHOTHERAPEUTIC AGENTS

COMMON ANTIDEPRESSANT DRUGS

Generic Name	Trade Name	Initial Adult Dose (mg/day)	Prescribing Limits * (mg/day)
Tricyclics			
Amitriptyline	Elavil, Emitrip, others	50–100	300
Desipramine	Pertofrane, Norpramin	100–200	300
Doxepin	Adapin, Sinequan	75	300
Imipramine	Janimine, Tofranil, others	75–200	300
Nortriptyline	Aventyl, Pamelor	75–100	150
Protriptyline	Vivactil	15–40	60
Trimipramine	Surmontil	75	300
MAO Inhibitors			
Isocarboxazid	Marplan	10–20	30
Phenelzine	Nardil	45	90

Tranylcypromine	Parnate	10–20	60
Second-Generation Agents			
Amoxapine	Asendin	100–150	600
Bupropion	Wellbutrin	200	450
Fluoxetine	Prozac	20	80
Maprotiline	Ludiomil	25–75	225
Sertraline	Zoloft	50	200
Trazodone	Desyrel	150	600

*Upper limits reflect dosages administered to patients with severe depression who are being treated as inpatients.
MAO = monoamine oxidase.
From Ciccone, CD: Pharmacology in Rehabilitation, ed 2. FA Davis, Philadelphia, 1996, p 86, with permission.

13

	SECOND-GENERATION ANTIDEPRESSANT DRUGS		
Drug	**Mechanism (Amine Selectivity)**	**Advantages**	**Disadvantages**
Buproprion	Appears to inhibit dopamine reuptake	Low sedative, anticholinergic, and cardiovascular side effects	May cause overstimulation (insomnia, tremor) and induce psychotic symptoms
Fluoxetine	Strong, selective inhibition of serotonin reuptake	Low sedative, anticholinergic, and cardiovascular side effects; helpful in obsessive-compulsive disorders	May cause anxiety, nausea, insomnia; long half-life can lead to accumulation
Maprotiline	Moderate inhibition of norepinephrine reuptake	Sedating; useful in agitation	Possibility of seizures; overdoses lethal; long half-life
Sertraline	Strong selective inhibition of serotonin reuptake	Similar to fluoxetine	Similar to fluoxetine
Trazodone	Slight inhibition of serotonin reuptake	Sedating; useful in agitation; lower relative risk of overdose	May induce or exacerbate arrhythmias
Amoxapine	Moderate inhibition of norepinephrine reuptake	Low sedative and anticholinergic activity; may have more rapid onset of action	Possibility of extrapyramidal side effects (tardive dyskinesia); overdoses lethal

From Ciccone, CD: Pharmacology in Rehabilitation, ed 2. FA Davis, Philadelphia, 1996, p 88, with permission.

SIDE EFFECTS OF ANTIDEPRESSANT DRUGS*

Drug	Sedation	Insomnia	Anticholinergic Effects	Orthostatic Hypotension
Tricyclic Drugs				
Amitriptyline	+++	0	+++	+++
Trimipramine	+++	0	+++	++
Desipramine	+	+	+	++
Doxepin	+++	0	++	+++
Imipramine	++	0	++	+++
Nortriptyline	++	0	+	++
Protriptyline	+	++	++	++
MAO Inhibitors				
Phenelzine	+	+	0	+++
Tranylcypromine	0	++	0	+++
Isocarboxazid	0	++	0	++
Second-Generation Drugs				
Amoxapine	++	0	+	++
Fluoxetine	0	++	0	0
Maprotiline	++	0	+	++
Trazodone	+++	0	0	+++
Bupropion	0	++	0	0

*Zero denotes no side effect, + a minor side effect, ++ a moderate side effect, +++ a major side effect.
Based on Potter, WZ, Rudorfer, MV, and Manji, H: Drug therapy: The pharmacologic treatment of depression. N Engl J Med 325:633, 1991. As appearing in Ciccone, CD: Pharmacology in Rehabilitation, ed 2. FA Davis, Philadelphia, 1996, p 90, with permission.

13

SIDE EFFECTS AND TOXICITY OF LITHIUM

Mild (Below 1.5 mEq/L)	Moderate (1.5–2.5 mEq/L)	Toxicity (2.5–7.0 mEq/L)
Metallic taste in mouth	Severe diarrhea	Nystagmus
Fine hand tremor (resting)	Nausea and vomiting	Coarse tremor
Nausea	Mild to moderate ataxia	Dysarthria
Polyuria	Incoordination	Fasciculations
Polydipsia	Dizziness, sluggishness, giddiness, vertigo	Visual or tactile hallucinations
Diarrhea or loose stools	Slurred speech	Oliguria, anuria
Muscular weakness or fatigue	Tinnitus	Confusion
	Blurred vision	Impaired consciousness
	Increasing tremor	Dyskinesia-chorea, athetoid movements
	Muscle irritability or twitching	Tonic-clonic convulsions
	Asymmetric deep tendon reflexes	Coma
	Increased muscle tone	Death

Based on Harris, E: Lithium. AJN 81(7):1312, 1981. As appearing in Ciccone, CD: Pharmacology in Rehabilitation, ed 2. FA Davis, Philadelphia, 1996, p 93, with permission.

ANTIPSYCHOTIC DRUGS CATEGORIZED BY SIDE EFFECTS*

Drug	Extra-pyramidal	Sedative	Anti-cholinergic
Group A			
Fluphenazine	S	W	W
Perphenazine	S	W–M	W–M
Prochlorperazine	S	M	W
Trifluoperazine	S	W	W
Chlorprothixene	S	W	W
Thiothixene	S	W	W
Haloperidol	S	W	W
Molindone	S	W	W
Loxapine	S	W	W
Group B			
Triflupromazine	M–S	M–S	S
Acetophenazine	M	M	W
Group C			
Chlorpromazine	W–M	S	M–S
Promazine	W	S	S
Mesoridazine	W	M–S	M
Thioridazine	W	S	S

*Side effects are classified as follows: S = Strong, M = Moderate, W = Weak. Drugs in group A tend to produce strong extrapyramidal effects but weak sedative and anticholinergic effects. Drugs in group C tend to produce moderate to strong sedative and anticholinergic side effects, but weak extrapyramidal effects. Drugs in group B tend to produce moderate to strong side effects in all three categories.

From Ciccone, CD: Pharmacology in Rehabilitation, ed 2. FA Davis, Philadelphia, 1996, p 99, with permission.

13

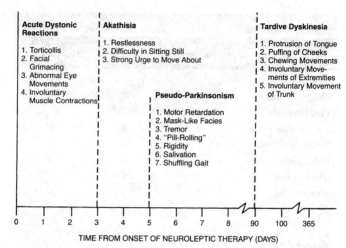

Acute Dystonic Reactions	Akathisia		Tardive Dyskinesia
1. Torticollis	1. Restlessness		1. Protrusion of Tongue
2. Facial Grimacing	2. Difficulty in Sitting Still		2. Puffing of Cheeks
3. Abnormal Eye Movements	3. Strong Urge to Move About		3. Chewing Movements
4. Involuntary Muscle Contractions			4. Involuntary Movements of Extremities
			5. Involuntary Movement of Trunk

Pseudo-Parkinsonism

1. Motor Retardation
2. Mask-Like Facies
3. Tremor
4. "Pill-Rolling"
5. Rigidity
6. Salivation
7. Shuffling Gait

TIME FROM ONSET OF NEUROLEPTIC THERAPY (DAYS)

0   1   2   3   4   5   6   7   8   90   100   365

Extrapyramidal side effects and their relative onset after beginning antipsychotic drug therapy.

ANTI-ANXIETY DRUGS: COMMON BENZODIAZEPINES

Generic Name	Trade Name	Antianxiety Dose (mg)*	Relative Half-Life
Alprazolam	Xanax	0.25–0.5 tid	Short–intermediate
Chlordiazepoxide	Librium, others	5–25 tid or qid	Long
Clorazepate	Tranxene, others	7.5–15 bid to qid	Long
Diazepam	Valium, others	15–30 od	Long
Halazepam	Paxipam	20–40 tid or qid	Long
Ketazolam	Loftran	15 od or bid	Long
Lorazepam	Alzapam, Ativan	1–3 bid or tid	Short–intermediate
Oxazepam	Serax	10–30 tid or qid	Short–intermediate
Prazepam	Centrax	10 tid	Long

*Doses refer to usual adult oral doses. Doses are often lower in elderly or debilitated patients.
From Ciccone, CD: Pharmacology in Rehabilitation, ed 2. FA Davis, Philadelphia, 1996, p 78, with permission.

13

COMMON SEDATIVE-HYPNOTIC DRUGS

Generic Name	Trade Name	Oral Adult Dose (mg)	
		Sedative	*Hypnotic*
Barbiturates			
Amobarbital	Amytal	30–50 bid or tid	65–200
Aprobarbital	Alurate	40 tid	40–160
Butabarbital	Butalan, Butisol, others	15–30 tid or qid	50–100
Pentobarbital	Nembutal	20 tid or qid	100
Phenobarbital	Solfoton	30–120 bid or tid	100–320
Secobarbital	Seconal	30–50 tid or qid	100
Benzodiazepines			
Estazolam	ProSom	—	1–2
Flurazepam	Dalmane, Durapam	—	15–30

Quazepam	Doral		7.5–15
Temazepam	Restoril		15–30
Triazolam	Halcion		0.125–0.25
Others			
Chloral hydrate	Noctec	250 tid	500–1000
Ethclorvynol	Placidyl		500–1000
Glutethimide	(Generic)		250–500
Promethazine	Phenergan (rectal)		25–50

From Ciccone, CD: Pharmacology in Rehabilitation, ed 2. FA Davis, Philadelphia, 1996, p 72, with permission.

13

PHARMACOKINETIC PROPERTIES OF BENZODIAZEPINE SEDATIVE-HYPNOTICS

Drug	Time to Peak Plasma Concentration (h)*	Relative Half-Life	Comments
Estazolam (ProSom)	0.5–1.6	Intermediate	Rapid oral absorption
Flurazepam (Dalmane)	0.5–1.0	Long	Long elimination half-life because of active metabolites
Quazepam (Doral)	2.0	Long	Daytime drowsiness more likely than with other benzodiazepines
Temazepam (Restoril)	2–3	Short–intermediate	Slow oral absorption
Triazolam (Halcion)	Within 2	Short	Rapid oral absorption

*Adult oral hypnotic dose.
From Ciccone, CD: Pharmacology in Rehabilitation, ed 2. FA Davis, Philadelphia, 1996, p 73, with permission.

KÜBLER-ROSS'S STAGES OF DYING

In 1969 Dr. Elisabeth Kübler-Ross published *On Death and Dying*. Since that date the renewed interest in the field of thanatology has led to many theories and models from dozens of volumes. However, in Kübler-Ross's first work, she described five stages of dying. They are not universally accepted but are an excellent conceptual model that can be used when working with patients with terminal conditions.

First Stage: Denial and Isolation

In this early period, patients may attempt to deny the diagnosis, shop for other doctors, or simply believe that they will defy the prognosis. Kübler-Ross considers it a healthy stage with great value as a buffer against the sudden realization of impending death. The isolation may arise from our inability to deal with such a person or their lack of desire to face challenges to the denial.

Second Stage: Anger

To understand this stage, Kübler-Ross suggests imagining how we would feel if all our plans and all our dreams collapsed, we were denied a future that we had saved for, or we were denied the chance to finish raising our children. The anger is coupled with resentment and may be expressed toward anyone near the patient. Anger may be most severe in patients who have had a lot of control over their lives. For them, the loss of control may be equally as disastrous as the death to come.

Third Stage: Bargaining

This is the period when the patient may attempt to deal with the medical team or supernatural forces. Kübler-Ross compares it to the childhood habit of seeking favors or privileges by swearing to be good, doing the dishes, or never hitting someone again. In a very real sense the child, like the patient, tries to gain control by offering something. In this stage patients may bargain for time, the use of body parts, or for life itself. The stage may be especially significant if patients reveal an inner guilt about themselves. It may be during this period that patients show that they will give up a behavior for which they feel they are now being punished.

Fourth Stage: Depression

This stage sets in as the patient realizes loss. Life is not what it was before the illness and never will be again. If accompanied by guilt and shame, this can be especially painful. Kübler-Ross suggests that it may be possible to alleviate some of the guilt and shame, when unrealistic, but otherwise this is a step toward acceptance. Depression, she says, may be functional and should not be denied by attempts to "look at the sunny side." Expressions of sorrow may be vital so that a patient may enter the final stage.

Continued on following page

Fifth Stage: Acceptance

Kübler-Ross says that those who have been given help through the previous stages will arrive at acceptance. They have expressed sorrow and anger and can now deal with the fate ahead. This, she says, is marked by a period of quiet expectation, during which the patient is tired and rests frequently. It is compared to the sleep of a newborn, but in reverse. As the patient finds peace and acceptance, there may be withdrawal from previous interests. Kübler-Ross says that some—a few—never reach this stage and fight to the end. She says that such patients reach a point where they can no longer fight; although they might never peacefully accept, they too reach a point of giving in.

BASED ON

Kübler-Ross, E: On Death and Dying. Macmillan, New York, 1969.

ELECTROMAGNETIC MODALITIES
The Electromagnetic Spectrum

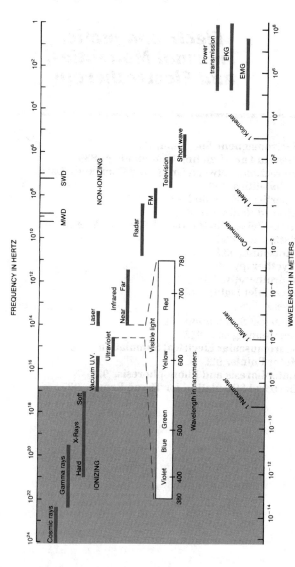

The electromagnetic spectrum.

Based on IES Lighting Handbook: The Standard Lighting Guide, ed 5. Illuminating Engineering Society, New York, 1972.

Physical Laws Relating to the Application of Electromagnetic Modalities

inverse square law: The intensity of the electromagnetic radiation received (RR) varies inversely with the square of the distance (D) from the source of the radiation. The following formula predicts the radiation received from a single source; it is not applicable to reflected radiation.

$$RR = \frac{\text{Radiation Source}}{D^2}$$

cosine law: Maximal radiation is applied when the source of radiation is at a right angle to the patient. The applied radiation is directly proportional to the cosine of the angle formed by the patient's body with the source of radiation.

Radiation	Wavelength (range in nm)*	Frequency (upper limit in Hz)
Electric power	0.5×10^{15}	60
Long-wave diathermy	$300 \times 10^9 - 30 \times 10^9$	10^6
Short-wave diathermy	$30 \times 10^9 - 3 \times 10^9$	10^7
Microwave	$1 \times 10^9 - 1.5 \times 10^9$	3×10^8
Long (far) infrared	15,000–1500	2.0×10^{13}
Short (near) infrared	1500–800	2.0×10^{14}
Visible light	800–400	3.75×10^{14}
Long (near) ultraviolet—UVA	400–280	7.5×10^{14}
Long (near) ultraviolet—UVB	315–280	9.0×10^{14}
Short (far) ultraviolet—UVC	280–230	1.03×10^{15}
Roentgen (x-rays)	120–0.14	5.9×10^{15}
Gamma	0.14–0.01	2.14×10^{18}

*Nanometer (nm) is equal to 10 angstrom (Å) or 10^{-7} cm.

14

INTERACTIONS BETWEEN DRUGS AND COMMONLY USED MODALITIES

Modality	Desired Therapeutic Effect	Drugs with Complementary/ Synergistic Effects	Drugs with Antagonistic Effects	Other Drug–Modality Interactions
Cryotherapy Cold/ice packs Ice massage Cold baths Vapocoolant sprays	Decreased pain, edema, and inflammation	Anti-inflammatory steroids (glucocorticoids); nonsteroidal anti-inflammatory analgesics (aspirin and similar NSAIDs)	Peripheral vasodilators may exacerbate acute local edema.	Some forms of cryotherapy may produce local vasoconstriction that temporarily impedes diffusion of drugs to the site of inflammation.
	Muscle relaxation and decreased spasticity	Skeletal muscle relaxants	Nonselective cholinergic agonists may stimulate the neuromuscular junction.	
Superficial and deep heat Local application Hot packs Paraffin Infrared	Decreased muscle/ joint pain and stiffness Decreased muscle spasms	NSAIDs; opioid analgesics; local anesthetics Skeletal muscle relaxants	Nonselective cholinergic agonists may stimulate the neuromuscular junction.	

Modality	Purpose	Interacting Drugs	Comments
Fluidotherapy Diathermy Ultrasound	Increased blood flow to improve tissue healing	Peripheral vasodilators	Systemic vasoconstrictors (e.g., α-1 agonists) may decrease perfusion of peripheral tissues.
Systemic heat Large whirlpool Hubbard tank	Decreased muscle/joint stiffness in large areas of the body	Opioid and nonopioid analgesics; skeletal muscle relaxants	Nonselective cholinergic agonists may stimulate the neuromuscular junction. Severe hypotension may occur if systemic hot whirlpool is administered to patients taking peripheral vasodilators and some antihypertensive drugs (e.g., α-1 antagonists, nitrates, direct-acting vasodilators, calcium channel blockers). *Continued on following page*

14

INTERACTIONS BETWEEN DRUGS AND COMMONLY USED MODALITIES (Continued)

Modality	Desired Therapeutic Effect	Drugs with Complementary/ Synergistic Effects	Drugs with Antagonistic Effects	Other Drug–Modality Interactions
Ultraviolet radiation	Increased wound healing	Various systemic and topical antibiotics	—	Antibacterial drugs generally increase cutaneous sensitivity to ultraviolet light (i.e., photosensitivity).
	Management of skin disorders (acne, rashes)	Systemic and topical antibiotics and anti-inflammatory steroids (glucocorticoids)	Many drugs may cause hypersensitivity reactions that result in skin rashes, itching.	Photosensitivity with antibacterial drugs.
Transcutaneous electrical nerve stimulation (TENS)	Decreased pain	Opioid and nonopioid analgesics	Opioid antagonists (naloxone).	—
Functional neuromuscular electrical stimulation	Increased skeletal muscle strength and endurance	—	Skeletal muscle relaxants.	—
	Decreased spasticity and muscle spasms	Skeletal muscle relaxants	Nonselective cholinergic agonists may stimulate the neuromuscular junction.	—

From Ciccone, CD: Pharmacology in Rehabilitation, ed 2. FA Davis, Philadelphia, 1996, pp. 601–602, with permission.

SUPERFICIAL HEAT MODALITIES

Hot Packs

Silica gel in a canvas cover is immersed in water that is typically between 165°–175°F (73.9°–79.4°C). The gel is typically applied as a source of conductive moist heat to the body part, using layerings of terry cloth toweling between the skin and hot pack.

Paraffin

In most clinical applications, paraffin is applied at temperatures between 113°–126°F (45°–52°C) for lower extremities and 126°–135°F (52.2°–57.2°C) for upper extremities. Paraffin melts rapidly at 130°F (54.4°C) and sterilizes at 200°F (93.9°C). For clinical use, paraffin is usually mixed using the following ratio: 7 parts paraffin : 1 part mineral oil. A small amount of oil of wintergreen is often added if the paraffin is used frequently.

Fluidotherapy

Small silicon or other solid particles are heated and suspended by circulating air at a temperature range of 115°–123°F (46.1°–50.6°C). Fluidotherapy is used to provide superficial dry convective heating to distal extremities.

FOR MORE INFORMATION

Hecox, B, Mehreteab, TA, and Weisberg, J: Physical Agents: A Comprehensive Text for Physical Therapists. Appleton & Lange, Norwalk, CT, 1994.

Lehmann, JF: Therapeutic Heat and Cold, ed 4. Williams & Wilkins, Baltimore, 1989.

Michlovitz, SL: Thermal Agents in Rehabilitation, ed 3. FA Davis, Philadelphia, 1995.

INFRARED RADIATION

Sources of Infrared Radiation

All bodies above absolute zero ($-273°C$) emit infrared radiation. The higher the temperature above absolute zero, the greater the emitted infrared radiation.

Nonluminous Sources of Infrared Radiation

These emit infrared via the heat generated in a high-resistance electrical coil. The coil heats and in turn heats a covering element that causes the generation of infrared radiation. This is primarily long wave radiation. Although these sources emit a dull glow, their primary source is nonluminous. These generators must be warmed before use.

Luminous Sources of Infrared Radiation

These are primarily incandescent lights that emit mostly short wave radiation. Emission is instantaneous.

Effects of Infrared Radiation

Exposure leads to capillary dilation, which causes an erythema. Infrared radiation also serves as a possible counterirritant.

TYPES OF INFRARED RADIATION AND PENETRATION DEPTHS		
Types	*Penetration*	*Source*
Visible spectrum, 390–760 nm	1–10 mm	Luminous
Near infrared (short wave), 770–1500 nm	1–10 mm	Luminous
Far infrared (long wave), 1500–12,000 nm	0.05–2 mm	Nonluminous

FOR MORE INFORMATION

Hecox, B, Mehreteab, TA, and Weisberg, J: Physical Agents: A Comprehensive Text for Physical Therapists. Appleton & Lange, Norwalk, CT, 1994.

Lehmann, JF: Therapeutic Heat and Cold, ed 4. Williams & Wilkins, Baltimore, 1989.

Michlovitz, SL: Thermal Agents in Rehabilitation, ed 2. FA Davis, Philadelphia, 1990.

TERMS RELATED TO THE USE OF THERMAL AGENTS

conductive heating (conduction): A method of heat transfer by successive molecular collisions. For example, paraffin and hot packs use this form of heating.

convective heating (convection): A method of heat transfer in which the heated molecules move from one place to another. For example, whirlpools and fluidotherapy use this form of heating.

first law of thermodynamics: A law of thermal physics which states that energy can neither be created nor destroyed but only transformed from one form to another. Heat for thermal modalitites is often released after energy transformations by chemical, mechanical, and electromagnetic systems.

14

heat transfer: The transfer of heat from higher to lower temperature molecules until a state of equilibrium is achieved. See also *conduction, radiation,* and *convection.*

heat of fusion: The heat required to change a substance from a liquid to a solid.

heat of vaporization: The heat required to change a substance from a solid to a gas.

quantity of heat: The amount of heat required to increase or decrease the temperature of a substance. The quantity of heat of a substance (Q) is determined by its specific heat capacity (S), mass (m), and amount of temperature change desired (T) according to the formula: $Q = SmT$.

radiant heating (radiation): A method of heat transfer produced by the propagation of energy through space or matter. For example, infrared lamps transfer heat in this manner.

reflex heating (consensual heating, remote heating, or the Landis-Gibbons reflex): A technique involving the application of heat to one area of the body that results in an increase in cutaneous circulation and other reactions in another area.

specific absorption rate (SAR): The rate of energy absorbed per unit mass of tissue (expressed in watts per kilogram).

specific heat capacity: The specific heat input required to raise the temperature of 1 g of a substance 1°C.

thermal conductivity: The ability of a substance to conduct heat.

TERMS RELATED TO THE USE
OF DIATHERMY

applicator: The electrode used to produce diathermy.

capacitance: The ability to store electric charge. A property of a structure that consists of two or more conductors separated by a dielectric. This arrangement permits the storage and release of electric charge. In the case of diathermy, the conductors are usually flat metal plates.

condenser (or capacitor) field diathermy: A form of short-wave diathermy in which the body part is positioned in an electric field generated by two oppositely charged condenser plates.

capacitor: A device capable of storing and releasing electric charge (see also *capacitance*).

diathermy: A deep-heating thermal agent that uses nonionizing electromagnetic energy from the radiofrequency portion of the electromagnetic spectrum.

dielectric: A nonconducting substance; an insulator. In the case of therapeutic diathermy, the patient's tissues serve as the dielectric.

direct-contact applicator: Microwave diathermy electrodes that are spaced 1 cm or less from the body.

director: In microwave diathermy, the electrode used to transmit microwave energy to the body. Microwave directors are typically circular or rectangular shaped.

eddy currents: In diathermy, these are the heat-producing currents in the body that are formed by a magnetic field applied externally.

electrode: A material through which a current flows (see also *applicator*).

induction (or coil) field diathermy: A form of short-wave diathermy in which the body part is placed within a fluctuating magnetic field generated by a single-induction field electrode.

magnetic field: A region in which force is exerted along a magnetic pole. Units are amperes per meter (A/m). In diathermy, magnetic fields are formed around eddy currents.

magnetron oscillator: A high-frequency electrical generator that is used to produce microwave radiation.

microwave diathermy (MWD): A modality that produces electromagnetic radiation with a frequency above 300 MHz and a wavelength shorter than 1 m. The electromagnetic energy is converted to heat in the body principally by dipole movement.

patient circuit: The part of a diathermy device that transfers electrical energy to the patient.

pulsed shortwave diathermy: Short-wave diathermy units that permit "on-off" cycles so that the energy is absorbed in the tissue without tissue temperature rise. These units are typically used for wound healing.

short-wave diathermy (SWD): A modality that produces electromagnetic energy by means of an oscillating electromagnetic field with a frequency between 10 and 100 MHz and a wavelength between 3 and 30 m.

FREQUENCIES USED IN DIATHERMY (FCC approved)		
Frequency	*Wavelength*	*Type of Diathermy*
13.56 MHz	22.0 m	Shortwave
27.12 MHz*	11.0 m	Shortwave
40.68 MHz	7.5 m	Shortwave
915 MHz	33.0 cm	Microwave
2450 MHz*	12.0 cm	Microwave

*Most widely used frequencies.

FOR MORE INFORMATION

Hecox, B, Mehreteab, TA, and Weisberg, J: Physical Agents: A Comprehensive Text for Physical Therapists. Appleton & Lange, Norwalk, CT, 1994.

Michlovitz, SL: Thermal Agents in Rehabilitation, ed 3. FA Davis, Philadelphia, 1995.

Therapeutic Microwave and Shortwave Diathermy: A Review of Thermal Effectiveness, Safe Use, and State of the Art: 1984. U.S. Department of Health and Human Services, Washington, DC, 1984.

TERMS RELATED TO THE USE
OF ULTRASOUND

attenuation: The combination of absorption and scattering of ultrasonic energy as it passes through a medium.

beam nonuniformity ratio (BNR): The ratio of the peak intensity of the ultrasound field to the spatial average intensity indicated on the ultrasound meter (see also *spatial average intensity*).

cavitation: A nonthermal effect of ultrasound in which gas- or vapor-filled cavities in biologic liquids are formed and collapsed by the compression and rarefaction cycles of ultrasound.

continuous-wave ultrasound: Acoustic energy from an ultrasound device is transmitted to the body part without interruption.

coupling agent: A commercially prepared agent that is used between the sound head (transducer) and the patient to enhance transmissivity. The most common coupling agents are thixotropic gels, mineral oil, glycerine, and degassed water.

direct contact procedure: The most common method of applying ultrasound. The sound head glides directly on the surface of the skin with the use of a coupling agent.

duty cycle: The term used in ultrasound to describe the time that sound waves are being emitted during one pulse period. Duty cycle is the duration of the pulse of sound waves in seconds divided by the pulse period. Duty cycle can also be expressed as a percentage.

effective intensity: See *spatial average intensity*.

effective radiating area (ERA): The area of the applicator that emits ultrasound, expressed in square centimeters (cm^2).

fluid cushion (or fluid-filled bag) procedure: An alternative to the immersion procedure for ultrasound treatment of areas that have irregular contours, particularly for a proximal body part. A thin-membraned bag is filled with a coupling agent and placed between the sound head and the body part (see also *immersion procedure*).

immersion procedure: A method of applying ultrasound where the body part is immersed in a fluid medium. Especially useful for treating small irregular surfaces such as the joints of the hands or feet.

phonophoresis: Use of ultrasound to deliver medications into body tissue. Hydrocortisone, dexamethasone, and lidocaine are the medications most commonly administered by this method.

piezoelectric effect (direct): The generation of an electrical voltage across a crystal when the crystal is compressed.

piezoelectric effect (indirect or reverse): The contraction or expansion of a crystal when voltage is applied to the crystal. In ultrasound the reverse piezoelectric effect is used to generate sound waves.

pulse duration: In pulsed ultrasound it is the time interval during which ultrasound is being emitted.

pulse period: In pulsed ultrasound it is the duration of one cycle (the sum of the time on and the time off).

pulse repetition rate: The repetition frequency of the ultrasonic waveform, expressed in pulses per second (pps).

pulsed average intensity (temporal peak intensity): The maximum output of energy that is produced during the "on" phase of a pulsed ultrasound cycle.

pulsed-wave ultrasound: Acoustic energy is transmitted to the body part with brief cyclical interruptions in transmission. Pulsed-wave ultrasound used to reduce the heating effects of ultrasound application.

reverse piezoelectric effect: See *piezoelectric effect.*

spatial average intensity: The ratio of the ultrasonic power to the effective radiating area (ERA) of the applicator, expressed in watts per square centimeter (W/cm^2). See also *effective radiating area (ERA).*

temporal peak intensity (pulsed average intensity): See *pulsed average intensity.*

ultrasonic frequency: The frequency of the ultrasound wave, expressed in hertz (Hz), kilohertz (kHz), or megahertz (MHz).

ultrasonic power: The average power emitted from the sound head during each cycle of the sound wave (expressed in watts).

ultrasonic transducer (sound head): A device, typically using a piezoelectric crystal, designed to convert electrical energy into ultrasonic energy.

ultrasound: Sound waves with a frequency of greater than 20,000 Hz. Therapeutic ultrasound is in the frequency range of 0.9–3 MHz.

FOR MORE INFORMATION

Hecox, B, Mehreteab, TA, and Weisberg, J: Physical Agents: A Comprehensive Text for Physical Therapists. Appleton & Lange, Norwalk, CT, 1994.

Michlovitz, SL: Thermal Agents in Rehabilitation, ed 3. FA Davis, Philadelphia, 1995.

U.S. Department of Health and Human Services: A Practitioner's Guide to the Ultrasonic Therapy Equipment Standard. HHS Publication FDA 85-8240, Washington, DC, 1985.

TERMS RELATED TO THE USE
OF CRYOTHERAPY

chemical cold pack: A reusable pack containing silica gel that is refrigerated at a temperature of approximately $10°-15°F$ ($-12.2°--9.4°C$). There are disposable cold packs that are not refrigerated but instead are activated by breaking an inner seal that mixes the chemicals within.

cryokinetics: A form of cryotherapy commonly used in the treatment of athletic injuries. Cold is applied, commonly by ice massage or immersion, followed by passive or active graded exercise.

cryotherapy (cold therapy): The therapeutic use of cold.

ice massage: The stroking of ice on a body part, primarily to anesthetize the skin. The ice is typically frozen in a cylindrical container, such as a paper cup, and held by the lower part of the cup or by a tongue depressor that is frozen into the center of the cup ("lollipop" technique). An ice cube held in a paper towel or gauze is also commonly used.

ice pack: A plastic bag filled with ice cubes or crushed ice.

ice towel: A towel that contains ice shavings.

quick icing: A technique developed by Margaret Rood in which several quick swipes of ice along an area are administered to facilitate a muscle contraction. This technique is primarily used in patients with central nervous system disorders.

RICE therapy: Cryotherapy combined with compression and elevation of the involved part to reduce or prevent pain, bleeding, and swelling. RICE is an acronym for *R*est, *I*ce, *C*ompression, and *E*levation.

vapocoolant spray: A method of quickly cooling the skin by the evaporation of a substance sprayed on the skin.

FOR MORE INFORMATION

Hecox, B, Mehreteab, TA, and Weisberg, J: Physical Agents: A Comprehensive Text for Physical Therapists. Appleton & Lange, Norwalk, CT, 1994.

Michlovitz, SL: Thermal Agents in Rehabilitation, ed 3. FA Davis, Philadelphia, 1995.

TERMS RELATED TO THE USE
OF HYDROTHERAPY

adhesion: The tendency of surface water molecules to adhere to molecules of other substances.

aquatherapy: The therapeutic use of exercise in water.

Archimedes' principle: A physical law stating that an object immersed in water experiences an upward force that is equal to the weight of the water displaced by the object.

bouyancy: The upward force of water acting on an immersed body that creates an apparent decrease in body weight.

cohesion: The tendency of water molecules to adhere to each other (see also *viscosity*).

contrast bath: A treatment technique to increase superficial blood flow by alternately placing the body part in very hot (105°–110°F, 40.6°–43.3°C) and very cold water (59°–68°F, 15°–20°C). Whirlpool tanks are typically used.

hydrostatic pressure: The amount of pressure exerted by water on an immersed object.

hydrotherapy: The therapeutic use of water.

moist air cabinet: A cabinet that encompasses approximately one half of the patient's body, which is either seated or supine. Water is heated to 103°–113°F (40°–45°C), and air is blown past the water, absorbing the moisture and heat and circulating it within the cabinet.

Pascal's law: A physical law stating that when a body is immersed in water and is at rest, the water will exert equal pressure on all surface areas of the body at a given depth.

peloid: Mineral mud is heated and applied to the body.

pressure gradient: The increase in hydrostatic pressure associated with the depth of immersion. The gradient results from the fact that pressure increases with density of a fluid, and density of water increases with depth.

sauna bath: A chamber made of wood in which stones or bricks are heated so that the room air, which is typically kept at low humidity, is raised to approximately 140°–176°F (60°–80°C) or higher. The hot and dry air promotes sweating and subsequent evaporation on the body. This treatment is commonly followed by a cold shower.

scotch douche: A shower of alternating hot (100°–110°F, 37.8°–43.3°C) and cold (80°–60°F, 26.7°–15.5°C) water.

sitz bath: A bath in which the pelvic and perineal areas are covered in water. Hot sitz baths require a temperature of 105°–115°F (40.5°–46°C). Cold sitz baths require a temperature of 35°–75°F (1.7°–24°C).

surface tension: The tendency of molecules located on the surface of a liquid to hold together and offer greater resistance.

viscosity: Resistance offered by a fluid to change of form or relative position of its particles due to attraction of molecules to each other.

Continued on following page

whirlpool: A modality used for warm, hot, or cold immersion therapy. Stainless steel or plastic tanks contain water that is thermostatically controlled and aerated to produce turbulence. The water temperature range for hot whirlpool treatments is approximately 103°–115°F (39.9°–46.1°C). For whole body immersion, the water temperature range is typically lower at 90°–102°F (32.2°–38.8°C). Whirlpool tanks come in various sizes, such as the "low boy" tank in which the patient can sit, or the "Hubbard" tank for full-body treatment.

FOR MORE INFORMATION

Hecox, B, Mehreteab, TA, and Weisberg, J: Physical Agents: A Comprehensive Text for Physical Therapists. Appleton & Lange, Norwalk, CT, 1994.

Michlovitz, SL: Thermal Agents in Rehabilitation, ed 3. FA Davis, Philadelphia, 1995.

ULTRAVIOLET LIGHT

EFFECTS OF DIFFERENT ULTRAVIOLET WAVELENGTHS
(approximate values)

Effect	Wavelength	Most Effective Wavelength
Erythema	250–297 nm	297 nm
Pigmentation	300–400 nm	340 nm
Antirachitic	240–300 nm	283 nm
Bactericidal	230–280 nm	245.3 nm
Carcinogenic	230–320 nm	300 nm
Antipsoriatic	280–400 nm	360 nm

14

Erythemal Doses

Definitions of Erythemal Doses

Two systems of classifying erythemal doses have been used. In one classification, the level where erythema, or reddening of the skin, first appears after UV exposure is called the *minimal erythemal dose* (MED). In the other system, the first level is called *first-degree erythema.* When the term MED is used, there will be three degrees of erythemal doses. When the minimum level of erythema is called *first-degree erythema,* there will be four degrees of erythemal doses.

suberythemal dose (SED): Ultraviolet exposure insufficient to cause reddening.

minimal erythemal dose (MED): (Also called *first-degree*) Slight reddening of skin, without desquamation; possible slight itching sensation.

first-degree erythemal (1D or E1): (Also called *second-degree*) More reddening than occurs with an MED and slight desquamation (peeling); itching and burning as with sunburn.

second-degree erythemal (2D or E2): (Also called *third-degree*) Marked reddening with considerable itching, burning, and desquamation (peeling) of epidermis, some edema; similar to severe sunburn.

third-degree erythemal (3D or E3): (Also called *fourth-degree*) Intense reaction with edema, swelling, blister formation.

CHARACTERISTICS OF ERYTHEMAL DOSES

Dose	Characteristic Effect	Appears	Disappears
SED	No visible reaction		
MED	Slight reddening	4–6 h	24 h
1D (2.5 × MED)	Mild sunburn	4–6 h	48 h
2D (5.0 × MED)	Severe sunburn	2 h	Several days
3D (10.0 × MED)	Edema and blistering	2 h	Several days

FOR MORE INFORMATION

Forster, A and Palastanga, N: Clayton's Electrotherapy: Theory and Practice, ed 9. Bailliere Tindall, New York, 1985.

Hecox, B, Mehreteab, TA, and Weisberg, J: Physical Agents: A Comprehensive Text for Physical Therapists. Appleton and Lange, Norwalk, CT, 1994.

LASERS

Physical Principles

Laser is an acronym for *l*ight *a*mplification by *s*timulated *e*mission *r*adiation. Lasers have three properties that distinguish them from incandescent and fluorescent light sources: *coherence, monochramaticity,* and a *collimated beam.*

Laser light can be transmitted into the tissue without alteration of its characteristic properties *(direct penetration)* or with alteration due to the hyperscopic absorption properties of the tissue *(indirect penetration).*

coherence: Refers to parallel waves that propagate either in the same phase *(temporal coherence)* or in the same direction *(spatial coherence).* These properties minimize divergence and make it possible to concentrate the light to a focused area.

monochramaticity: Refers to the specificity of light to a single defined wavelength. Laser light therefore has higher purity than most other light sources.

collimated beam: Refers to light beams with minimal divergence or moving apart of photons.

Types of Lasers Used in Physical Therapy

Lasers can be classified as high power or low power. Only low-power lasers (i.e., laser light with average power less than 1 mW) are available for physical therapy treatments. Low-power laser systems in use include the helium-neon (HeNe) laser and the gallium arsenide (GaAs) laser.

HeNe LASER. The most popular of laser modalities for physical therapy use, the laser light in this device is produced in a vacuum chamber filled with atoms of helium and neon gases. Electrical stimulation of these gases causes the emission of radiation at a wavelength of 632.8 nm (within the red band of visible light). The light is amplified and directed to the tip of a hand-held fiber optic wand that applies the laser beam in a pulsed or continuous mode to the tissue to be stimulated. Penetration of this laser light is to a depth of 0.8 mm (direct) or 10 mm–15 mm (indirect).

GaAs LASER. The first "semiconductor" laser, the GaAs laser is produced in a diode comprised of a thin coating of zinc on gallium arsenide, which allows electric current to pass in only one direction. The reaction at the gallium arsenide-zinc junction produces laser light at a wavelength of 910 nm (within the infrared or invisible spectrum). The energy is delivered in the pulsed mode and has a reported depth of tissue penetration of 5 cm (indirect).

Continued on following page

Food and Drug Administration Classification of Low-Power Lasers

Although their use in medicine is expanding, low-power lasers (cold lasers) as of 1995 are classified by the U.S. Food and Drug Administration (FDA) as Class III medical devices for approved experimental use. Therefore, practitioners must obtain an investigational device exemption from the FDA (FDA regulation 812.2[b]) prior to use.

FOR MORE INFORMATION

Forster, A and Palastanga, N: Clayton's Electrotherapy: Theory and Practice, ed 9. Bailliere Tindall, New York, 1985.

Hecox, B, Mehreteab, TA, and Weisberg, J: Physical Agents: A Comprehensive Text for Physical Therapists. Appleton & Lange, Norwalk, CT, 1994.

McCulloch, JM, Kloth, LC, and Feeder, JA: Wound Healing: Alternatives in Management, ed 2. FA Davis, Philadelphia, 1994.

Michlovitz, SL: Thermal Agents in Rehabilitation, ed 3. FA Davis, Philadelphia, 1995.

TERMS RELATED TO THE USE OF
ELECTRICAL STIMULATION

alternating current (AC): Uninterrupted bidirectional flow of charged particles (current) that may either be symmetrical or asymmetrical with reference to the baseline. See also *direct current.*

beat: A type of amplitude modulation resulting from the intersection and temporal summation of two or more sine waves of slightly different frequencies. See also *modulations of alternating current.*

burst: A finite series of pulses or cycles of AC delivered at an identified frequency, amplitude, or duration. See also *modulations of pulsed current.*

constant (or regulated) current stimulator: Instrument that provides current flowing at the same amplitude regardless of the impedance.

constant (or regulated) voltage stimulator: Instrument that provides a constant voltage regardless of the impedance.

direct current (DC): Continuous unidirectional flow of charged particles (current), the direction of which is determined by the polarity. See also *alternating current.*

electrical muscle stimulation (EMS): The use of electrical stimulation for direct activation of denervated muscle.

electrical stimulation for tissue repair (ESTR): Use of electrical stimulation for reducing inflammation and enhancing tissue healing by various means, including controlling edema, administering pharmacologic agents iontophoretically, or improving vascular status.

faradic: A type of pulsed current generated by rotating a coiled wire in a magnetic field that produces an asymmetrical biphasic pulsed waveform. It is not synonymous with AC.

galvanic: Uninterrupted current that is synonymous with DC.

high-voltage pulsed current (HVPC): Stimulation current produced by high-driving voltage (greater than 150 V), monophasic waveform, and phase duration typically less than 100 μs.

low-intensity direct current (LIDC): Therapeutic use of direct current of less than 1 mA.

modulations of alternating current: See *modulations of pulsed current.*

modulations of pulsed current: Variations imposed on pulsed and/or alternating current; may include:

> **amplitude modulations:** Variations in the peak amplitude in a series of pulses or cycles.
>
> **pulse duration or phase modulations:** Variations in pulse duration or phase in a series of pulses or cycles.
>
> **frequency modulations:** Variations in frequency in a series of pulses or cycles.
>
> **ramp (surge) modulations:** Cyclical, sequential increases or decreases in pulsed or alternating current that typically occur as a

Continued on following page

14

result of changing the phase duration or amplitude of the pulse or cycle.

timing modulations: Variations in the delivery pattern of a series of pulses or alternating current. See also *train, burst, beat,* and *duty cycle.*

neuromuscular electrical stimulation (NMES): The application of electrical current to elicit a muscle contraction through stimulation of the intact peripheral nerve. The FDA has approved NMES devices for the treatment of disuse atrophy, increase and maintenance of range of motion, and muscle re-education. Other areas of clinical use include spasticity management, orthotic substitution, and augmentation of motor recruitment in healthy muscle. NMES is further classified according to "low frequency" (1–1000 pps), "medium (middle) frequency" (1,000–10,000 pps), and "high frequency" (greater than 10,000 pps) modes.

pulsed current (pulsatile or interrupted current): Unidirectional or bidirectional flow of charged particles (current) that periodically cease to flow for a finite period. A pulsed current may be *monophasic* (deviating from baseline in one direction) or *biphasic* (deviating from baseline in one direction and then the opposite direction). See also *modulation of pulsed current.*

train: A continuous repetitive sequence of pulses or cycles of AC. See also *modulations of alternating current.*

transcutaneous electrical nerve stimulation (TENS): The application of controlled, low-voltage electrical pulses to the nervous system by passing electricity through the skin via electrodes.

FOR MORE INFORMATION

Electrotherapeutic Terminology in Physical Therapy. Section on Clinical Electrophysiology and the American Physical Therapy Association, Alexandria, VA, 1990.

Gersh, MR: Electrotherapy in Rehabilitation. FA Davis, Philadelphia, 1992.

"TRADITIONAL" DESIGNATIONS OF SELECTED WAVEFORMS

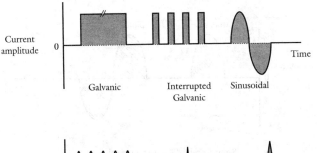

Current amplitude

Galvanic   Interrupted Galvanic   Sinusoidal

Time

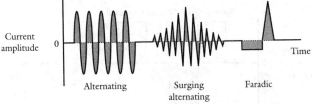

Current amplitude

Alternating   Surging alternating   Faradic

Time

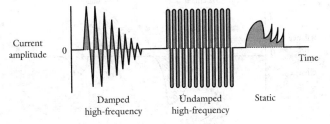

Current amplitude

Damped high-frequency   Undamped high-frequency   Static

Time

Each graph shows changes in current amplitude over time.

From Robinson, AJ and Snyder-Mackler, L (eds): Clinical Electrophysiology: Electrotherapy and Electrophysiologic Testing, ed 2. Williams & Wilkins, Baltimore, 1995, p 10, with permission.

CHARACTERISTICS OF PULSED OR ALTERNATING CURRENT WAVEFORMS

Phase-Dependent Characteristics

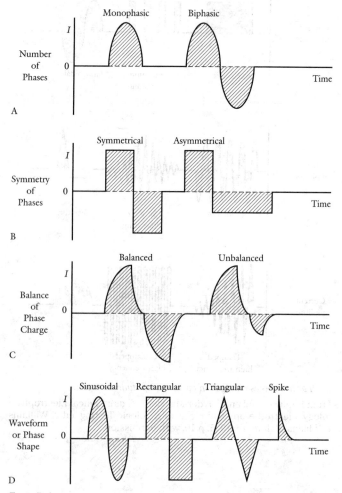

From Robinson, AJ and Snyder-Mackler, L (eds): Clinical Electrophysiology: Electrotherapy and Electrophysiologic Testing, ed 2. Williams & Wilkins, Baltimore, 1995, p 18, with permission.

Descriptions of Selected Pulsed Current Waveforms

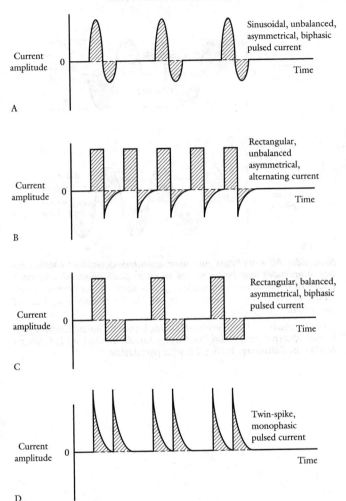

Graphical representation of several common forms of pulsed current labeled with appropriate "descriptive" designation. The waveform represented in (B) has been called faradic current in (D) has been called high volt Galvanic.

From Robinson, AJ and Snyder-Mackler, L (eds): Clinical Electrophysiology: Electrotherapy and Electrophysiologic Testing, ed 2. Williams & Wilkins, Baltimore, 1995, p 20, with permission.

Amplitude-Dependent Characteristics of Sinusoidal Waveforms

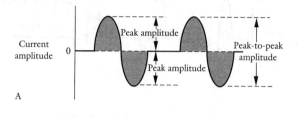

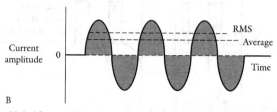

Sinusoidal AC waveforms and their amplitude-dependent characteristics. Amplitudes may be expressed as either peak amplitudes for each phase or peak-to-peak amplitude (A). Alternatively, root mean square (RMS) or average amplitudes can be used to describe the magnitude of currents or voltage (B).

From Robinson, AJ and Snyder-Mackler, L (eds): Clinical Electrophysiology: Electrotherapy and Electrophysiologic Testing, ed 2. Williams & Wilkins, Baltimore, 1995, p 22, with permission.

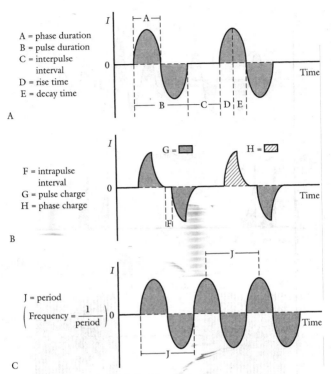

A = phase duration
B = pulse duration
C = interpulse interval
D = rise time
E = decay time

A

F = intrapulse interval
G = pulse charge
H = phase charge

B

J = period

$$\left(\text{Frequency} = \frac{1}{\text{period}} \right)$$

C

Time-dependent characteristics of pulsed or AC waveforms.

From Robinson, AJ and Snyder-Mackler, L (eds): Clinical Electrophysiology: Electrotherapy and Electrophysiologic Testing, ed 2. Williams & Wilkins, Baltimore, 1995, p 23, with permission.

"COMMERCIAL" DESIGNATIONS OF PULSED OR ALTERNATING CURRENT WAVEFORMS

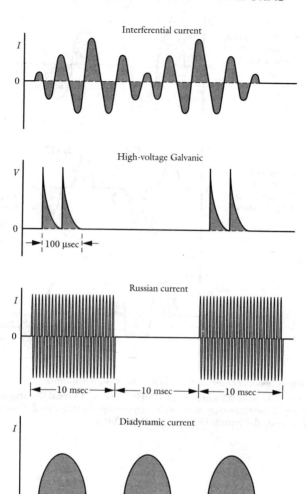

"Commercial" designations of selected electrical currents available from certain contemporary stimulators. Graphs show either changes in current amplitude over time or changes in voltage amplitude over time.

From Robinson, AJ and Snyder-Mackler, L (eds): Clinical Electrophysiology: Electrotherapy and Electrophysiologic Testing, ed 2. Williams & Wilkins, Baltimore, 1995, p 11, with permission.

COMMON STIMULATION CHARACTERISTICS FOR ELECTROANALGESIA					
Mode of Stimulation	Phase Duration (μs)	Frequency (pps,bps, or beat/s)	Amplitude	Duration of Treatment	Duration of Analgesia
Subsensory-level stimulation	Not specified	<3	< 1 mA/cm^2	Not known	Not known
Sensory-level stimulation	2–50	50–100	Perceptible tingling	20–30 min	Little residual posttreatment
Motor-level stimulation	>150	2–4	Strong visible muscle contraction	30–45 min	Hours
Noxious-level stimulation	≤1 msec, up to 1 sec	1–5 or >100	Noxious; below motor threshold	Seconds to minutes	Hours

From Robinson, AJ and Snyder-Mackler, L (eds): Clinical Electrophysiology: Electrotherapy and Electrophysiologic Testing, ed 2. Williams & Wilkins, Baltimore, 1995, p 288, with permission.

COMMONLY USED MODES OF TENS STIMULATION			
Mode	Intensity (pulse amplitude)	Frequency (pulse rate)	Commonly Used Durations (pulse width)
High rate—conventional TENS	Comfortable paresthesia	>50 pps (typically 75–100 pps)	<200 μs
Low rate-acupuncture-like (LRAT)	Motor threshold	<10 pps (typically 1–4 pps)	200–300 μs
Brief, intense TENS	Muscle fasciculations or tetany	150 pps	>150 μs

Based on Gersh, MR: Electrotherapy in Rehabilitation. FA Davis, Philadelphia, 1992, p 174.

WAVEFORMS USED FOR ELECTROANALGESIA INCLUDING TENS

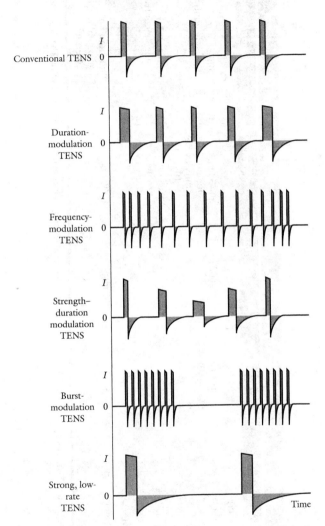

A sample of different types of pulse patterns used by clinical and portable TENS units.

From Robinson, AJ and Snyder-Mackler, L (eds): Clinical Electrophysiology: Electrotherapy and Electrophysiologic Testing, ed 2. Williams & Wilkins, Baltimore, 1995, p 289, with permission.

NEUROMUSCULAR ELECTRICAL STIMULATION (NMES)

Muscle Dysfunction	Phase Duration	Pulse Duration	Frequency	Amplitude
Innervated Muscle				
1. Neuromuscular electrical stimulation	1–300 μs or burst up to 10 ms	2–600 μs	30–50 pps or until fusion (duty cycle: 1:10–1:1)	Sufficient for muscle contraction
2. Functional electrical stimulation	1–300 μs	2–600 μs	>fusion frequency (duty cycle ≤1.7)	Sufficient for muscle contraction
Denervated Muscle				
1. Electrical muscle stimulation	>0.5 ms	1 ms	1–30 pps	Sufficient for maximal tension to tolerance

Based on Electrotherapeutic Terminology in Physical Therapy. Section on Clinical Electrophysiology and the American Physical Therapy Association, Alexandria, VA, 1990, pp 33–34.

WAVEFORMS USED FOR NEUROMUSCULAR ELECTRICAL STIMULATION

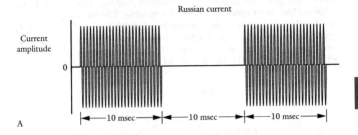

Russian current

A

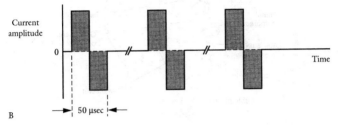

Rectangular, symmetric, biphasic pulsed current

B

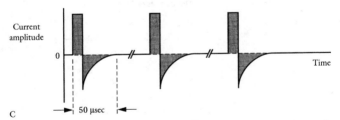

Rectangular, asymmetric, biphasic pulsed current

C

Examples of currents used with commercially available stimulators designed for neuromuscular electrical stimulation.

From Robinson, AJ and Snyder-Mackler, L (eds): Clinical Electrophysiology: Electrotherapy and Electrophysiologic Testing, ed 2. Williams & Wilkins, Baltimore, 1995, p 64, with permission.

MOTOR POINTS

Motor points are sites on the skin surface where the underlying muscle can be electrically stimulated to contract by lower levels of electricity than are needed in surrounding areas. The motor point overlies the innervation zone(s) of a muscle. The motor point is often used as a placement site for surface electrodes used to stimulate muscle. The accompanying figures should be considered only as approximate locations of motor points for major muscle groups. The exact location, extent, and number of motor points can vary.

Motor Points of Face

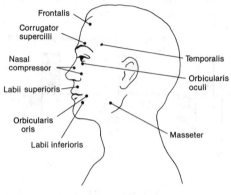

Motor Points of Face

Motor Points of Anterior Body

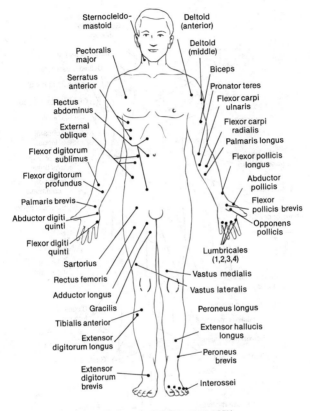

Sternocleido-mastoid
Deltoid (anterior)
Pectoralis major
Deltoid (middle)
Serratus anterior
Biceps
Rectus abdominus
Pronator teres
External oblique
Flexor carpi ulnaris
Flexor digitorum sublimus
Flexor carpi radialis
Flexor digitorum profundus
Palmaris longus
Palmaris brevis
Flexor pollicis longus
Abductor digiti quinti
Abductor pollicis
Flexor digiti quinti
Flexor pollicis brevis
Sartorius
Opponens pollicis
Rectus femoris
Lumbricales (1,2,3,4)
Adductor longus
Vastus medialis
Gracilis
Vastus lateralis
Tibialis anterior
Peroneus longus
Extensor digitorum longus
Extensor hallucis longus
Extensor digitorum brevis
Peroneus brevis
Interossei

MOTOR POINTS OF ANTERIOR BODY

Continued on following page

Motor Points   **921**

Motor Points of Posterior Body

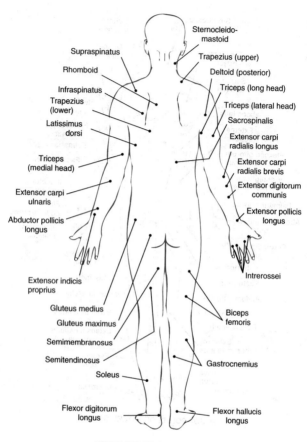

MOTOR POINTS OF POSTERIOR BODY

FOR MORE INFORMATION

Coers, C and Woolf, AL: The Innervation of Muscle: A Biopsy Study. Charles C. Thomas, Springfield, IL, 1959.

Walthard, KM and Tchicaloff, M: Motor points. In Licht, SH (ed): Electrodiagnosis and Electromyography, ed 3. Waverly Press, Baltimore, 1971.

IONTOPHORESIS AND PHONOPHORESIS

OPTIMAL CURRENT VARIABLES DURING IONTOPHORESIS	
Type:	DC
Amplitude:	1.0–4.0 mA
Duration:	20–40 min
Total Current Dosage:	40–80 mA/min

From Robinson, AJ and Snyder-Mackler, L (eds): Clinical Electrophysiology: Electrotherapy and Electrophysiologic Testing, ed 2. Williams & Wilkins, Balitmore, 1995, p 339, with permission.

SUMMARY OF REACTIONS AT THE ANODE AND CATHODE IN IONTOPHORESIS	
Cathode	*Anode*
Attraction of (+) ions	Attraction of (−) ions
Alkaline reaction by formation of NaOH	Acid reaction by formation of HCl
Increased density of proteins (sclerotic)	Decreased density of proteins (sclerolytic)
Increased nerve excitability via depolarization	Decreased nerve excitability via hyperpolarization (anode blockade)

From Robinson, AJ and Snyder-Mackler, L (eds): Clinical Electrophysiology: Electrotherapy and Electrophysiologic Testing, ed 2. Williams & Wilkins, Balitmore, 1995, p 340, with permission.

DRUGS USED WITH IONTOPHORESIS AND PHONOPHORESIS

Drug	Principal Indication(s)	Treatment Rationale	Iontophoresis	Phonophoresis
Acetic acid	Calcific tendinitis	Acetate is believed to increase solubility of calcium deposits in tendons and other soft tissues.	2%–5% aqueous solution from negative pole	—
Calcium chloride	Skeletal muscle spasms	Calcium stabilizes excitable membranes; appears to decrease excitability threshold in peripheral nerves and skeletal muscle.	2% aqueous solution from positive pole	—
Dexamethasone	Inflammation	Synthetic steroidal anti-inflammatory agent	4 mg/mL in aqueous solution from negative pole	0.4% ointment
Hydrocortisone	Inflammation	Anti-inflammatory steroid	0.5% ointment from positive pole	0.5%–1.0% ointment

Iodine	Adhesive capsulitis and other soft-tissue adhesions; microbial infections	Iodine is a broad-spectrum antibiotic, hence its use in infections, etc.; the sclerolytic actions of iodine are not fully understood.	5%–10% solution or ointment from negative pole	10% ointment
Lidocaine	Soft-tissue pain and inflammation (e.g., bursitis, tenosynovitis)	Local anesthetic effects healing	4%–5% solution or ointment from positive pole	5% ointment
Magnesium sulfate	Skeletal muscle spasms; myositis	Muscle relaxant effect may be caused by decreased excitability of the skeletal muscle membrane and decreased transmission at the neuromuscular junction.	2% aqueous solution or ointment from positive pole	2% ointment
Hyaluronidase	Local edema (subacute and chronic stage)	Appears to increase permeability in connective tissue by hydrolyzing hyaluronic acid, thus decreasing encapsulation and allowing dispersion of local edema.	Reconstitute with 0.9% sodium chloride to provide a 150 µg/mL solution from positive pole	—

14

Continued on following page

DRUGS USED WITH IONTOPHORESIS AND PHONOPHORESIS (Continued)

Drug	Principal Indication(s)	Treatment Rationale	Iontophoresis	Phonophoresis
Salicylates	Muscle and joint pain in acute and chronic conditions (e.g., overuse injuries, rheumatoid arthritis)	Aspirin-like drugs with analgesic and anti-inflammatory effects.	10% trolamine salicylate ointment or 2%–3% sodium salicylate solution from negative pole	10% trolamine salicylate ointment or 3% sodium salicylate ointment
Tolazoline hydrochloride	Indolent cutaneous ulcers	Increases local blood flow and tissue healing by inhibiting vascular smooth muscle contraction.	2% aqueous solution from positive pole	—
Zinc oxide	Skin ulcers, other dermatologic disorders	Zinc acts as a general antiseptic; may increase tissue healing.	20% ointment from positive pole	20% ointment

From Ciccone, CD: Pharmacology in Rehabilitation, ed 2. FA Davis, Philadelphia, 1996, pp 598–599, with permission.

COMMONLY USED ELECTRICAL STIMULATION SETTINGS FOR TISSUE REPAIR

Application	Type of Current	Phase Duration (μs)	Amplitude	Treatment Duration
Edema control	Pulsed or burst-mod AC	>100	Rhythmic muscle contraction	*
	High-voltage, pulsed monophasic, negative polarity	2–50	90% of motor threshold	30 min every 4 h
Improve vascular status	Pulsed or burst-mod AC	>2	Sensory level	10 min
	Pulsed or burst-mod AC	>100	>10% MVC	1–2 h bid
Wound healing	DC	NA	<1 mA	45 min
	pulsed	2–150	<Motor threshold	

*Undetermined.

NA = not applicable.

MVC = maximal voluntary contraction.

From Robinson, AJ and Snyder-Mackler, L (eds): Clinical Electrophysiology: Electrotherapy and Electrophysiologic Testing, ed 2. Williams & Wilkins, Baltimore, 1995, p 317, with permission.

S·E·C·T·I·O·N ① ⑤

Massage and Soft-Tissue Techniques

15

MASSAGE

A review of the literature on massage reflects the very inexact nature of the field. The definitions and categories given below are by no means universal. Massage strokes are listed in the order of increasing vigor.

stroking (effleurage): Passing of the hands over a large body area with constant pressure.

> **superficial effleurage:** Extremely light form, using palms of hands, described as little more than a caress.

> **deep effleurage:** Strong enough stroking to evoke a mechanical as well as reflex effect on muscles.

compression: Use of intermittent pressure to lift, roll, press, squeeze, and stretch tissue and to hasten venous and lymphatic flow.

kneading (petrissage): Hands take a large fold of skin and underlying tissue and forcefully roll, raise, and squeeze it.

> **pinching (placement):** Pinching using thumb and index finger.

> **rolling (roulement):** Rolling of muscle belly.

> **wringing:** Like wringing a towel.

> **fulling:** Rippling of deeper muscle caused by asynchronous movement of hands.

> **fist kneading:** Compression via knuckles of a partially closed fist.

> **digital kneading:** Use of a single finger or three fingers positioned triangularly.

friction: Firm contact over a limited area to loosen adherent tissue.

> **crushing (ecrasement):** Localized and vigorous.

> **tearing (dilaceration):** Intense deep pressure, like connective tissue massage.

> **pleating (pleissate):** Ends of finger perpendicular to veins.

> **sawing (sciage):** Rapid and deep transverse movement of the ulnar border.

> **come-and-go:** Reciprocal movement of the two index fingers or the thumbs.

vibration and shaking: Hands are kept in contact with the patient, and movement originates with the therapist's body and is transmitted to the patient via the therapist's outstretched arms. Shaking (secousses) is characterized by the alternate flexion and extension of the therapist's elbows, whereas in vibration the elbows remain fully extended.

> **point vibration:** Use of a single digit.

> **percussion:** Brief, brisk, rapid contacts reciprocally applied with relaxed wrists.

> **tapping (tapotement):** Rapid series of blows, hands parallel and partially flexed, with the ulnar borders of the hand striking the patient. Sometimes *tapping* is used to describe percussion with the fingertips.

hammering (martelage): Soft percussion with the ulnar edges of the hand of the slightly flexed last four fingers, so that the little finger strikes first.

clapping (claquement): Use of fingers, palm, and thumb to form a concave surface.

hacking (hachure): Chopping strokes made by the ulnar surface hitting the patient; more vigorous than tapping.

beating (frappement): Striking with half-closed fists so that the ulnar side of the hand makes contact.

FOR MORE INFORMATION

Tappan, F: Healing Massage Techniques: Holistic, Classic and Emerging Methods. Appleton & Lange, East Norwalk, CT, 1988.

Wood, EC: Beard's Massage Principles and Treatment, ed 3. WB Saunders, Philadelphia, 1981.

15

SOFT-TISSUE MOBILIZATION TECHNIQUES

bending: The muscle belly is held by approximating both thumb and index fingers in a triangular shape. Alternating compressive and distractive forces are applied to the muscle belly working towards the tendinous insertion.

C-stroke: While stabilizing with one hand, the index, middle, and ring fingers (interphalangeals flexed) of the other hand draw the skin away in a C-fashion.

clearing: A rhythmical, rolling stroke, with successively increasing pressure. This technique is typically applied using the fingertips, movements of which are coordinated with the patient's expirations.

cross-fiber: Deep pressure applied perpendicularly to muscle tendon or fascia using fingertips.

deep perpendicular: With two middle fingers held together overlapping the index fingers, the therapist starts at the lateral border of the muscle and pushes toward the muscle belly while maintaining pressure.

distraction: Stretching of soft tissue using both hands to mobilize a joint or bony segment of the body.

forearm inhibition: Proximal one third of forearm is slowly swept longitudinally or laterally across the muscle in a repetitive motion. Strokes are typically synchronized with the patient's expirations when applied to the paraspinal musculature.

inhibitive kneading: Using both hands with fingertips slightly flexed on either side of the muscle belly, the therapist alternately applies upward and downward rolling pressure.

release: Application of slow, firm, and deep pressure across a muscle belly using fingertips of one hand (or one hand placed over the other). Pressure is often held for an extended period.

skin rolling: Fingertips of both hands are placed in a V-pattern with both thumbs and index fingers touching. The thumbs are gently, but firmly pushed towards the index fingers, rolling the superficial skin layers toward the index fingers. This technique is typically applied to lumbar paraspinal muscles.

sweep: Sweeping motion with applied pressure along the length of a muscle held in either a stretched or shortened position. Contact is made by either the thumb, fingers (either singularly or in combination), knuckles, or forearm.

FOR MORE INFORMATION

Mottice, M, et al: Soft Tissue Mobilization Techniques. JEMD Publications, North Canton, OH, 1986.

TRIGGER POINTS

Many treatment techniques require the location of trigger points. Travell first described these points when she stated that the "trigger area is simply derived from the fact that if you do something at one place, which we call the trigger, then something else happens in another place, which we call the reference or the target. It implies that some relationship exists between two different topographic areas."

The diagrams on pages 934–943 are based on Travell's publications. The trigger points are said to be hypersensitive areas. In response to pressure, needling, extreme heat or cold, or stretch, these areas give rise to pain referred elsewhere.

FOR MORE INFORMATION

Travell, JG: Pain Mechanisms in Connective Tissues, Transactions of the Second Conference of the Josiah Macy Jr. Foundation, New York, 1951.

Travell, JG and Rinzler, SH: The Myofascial Genesis of Pain. Postgraduate Medicine 11:425, 1952.

Travell, JG and Simons, DG: Myofascial Pain and Dysfunction: The Trigger Point Manual. Williams & Wilkins, Baltimore, 1983.

Travell, JG and Simons, DG: Myofascial Pain and Dysfunction: The Lower Extremities, Volume 2. Williams & Wilkins, Baltimore, 1992.

15

Trigger Points of the Head and Neck

Sternomastoid

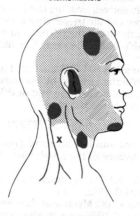

Temporalis

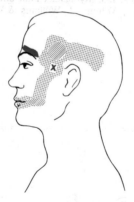

✗ = Trigger point

▮ = Most common areas of referred pain

▨ = Secondary areas where pain may be felt

▦ = Tertiary areas where pain may be felt

Splenius capitis

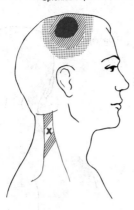

Masseter

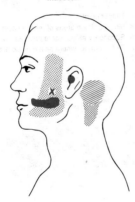

✗ = Trigger point
⬛ = Most common areas of referred pain
▨ = Secondary areas where pain may be felt
▧ = Tertiary areas where pain may be felt

Continued on following page

Trigger Points of the Head and Neck (Continued)

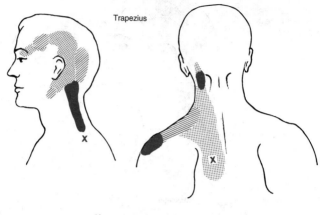

Trapezius

✗ = Trigger point

■ = Most common areas of referred pain

▨ = Secondary areas where pain may be felt

▦ = Tertiary areas where pain may be felt

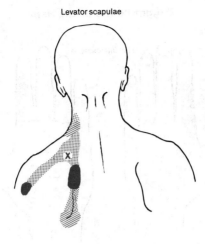

Levator scapulae

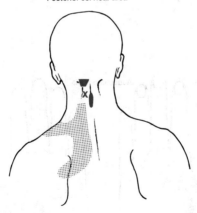

Posterior cervical area

✗ = Trigger point
■ = Most common areas of referred pain
▨ = Secondary areas where pain may be felt
▩ = Tertiary areas where pain may be felt

Continued on following page

Trigger Points of the Hand

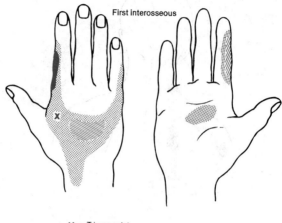

First interosseous

✖ = Trigger point
⬛ = Most common areas of referred pain
▨ = Secondary areas where pain may be felt
▦ = Tertiary areas where pain may be felt

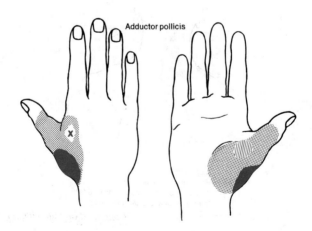

Adductor pollicis

✖ = Trigger point
⬛ = Most common areas of referred pain
▨ = Secondary areas where pain may be felt
▦ = Tertiary areas where pain may be felt

Trigger Points of the Trunk and Upper Extremities

Sternal area

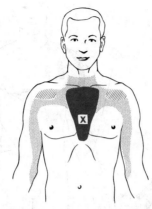

✗ = Trigger point
■ = Most common areas of referred pain
▨ = Secondary areas where pain may be felt
▨ = Tertiary areas where pain may be felt

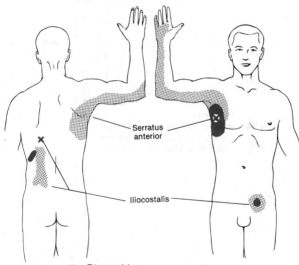

Serratus anterior

Iliocostalis

✗ = Trigger point
■ = Most common areas of referred pain
▨ = Secondary areas where pain may be felt
▨ = Tertiary areas where pain may be felt

Continued on following page

Trigger Points   **939**

Trigger Points of the Trunk and Extremities

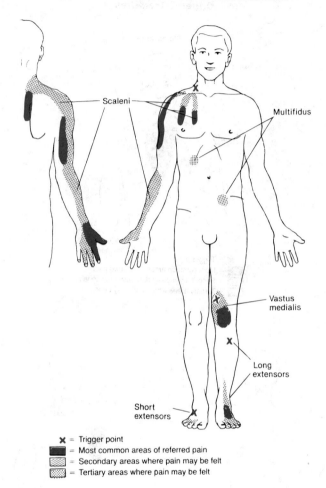

Scaleni

Multifidus

Vastus medialis

Long extensors

Short extensors

x = Trigger point
◼ = Most common areas of referred pain
▨ = Secondary areas where pain may be felt
▨ = Tertiary areas where pain may be felt

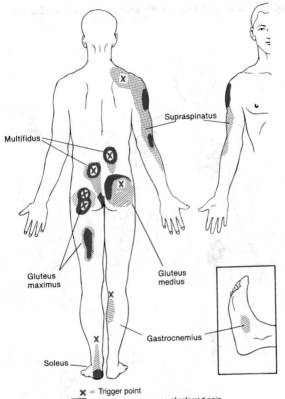

Multifidus

Supraspinatus

Gluteus
maximus

Gluteus
medius

Gastrocnemius

Soleus

X = Trigger point
= Most common areas of referred pain
= Secondary areas where pain may be felt
= Tertiary areas where pain may be felt

Continued on following page

15

Trigger Points of the Trunk and Extremities (Continued)

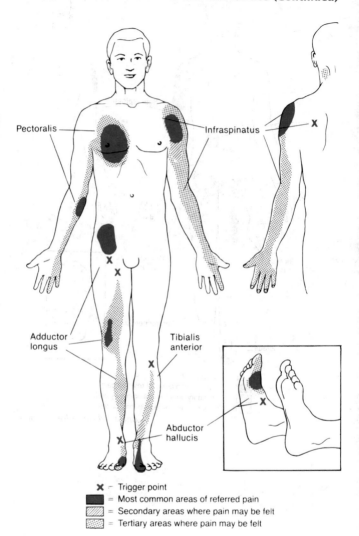

Pectoralis

Infraspinatus

Adductor longus

Tibialis anterior

Abductor hallucis

X = Trigger point
■ = Most common areas of referred pain
▨ = Secondary areas where pain may be felt
▧ = Tertiary areas where pain may be felt

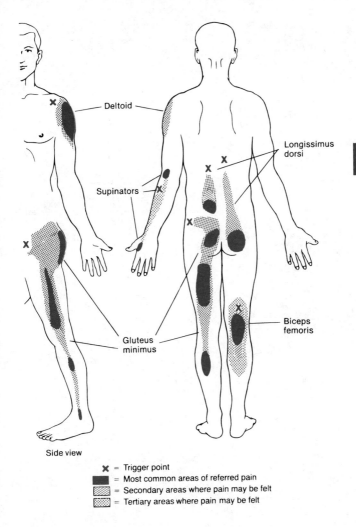

Deltoid

Longissimus dorsi

Supinators

Biceps femoris

Gluteus minimus

Side view

✖ = Trigger point
▮ = Most common areas of referred pain
▨ = Secondary areas where pain may be felt
▨ = Tertiary areas where pain may be felt

General Medicine
(Including Oncology)

16

COMMON LABORATORY TESTS

NORMAL LABORATORY VALUES FROM THE MASSACHUSETTS GENERAL HOSPITAL

BLOOD, PLASMA, OR SERUM VALUES

Determination	Reference Range		Minimal ml Required	Note
	Conventional	SI		
Acetoacetate plus acetone	Negative		1–B	
Aldolase	1.3–8.2 U/L	22–137 nmol·s⁻¹/L	2–S	Use unhemolyzed serum.
Ammonia	12–55 µmol/L	12–55 µmol/L	2–B	Collect in heparinized tube; deliver *immediately* packed in ice.
Amylase	53–123 U/L	884–2050 nmol·s⁻¹/L	1–S	
Ascorbic acid	0.4–1.5 mg/dl	23–85 µmol/L	7–B	Collect in heparinized tube before any food is given.
Bilirubin	Direct: up to 0.4 mg/dl Total: up to 1.0 mg/dl	Up to 7 µmol/L Up to 17 µmol/L	1–S	
Blood volume	8.5–9.0% of body weight in kilograms	80–85 ml/kg		
Calcium	8.5–10.5 mg/dl (slightly higher in children)	2.1–2.6 mmol/L	1–S	
Carbamazepine	4.0–12.0 µg/ml	17–51 µmol/L		
Carbon dioxide content	24–30 mEq/L	24–30 mmol/L	1–S	Fill tube to top.

Carbon monoxide	<5% of total hemoglobin	3 – B	Fill tube to top.
Carotenoids	0.8–4.0 µg/ml	1.5 – 7.4 µmol/L	3 – S	Vitamin A may be done on same specimen.
Ceruloplasmin	23–43 mg/dl	1.5–2.9 µmol/L	2 – S	
Chloramphenicol	10–20 µg/ml	31–62 µmol/L	0.2 – S	
Chloride	100–108 mmol/L	100–108 mmol/L	1 – S	
Copper	Total: 70–150 µg/dl	11–24 µmol/L	1 – S	
Creatine kinase (CK)	Female: 10–79 U/L	167–1317 nmol·s⁻¹/L	1 – S	
	Male: 17–148 U/L	283–2467 nmol·s⁻¹/L		
CK isoenzymes	5% MB or less		0.2 – S	
Creatinine	0.6–1.5 mg/dl	53–133 µmol/L	1 – S	
Ethanol	0 mg/dl	0 mmol/L	2 – B	Collect in oxalate and refrigerate.
Glucose	Fasting: 70–110 mg/dl	3.9–5.6 mmol/L	1 – P	Collect with oxalate-fluoride mixture.
Iron	50–150 µg/dl (higher in males)	9.0–26.9 µmol/L	1 – S	
Iron-binding capacity	250–410 µg/dl	44.8–73.4 µmol/L	1 – S	
Lactic acid	0.5–2.2 mmol/L	0.5–2.2 mmol/L	2 – B	Collect with oxalate-fluoride mixture; deliver *immediately* packed in ice.
Lactic dehydrogenase	45–90 U/L	750–1500 nmol·s⁻¹/L	1 – S	Unsuitable if hemolyzed.
Lead	50 µg/dl or less*	Up to 2.4 µmol/L	2 – B	Collect with oxalate-fluoride mixture.

Continued on following page

* Blood lead levels much lower than this are of concern in children.
Abbreviations used: SI = Système International d'Unités; P = plasma; S = serum; B = blood; and U = urine.

16

NORMAL LABORATORY VALUES FROM THE MASSACHUSETTS GENERAL HOSPITAL (Continued)

BLOOD, PLASMA, OR SERUM VALUES

Determination	Reference Range		Minimal ml Required	Note
	Conventional	SI		
Lipase	4–24 U/dl	667–4001 nmol·s^{-1}/L	1–S	
Lipids				
Cholesterol	120–220 mg/dl	3.10–5.69 mmol/L	1–S	Fasting.
Triglycerides	40–150 mg/dl	0.4–1.5 g/L	1–S	Fasting.
Lipoprotein electrophoresis (LEP)			2–S	Fasting; do not freeze serum.
Lithium	0.5–1.5 mEq/L	0.5–1.5 mmol/L	1–S	
Magnesium	1.5–2.0 mEq/L	0.8–1.3 mmol/L	1–S	
5'-Nucleotidase	1–11 U/L	17–183 nmol·s^{-1}/L	1–S	
Osmolality	280–296 mOsm/kg H$_2$O	280–296 mmol/kg	1–S	
Oxygen saturation (arterial)	96–100%	0.96–1.001	3–B	Deliver in sealed heparinized syringe packed in ice.
P$_{CO_2}$	35–45 mm Hg	4.7–6.0 kPa	2–B	Collect and deliver in sealed heparinized syringe.
pH	7.35–7.45	Same	2–B	Collect without stasis in sealed heparinized syringe; deliver packed in ice.

Po$_2$	75–100 mm Hg (dependent on age) while breathing room air	10.0–13.3 kPa	2–B
	Above 500 mm Hg while on 100% O$_2$		
Phenobarbital	15–50 µg/ml	65–215 µmol/L	1–S
Phenylalanine	0–2 mg/dl	0–120 µmol/L	0.4–S
Phenytoin	Therapeutic level: 5–20 µg/ml	19.8–79.5 µmol/L	1–S
Phosphatase (acid) Prostatic	0–0.8 U/L	0–13.3 nmol·s^{-1}/L	1–S Must always be drawn just before analysis or stored as frozen serum; avoid hemolysis.
Phosphatase (alkaline)	13–39 U/L; infants and adolescents up to 104 U/L	217–650 nmol·s^{-1}/L; up to 1.26 µmol·s^{-1}/L	1–S
Phosphorus (inorganic)	3.0–4.5 mg/dl (infants in 1st year up to 6.0 mg/dl)	1.0–1.5 mmol/L	1–S
Potassium	3.5–5.0 mEq/L	3.5–5.0 mmol/L	1–S Serum must be separated promptly from cells.
Primidone	Therapeutic level: 4–12 µg/ml	18–55 µmol/L	1–S
Procainamide	4–10 µg/ml	17–42 µmol/L	1–S
Protein: Total	6.0–8.4 g/dl	60–84 g/L	1–S
Albumin	3.5–5.0 g/dl	35–50 g/L	1–S

Continued on following page

Abbreviations used: SI = Système International d'Unités; P = plasma; S = serum; B = blood; and U = urine.

16

NORMAL LABORATORY VALUES FROM THE MASSACHUSETTS GENERAL HOSPITAL (Continued)

BLOOD, PLASMA, OR SERUM VALUES

Determination	Reference Range		Minimal ml Required	Note
	Conventional	SI		
Globulin	2.3–3.5 g/dl	23–35 g/L		Globulin equals total protein minus albumin.
Electrophoresis	% of total protein		1–S	Quantitation by densitometry.
Albumin	52–68			
Globulin:				
α_1	4.2–7.2			
α_2	6.8–12			
β	9.3–15			
γ	13–23			
Pyruvic acid	0–0.11 mEq/L	0–0.11 mmol/L	2–B	Collect with oxalate-fluoride; deliver *immediately* packed on ice.
Quinidine	1.2–4.0 μg/ml	3.7–12.3 μmol/L	1–S	
Salicylate	100–200 mg/L	724–1448 μmol/L	2–P	
Sodium	135–145 mEq/L	135–145 mmol/L	1–S	
Sulfonamide	5–15 mg/dl		2–P	
Transaminase (AST or SGOT) (ALT or SGPT)	7–27 U/L 1–21 U/L	117–450 nmol·s⁻¹/L 17–350 nmol·s⁻¹/L	1–S	

Determination	Reference Range		Minimal Quantity Required	Note
	Conventional	SI		
Urea nitrogen (BUN)	8–25 mg/dl	2.9–8.9 mmol/L	1–S	
Uric acid	3.0–7.0 mg/dl	0.18–0.42 mmol/L	1–S	
Vitamin A	0.15–0.6 µg/ml	0.5–2.1 µmol/L	3–S	

URINE VALUES

Determination	Reference Range		Minimal Quantity Required	Note
	Conventional	SI		
Acetone plus acetoacetate (quantitative)	0	0 mg/L	2 ml	
Amylase	0–375 U/L	0–6251 nmol·s^{-1}/L		
Calcium	300 mg/d or less	7.5 mmol/L	24-h specimen	Collect in special bottle with 10 ml of concentrated HCl.
Catecholamines Epinephrine Norepinephrine	<20 µg/d <100 µg/d	<109 nmol/d <590 nmol/d	24-h specimen	Collect with 10 ml of concentrated HCl (pH should be 2.0–3.0).
Chorionic gonadotropin	0	0 arb Units	First morning voiding	
Copper	0–100 µg/d	0–1.6 µmol/d	24-h specimen	

Continued on following page

Abbreviations used: SI = Système International d'Unités; P = plasma; S = serum; B = blood; and U = urine.

16

NORMAL LABORATORY VALUES FROM THE MASSACHUSETTS GENERAL HOSPITAL (Continued)

URINE VALUES

Determination	Reference Range		Minimal Quantity Required	Note
	Conventional	SI		
Coproporphyrin	50–250 μg/d Children <80 lb (36 kg): 0–75 μg/d	80–380 nmol/d 0–115 nmol/d	24-h specimen	Collect with 5 g of sodium carbonate.
Creatine	<100 mg/day or <6% of creatinine. In pregnancy, up to 12%. In children <1 y, may equal creatinine; in older children, up to 30% of creatinine	<0.75 mmol/d	24-h specimen	Order serum creatinine also.
Creatinine	15–25 mg·kg/d	0.13–0.22 mmol·kg^{-1}/d	24-h specimen	
Cystine or cysteine	0	0	10 ml	Qualitative.
Hemoglobin and myoglobin	0		Freshly voided sample	Chemical examination with benzidine.
5-Hydroxyindole-acetic acid	2–9 mg/d (women lower than men)	10–45 μmol/d	24-h specimen	
Lead	0.08 μg/ml or 120 μg or less per day	0.39 μmol/L or less	24-h specimen	Collect in special bottle with 10 ml of concentrated HCl.

Phosphorus (inorganic)	Varies with intake; average 1 g/d	32 mmol/d	24-h specimen	Collect in special bottle with 10 ml of concentrated HCl.
Porphobilinogen	0	0	10 ml	Use freshly voided urine.
Protein: Quantitative	<165 mg/24 h	<0.16 g/d	24-h specimen	

Steroids:

17-Ketosteroids

Age	Male (mg/d)	Female (mg/d)		
10	1–4	1–4		
20	6–21	4–16		
30	8–26	4–14		
50	5–18	3–9		
70	2–10	1–7		

Male (µmol/d)	Female (µmol/d)	
3–14	3–14	24-h specimen
21–73	14–56	Not valid if patient is receiving meprobamate.
28–90	14–49	
17–62	10–31	
7–35	3–24	

17-Hydroxysteroids	3–8 mg/d (women lower than men)	8–22 µmol/d as tetrahydrocortisol	24-h specimen	Keep cold; chlorpromazine and related drugs interfere with assay.
Sugar: Quantitative glucose	0	0 mmol/L	24-h or other timed specimen	
Urobilinogen	Up to 1.0 Ehrlich U	To 1.0 arb Units	2-h specimen (1–3 PM)	
Uroporphyrin	0–30 µg/d	<36 nmol/d	See Coproporphyrin	
Vanillylmandelic acid (VMA)	Up to 9 mg/24 h	Up to 45 µmol/d	24-h specimen	Collect as for catecholamines.

Continued on following page

Abbreviations used: SI = Système International d'Unités; P = plasma; S = serum; B = blood; and U = urine.

16

NORMAL LABORATORY VALUES FROM THE MASSACHUSETTS GENERAL HOSPITAL (Continued)

SPECIAL ENDOCRINE TESTS

Determination	Reference Range		Minimal ml Required	Note
	Conventional	SI		
Steroid Hormones				
Aldosterone	Excretion: 5–19 μg/24 h	14–53 mmol/d	5/d	Keep specimen cold.
	Supine: 48 ± 29 pg/ml	133 ± 80 pmol/L	3–S,P	Fasting, at rest, 210-mEq Na diet.
	Upright: (2 h) 65 ± 23 pg/ml	180 ± 64 pmol/L		Upright, 2 h, 210-mEq Na diet.
	Supine: 107 ± 45 pg/ml	279 ± 125 pmol/L		Fasting, at rest, 110-mEq Na diet.
	Upright: (2 h) 239 ± 123 pg/ml	663 ± 341 pmol/L		Upright, 2 h, 110-mEq Na diet.
	Supine: 175 ± 75 pg/ml	485 ± 208 pmol/L		Fasting, at rest, 10-mEq Na diet.
	Upright: (2 h) 532 ± 228 pg/ml	1476 ± 632 pmol/L		Upright, 2 h, 10-mEq Na diet.
Cortisol	8 AM: 5–25 μg/dl	0.14–0.69 μmol/L	1–P	Fasting.
	8 PM: <10 μg/dl	0–0.28 μmol/L	1–P	At rest.
	4-h ACTH test: 30–45 μg/dl	0.83–1.24 μmol/L	1–P	20 U ACTH IV per 4 h.
	Overnight suppression test:	<0.14 nmol/L	1–P	8 AM sample after 0.5 mg
	<5 μg/dl			dexamethasone at midnight.
	Excretion: 20–70 μg/24 h	55–193 nmol/d	2–day	Keep specimen cold.
Dehydroepiandro-sterone (DHEA)	Male: 0.5–5.5 ng/ml	1.7–19 nmol/L	2–S,P	
	Female: 1.4–8.0 ng/ml	4.9–28 nmol/L		Adult.
	0.3–4.5 ng/ml	1.0–15.6 nmol/L		Postmenopausal.
Dehydroepiandro-sterone sulfate (DHEAS)	Male: 151–446 μg/ml	3.9–11.4 μmol/L	2–S,P	Adult.
	Female: 84–433 μg/ml	2.2–11.1 μmol/L		
	1.7–177 μg/ml	0.04–4.5 μmol/L		Postmenopausal.

	Conventional	SI	Specimen	Notes
11-Deoxycortisol	Responsive: >7.5 µg/dl	>0.22 µmol/L	1–P	8 AM sample preceded by metyrapone 4.5 g orally per 24 h or by single 2.5-g dose orally at midnight.
Estradiol	Male: <50 pg/ml Female: 23–361 pg/ml <30 pg/ml <20 pg/ml	<184 pmol/L 84–1325 pmol/L <110 pmol/L <73 pmol/L	5–S,P	Adult. Postmenopausal. Prepubertal.
Progesterone	Male: <1.0 ng/ml Female: 0.2–0.6 ng/ml 0.3–3.5 ng/ml 6.5–32.2 ng/ml	<3.2 nmol/L 0.6–1.9 nmol/L 0.95–11 nmol/L 21–108 nmol/L	5–S,P	Follicular phase. Midcycle peak. Postovulatory phase.
Testosterone	Adult male: 300–1100 ng/dl Adolescent male: >100 ng/dl Female: 25–90 ng/dl	10.4–38.1 nmol/L >3.5 nmol/L 0.87–3.12 nmol/L	1–P	AM sample.
Unbound testosterone	Adult male: 3.06–24 ng/dl Adult female: 0.09–1.28 ng/dl	106–832 pmol/L 3.1–44.4 pmol/L	2–P	AM sample.
Polypeptide Hormones				
ACTH	15–70 pg/ml	3.3–15.4 pmol/L	5–P	Place specimen on ice and send promptly to laboratory. Use EDTA tube only.
Calcitonin	Male: 0–14 pg/ml Female: 0–28 pg/ml >100 pg/ml in medullary carcinoma	0–4.1 pmol/L 0–8.2 pmol/L >29.3 pmol/L	5–S	Test done only on known or suspected cases of medullary carcinoma of the thyroid.

Continued on following page

16

Abbreviations used: SI = Système International d'Unités; P = plasma; S = serum; B = blood; and U = urine.

SPECIAL ENDOCRINE TESTS

Determination	Reference Range		Minimal ml Required	Note
	Conventional	SI		
Follicle-stimulating hormone	Male: 3–18 mU/ml	3–18 arb Units	5–S,P	Same sample may be used for LH;
	Female: 4.6–22.4 mU/ml	4.6–22.4 arb Units		Pre- or postovulatory
	13–41 mU/ml	13–41 arb Units		Midcycle peak
	30–170 mU/ml	30–170 arb Units		Postmenopausal
Growth hormone	<5 ng/ml	<233 pmol/L	1–S	Fasting, at rest.
	Children: >10 ng/ml	>465 pmol/L		After exercise.
	Male: <5 ng/ml	<233 pmol/L		
	Female: Up to 30 ng/ml	0–1395 pmol/L		
	Male: <5 ng/ml	<233 pmol/L		After glucose load.
	Female: <5 ng/ml	<233 pmol/L		
Insulin	6–26 μU/ml	43–187 pmol/L	1–S	Fasting.
	<20 μU/ml	<144 pmol/L		During hypoglycemia.
	Up to 150 μU/ml	0–1078 pmol/L		After glucose load.
Luteinizing hormone	Male: 3–18 mU/ml	3–18 arb Units	5–S,P	Pre- or postovulatory.
	Female: 2.4–34.5 mU/ml	2.4–34.5 arb Units		Midcycle peak.
	43–187 mU/ml	43–187 arb Units		Postmenopausal.
	30–150 mU/ml	30–150 arb Units		
Parathyroid hormone	<25 pg/ml	<2.94 pmol/L	5–P	Keep blood on ice, or plasma must be frozen if it is to be sent any distance; AM sample.
Prolactin	2–15 ng/ml	0.08–6.0 nmol/L	2–S	
Renin activity	Supine: 1.1 ± 0.8 ng/ml/h	0.9 ± 0.6 nmol·L/h	4–P	EDTA tubes, on ice; normal diet.

Somatomedin C (Sm-C, ICF-1)	Upright: 1.9 ± 1.7 ng·ml/h	1.5 ± 1.3 nmol·L/h		
	Supine: 2.7 ± 1.8 ng·ml/h	2.1 ± 1.4 nmol·L/h		
	Upright: 6.6 ± 2.5 ng·ml/h	5.1 ± 1.9 nmol·L/h		Low Na diet.
	Diuretics: 10.0 ± 3.7 ng·ml/h	7.7 ± 2.9 nmol·L/h	2–P	Low Na diet.
	0.08–2.8 U/ml	0.08–2.8 arb Units		Prepubertal.
	0.9–5.9 U/ml	0.9–5.9 arb Units		During puberty.
	0.34–1.9 U/ml	0.34–1.9 arb Units		Adult males.
	0.45–2.2 U/ml	0.45–2.2 arb Units		Adult females.
Thyroid Hormones				
Thyroid-stimulating hormone (TSH)	0.5–5.0 µU/ml	0.5–5.0 mU/L	2–S	
Thyroxine-binding globulin capacity	15–25 µg T_4/dl	193–322 nmol/L.	2–S	
Total triiodothyronine by radioimmunoassay (T_3)	75–195 ng/dl	1.16–3.00 nmol/L	2–S	
Reverse diiodothyronine (rT_3)	13–53 ng/ml	0.2–0.8 nmol/L	2–S	
Total thyroxine by radioimmunoassay (T_4)	4–12 µg/dl	52–154 nmol/L	1–S	
T_3 resin uptake	25%–35%	0.25–0.35	2–S	
Free thyroxine index (FT_4I)	1–4		2–S	EDTA plasma.

Continued on following page

Abbreviations used: SI = Système International d'Unités; P = plasma; S = serum; B = blood; and U = urine.

HEMATOLOGIC VALUES

Determination	Reference Range		Minimal ml Required	Note
	Conventional	SI		
Coagulation Factors				
Factor I (fibrinogen)	0.15–0.35 g/dl	4.0–10.0 μmol/L	4.5 – P	Collect in vacuum tube containing sodium citrate.
Factor II (prothrombin)	60 %–140%	0.60–1.40	4.5–P	Collect in plastic tubes with 3.8% sodium citrate.
Factor V (accelerator globulin)	60 %–140%	0.60–1.40	4.5–P	Collect as for factor II.
Factor VIII–X (proconvertin-Stuart)	70 %–130%	0.70–1.30	4.5–P	Collect as for factor II.
Factor X (Stuart factor)	70 %–130%	0.70–1.30	4.5–P	Collect as for factor II.
Factor VIII (antihemophilic globulin)	50 %–200%	0.50–2.0	4.5–P	Collect as for factor II.
Factor IX (plasma thromboplastic cofactor)	60 %–140%	0.60–1.40	4.5–P	Collect as for factor II.
Factor XI (plasma thromboplastic antecedent)	60 %–140%	0.60–1.40	4.5–P	Collect as for factor II.

Test	Conventional	SI	Specimen	Collection
Factor XII (Hageman factor)	60%–140%	0.60–1.40	4.5–P	Collect as for factor II.
Coagulation Screening Tests				
Bleeding time	3–9.5 min	180–570 s		
Prothrombin time	<2-s deviation from control	<2-s deviation from control	4.5–P	Collect in vacuum tube containing 3.8% sodium citrate.
Partial thromboplastin time (activated)	25–38 s	25–38 s	4.5–P	Collect in vacuum tube containing 3.8% sodium citrate.
Whole-blood clot lysis	No clot lysis in 24 h	0/d	2.0 whole blood	Collect in sterile tube and incubate at 37°C.
Fibrinolytic Studies				
Euglobin lysis	No lysis in 2 h	0 (in 2 h)	4.5–P	Collect as for factor II.
Fibrinogen split products	Negative reaction at >1:4 dilution	0 (at >1:4 dilution)	4.5–S	Collect in special tube containing thrombin and aminocaproic acid.
Thrombin time	Control ±5 s	Control ±5 s	4.5–P	Collect as for factor II.
"Complete" Blood Count				
Hematocrit	Male: 45%–52% Female: 37%–48%	0.45–0.52 0.37–0.48	1–B	Use EDTA as anticoagulant; the seven listed tests are performed automatically on the Ortho ELT 800, which directly determines
Hemoglobin	Male: 13–18 gm/dl Female: 12–16 g/dl	8.1–11.2 mmol/L 7.4–9.9 mmol/L		

Continued on following page

Abbreviations used: SI = Système International d'Unités; P = plasma; S = serum; B = blood; and U = urine.

16

NORMAL LABORATORY VALUES FROM THE MASSACHUSETTS GENERAL HOSPITAL (Continued)

HEMATOLOGIC VALUES

Determination	Reference Range		Minimal ml Required	Note
	Conventional	SI		
Leukocyte count	4300–10,800/μL	4.3–10.8 × 10⁹/L		cell counts, Hb (as the
Erythrocyte count	4.2–5.9 million/μL	4.2–5.9 × 10¹²/L		cyanmethemoglobin derivative), and MCV, and computes Hct, MCH, and MCHC.
MCV	86–98 μm³/cell	86–98 fl (femtoliter)		MCV = mean corpuscular volume.
MCH	27–32 pg	1.7–2.0 pg/cell		MCH = mean corpuscular hemoglobin.
MCHC	32%–36%	0.32–0.36		MCHC = mean corpuscular hemoglobin concentration.
ESR	Male:1–13 mm/h	1–13 mm/h	5–B	Use EDTA as anticoagulant.
	Female: 1–20 mm/h	1–20 mm/h		
Erythrocyte Enzymes				
Glucose-6-phosphate dehydrogenase	5–15 Ug Hb	5–15 Ug	9–B	Use special anticoagulant (ACD solution).
Pyruvate kinase	13–17 Ug Hb	13–17 Ug	8–B	Use special anticoagulant (ACD solution).
Ferritin (serum) Iron deficiency	0–12 ng/ml (borderline: 13–20)	0–4.8 nmol/L (borderline: 5.2–8)		

	Conventional	SI	Notes
Iron excess	>400 ng/L	>160 nmol/L	
Folic acid			
Normal	>3.3 ng/ml	>7.3 nmol/L	1−S
Borderline	2.5−3.2 ng/ml	5.75−7.39 nmol/L	1−S
Haptoglobin	40−336 mg/dl	0.4−3.36 g/L	1−S
Hemoglobin Studies			
Electrophoresis for abnormal Hb			5−B Collect with anticoagulant.
Electrophoresis for A₂ Hb	1.5%−3.5% (borderline: 0.3%−3.5%)	0.015−0.035 (borderline: 0.03−0.035)	5−B Use oxalate as anticoagulant.
Fetal Hb	<2%	<0.02	5−B Collect with anticoagulant.
Met- and sulf-Hb	0	0	5−B Use heparin as anticoagulant.
Serum Hb	2−3 mg/dl	1.2−1.9 μmol/L	2−S
Thermolabile Hb	0	0	1−B Any anticoagulant.
Lupus anticoagulant	0	0	4.5−P Collect as for factor II.
LE (lupus erythematosus) cell preparation			
Hargraves method	0	0	5−B Use heparin as anticoagulant.
Barnes method	0	0	5−B Use defibrinated blood.
Leukocyte alkaline phosphatase: Qualitative method	Males: 33−188 U Females: (off contraceptive pill): 30−160 U	33−188 U 30−160 U	Smear-B

Continued on following page

Abbreviations used: SI = Système International d'Unités; P = plasma; S = serum; B = blood; and U = urine.

16

NORMAL LABORATORY VALUES FROM THE MASSACHUSETTS GENERAL HOSPITAL (Continued)

HEMATOLOGIC VALUES

Determination	Reference Range		Minimal ml Required	Note
	Conventional	SI		
Muramidase (lysozyme)	Serum: 3–7 μg/ml Urine: 0–2 μg/ml	3–7 mg/L 0–2 mg/L	1–S 1–U	
Osmotic fragility of erythrocytes	Increased if hemolysis occurs in >0.5% NaCl; decreased if hemolysis is incomplete in 0.3% NaCl		5–B	Use heparin as anticoagulant.
Peroxide hemolysis	<10%	<0.10	6–B	Use EDTA as anticoagulant.
Platelet count	150,000–350,000/μL	150–350 × 10⁹/L	0.5–B	Use EDTA as anticoagulant. Counts are performed on Clay Adams Ultraflow. Low counts are confirmed by hand counting.
Platelet Function Tests				
Clot retraction	50%–100%/2 h	0.50–1.00/2 h	4.5–P	Collect as for factor II.
Platelet aggregation	Full response to ADP, epinephrine, and collagen	1.0	18–P	Collect as for factor II.
Platelet factor 3	33–57 s	33–57 s	4.5–P	Collect as for factor II.
Reticulocyte count	0.5%–2.5% RBCs	0.005–0.025	0.1–B	
Vitamin B₁₂	205–876 pg/ml (borderline: 140–204)	150–674 pmol/L (borderline: 102.6–149)	12–S	

CEREBROSPINAL FLUID VALUES

Determination	Reference Range		Minimal ml Required	Note
	Conventional	SI		
Bilirubin	0	0 μmol/L	2	
Cell count	0–5 mononuclear cells		0.5	
Chloride	120–130 mEq/L	120–130 mmol/L	0.5	20 mEq/L Higher than serum chloride.
Colloidal gold	0000000000–0001222111	Same	0.1	
Albumin	Mean: 29.5 mg/dl ± 2 SD: 11–48 mg/dl	0.295 g/L 0.11–0.48	2.5	
IgG	Mean: 4.3 mg/dl ± 2 SD: 0–8.6 mg/dl	0.043 g/L 0–0.086		
Glucose	50–75 mg/dl	2.8–4.2 mmol/L	0.5	30%–50% Less than blood glucose.
Pressure (initial)	70–180 mm H₂O	70–180 arb Units		
Protein:				
Lumbar	15–45 mg/dl	0.15–0.45 g/L	1	
Cisternal	15–25 mg/dl	0.15–0.25 g/L	1	
Ventricular	5–15 mg/dl	0.05–0.15 g/L	1	

Continued on following page

Abbreviations used: SI = Système International d'Unités; P = plasma; S = serum; B = blood; and U = urine.

16

NORMAL LABORATORY VALUES FROM THE MASSACHUSETTS GENERAL HOSPITAL (Continued)

MISCELLANEOUS VALUES

Determination	Reference Range		Minimal ml Required	Note
	Conventional	SI		
Carcinoembryonic antigen (CEA)	0–2.5 ng/ml	0–2.5 µg/L	20–P	Must be sent on ice.
Chylous fluid				Use fresh specimen.
Digitoxin	9–25 µg/L	11.8–32.8 nmol/L	1–S	Medication with digitoxin or digitalis.
Digoxin	0.9–2.0 ng/ml	1.15–2.56 nmol/L.	1–S	
Gastric analysis	Basal:			
	Females 2.0 ± 1.8 mEq/h	0.6 ± 0.5 µmol/s		
	Males 3.0 ± 2.0 mEq/h	0.8 ± 0.6 µmol/s		
	Maximal (after histalog or gastrin):			
	Females 16 ± 5 mEq/h	4.4 ± 1.4 µmol/s		
	Males 23 ± 5 mEq/h	6.4 ± 1.4 µmol/s		
Gastrin-1	0–200 pg/ml	0–95 pmol/L	4–P	Heparinized sample.

Immunologic Tests			
α-Fetoglobulin	Undetectable in normal adults		
α₁-Antitrypsin	85–213 mg/dl	0.85–2.13 g/L	2–S
antinuclear antibodies	Negative at a 1:8 dilution of serum		10–B 2–S
Anti-DNA antibodies	Negative at a 1:10 dilution of serum		2–S
Bence-Jones protein	Abnormal if present		50–U
Complement, total hemolytic	150–250 U/ml		10–B
C3	Range: 83–177 mg/dl	0.83–1.77 g/L	2–S
C4	Range: 15–45 mg/dl	0.15–0.45 g/L	2–S
Rheumatoid factor	<60 IU/ml		10 ml Clotted blood
Immunoglobulins			
IgG	639–1349 mg/dl	6.39–13.49 g/L	2–S
IgA	70–312 mg/dl	0.7–3.12 g/L	2–S
IgM	86–352 mg/dl	0.86–3.52 g/L	2–S
Viscosity	1.4–1.8 relative viscosity units		10–B
Iontophoresis	Children: 0–40 mEq Na/L	0–40 mmol/L	2–S
	Adults: 0–60 mEq Na/L	0–60 mmol/L	2–S

Send to laboratory promptly.

Must be sent on ice.

Fasting sample preferred.

Expressed as the relative viscosity of serum compared with water.

Value given in terms of sodium.

Continued on following page

Abbreviations used: SI = Système International d'Unités; P = plasma; S = serum; B = blood; and U = urine.

16

NORMAL LABORATORY VALUES FROM THE MASSACHUSETTS GENERAL HOSPITAL (Continued)

MISCELLANEOUS VALUES

Determination	Reference Range		Minimal ml Required	Note
	Conventional	SI		
Stool fat	<5 gm in 24 h or <4% of measured fat intake in 3-d period	<5 g/d	24-h or 3-day specimen	
Stool nitrogen	<2 g/d or 10% of urinary nitrogen	<2 g/d	24-h or 3-day specimen	
Synovial fluid Glucose	Not <20 mg/dL lower than simultaneously drawn blood sugar	See blood glucose	1 ml of fresh fluid	Collect with oxalate-floride mixture.
D-Xylose absorption	5–8 g/5 h in urine (40 mg/dl in blood after 2 h of ingestion of 25 g D-xylose)	33–53 mmol (2.7 mmol/L)	5–U 5–B	Administer 25 g of D-xylose orally.

Abbreviations used: SI = Système International d"Unités; P = plasma; S = serum; B = blood; and U = urine.
As appearing in The Merck Manual, ed 16. Merck & Co., Rahway, NJ, 1992, pp 2580–2591, with permission. Based on N Engl J Med 314(1): 39–49, January 2, 1986, and 315(25): 1606, December 18, 1986.

COMMON LABORATORY TESTS AND THEIR DISEASE ASSOCIATIONS

Laboratory Test	Increase	Decrease
Acid phosphatase	Prostatic carcinoma, postprostatic massage, prostatitis, myocardial infarction, excess platelet destruction, bone disease, liver disease	
Alanine aminotransferase (ALT or SGPT)	Hepatitis, cirrhosis, liver metastases, obstructive jaundice, infectious mononucleosis, hepatic congestion, pancreatitis, renal disease, ethanol ingestion	Pyridoxine (vitamin B_6) deficiency
Albumin	Dehydration, diabetes insipidus	Overhydration, malnutrition, malabsorption, nephrosis, hepatic failure, burns, multiple myeloma, metastatic carcinomas
Alkaline phosphatase	Bone growth, bone metastases, Paget's disease, rickets, healing fracture, hyperparathyroidism, hepatic disease, obstructive jaundice, hepatic metastases, pulmonary infarction, heart failure, pregnancy	Pernicious anemia, hypoparathyroidism, hypophosphatasia
α-Fetoprotein	Hepatoma, testicular tumor, hepatitis	
Amylase	Pancreatitis, GI obstruction, mesenteric thrombosis and infarction, macroamylasemia, parotitis, mumps, renal disease, ruptured tubal pregnancy, lung carcinoma, acute ethanol ingestion, postoperative abdominal surgery	Marked pancreatic destruction

Continued on following page

16

COMMON LABORATORY TESTS AND THEIR DISEASE ASSOCIATIONS (Continued)

Laboratory Test	Increase	Decrease
Aspartate aminotransferase (AST or SGOT)	Myocardial infarction, heart failure, myocarditis, pericarditis, myositis, muscular dystrophy, trauma, hepatic disease, pancreatitis, renal infarct, eclampsia, neoplasia, cerebral damage, seizures, hemolysis, ethanol intake	Pyridoxine (vitamin B_6) deficiency, terminal stage of liver disease
Bilirubin	Hepatic disease, obstructive jaundice, hemolytic anemia, pulmonary infarct, Gilbert's disease, Dubin-Johnson syndrome, neonatal jaundice	
Calcium	Hyperparathyroidism, bone metastases, myeloma, sarcoidosis, hyperthyroidism, hypervitaminosis D, malignancy without bone metastases, milk-alkali syndrome	Hypoparathyroidism, renal failure, malabsorption, pancreatitis, hypo-albuminemia, vitamin D deficiency, overhydration
Cholesterol	Hypothyroidism, obstructive jaundice, nephrosis, diabetes mellitus, pancreatitis, pregnancy, familial factors	Hyperthyroidism, infection, malnutrition, heart failure, malignancies, severe liver damage (due to chemicals, drugs, hepatitis)
HDL cholesterol	Vigorous exercise, increased clearance of triglyceride (VLDL), moderate ethanol consumption, insulin, estrogens	Starvation, obesity, cigarette smoking, diabetes mellitus, hypothyroidism, liver disease, nephrosis, uremia

Creatine kinase	Myocardial infarction, muscle disease, burns, chest trauma, collagen-vascular disease, meningitis, drugs (e.g., lovastatin), burns, status epilepticus, brain infarction, hyperthermia, postoperative increase	
Creatinine	Renal failure, urinary obstruction, dehydration, hyperthyroidism, diet, muscle disease	Aging
Glucose	Diabetes mellitus, IV glucose, thiazides, corticosteroids, pheochromocytoma, hyperthyroidism, Cushing's syndrome, acromegaly, brain damage, hepatic disease, nephrosis, hemochromatosis, stress (e.g., emotion, burns, shock, anesthesia), acute or chronic pancreatitis, Wernicke's encephalopathy (vitamin B_1 deficiency), epinephrine, estrogens, ethanol, phenytoin, propranolol, chronic hypervitaminosis A	Excess insulin, insulinoma, Addison's disease, myxedema, hepatic failure, malabsorption, pancreatitis, glucagon deficiency, extrapancreatic tumors, early diabetes mellitus, postgastrectomy, autonomic nervous system disorders, idiopathic leucine sensitivity, enzyme diseases (von Gierke's disease, fructose intolerance), oral hypoglycemic medications (factitious), malnutrition, alcoholism

Continued on following page

HDL = high-density lipoprotein; VLDL = very low density lipoprotein.

16

COMMON LABORATORY TESTS AND THEIR DISEASE ASSOCIATIONS (Continued)

Laboratory Test	Increase	Decrease
Lactate dehydrogenase (LDH)	Myocardial infarction, pulmonary infarction, hemolytic anemia, pernicious anemia, leukemia, lymphoma, other malignancies, hepatic disease, renal infarction, seizures, cerebral damage, trauma, sprue	
Lipase	Same as amylase (except not in parotitis, mumps), macroamylasemia	
Magnesium	Renal disease, excess Mg (IV or po)	Diarrhea, malabsorption, renal tubular acidosis, acute tubular necrosis, chronic glomerulonephritis, drugs (diuretics, antibiotics), aldosteronism, hyperthyroidism, hypercalcemia, uncontrolled diabetes, nutritional deficit
Phosphorus	Renal failure, hypoparathyroidism, diabetic acidosis, acromegaly, hyperthyroidism, high phosphate intake (IV or po) vitamin D intoxication, lactic acidosis, cell lysis, leukemia, volume contraction, spurious, prolonged refrigeration of sample, heparin sodium contamination, hyperbilirubinemia, hyperlipidemia, dysproteinemia	Hyperparathyroidism, osteomalacia, rickets, Fanconi's syndrome, cirrhosis, hypokalemia, excess IV glucose, respiratory alkalosis, dietary deprivation, P-binding

Potassium	Hyperkalemic acidosis, diabetic acidosis, hypoadrenalism, hereditary hyperkalemia, hemolysis, myoglobinuria, K-retaining diuretic, ACE inhibitors, large exogenous K load, renal tubular defect, thrombocytosis	antacid, alcoholism, gout, hemodialysis
		Cirrhosis, malnutrition, vomiting, metabolic alkalosis, diarrhea, nephrosis, diuretics, hyperadrenalism, familial periodic paralysis, ectopic ACTH excess, β-hydroxylase deficiency
Sodium	Dehydration, diabetes insipidus, excessive salt ingestion, diabetes mellitus with diuresis, diuretic phase of acute tubular necrosis, hypercalcemic nephropathy with diuresis, "essential" hypernatremia due to hypothalamic lesions	Excess antidiuretic hormone, nephrosis, hypoadrenalism, myxedema, heart failure, diarrhea, vomiting, diabetic acidosis, diuretics, adrenocortical insufficiency, spurious (serum osmolality is normal or increased—avoid by using direct-reading potentiometry with ion-selective electrode); hyperlipidemia (serum Na decreases by 1 mmol/L per every 4.6 g/L increase in lipid), hyperglycemia (serum

Continued on following page

ACE = angiotensin converting enzyme; ACTH = adrenocorticotropin.

16

	COMMON LABORATORY TESTS AND THEIR DISEASE ASSOCIATIONS (Continued)	
Laboratory Test	*Increase*	*Decrease*
Sodium		Na decreases 3 mEq/L per every 100 mg/dl increase of serum glucose), mannitol, hyperproteinemia (e.g., multiple myeloma)
Total protein	Multiple myeloma, myxedema, lupus, sarcoidosis, diabetes insipidus, dehydration, collagen disease	Burns, cirrhosis, malnutrition, nephrosis, malabsorption, overhydration, GI protein loss
Triglyceride	Nephrosis, cholestasis, pancreatitis, cirrhosis, diabetes mellitus, hepatitis, dietary excess, hereditary	Malnutrition
Urea nitrogen	Renal disease, dehydration, GI bleeding, leukemia, heart failure, shock, postrenal azotemia, any obstruction of urinary tract (BUN: creatinine > 10 : 1), acute myocardial infarction	Hepatic failure, overhydration, pregnancy, acromegaly, diet, IV feedings only

| Uric acid | Gout, renal failure, diuretic therapy, leukemia, lymphoma, polycythemia, acidosis, psoriasis, hypothyroidism, eclampsia, multiple myeloma, pernicious anemia, tissue necrosis, inflammation, 25% of relatives of patients with gout, cancer chemotherapy (e.g., nitrogen mustards, vincristine, mercaptopurine), hemolytic anemia, sickle cell anemia, high-protein weight-reduction diet, lead poisoning, Lesch-Nyhan syndrome, polycystic kidneys, calcinosis universalis and circumscripta, hypoparathyroidism, sarcoidosis, elevated serum triglycerides | Uricosuric drugs, allopurinol, Wilson's disease, large doses of vitamin C, Fanconi's syndrome, xanthinuria |

ACE = angiotensin converting enzyme; ACTH = adrenocorticotropin; BUN = blood urea nitrogen; HDL = high-density lipoprotein; VLDL = very low density lipoprotein.

As appearing in The Merck Manual, ed 16. Merck & Co, Rahway, NJ, 1992, pp 2575–2578. Based on material appearing in Wallach, J: Interpretation of Diagnostic Tests, ed 4. Little, Brown, Boston, 1986, pp 41–96, with permission.

URINE AND BLOOD CHANGES IN ELECTROLYTES, pH, AND VOLUME IN VARIOUS CONDITIONS

Measurement	Pulmonary Emphysema	Congestive Heart Failure	Excessive Sweating	Diarrhea	Pyloric Obstruction	Dehydration	Starvation	Malabsorption	Salicylate Intoxication	Primary Aldosteronism	Adrenal Cortical Insufficiency	Diabetes Insipidus	Diabetic Acidosis	Thiazide Administration	Renal Tubular Acidosis	Chronic Renal Failure	Acute Renal Failure
Blood sodium	N	N or D	D	D	D	I	N	D	N	I	D	N or I	D	D	D	D	D
Potassium	N	N	N	D	D	N	D	D	N or D	D	I	N	N or I	D	D	N or D	I
Bicarbonate	I	N	N	D	I	N or D	D	N or D	D	I	N or D	N	D	D	D	D	D

Chloride	D	D	D	D	D	I	N	N	I	D	D	I	D or N	I
Volume	N or I	I	N	D	D	D	N or D	D	N	N	D	D	V	I
Urine sodium	D	D	D	D	D	I	N or I	D	I	D	I	I	I	D
Potassium	N	N	N	N or D	N	I	I or N	D	N or I	I	N or D	I	I	D
pH	D	N	N	D	I	D	D	N or D	I	N or D	N or I	I	I	N or I
Volume	N	D	N	D	D	D	I	N	N	I	N or D	I	V*	D

*Usually increased.

N = normal; D = decreased; I = increased; V = variable.

As appearing in The Merck Manual, ed 16. Merck & Co., Rahway, NJ, 1992, p 2579. Based on Wallach, J: Interpretation of Diagnostic Tests, ed 4. Little, Brown, Boston, 1986, with permission.

16

SMOKING ADJUSTMENTS FOR HEMOGLOBIN AND HEMATOCRIT CUT POINTS FOR ANEMIA		
Smoking Status	Hb (g/dl)	Hct (%)
Nonsmoker	0.0	0.0
Smoker (all)	+0.3	+1.0
0.5–<1.0 packs/d	+0.3	+1.0
1.0–2.0 packs/d	+0.5	+1.5
>2.0 packs/d	+0.7	+2.0

From Centers for Disease Control: Reference criteria for anemia screening. MMWR 38:400, 1989, with permission.

BACTERIAL INFECTIONS

TYPES OF BACTERIA

Type	Principal Features	Common Examples
Gram-positive bacilli	Generally rod shaped; retain color when treated by Gram's method of staining	*Bacillus anthracis, Clostridium tetani*
Gram-negative bacilli	Rod shaped; do not retain color of Gram's method	*Escherichia coli, Klebsiella pneumoniae, Pseudomonas aeruginosa*
Gram-positive cocci	Generally spherical or ovoid in shape; retain color of Gram's method	*Staphylococcus aureus, Streptococcus pneumoniae*
Gram-negative cocci	Spherical or ovoid; do not retain color of Gram's method	*Neisseria gonorrhoeae* (gonococcus), *Neisseria meningitidis* (meningococcus)
Acid-fast bacilli	Rod shaped; retain color of certain stains even when treated with acid	*Mycobacterium leprae, Mycobacterium tuberculosis*
Spirochetes	Slender, spiral shape; able to move about without flagella (intrinsic locomotor ability)	Lyme disease agent; *Treponema pallidum* (syphilis)
Acitinomycetes	Thin filaments that stain positively by Gram's method	*Actinomyces israeli; Nocardia*
Others: Mycoplasmas	Spherical; lack the rigid, highly structured cell wall found in most bacteria	*Mycoplasma pneumoniae*
Rickettsias	Small, gram-negative bacteria	*Rickettsia typhi, Rickettsia rickettsii*

From Ciccone, CD: Pharmacology in Rehabilitation, ed 2. FA Davis, Philadelphia, 1996, p 503, with permission.

16

COMMON ANTIMICROBIAL DRUGS

DRUGS USED TO INHIBIT BACTERIAL CELL MEMBRANE SYNTHESIS

Penicillins	Cephalosporins	Other Agents
Natural penicillins	First-generation cephalosporins	Aztreoman (Azactam)
Penicillin G (Bicillin, Wycillin, many others)	Cefadroxil (Duricef, Ultracef)	Bacitracin (Bacitracin ointment)
Penicillin V (Beepen-VK, V-Cillin K, others)	Cefazolin (Ancef, Kefzol)	Colistin (Coly-Mycin S)
Penicillinase-resistant penicillins	Cephalexin (Keflex, Keftab)	Cycloserine (Seromycin)
Cloxacillin (Cloxapen, Tegopen)	Cephalothin (Keflin)	Imipenem/cilastatin (Primaxim)
Dicloxacillin (Cynapen, Pathocil)	Cephapirin (Cefadyl)	Polymyxin B (generic)
Methicillin (Staphcillin)	Cephradine (Anspor, Velosef)	Vancomycin (Vancocin I.V., Vancoled)
Nafcillin (Unipen)	Second-generation cephalosporins	
Oxacillin (Bactocill, Prostaphlin)	Cefaclor (Ceclor)	
Aminopenicillins	Cefamandole (Mandol)	
Amoxicillin (Amoxil, Polymox, others)	Cefmetazole (Zefazone)	
Ampicillin (Omnipen, Polycillin, others)	Cefonicid (Monocid)	
Bacampicillin (Spectrobid)	Ceforanide (Precef)	
Cyclacillin (Cyclapen-W)	Cefotetan (Cefotan)	
	Cefoxitin (Mefoxin)	

Extended-spectrum penicillins
Azlocillin (Azlin)
Carbenicillin (Geocillin, Geopen, Pyopen)
Mezlocillin (Mezlin)
Piperacillin (Pipracil)
Ticarcillin (Ticar)

Cefprozil (Cefzil)
Cefuroxime (Kefurox, Zinacef)
Third-generation cephalosporins
Cefixime (Suprax)
Cefoperazone (Cefobid)
Cefotaxime (Claforan)
Ceftazidime (Fortaz, Tazicef)
Ceftizoxime (Cefizox)
Ceftriaxone (Rocephin)
Moxalactam (Moxam)

From Ciccone, CD: Pharmacology in Rehabilitation, ed 2. FA Davis, 1996, p 509, with permission.

16

DRUGS USED TO TREAT COMMON INFECTIONS CAUSED BY GRAM-POSITIVE BACILLI

Bacillus	Disease	Primary Agent(s)	Alternative Agent(s)
Bacillus anthracis	Anthrax; pneumonia	Penicillin G	Erythromycin; a tetracycline; a cephalosporin; chloramphenicol
Clostridium	Gas gangrene	Penicillin G	A cephalosporin; clindamycin; imipenem; chloramphenicol; a tetracycline
Clostridium tetani	Tetanus	Penicillin G	A tetracycline; erythromycin
Corynebacterium diphtheriae	Pharyngitis; laryngotracheitis; pneumonia; other local lesions	Penicillin G	Erythromycin, a cephalosporin; clindamycin; rifampin
Corynebacterium species	Endocarditis; infections in various other tissues	Penicillin G ± an aminoglycoside; vancomycin	Rifampin + penicillin G; ampicillin-sulbactam
Listeria monocytogenes	Bacteremia; meningitis	Ampicillin or penicillin G ± gentamicin	Trimethoprim-sulfamethoxazole; chloramphenicol; erythromycin; a tetracycline

Based on Sande, MA, Kapusnik-Uner, JE, and Mandell, GL: Chemotherapy of microbial diseases. In Gilman, AG, et al (eds): The Pharmacological Basis of Therapeutics, ed 8. Pergamon Press, New York, 1990.

DRUGS USED TO TREAT COMMON INFECTIONS CAUSED BY GRAM-NEGATIVE BACILLI

Bacillus	Disease	Primary Agent(s)	Alternative Agent(s)
Acinetobacter	Infections in various tissues; hospital-acquired infections	An aminoglycoside; imipenem	A cephalosporin
Bacteroides fragilis	Abscesses (brain, lung, intra-abdominal); bacteremia; empyema; endocarditis	Clindamycin; metronidazole	Cefoxitin or cefotetan; chloramphenicol; imipenem; other combinations
Bacteroides species	Abscesses (brain, lung); oral disease; sinusitis	Clindamycin; penicillin G	Cefoxitin; cefotetan or ceftizoxime; metronidazole; chloramphenicol; erythromycin; a tetracycline
Escherichia coli	Bacteremia; urinary tract infections; infections in other tissues	Ampicillin ± an aminoglycoside; trimethoprim-sulfamethoxazole; other combinations	An aminoglycoside; a cephalosporin; aztreonam; nitrofurantoin; a tetracycline
Flavobacterium meningosepticum	Meningitis	Vancomycin	Trimethoprim-sulfamethoxazole; rifampin
Fusobacterium nucleatum	Genital infections; gingivitis; lung abscesses; ulcerative pharyngitis	Penicillin G; clindamycin	A cephalosporin; metronidazole; chloramphenicol; erythromycin; a tetracycline

Continued on following page

	DRUGS USED TO TREAT COMMON INFECTIONS CAUSED BY GRAM-NEGATIVE BACILLI (Continued)		
Bacillus	**Disease**	**Primary Agent(s)**	**Alternative Agent(s)**
Klebsiella pneumoniae	Pneumonia; urinary tract infection	A cephalosporin ± an aminoglycoside	Mezlocillin or piperacillin; aztreonam; imipenem; trimethoprim-sulfamethoxazole
Legionella pneumophila	Legionnaires' disease	Erythromycin ± rifampin	Ciprofloxacin; trimethoprim-sulfamethoxazole
Pasteurella multocida	Abscesses; bacteremia; meningitis; wound infections (animal bites)	Penicillin G	A cephalosporin; a tetracycline; amoxicillin
Proteus mirabilis	Urinary tract and other infections	Ampicillin or amoxicillin	An aminoglycoside; a cephalosporin
Proteus, other species	Urinary tract and other infections	An aminoglycoside; a cephalosporin	A broad-spectrum penicillin; aztreonam; imipenem
Pseudomonas aeruginosa	Bacteremia; pneumonia; urinary tract infection	A broad-spectrum penicillin ± an aminoglycoside	An aminoglycoside; a cephalosporin; ticarcillin; aztreonam; imipenem
Streptobacillus moniliformis	Abscesses; bacteremia; endocarditis	Penicillin G	Streptomycin; a tetracycline; chloramphenicol; erythromycin

Based on Sande, MA, Kapusnik-Uner, JE, and Mandell, GL: Chemotherapy of microbial diseases. In Gilman, AG, et al (eds): The Pharmacological Basis of Therapeutics, ed 8. Pergamon Press, New York, 1990.

Gram-Positive Coccus	Disease	Primary Agent(s)	Alternative Agent(s)
Staphylococcus aureus	Abscesses; bacteremia; endocarditis; meningitis; osteomyelitis; pneumonia	Penicillin G (or a penicillinase-resistant penicillin); vancomycin	A cephalosporin; clindamycin; erythromycin; other combinations
Streptococcus agalactiae (group B)	Meningitis; septicemia	Ampicillin or penicillin G ± an aminoglycoside	A cephalosporin; chloramphenicol; erythromycin
Streptococcus bovis	Bacteremia; endocarditis	Penicillin G ± streptomycin or gentamicin	A cephalosporin; vancomycin
Streptococcus faecalis	Bacteremia; endocarditis; urinary tract infection	Ampicillin; penicillin G	Gentamicin; streptomycin; vancomycin
Streptococcus pneumoniae	Arthritis; otitis; pneumonia; sinusitis	Penicillin G or V	A cephalosporin; erythromycin; chloramphenicol; clindamycin; trimethoprim-sulfamethoxazole
Streptococcus pyogenes	Bacteremia; cellulitis; pharyngitis; pneumonia; scarlet fever; other local and systemic infections	Penicillin G or V	A cephalosporin; erythromycin; vancomycin

Continued on following page

16

DRUGS USED TO TREAT COMMON INFECTIONS CAUSED BY GRAM-POSITIVE AND GRAM-NEGATIVE COCCI (Continued)

Gram-Positive Coccus	Disease	Primary Agent(s)	Alternative Agent(s)
Streptococcus (anaerobic species)	Bacteremia; brain and other abscesses; endocarditis; sinusitis	Penicillin G	A cephalosporin; clindamycin; chloramphenicol; erythromycin
Streptococcus (*viridans* group)	Bacteremia; endocarditis	Penicillin G ± streptomycin or gentamicin	A cephalosporin; vancomycin
Neisseria gonorrhoeae (gonococcus)	Arthritis-dermatitis syndrome; genital infections	Ampicillin or amoxicillin + probenecid; penicillin G	Cefoxitin or cefotaxime; a tetracycline; trimethoprim-sulfamethoxazole; ciprofloxacin; erythromycin; spectinomycin
Neisseria meningitidis (meningococcus)	Bacteremia; meningitis	Penicillin G	A cephalosporin; chloramphenicol

Based on Sande, MA, Kapusnik-Uner, JE, and Mandell, GL: Chemotherapy of microbial diseases. In Gilman, AG, et al (eds): The Pharmacological Basis of Therapeutics, ed 8. Pergamon Press, New York, 1990.

DRUGS USED TO TREAT INFECTIONS CAUSED BY ACID-FAST BACILLI, SPIROCHETES, ACTINOMYCETES, AND OTHER MICROORGANISMS

Microorganism	Disease	Primary Agent(s)	Alternative Agent(s)
Acid-fast bacillus			
Mycobacterium leprae	Leprosy	Dapsone + rifampin	Clofazimine
Mycobacterium tuberculosis	Pulmonary, renal, meningeal, and other tuberculosis infections	Isoniazid + rifampin + pyrazinamide	Ethambutol (added to the primary drugs); streptomycin (added to the primary drugs)
Spirochetes			
Treponema pallidum	Syphilis	Penicillin G	Ceftriaxone; a tetracycline
Leptospira	Meningitis	Penicillin G	A tetracycline
Borrelia burgdorferi	Lyme disease	A tetracycline	Penicillin G; ceftriaxone
Actinomycetes			
Actinomyces israelii	Cervicofacial, abdominal, thoracic, and other lesions	Penicillin G or ampicillin	A tetracycline; erythromycin

Continued on following page

16

985

DRUGS USED TO TREAT INFECTIONS CAUSED BY ACID-FAST BACILLI, SPIROCHETES, ACTINOMYCETES, AND OTHER MICROORGANISMS (Continued)

Microorganism	Disease	Primary Agent(s)	Alternative Agent(s)
Nocardia	Brain abscesses; pulmonary and other lesions	A sulfonamide; trimethoprim-sulfamethoxazole	Minocycline ± a sulfonamide
Other microorganisms *Chlamydia trachomatis*	Blennorrhea; lymphogranuloma venereum; nonspecific urethritis trachoma	A tetracycline; doxycycline	Erythromycin; a sulfonamide
Mycoplasma pneumoniae	"Atypical" pneumonia	Erythromycin; a tetracycline	—
Rickettsia	Q fever; rickettsialpox; Rocky Mountain spotted fever; typhus fever, other diseases	Chloramphenicol; a tetracycline	—

Based on Sande, MA, Kapusnik-Uner, JE, and Mandell, GL: Chemotherapy of microbial diseases. In Gilman, AG, et al (eds): The Pharmacological Basis of Therapeutics, ed 8. Pergamon Press, New York, 1990.

DRUGS USED TO INHIBIT BACTERIAL PROTEIN SYNTHESIS				
Aminoglycosides	Erythromycins	Tetracyclines	Other Agents
Amikacin (Amikin)	Erythromycin (ERYC, E-Mycin, others)	Demeclocycline (Declomycin)	Chloramphenicol (Chloromycetin)
Gentamicin (Garamycin)	Erythromycin estolate (Ilosone)	Doxycycline (Doxy, Vibramycin, others)	Clindamycin (Cleocin)
Kanamycin (Kantrex)	Erythromycin ethylsuccinate (E.E.S., EryPed)	Minocycline (Minocin)	Ethionamide (Trecator-SC)
Neomycin (generic)	Erythromycin gluceptate (Ilotycin)	Oxytetracycline (Terramycin)	Lincomycin (Lincocin)
Netilmicin (Netromycin)	Erythromycin lactobionate (Erythrocin)	Tetracycline (Achromycin V, Sumycin, many others)	
Streptomycin (generic)	Erythromycin stearate (Erythrocin, Wyamycin-S)		
Tobramycin (Nebcin)			

From Ciccone, CD: Pharmacology in Rehabilitation, ed 2. FA Davis, Philadelphia, 1996, p 516, with permission.

16

987

DRUGS USED TO INHIBIT BACTERIAL DNA/RNA SYNTHESIS AND FUNCTION

Fluoroquinolones	Sulfonamides	Others
Ciprofloxacin (Cipro)	Sulfacytine (Renoquid)	Aminosalicylic acid (Tubasal)
Enoxacin (Penetrex)	Sulfadiazine (Silvadene)	Clofazimine (Lamprene)
Lomefloxacin (Maxaquin)	Sulfamethizole (Thiosulfil Forte)	Dapsone (Avlosulfon)
Norfloxacin (Noroxin)	Sulfamethoxazole (Gantanol)	Ethambutol (Myambutol)
Ofloxacin (Floxin)	Sulfisoxazole (Gantrisin)	Metronidazole (Flagyl, Protostat, others)
		Rifampin (Rifadin, Rimactane)
		Trimethoprim (Proloprim, Trimpex)

From Ciccone, CD: Pharmacology in Rehabilitation, ed 2. FA Davis, Philadelphia, 1996, p 519, with permission.

VIRUSES

COMMON VIRUSES AFFECTING HUMANS

Family	Virus	Related Infections
DNA viruses		
Adenoviridae	Adenovirus, types 1–33	Respiratory tract and eye infections
Hepatitis B	Hepatitis B virus	Hepatitis B
Herpesviridae	Cytomegalovirus	Cytomegalic inclusion disease (i.e., widespread involvement of virtually any organ, especially the brain, liver, lung, kidney, and intestine)
	Epstein-Barr virus	Infectious mononucleosis

Family	Virus	Related Infections
	Herpes simplex, types 1 and 2	Local infections of oral, genital, and other muco-cutaneous areas; systemic infections
	Varicella-zoster virus	Chickenpox; herpes zoster (shingles); other systemic infections
Poxviridae	Smallpox virus	Smallpox
RNA viruses		
Arenaviridae	Human respiratory virus	Respiratory tract infection
Hepatitis A	Hepatitis A virus	Hepatitis A
Orthomyxoviridae	Influenza virus, types A, B, and C	Influenza
Paramyxoviridae	Measles virus	Measles
	Mumps virus	Mumps
	Respiratory syncytial virus	Respiratory tract infection in children
Picornaviridae	Polioviruses	Poliomyelitis
	Rhinovirus, types 1–89	Common cold
Retroviridae	Human immuno-deficiency virus (HIV)	AIDS
Rhabdoviridae	Rabies virus	Rabies
Togaviridae	*Alphavirus*	Encephalitis
	Rubella virus	Rubella

AIDS = acquired immunodeficiency disease.
From Ciccone, CD: Pharmacology in Rehabilitation, ed 2. FA Davis, Philadelphia, 1996, p 529, with permission.

16

	METHODS OF TRANSMISSION OF SOME COMMON COMMUNICABLE DISEASES		
Disease	How Agent Leaves the Body	How Organisms May Be Transmitted	Method of Entry into the Body
Acquired immunodeficiency syndrome (AIDS)	Blood, semen, or other body fluids, including breast milk	Inoculation by use of contaminated needles or by direct contact so that infected body fluids can enter the body	Transplacentally to embryo or fetus Nursing at breast
Cholera	Excreta from intestinal tract	As in typhoid fever	As in typhoid fever
Diphtheria	Sputum and discharges from nose and throat Skin lesions	Direct contact Droplet infection from patient coughing Hands of nurse Articles used by and about patient	Through mouth to throat or nose to throat
Gonococcal disease	Lesions Discharges from infected mucous membranes	Direct contact as in sexual intercourse Towels, bathtubs, toilets, etc. Hands of infected persons soiled with their own discharges Hands of attendant	Directly onto mucous membrane Through breaks in membrane

Hepatitis A, viral	Feces	As in typhoid fever	As in typhoid fever, rarely by blood transfusion
Hepatitis B, viral and delta hepatitis	Blood and serum-derived fluids, including semen and vaginal fluids	Contact with blood and body fluids	Transfusion Exposure to body fluids including hetero- or homosexual intercourse
Hepatitis C	Blood	Transfusion Parenteral drug use Laboratory exposure to blood Health care workers exposed to blood, e.g., dentists and their assistants, and clinical and laboratory staff	Infected blood Contaminated needles
Hookworm	Feces	Direct contact with soil polluted with feces Eggs in feces hatch in sandy soil Feces may also contaminate food	Larvae enter through breaks in skin, especially skin of feet, and after devious passage through the body settle in the intestine
Influenza	As in pneumonia	As in pneumonia	As in pneumonia

Continued on following page

METHODS OF TRANSMISSION OF SOME COMMON COMMUNICABLE DISEASES (Continued)

Disease	How Agent Leaves the Body	How Organisms May Be Transmitted	Method of Entry into the Body
Leprosy	Uncertain, may be from lesions Bacilli found in nodules that may break down, forming lesions	Uncertain, probably nasal discharges of untreated patients	Uncertain, probably via upper respiratory tract and broken skin
Measles (rubella)	As in streptococcal sore throat	As in streptococcal sore throat	As in streptococcal sore throat
Meningitis, meningococcal	Discharges from nose and throat	Direct contact Hands of nurse or attendant. Articles used by and about patient Flies	Mouth and nose
Mumps	Discharges from infected glands and mouth	Direct contact with persons affected	Mouth and nose
Ophthalmia neonatorum (gonococcal infection of eyes of newborn)	Purulent dischages from the eye	Direct contact with infected areas as vagina of infected mother during birth Other infected babies Hands of doctor or nurse Linens	Directly on the conjunctiva

Pneumonia	Sputum and discharges from nose and throat	Direct contact Hands of nurse Articles used by and about patient	Through mouth and nose to lungs
Poliomyelitis	Discharges from nose and throat, and via feces	Direct contact Hands of nurse or attendant Rarely in milk	Through mouth and nose
Rubeola	Secretions from nose and throat	Droplet spread from nose or throat by direct contact with nasal or throat secretions Airborne spread is possible	Through mouth and nose
Streptococcal sore throat	Discharges from nose and throat Skin lesions	Direct contact Hands of nurse Articles used by and about patient	Through mouth and nose
Syphilis	Infected tissues Lesions Blood Transfer through placenta to fetus	Direct contact Kissing or sexual intercourse Contaminated needles and syringes	Directly into blood and tissues through breaks in skin or membrane Contaminated needles and syringes
Tetanus	Excreta from infected herbivorous animals and man	Soil, especially that with manure or feces in it Dust, etc. Articles used about stables	Directly into bloodstream through wounds (organism is an anaerobe and prefers deep, incised wound)

Continued on following page

16

METHODS OF TRANSMISSION OF SOME COMMON COMMUNICABLE DISEASES (Continued)

Disease	How Agent Leaves the Body	How Organisms May Be Transmitted	Method of Entry into the Body
Trachoma	Discharges from infected eyes	Direct contact Hands, towels, handkerchiefs	Directly on conjunctiva
Tuberculosis, bovine		Milk from infected cow	As in tuberculosis, human
Tuberculosis, human	Sputum Lesions Feces	Direct contact such as kissing Droplet infection from a person coughing with mouth uncovered Sputum from mouth to fingers, thence to food and other things Soiled dressings	Through mouth to lungs and intestines From intestines via lymph channels to lymph vessels and to tissues
Typhoid fever	Feces and urine	Direct contact with food, water, articles, or insects contaminated with feces, or urine from patients	Through mouth via infected food or water and thence to intestinal tract
Whooping cough	Discharges from respiratory tract	Direct contact with persons affected	Mouth and nose

From Thomas, CL, (ed): Taber's Cyclopedic Medical Dictionary, ed 17. FA Davis, Philadelphia, 1993, pp 426–428, with permission.

FOR MORE INFORMATION

Garner, JS and Simmons, BP: CDC guidelines for isolation precautions in hospitals. Infection Control 4:258, 1983.

ISOLATION PRECAUTIONS FOR HOSPITALS

Draft of Guidelines for Isolation Precautions in Hospitals appeared as a notice in the Federal Register, Vol 59, no. 214, November 7, 1994, pages 55552–55570. This Center for Disease Control and Prevention guideline is intended to update and replace previously published CDC Guideline for Isolation Precautions in Hospitals. The table that follows contains the recommendations of the Hospital Infection Control Practices Advisory Committee (HICPAC).

GUIDELINES FOR ISOLATION PRECAUTIONS

CATEGORY IA RECOMMENDATIONS. Strongly recommended for all hospitals. The recommendations are strongly supported by well-designed experimental or epidemiological studies.

CATEGORY IB RECOMMENDATIONS. Strongly recommended for all hospitals and viewed as effective by experts in the field and a consensus of HICPAC. The recommendations are based on strong rationales and suggestive evidence, even though definitive scientific studies have not been done.

CATEGORY II RECOMMENDATIONS. Suggested for implementation in many hospitals. Recommendations may be supported by suggestive clinical or epidemiological studies, a strong theoretical rationale, or definitive studies applicable to some but not all hospitals.

Type of Precaution	Description	Indication	Classification of the Recommendation
Standard Precautions	The primary strategy for successful nosocomial infection control. Synthesizes the major features of Universal (blood and body fluid) Precautions and Body Substance Isolation	For the care of all patients receiving care in hospitals regardless of diagnosis or presumed infection status.	IB

Continued on following page

GUIDELINES FOR ISOLATION PRECAUTIONS (Continued)

Type of Precaution	Description	Indication	Classification of the Recommendation
Hand washing	Plain nonantimicrobial soap. After touching blood, body fluids, secretions, excretions, and contaminated items. After removal of gloves and between patient contacts.	As per standard precautions	IB, II
Gloves	Clean nonsterile gloves. When touching blood, body fluids, secretions, excretions, and contaminated items. When touching mucous membranes and nonintact skin.	As per standard precautions	IB
Mask, eye protection, face shield	Protects mucous membranes of the eyes, nose, and mouth.	As per standard precautions and during activities that are likely to generate splashes or sprays of blood, body fluids, secretions, and excretions	IB

Gown	Clean nonsterile gown protects skin and prevents soiling of clothing.	As per standard precautions and during activities that are likely to generate splashes or sprays of blood, body fluids, secretions, and excretions	IB
Patient-care equipment	Used patient-care equipment soiled with blood, body fluids, secretions, and excretions are handled in a manner that prevents skin and mucous membrane exposure, contamination of clothing, and transfer of microorganisms to patients and others.	As per standard precautions	IB
Linen	Used linen soiled with blood, body fluids, secretions, and excretions are handled in a manner that prevents skin and mucous membrane exposure, contamination of clothing, and transfer of microorganisms to patients and others.	As per standard precautions	IB
Occupational health and blood-borne pathogens	Proper use and disposable procedures are followed to prevent injuries when using needles, scalpels, and other sharp instruments.	As per standard precautions	IB

16

Continued on following page

GUIDELINES FOR ISOLATION PRECAUTIONS (Continued)

Type of Precaution	Description	Indication	Classification of the Recommendation
	Mouthpieces, resuscitation bags, or other ventilation devices are used when possible as an alternative to mouth-to-mouth resuscitation.		
Patient placement	Private-room placement for patients who may contaminate their environments.	For patients who do not (or cannot be expected to) assist in maintaining appropriate hygiene or environmental control	IB
Airborne Precautions	Used in addition to standard precautions to reduce the risk of airborne transmission of infectious agents.	For patients known or suspected to be infected with microorganisms transmitted by airborne droplets (5 microns or smaller) traveling in air currents.	IB
Patient placement	Private room with monitored negative air pressure, minimum of six air changes per day and high-efficiency filtration of room air. Patient confined to room with door closed.	As per airborne precautions	IB

Respiratory protection	Respiratory protection is worn for patients known or suspected of infectious tuberculosis.	As per airborne precautions	IB
Patient transport	Patient transport should be limited to essential purposes only; patient is masked when transported out of room.	As per airborne precautions	IB
Droplet Precautions	Used in addition to standard precautions to reduce the risk of droplet transmission of infectious microorganisms	Patients known or suspected of being infected with microorganisms transmitted by droplets larger than 5 microns as during coughing, sneezing, or direct contact with conjunctivae or mucous membranes of the nose or mouth	IB
Patient placement	Private room, or if unavailable, in a room with cohort infected with the same microorganism; at least 3 ft of separation maintained between infected patient and other patients and visitors.	As per droplet precautions	IB

16

Continued on following page

GUIDELINES FOR ISOLATION PRECAUTIONS (Continued)

Type of Precaution	Description	Indication	Classification of the Recommendation
Mask	Mask is worn when working within 3 ft of infected patient.	As per droplet precautions	IB
Patient transport	Patient transport should be limited to essential purposes only; patient is masked when transported out of room.	As per droplet precautions	IB
Contact Precautions	Used in addition to standard precautions to reduce the risk of transmission of microorganisms by direct or indirect contact (e.g., skin to skin or skin to object).	Patients known or suspected to be infected or colonized with microorganisms that can be transmitted by direct contact or indirect contact	IB
Patient placement	Private room, or if unavailable, in a room with a cohort infected with the same microorganism.	As per contact precautions	IB

Gloves and hand washing	Gloves changed after having contact with infective material; gloves removed before leaving patient room and hands washed immediately with antimicrobial agent.	IB
Gown	Gown is worn before entering room and removed before leaving the room.	IB
Patient transport	Transport limited to essential purposes.	As per contact precautions	IB
Environmental control	Daily cleaning of patient-care items, bedside equipment, and frequently touched surfaces.	As per contact precautions	IB
Patient-care equipment	Noncritical patient-care equipment and items such as stethoscopes, sphygmomanometers, commodes, and thermometers are used for a single patient when possible.	As per contact precautions	IB

16

CLINICAL SYNDROMES OR CONDITIONS WARRANTING PRECAUTIONS TO PREVENT TRANSMISSION OF PATHOGENS (PENDING CONFIRMATION OF DIAGNOSIS)

Clinical Syndrome or Condition	Potential Pathogens	Types of Precautions
Diarrhea		
Acute diarrhea with a likely infectious cause in an incontinent or diapered patient.	Enteric pathogens	Contact precautions
Diarrhea in an adult with a history of broad spectrum or long-term antibiotics	*Clostridium difficile*	Contact precautions
Meningitis	*Neisseria meningitidis*	Droplet precautions
Respiratory Infections		
Cough, fever, or upper lobe pulmonary infiltrate in an HIV-negative patient and in patients with a low risk for HIV infection	*Mycobacterium tuberculosis*	Airborne precautions
Cough, fever, or pulmonary infiltrate in any lung location in an HIV-infected patient and in patients at high risk for HIV infection	*Mycobacterium tuberculosis*	Airborne precautions

Clinical syndrome or condition	Potential pathogens	Precautions
Paroxysmal or severe persistent cough during periods of pertussis activity	*Bordetella pertussis*	Droplet precautions
Respiratory infections, particularly bronchiolitis and croup, in infants and young children	Respiratory syncytial parainfluenza virus	Contact precautions

Risk of Multidrug-Resistant Microorganisms

History of infection or colonization with multidrug-resistant organisms	Resistant bacteria	Contact precautions
Skin, wound, or urinary tract infection in a patient with a recent hospital or nursing home stay in a facility where multidrug-resistant organisms are prevalent	Resistant bacteria	Contact precautions

Skin or Wound Infection

Abscess or draining wound that cannot be covered	*Staphylococcus aureus*, group A streptococcus	Contact precautions

Based on Guidelines for Isolation Precautions in Hospitals. Federal Register, Vol 59, no 214, November 7, 1994, pp 55552–55570.

16

Synopsis of Types of Precautions as in Draft Guidelines and Patients Requiring the Precautions

Standard Precautions

Use standard precautions for the care of all patients.

Airborne Precautions

In addition to standard precautions, use airborne precautions for patients known or suspected to have serious illnesses transmitted by airborne droplets. Examples of such illnesses are: measles, varicella (including disseminated zoster), and tuberculosis.

Droplet Precautions

In addition to standard precautions, use droplet precautions for patients known or suspected to have serious illnesses transmitted by large particle droplets. Examples of such illnesses are:

1. Invasive *Haemophilus influenzae type b*, including meningitis, pneumonia, epiglottitis, and sepsis.
2. Invasive *Neisseria meningitides*, including meningitis, pneumonia, and sepsis.
3. Invasive multidrug-resistant *Streptococcus pneumoniae*, including meningitis, pneumonia, sinusitis, and otitis media.
4. Other serious bacterial respiratory infections spread by droplet transmission, including:
   a. Diphtheria (pharyngeal)
   b. Mycoplasma pneumonia
   c. Pneumonic plague
   d. Streptococcal pharyngitis, pneumonia, or scarlet fever in infants and young children
5. Serious viral infections spread by droplet transmission, including adenovirus, influenza, mumps, parvo virus B19, rubella

Contact Precautions

In addition to standard precautions, use contact precautions for patients known or suspected to have serious illnesses easily transmitted by direct patient contact or by contact with items in the patient's environment. Examples of such illnesses are:

1. Gastrointestinal, respiratory, skin, or wound infections or colonization with multidrug-resistant bacteria judged by infection control programs to be of special clinical epidemiologic significance based on current state, regional, or national recommendations.
2. Enteric infections with a low infectious dose or prolonged environmental survival, including: *clostridium difficile,* for diapered or incontinent patients: enterohemorrhagic *escherichia coli* O 157:H7, *shigella,* hepatitis A, or rotavirus.
3. Respiratory syncytial virus, parainfluenza virus, or enteroviral infections in infants and young children.
4. Skin infections that are highly contagious or that may occur on dry skin, including: diphtheria (cutaneous), herpes simplex (neonatal or mucocutaneous), impetigo, major (noncontaminated) abscesses, cellulitis, or decubiti, pediculosis, scabies, staphylococcal furunculosis in infants and young children, staphylococcal scaled skin syndrome, zoster (disseminated or in the immunocompromised host)
5. Viral hemorrhagic conjunctivitis
6. Viral hemorrhagic fevers (Lassa fever or Marburg virus)

16

FROM

Draft Guidelines for Isolation Precautions in Hospitals: Federal Register, Vol 59, no 214, November 7, 1994.

METHODS OF DISINFECTION

Method	Concentration or Temperature	Use	Limitations
Moist heat Autoclaving	250°–270°F (121°–132°C)	Sterilize instruments not harmed by heat and water pressure.	Moisture will not permeate some materials. Cannot be used for heat-sensitive items.
Boiling water	212°F (100°C)	Kill non-spore-forming pathogenic organisms.	Does not kill spores. Probably not effective against hepatitis virus.
Radiation Ultraviolet light		Air and surface disinfection.	Penetrates poorly. Harmful to unprotected skin and eyes.
Ionizing		Sterilize medicines, some plastics, sutures, and biologicals.	Expensive. May alter the medicine or material.

Filtration			
Membrane		Water purification.	Slow and expensive.
Fiberglass filters		Air disinfection.	Only cleans incoming air; does not prevent recontamination.
Physical cleaning			
Ultrasonic		Disinfect instruments.	Aids in cleaning but not effective alone.
Washing		Disinfect hands and surfaces.	Does not remove all organisms.
Chemicals			
Alcohols	70%–90%	Skin degerming.	Sometimes irritating. Does not kill spores.
Chlorines	100–200 ppm	Water disinfection. Food surface sanitization.	Inactivated by inorganic matter. Does not kill spores. Ineffective at certain pH values.

Continued on following page

METHODS OF DISINFECTION (Continued)

Method	Concentration or Temperature	Use	Limitations
Iodines, tincture	2%	Skin degerming.	Not sporicidal. Sometimes irritating.
Iodines, iodophors	74–450 ppm	General disinfectant.	Not sporicidal.
Phenols	1%–4%	General disinfectant.	Ineffective against some bacteria.
Quaternary ammonia compounds, tincture	0.1%	Skin degerming.	Neutralized by soap. Not sporicidal.
Quaternary ammonia compounds, aqueous	Diluted 1 part:750 parts	General disinfectant.	May be incompatible with some water. Ineffective against some bacteria.
Mercurials	0.1%	Skin degerming.	Slow acting. May be irritating.

Formaldehyde (formalin)	5%	Drastic disinfection.	Irritating, corrosive.
Glutaraldehyde	2%	Instrument sterilization.	Irritates mucous membranes. Unstable.
Germicidal soaps (hexachlorophene)	2%–3%	Skin degerming.	Bacteriostatic rather than bactericidal.
Gaseous Ethylene oxide	450 mg/L of air	Sterilization of heat-sensitive materials or those that must be kept dry.	Temperature, time, humidity critical. Treated materials need to air for varying periods of time (depending on composition) following treatment.
Formaldehyde gas		Fumigation. Sterilization of heat-sensitive materials.	Irritating, corrosive, toxic.

From Benarde, MA (ed:) Disinfection: A Treatise. Marcel Dekker Inc, New York, NY, 1970, with permission.

16

COMMONLY ABUSED DRUGS

Drug(s)	Classification/Action	Route/Method of Administration	Effect Desired by User	Principal Adverse Effects
Alcohol	Sedative-hypnotic	Oral, from various beverages (wine, beer, other alcoholic drinks)	Euphoria; relaxed inhibitions; decreased anxiety; sense of escape	Physical dependence; impaired motor skills; chronic degenerative changes in brain, liver, and other organs
Barbiturates Nembutal Seconal Others	Sedative-hypnotic	Oral or injected (IM, IV)	Relaxation and a sense of calmness; drowsiness	Physical dependence; possible death from overdose; behavior changes (irritability, psychosis) following prolonged use

Benzodiazepines Valium Librium Others	Similar to barbiturates	Similar to barbiturates	Similar to barbiturates	Similar to barbiturates
Caffeine	CNS stimulant	Oral, from coffee, tea, other beverages	Increased alertness; decreased fatigue; improved work capacity	Sleep disturbances; irritability; nervousness; cardiac arrhythmias
Cocaine	CNS stimulant (when taken systemically)	"Snorted" (absorbed via nasal mucosa); smoked (in crystalline form)	Euphoria; excitement; feelings of intense pleasure and well-being	Physical dependence; acute CNS and cardiac toxicity; profound mood swings
Cannabinoids Hashish Marijuana	Psychoactive drugs with mixed (stimulant and depressant) activity	Smoked; may also be eaten	Initial response: euphoria, excitement, increased perception; later response: relaxation, stupor, dreamlike state	Heavy use may lead to endocrine changes (decreased testosterone in males) and changes in respiratory function similar to chronic cigarette smoking

Continued on following page

16

COMMONLY ABUSED DRUGS (Continued)

Drug(s)	Classification/Action	Route/Method of Administration	Effect Desired by User	Principal Adverse Effects
Narcotics Demerol Morphine Heroin Others	Natural and synthetic opioids; analgesics	Oral or injected (IM, IV)	Relaxation; euphoria; feelings of tranquility; prevent onset of opiate withdrawal	Physical dependence; respiratory depression; high potential for death due to overdose
Nicotine	CNS toxin: produces variable effects via somatic and autonomic nervous system interaction	Smoked or absorbed from tobacco products (cigarettes, cigars, chewing tobacco)	Relaxation; calming effect; decreased irritability	Physical dependence; possible carcinogen; associated with pathologic changes in respiratory function during long-term tobacco use
Psychedelics LSD Mescaline Phencyclidine (PCP) Psilocybin	Hallucinogens	Oral; may also be smoked or inhaled	Altered perception and insight; distorted senses; disinhibition	Severe hallucinations; panic reaction; acute psychotic reactions

CNS = central nervous system; LSD = lysergic acid diethylamide.

From Ciccone, CD: Pharmacology in Rehabilitation, ed 2. FA Davis, Philadelphia, 1996, pp 606–607, with permission.

DIABETES

COMPARISON OF TYPE I INSULIN-DEPENDENT DIABETES MELLITUS AND TYPE II NON-INSULIN-DEPENDENT DIABETES MELLITUS

	Type I	Type II
Age at onset	Usually under 30.	Usually over 40
Type of onset	Abrupt	Gradual
Body weight	Normal	Obese—80%
HLA association	Positive	Negative
Insulin in blood	Little to none	Some usually present
Islet cell antibodies	Present at onset	Absent
Symptoms	Polyuria, polydipsia, polyphagia, weight loss, ketoacidosis	Polyuria, polydipsia, pruritus, peripheral neuropathy
Control	Insulin and diet	Diet (sometimes only diet control), hypoglycemic agents, sometimes insulin
Vascular and neural changes	Eventually develop	Usually develops
Stability of condition	Fluctuates, difficult to control	Fairly stable, usually easy to control
Prevalence	0.2%–0.3%	2%–4%

From Thomas, CL (ed): Taber's Cyclopedic Medical Dictionary, ed 17. FA Davis, Philadelphia, 1993, p 535, with permission.

16

INSULIN PREPARATIONS

Type of Insulin	Effects (h)			Examples*	
	Onset	Peak	Duration	Animal	Human
Rapid acting					
Regular insulin	0.5–1	2–4	5–7	Regular Iletin I	Humulin R
				Regular Iletin II	Novolin R
				Velosulin	Velosulin Human
Prompt insulin	1–3	2–8	12–16	Semilente Insulin	—
zinc				Semilente Iletin I	
Intermediate acting					
Isophane insulin	3–4	6–12	18–28	Insulatard NPH	Humulin N
				NPH Insulin	Insulatard NPH
					Human

Insulin zinc	1–3	8–12	18–28	NPH Iletin I NPH Iletin II Lente Insulin Lente Iletin I Lente Iletin II	Novolin N Humulin L Novolin L
Long acting					
Extended insulin zinc	4–6	18–24	36	Ultralente Insulin Ultralente Iletin I	—
Protamine zinc insulin	4–6	14–24	36	Protamine Zinc and Iletin I Protamine Zinc and Iletin II	—

*Examples are trade names of preparations derived from animal sources (beef, pork, or mixed beef and pork) and synthetic human insulin derived from recombinant DNA techniques.

From Ciccone, CD: Pharmacology in Rehabilitation, ed 2. FA Davis, Philadelphia, 1996, p 487, with permission.

16

ORAL HYPOGLYCEMIC AGENTS

Generic Name	Trade Name	Time to Peak Plasma Concentration (h)	Duration of Effect (h)
Acetohexamide	Dymelor	1–3	12–24
Chlorpropamide	Diabinese, Glucamide	2–4	24–48
Glipizide	Glucotrol	1–3	12–24
Glyburide	DiaBeta, Micronase	4	24
Tolazamide	Tolamide, Tolinase	3–4	10
Tolbutamide	Oramide, Orinase	3–4	6–12

From Ciccone, CD: Pharmacology in Rehabilitation, ed 2. FA Davis, Philadelphia, 1996, p 490, with permission.

DIABETIC AND HYPOGLYCEMIC COMAS

	Diabetic Coma	*Hypoglycemic Coma*
Onset	Gradual	Often sudden
History	Often of acute infection in a diabetic or insufficient insulin intake. Previous history of diabetes may be absent.	Recent insulin injection, inadequate meal, or excessive exercise after insulin
Skin	Flushed, dry	Pale, sweating
Tongue	Dry or furred	Moist
Breath	Smell of acetone	Acetone odor rare
Thirst	Intense	Absent
Respiration	Deep (air hunger) (Kussmaul)	Shallow
Vomiting	Common	Rare
Pulse	Rapid, feeble	Full and bounding
Eyeball Tension	Low	Normal
Urine	Sugar and acetone present	No sugar or acetone, unless bladder has not been emptied for some hours
Blood Sugar	Raised (over 200 mg/dl)	Subnormal (20–50 mg/dl)
Blood Pressure	Low	Normal
Abdominal Pain	Common and often acute	Absent

16

From Thomas, CL (ed): Taber's Cyclopedic Medical Dictionary, ed 17. FA Davis, Philadelphia, 1993, p 424, with permission.

FOR MORE INFORMATION

Diabetes Mellitus, ed 8. Lilly Research Laboratory, Indianapolis, Indiana, 1980.

Jarrett, RJ: Diabetes Mellitus. PGS Publishers, Littleton, Massachusetts, 1980.

Sussman, KE, Druznin, B and James, WE: A Clinical Guide to Diabetes Mellitus. Liss, New York, 1987.

CANCER INCIDENCE AND DEATHS

LEADING SITES OF CANCER INCIDENCE AND DEATH—1994 ESTIMATES

Rank	Cancer Incidence*		Cancer Deaths	
	Male	Female	Male	Female
1	Prostate 200,000	Breast 182,000	Lung 94,000	Lung 59,000
2	Lung 100,000	Colon/Rectum 74,000	Prostate 38,000	Breast 46,000
3	Colon/Rectum 75,000	Lung 72,000	Colon/Rectum 27,800	Colon/Rectum 28,200
4	Bladder 38,000	Uterus 46,000	Pancreas 12,400	Ovary 13,600
5	Lymphoma 29,400	Ovary 24,000	Lymphoma 12,100	Pancreas 13,500

6	Oral 19,800	Lymphoma 23,500	Leukemia 10,500	Lymphoma 10,650
7	Melanoma 17,000	Melanoma 15,000	Stomach 8,400	Uterus 10,500
8	Kidney 17,000	Pancreas 14,000	Esophagus 7,800	Leukemia 8,600
9	Leukemia 16,200	Bladder 13,200	Liver 7,200	Liver 6,000
10	Stomach 15,000	Leukemia 12,400	Bladder 7,000	Brain 5,800
11	Pancreas 13,000	Kidney 10,600	Brain 6,800	Stomach 5,600
12	Larynx 9,800	Oral 9,800	Kidney 6,800	Multiple myeloma 4,800
All sites†	632,000	576,000	283,000	255,000

*Excluding basal and squamous cell skin cancer and in situ carcinomas except bladder.

†Including sites not listed in the table.

From Boring, CC, et al: Cancer statistics, 1994. CA 4:7, 1994.

1996 ESTIMATED CANCER INCIDENCE BY SITE AND SEX

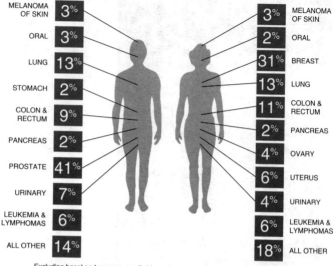

MELANOMA OF SKIN	3%		3%	MELANOMA OF SKIN
ORAL	3%		2%	ORAL
			31%	BREAST
LUNG	13%		13%	LUNG
STOMACH	2%		11%	COLON & RECTUM
COLON & RECTUM	9%		2%	PANCREAS
PANCREAS	2%		4%	OVARY
PROSTATE	41%		6%	UTERUS
URINARY	7%		4%	URINARY
LEUKEMIA & LYMPHOMAS	6%		6%	LEUKEMIA & LYMPHOMAS
ALL OTHER	14%		18%	ALL OTHER

Excluding basal and squamous cell skin cancers and in situ carcinoma except bladder.

1996 ESTIMATED CANCER DEATHS BY SITE AND SEX

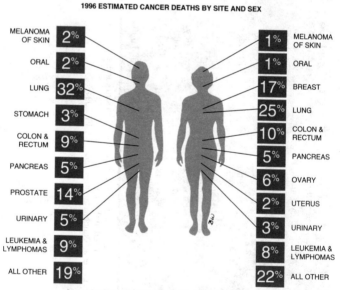

MELANOMA OF SKIN	2%		1%	MELANOMA OF SKIN
ORAL	2%		1%	ORAL
			17%	BREAST
LUNG	32%		25%	LUNG
STOMACH	3%		10%	COLON & RECTUM
COLON & RECTUM	9%		5%	PANCREAS
PANCREAS	5%		6%	OVARY
PROSTATE	14%		2%	UTERUS
URINARY	5%		3%	URINARY
LEUKEMIA & LYMPHOMAS	9%		8%	LEUKEMIA & LYMPHOMAS
ALL OTHER	19%		22%	ALL OTHER

Cancer Statistics, 1995, American Cancer Society, New York, N.Y.

From Thomas, CL (ed): Taber's Cyclopedic Medical Dictionary, ed 18. FA Davis, Philadelphia, 1997, p 294, with permission.

STAGING PROCEDURES FOR ORGAN-SPECIFIC NEOPLASIA

Organ System	Lesion	Clinical Testing	Tissue Diagnosis	Special Procedures	Testing: Clinical/Pathology
Lung	Solitary nodule	History and physical Chest x-ray CT scan	Sputum cytology Bronchoscopy and biopsy Percutaneous needle aspiration cytology	Lung biopsy Pleural biopsy (if effusion present)	Gallium scan Mediastinoscopy
	Multiple mass	History and physical with rectal examination	Percutaneous needle aspiration cytology	Lung biopsy	Metastatic, no further staging required
Breast	Single mass	History and physical Mammogram if palpable lesion present History and physical Mammogram Xerogram	Needle aspiration Excisional biopsy	Estrogen receptor assay Progesterone receptor assay Oncogene (Her-2-[neu]) Cathepsin D	Liver scan Bone scan Brain CT scan
Lymphoid	Adenopathy	History and physical Chest x-ray (hilar/ mediastinal nodes) Abdominal flat plate (splenomegaly)	Excisional biopsy	Lymphocyte Ig phenotyping Ig gene rearrangement studies Cytogenetics	US Gallium scan IVU Abdominal CT scan Liver-spleen scan

Continued on following page

16

STAGING PROCEDURES FOR ORGAN-SPECIFIC NEOPLASIA (Continued)

Organ System	Lesion	Clinical Testing	Tissue Diagnosis	Special Procedures	Testing; Clinical/Pathology
	Splenomegaly	History and physical Blood counts	Bone marrow aspiration and biopsies		Bone scan Bone marrow biopsies *and* aspiration Laparoscopy Laparotomy and splenectomy Proceed as above Peripheral blood for B and T lymphocytes Total protein Serum protein electrophoresis
GI	Esophageal mass or stricture	Chest x-ray Barium swallow	Esophagoscopy with brushing, cytology, and biopsy		CT scan Bronchoscopy Mediastinoscopy
	Gastric mass	Upper GI barium series (double contrast)	Gastroscopy with brushing, cytology, and biopsy		Liver scan Chest x-ray

Site	Finding				
	Pancreatic mass	US CT scan	Duodenal drainage for cytology Cannulation of ampulla of Vater for cytology	Percutaneous cholangiogram; ERCP	Liver scan Arteriogram Laparotomy and biopsy
GI	Liver mass	Liver scan α-fetoprotein		Peritoneoscopy and biopsy	Arteriogram Laparotomy
	Liver: multiple masses	Liver scan Chest x-ray Mammogram if palpable mass present Pancreatic US	Percutaneous biopsy	Peritoneoscopy and biopsy	Laparotomy
Testis	Mass	Chest x-ray IVU α-fetoprotein scan β-human chorionic gonadotropin	High inguinal orchiectomy	α-fetoprotein β-human chorionic gonadotropin	IVU Lymphangiogram Abdominal CT
					Laparotomy
Pelvis (cervix, endometrium, ovaries)	Mass	Pelvic examination under anesthesia Pelvic US Barium enema CT scan	Laparotomy	CEA Bast antigen (CA-125) for ovarian cancer	Laparotomy Abdominal CT scan

CEA = carcinoembryonic antigen; CT = computed tomography; ERCP = endoscopic retrograde cholangiopancreatography; GI = gastrointestinal; Ig = immunoglobulin; IVU = intravenous urography; US = ultrasound.
From The Merck Manual, ed 16. Merck & Co, Rahway, NJ, 1992, pp 1271–1272, with permission.

16

BRAIN TUMORS

Classification of Brain Tumors

Proposed Revision of 1979 World Health Organization Classification of Central Nervous System Tumors (1990)

I. Tumors of neuroepithelial tissue

Astrocytic	astrocytoma, anaplastic astrocytoma, glioblastoma multiforme, pilocytic astrocytoma, pleomorphic xanthoastrocytoma, subependymal giant cell astrocytoma
Oligodendroglial	oligodendroglioma, anaplastic (malignant) oligodendroglioma
Ependymal	ependymoma, anaplastic (malignant) ependymoma, myxopapillary ependymoma, subependymoma
Mixed gliomas	mixed oligoastrocytoma, anaplastic (malignant) oligoastrocytoma
Choroid plexus tumors	choroid plexus papilloma, choroid plexus carcinoma
Neuroepithelial tumors of uncertain origin	astroblastoma, polar spongioblastoma, gliomatosis cerebri
Neuronal and mixed neuronal-glial tumors	gangliocytoma, dysplastic gangliocytoma of the cerebellum, desmoplastic infantile ganglioglioma, dysembryoplastic neuroepithelial tumor, ganglioglioma, anaplastic (malignant) ganglioglioma
Pineal tumors	pineocytoma, pineoblastoma
Embryonal tumors	medulloepithelioma, neuroblastoma (variant: ganglioneuroblastoma), ependymoblastoma, retinoblastoma primitive neuroectodermal tumors
	medulloblastoma, cerebral and spinal primitive neuroectodermal tumors

II. Tumors of cranial and spinal nerves

Schwannoma	(synonymous with neurolemmoma, neurinoma)

Neurofibroma

Malignant peripheral nerve
    sheath tumor

III. Tumors of the Meninges

Meningothelial cells	meningoma
	  histologic types: meningothe-
	  lial (syncytial), transitional/
	  mixed, fibrous (fibroblastic),
	  psammomatous, angiomatous,
	  microcystic, secretory, clear
	  cell, choroid, lymphoplasma-
	  cyte-rich, metaplastic variants
	  (xanthomatous, myxoid, os-
	  seous, chondroid)
	atypical meningoma
	anaplastic (malignant)
	meningoma

Mesencymal, non-
  meningothelial tumors
	benign
	  oseocartilagenous, lipoma, fi-
	  brous histiocytoma, others
	malignant
	  mesenchymal chondrosar-
	  coma, malignant fibrous histio-
	  cytoma, rhabdomyosarcoma,
	  meningeal sarcomatosis, other

Primary melanocytic lesions	diffuse melanosis, melanocy- toma, malignant melanoma
Tumors of uncertain origin	hemangiopericytoma, capillary hemangioblastoma

IV. Hemopoietic neoplasms
    Malignant lymphomas
    Plasmacytoma
    Granulocytic sarcoma
    Others

V. Germ cell tumors
    Germinoma
    Embryonal carcinoma
    Yolk sac tumor—endodermal sinus tumor
    Choriocarcinoma
    Teratoma
    Mixed germ cell tumors

VI. Cysts and tumorlike lesions
    Rathke's cleft-cyst
    Epidermoid cyst
    Dermoid cyst
    Colloid cyst of third ventricle
    Enterogenous cyst—neuroenteric cyst
    Neuroglial cyst
    Other cysts

16

Continued on following page

Lipoma
Granular cell tumor—choriostoma, pituicytoma
Hypothalamic neuronal hamartoma
Nasal glial heterotopias
VII. Tumors of the anterior pituitary
Pituitary adenoma
Pituitary carcinoma
VIII. Local extensions from regional tumors
Craniopharyngioma—variants: adamantinomatous, squamous papillary
Paraganglioma—chemodectoma
Chordoma
Chondrosarcoma
Adenoid cystic carcinoma—cylindroma
Others
IX. Metastic tumors
Subcategorizations of metastatic tumors have not been attempted, primarily because of the large variety of tumors that can metastasize from the central nervous system (CNS). Most of these originate from breast and lung tissue, with many also originating from cutaneous malignant melanomas.)

Facts about Tumors of the Central Nervous System

1. Approximately 15% of patients have a family history of cancer. Anaplastic astrocytoma and glioblastoma multiforme are the most frequently occurring brain tumors in adults.
2. Brain tumors are the fourth most frequent cause of cancer-related deaths in middle-aged men and the second most common cause of cancer deaths in children.
3. A relationship between oncogenes and CNS tumor type is emerging.
4. Chemical and industrial agents associated with the development of CNS tumors but for which data are inconclusive include aromatic hydrocarbons, hydrazines, bis (chloromethyl) ether, vinyl chloride, and acrylonitrile.
5. Viruses associated with brain tumors include progressive multifocal leukoencephalopathy leading to astrocytomas; Epstein-Barr virus leading to primary CNS lymphoma.
6. Other factors associated with CNS tumors include hormones (meningiomas, particularly during pregnancy); alcohol; tobacco; radiation; trauma.

FOR MORE INFORMATION

Fields, WS: Brain tumours: Morphological aspects and classification. Brain Pathol 3:251, 1993.
Gonzales, MF: Classification and pathogenesis of brain tumors. In Kaye, AH and Laws, ER (eds): Brain Tumors: An Encyclopedic Approach. Churchill Livingstone, New York, 1995, pp 31–45.
Kleihues, P: The new classification of brain tumours. Brain Pathol 3:225, 1993.
Salcman, M: Globastoma and malignant astrocytoma. In Kaye, AH and Laws, ER (eds): Brain Tumors: An Encyclopedic Approach. Churchill Livingstone, New York, 1995, pp 449–477.

CANCER TREATMENT

Recommendations for Cancer Screening

STATEMENT OF THE AMERICAN CANCER SOCIETY REGARDING SCREENING PROCEDURES	
Procedure	**Position Statement**
For males and females of any age:	
Chest x-ray Sputum cytology	Not recommended on a routine basis
For males and females:	
Stool examination for occult blood	Yearly after age 50
Rectal examination	Yearly after age 40
Proctoscopic examination	Every 3 y after age 50
For females:	
Pelvic examination	Every 3 y between ages 20 and 40; then yearly
Papanicolaou (Pap) smear	Every 3 y between ages 20 and 65
Breast self-examination	Monthly after age 20
Breast physical examination	Every 3 y between ages 20 and 40; then yearly
Mammography	Initial baseline examination between ages 35 and 40; every 1–2 y from age 40–49; and yearly after age 50

As appearing in The Merck Manual, ed 16. Merck & Co, Rahway, NJ, 1992, p 1270. Based on CA—A Cancer Journal for Clinicians 40(2):79, March/April 1990, and Professional Education Publication #3347.01; used with permission of the American Cancer Society, Inc.

16

Common Drugs Used in Cancer Therapy

ANTIEMETIC DRUGS

Agent	Usual Adult Dosage (mg)	Route of Administration	Frequency
Antidopaminergics			
Chlorpromazine	10–25	Oral	q 4–6 h
	50–100	Rectal	q 6–8 h
	25	IM	q 3–4 h
Droperidol	2.5–10	IM	Once, for premedication
	1.25–5	IV	Once
Fluphenazine	1.25	Oral	q 6–8 h
	1.25	IM	q 6–8 h
Haloperidol	1–5	Oral	bid
	1–5	IM	bid
Metoclopramide	10	Oral	qid ½ h before meals and at bedtime
	10	IV	Once
Perphenazine	8–16	Oral	Daily in divided doses
	5	IM or IV	Only as necessary

Prochlorperazine	5–10	Oral	tid or qid
	25	Rectal	bid
	5–10	IM	q 3–4 h
Thiethylperazine	10	Oral	Once daily to tid
	10	Rectal	Once daily to tid
	10	IM	Once daily to tid
Triflupromazine	20–30	Oral	Daily
	5–15	IM	q 4 h
	1–3	IV	Daily
Ondansetron	8–12	IV	q 4 h for 3 doses
Antihistamines			
Buclizine	50	Oral	bid
Cyclizine	50	Oral	qid
	50	IM	q 4–6 h
Dimenhydrinate	50	Oral	q 4 h
	50	IM or IV	q 4 h
Hydroxyzine	25–100	Oral	tid or qid
	25–100	IM	q 4–6 h

Continued on following page

16

ANTIEMETIC DRUGS (Continued)

Agent	Usual Adult Dosage (mg)	Route of Administration	Frequency
Meclizine	25–50	Oral	Once daily
Promethazine	10–25	Oral	bid
	12.5–50	Rectal	bid
	12.5–25	IM	q 4–8 h
Anticholinergics			
Scopolamine	0.3–1.0	Oral	Before travel
	1 adhesive unit	Topical	Before travel
Miscellaneous			
Benzquinamide	50	IM	q 3–4 h
	25	IV	1st dose only
Dronabinol	5–15 mg/m²	Oral	q 2–4 h beginning 1–12 h before chemotherapy and continuing 8–24 h after therapy
Diphenidol	25–50	Oral	q 4 h
Trimethobenzamide	250	Oral	tid or qid
	200	Rectal	tid or qid
	200	IM	tid or qid

From Merck Manual, ed 16. Merck & Co, Rahway, NJ, p 1282, with permission.

ALKYLATING AGENTS

Generic Name	Trade Name	Primary Antineoplastic Indication(s)*	Common Adverse Effects
Busulfan	Myleran	Chronic myelocytic leukemia	Blood disorders (anemia, leukopenia, thrombocytopenia); metabolic disorders (hyperuricemia, fatigue, weight loss, other symptoms)
Carmustine	BCNU, BiCNU	Primary brain tumors; Hodgkin's disease; non-Hodgkin's lymphomas; multiple myeloma	Blood disorders (thrombocytopenia, leukopenia); GI distress (nausea, vomiting); hepatotoxicity; pulmonary toxicity
Chlorambucil	Leukeran	Chronic lymphocytic leukemia; Hodgkin's disease; non-Hodgkin's lymphomas	Blood disorders (leukopenia, thrombocytopenia, anemia); skin rashes/itching; pulmonary toxicity; seizures
Cisplatin†	Platinol	Carcinoma of bladder, ovaries, testicles, and other tissues	Nephrotoxicity; GI distress (nausea, vomiting); neurotoxicity (cranial and peripheral nerves); hypersensitive reactions (e.g., flushing, respiratory problems, tachycardia) *Continued on following page*

16

ALKYLATING AGENTS (Continued)

Generic Name	Trade Name	Primary Antineoplastic Indication(s)*	Common Adverse Effects
Cyclophosphamide	Cytoxan, Neosar	Acute and chronic lymphocytic leukemia; acute and chronic myelocytic leukemia; carcinoma of ovary, breast; Hodgkin's disease; non-Hodgkin's lymphoma; multiple myeloma	Blood disorders (anemia, leukopenia, thrombocytopenia); GI distress (nausea, vomiting, anorexia); bladder irritation; hair loss; cardiotoxicity; pulmonary toxicity
Decarbazine	DTIC-Dome	Malignant melanoma; refractory Hodgkin's lymphoma	GI distress (nausea, vomiting, anorexia); blood disorders (leukopenia, thrombocytopenia)
Lomustine	CeeNU	Brain tumors; Hodgkin's disease	Blood disorders (anemia, leukopenia); GI disorders (nausea, vomiting)
Mechlorethamine	Mustargen, Nitrogen mustard	Bronchogenic carcinoma; chronic leukemia; Hodgkin's disease; non-Hodgkin's lymphomas	Blood disorders (anemia, leukopenia, thrombocytopenia); GI distress (nausea, vomiting); CNS effects (headache, dizziness, convulsions); local irritation at injection site
Melphalan	Alkeran	Ovarian carcinoma; multiple myeloma	Blood disorders (leukopenia, thrombocytopenia); skin rashes/itching

Procarbazine†	Matulane	Hodgkin's disease	Blood disorders (leukopenia, thrombocytopenia); GI distress (nausea, vomiting); CNS toxicity (mood changes, incoordination, motor problems)
Streptozocin	Zanosar	Pancreatic carcinoma	Nephrotoxicity; GI distress (nausea, vomiting); blood disorders (anemia, leukopenia, thrombocytopenia); local irritation at injection site
Thiotepa	—	Carcinoma of breast, ovary, and bladder; Hodgkin's disease	Blood disorders (anemia, leukopenia, thrombocytopenia, pancytopenia)
Uracil mustard	—	Chronic lymphocytic leukemia; chronic myelocytic leukemia; non-Hodgkin's lymphoma	Blood disorders (anemia, leukopenia, thrombocytopenia); GI distress (nausea, vomiting, diarrhea, anorexia)

*Only the indications listed in the U.S. product labeling are included here. Many anticancer drugs are used for additional types of neoplastic disease.
†These drugs are not classified chemically as alkylating agents (i.e., they do not produce an "alkyl" group). However, they appear to form cross-links within DNA similar to alkylating drugs; hence their inclusion here.
From Ciccone, CD: Pharmacology in Rehabilitation, ed 2. FA Davis, 1996, pp 569–570, with permission.

16

ANTINEOPLASTIC ANTIBIOTICS

Generic Name	Trade Name	Primary Antineoplastic Indication(s)*	Common Adverse Effects
Bleomycin	Blenoxane	Carcinoma of head, neck, cervical region, skin, penis, vulva, and testicle; Hodgkin's disease; non-Hodgkin's lymphoma	Pulmonary toxicity (interstitial pneumonitis); skin disorders (rashes, discoloration); mucosal lesions; fever; GI distress; general weakness and malaise
Dactinomycin	Cosmegen	Carcinoma of testicle and endometrium; carcinosarcoma of kidney (Wilms' tumor); Ewing's sarcoma; rhabdomyosarcoma	Blood disorders (leukopenia, thrombocytopenia, others); GI distress (nausea, vomiting, anorexia); mucocutaneous lesions; skin disorders (rashes, hair loss); local irritation at injection site
Daunorubicin	Cerubidine	Several forms of acute leukemia	Blood disorders (anemia, leukopenia, thrombocytopenia); cardiotoxicity (arrhythmias, congestive heart failure); GI distress (nausea, vomiting, GI tract ulceration); hair loss

Doxorubicin	Adriamycin RDF	Acute leukemias; carcinoma of bladder, breast, ovary, thyroid, and other tissues; Hodgkin's disease; non-Hodgkin's lymphoma; several sarcomas	Similar to daunorubicin
Idarubicin	Idamycin	Acute myelocytic leukemia	Similar to daunorubicin
Mitomycin	Mutamycin	Carcinoma of stomach and pancreas; chronic myelocytic leukemia	Blood disorders (leukopenia, thrombocytopenia); GI distress (nausea, vomiting, GI irritation and ulceration); nephrotoxicity; pulmonary toxicity
Plicamycin	Mithracin	Testicular carcinoma	Blood disorders (leukopenia, thrombocytopenia); GI distress (nausea, vomiting, diarrhea, GI tract irritation); general weakness and malaise

*Only the indications listed in the U.S. product labeling are included here. Many anticancer drugs are used for additional types of neoplastic disease.
From Ciccone, CD: Pharmacology in Rehabilitation, ed 2. FA Davis, 1996, p 573, with permission.

16

ANTINEOPLASTIC HORMONES

Types of Hormones	Primary Antineoplastic Indication(s)*	Common Adverse Effects
Adrenocorticosteroids Prednisone Prednisolone	Acute lymphoblastic leukemia; chronic lymphocytic leukemia; Hodgkin's disease	Adrenocortical suppression; general catabolic effect on supporting tissues
Androgens Fluoxymesterone Methyltestosterone Testolactone Testosterone	Advanced, inoperable breast cancer in postmenopausal women	Masculinization in women
Antiandrogens Flutamide	Inhibits the cellular uptake and effects of androgens in advanced metastatic prostate cancer	Nausea, vomiting, diarrhea; decreased sex drive

Drug	Indications	Adverse effects
Estrogens Chlorotrianisene Diethylstilbestrol Estradiol Others	Advanced, inoperable breast cancer in selected men and postmenopausal women; advanced, inoperable prostate cancer in men	Cardiovascular complications (including stroke and heart attack—especially in men); many other adverse effects
Antiestrogens Tamoxifen	Acts as an estrogen antagonist to decrease the recurrence of cancer following mastectomy or to reduce tumor growth in advanced stages of breast cancer	Nausea, vomiting, hot flashes (generally well tolerated relative to other antineoplastic hormones)
Gonadotropin-releasing hormone drugs Leuprolide Goserelin	Work by negative feedback mechanisms to inhibit testosterone production; used primarily in advanced prostate cancer	Hot flashes; bone pain; CNS effects (e.g., headache, dizziness); GI disturbances (nausea, vomiting)

*Administration of hormonal agents in neoplastic disease is frequently palliative—that is, these drugs may offer some relief of symptoms but are not curative. Also, hormones are usually combined with other antineoplastic drugs or are used as an adjuvant to surgery and radiation treatment.
From Ciccone, CD: Pharmacology in Rehabilitation, ed 2. FA Davis, Philadelphia, 1996, p 574, with permission.

16

OTHER ANTICANCER DRUGS

Drugs(s)	Primary Antineoplastic Indication(s)*	Common Adverse Effects
Interferons		
Interferon alfa-2a (Roferon-A) Interferon alfa-2b (Intron-A)	Hairy cell leukemia, Kaposi's sarcoma, chronic myelocytic leukemia, renal and bladder cancers	Flulike syndrome (mild fever, chills, malaise)
Plant alkaloids		
Vinblastine (Velban, Velsar)	Carcinoma of breast, testes, other tissues; Hodgkin's disease; non-Hodgkin's lymphoma; Kaposi's sarcoma	Blood disorders (primarily leukopenia); GI distress (nausea, vomiting); hair loss; central and peripheral neuropathies; local irritation at injection site
Vincristine (Oncovin, Vincasar)	Acute lymphocytic leukemia; neuroblastoma; Wilms' tumor; Hodgkin's disease; non-Hodgkin's lymphoma, Ewing's sarcoma	Neurotoxicity (peripheral neuropathies, CNS disorders); hair loss; local irritation at injection site
Miscellaneous agents		
Asparaginase (Elspar)	Acute lymphocytic leukemia	Allergic reactions; renal toxicity; hepatic toxicity; delayed hemostasis; CNS toxicity (fatigue, mood changes); GI distress (nausea, vomiting); pancreatitis

Drug	Indication	Side Effects
Etoposide (VePesid)	Carcinoma of lung, testes	Blood disorders (anemia, leukopenia, thrombocytopenia); GI distress (nausea, vomiting); hypotension, allergic reactions; hair loss; neurotoxicity (peripheral neuropathies, CNS effects)
Hydroxyurea (Hydrea)	Carcinoma of the ovaries, head/neck region, other tissues; chronic myelocytic leukemia; melanomas	Blood disorders (primarily leukopenia); GI distress (nausea, vomiting, anorexia, GI tract irritation and ulceration); skin rashes
Mitotane (Lysodren)	Suppresses adrenal gland; used primarily to treat adrenocortical carcinoma	GI distress (nausea, vomiting, diarrhea, anorexia); CNS toxicity (lethargy, fatigue, mood changes); skin rashes

*Only the indications listed in the U.S. product labeling are included here. Many anticancer drugs are used for additional types of neoplastic disease. From Ciccone, CD: Pharmacology in Rehabilitation, ed 2. FA Davis, Philadelphia, 1996, p 576, with permission.

16

ANTIMETABOLITES

Generic Name	Trade Name	Primary Antineoplastic Indication(s)*	Common Adverse Effects
Cytarabine	Cytosar-U	Several forms of acute and chronic leukemia; non-Hodgkin's lymphoma	Blood disorders (anemia, megaloblastosis, reticulocytopenia, others); GI distress (nausea, vomiting); skin rashes; hair loss
Floxuridine	FUDR	Carcinoma of the GI tract and liver	GI disorders (nausea, vomiting, anorexia); skin disorders (discoloration, rashes, hair loss)
Fluorouracil	Adrucil	Carcinoma of colon, rectum, stomach, and pancreas	GI distress (anorexia, nausea); blood disorders (anemia, leukopenia, thrombocytopenia); skin disorders (rashes, hair loss)
Mercaptopurine	Purinethol	Acute lymphocytic and myelocytic leukemia; chronic myelocytic leukemia	Blood disorders (anemia, leukopenia, thrombocytopenia); GI distress (nausea, anorexia); hepatotoxicity
Methotrexate	Folex, Mexate	Acute lymphocytic leukemia; meningeal leukemia; carcinoma of head and neck region, lung; non-Hodgkin's lymphoma	Blood disorders (anemia, leukopenia, thrombocytopenia); GI distress (including ulceration of GI tract); skin disorders (rashes, photosensitivity, hair loss); hepatotoxicity; CNS effects (headaches, drowsiness, fatigue)
Thioguanine	Lanvis	Acute lymphocytic leukemia; acute and chronic myelocytic leukemia	Blood disorders (anemia, leukopenia, thrombocytopenia); GI distress (nausea, vomiting); hepatotoxicity

*Only the indications listed in the U.S. product labeling are included here. Many anticancer drugs are used for additional types of neoplastic disease.
From Ciccone, CD: Pharmacology in Rehabilitation, ed 2. FA Davis, 1996, p 572, with permission.

FREQUENTLY USED COMBINATION CHEMOTHERAPY REGIMENS

Type of Cancer	Therapy	Components of Therapy Regimen
Breast	FAC	5-Fluorouracil, doxorubicin (Adriamycin), cyclophosphamide (Cytoxan)
	CMF	Cyclophosphamide (Cytoxan), methotrexate, 5-fluorouracil
	Cooper's regimen (CVFMP)	5-Fluorouracil, methotrexate, vincristine (Oncovin), cyclophosphamide (Cytoxan), prednisone
Hodgkin's disease	MOPP	Mustargen (mechlorethamine), Oncovin (vincristine), procarbazine, prednisone
	ABVD	Doxorubicin (Adriamycin), bleomycin (Blenoxane), vinblastine (Velban), dacarbazine (DTIC)
Leukemia	OAP	Oncovin, Ara-C (cytarabine). prednisone
	COAP	Cyclophosphamide, Oncovin (vincristine), Ara-C (cytarabine), prednisone
	Ad-OAP	Adriamycin (doxorubicin), Oncovin (vincristine), Ara-C (cytarabine), prednisone
Multiple myeloma	VBAP	Vincristine, BCNU (carmustine), Adriamycin (doxorubicin), prednisone
	VCAP	Vincristine, Cytoxan (cyclophosphamide), Adriamycin (doxorubicin), prednisone
Non-Hodgkin's lymphoma	CHOP	Cytoxan (cyclophosphamide), doxorubicin,* Oncovin, prednisone
	COP	Cytoxan (cyclophosphamide), Oncovin (vincristine), prednisone
Testicular tumors	VB-3	Vinblastine (Velban), bleomycin (Blenoxane)

*The H in this regimen refers to hydroxyldaunorubicin, the chemical synonym for doxorubicin.
Based on Moraca-Sawicki, AM: Antineoplastic chemotherapy. In Kuhn: Pharmacotherapeutics: A Nursing Process Approach, ed 3. FA Davis, Philadelphia, 1994, p 1225, with permission.

16

IMMUNOSUPPRESSIVE DRUGS

COMMON IMMUNOSUPPRESSIVE DRUGS

Generic Name	Trade Name(s)	Prevention or Treatment of Transplant Rejection	Primary Indications* — Diseases with an Autoimmune Response
Antibodies	Names vary according to specific lymphocyte targets	Bone marrow, other organ transplants	Idiopathic thrombocytic purpura, other hemolytic disorders
Azathioprine	Imuran	Kidney, heart	Rheumatoid arthritis, inflammatory bowel disease, myasthenia gravis, systemic lupus erythematosus (SLE), others
Cyclophosphamide	Cytoxan	Bone marrow	Rheumatoid arthritis, multiple sclerosis, SLE, dermatomyositis, glomerulonephritis, hematologic disorders

Myoglobin (a muscle protein) into circulation causing kidney failure.

Rhamido

Cyclosporine	Sandimmune	Kidney, liver, heart, lung, pancreas, bone marrow	Psoriasis, rheumatoid arthritis, inflammatory bowel disease, glomerulonephritis, others
Glucocorticoids	S-2	Heart, kidney, liver, bone marrow	Multiple sclerosis, rheumatoid arthritis, SLE, inflammatory bowel disease, hemolytic disorders, others
Methotrexate	Folex, Mexate, Rheumatrex	—	Rheumatoid arthritis, psoriasis
Sulfasalazine	Azulfidine, others	—	Rheumatoid arthritis, inflammatory bowel disease
Tacrolimus	Prograf	Liver	—

*Indications vary considerably and many indications listed here are not in the U.S. product labeling for each drug; optimal use of these drugs alone or in combination with each other continues to be investigated.

From Ciccone, CD: Pharmacology in Rehabilitation, ed 2. FA Davis, 1996, p 588, with permission.

16

GLUCOCORTICOIDS USED AS IMMUNOSUPPRESSIVE DRUGS	
Betamethasone (Celestone)	Methylprednisolone (Medrol)
Corticotropin (Acthar)	Paramethasone (Haldrone)
Cortisone (Cortone)	Prednisolone (Hydeltrasol, Predate)
Dexamethasone (Decadron)	Prednisone (Deltasone)
Hydrocortisone (Cortef)	Triamcinolone (Aristocort)

*Common trade names are shown in parentheses.

From Ciccone, CD: Pharmacology in Rehabilitation, ed 2. FA Davis, Philadelphia, 1996, p 591, with permission.

ORGAN TRANSPLANTS

Systemic Effects of Organ Failures Associated with Organ Transplants

Decreased peripheral oxygenation
Hypertension
Pulmonary congestion
Poor diaphragmatic excursion
Limited chest wall compliance
Anemia
Increased release of calcium ions from bone
Increased risk of infection
Muscle degradation and fiber loss
Peripheral neuropathies
Altered abdominal mechanics
Generalized muscle weakness and deconditioning

Common Side Effects of Drugs Frequently Used in Transplantation

Steroids

Increased serum cholesterol
Mood swings
Weight gain
Hyperglycemia
Muscle weakness
Loss of connective tissue compliance
Bruising

Cyclosporine

Hypertension
Disease of central nervous system white matter (usually transient)
Tremors

Symptoms Commonly Associated with Transplants

Liver Transplants

Fragile skin continuity
Easy bruising and bleeding
Encephalopathy
Weak abdominal musculature
Poor breathing patterns
Low back pain

Renal Transplants

Orthostatic hypotension (due to antihypertensive medication)
Osteopenia, osteodystrophy
Hypoglycemia (diabetics)
Hypertension
Muscle fiber loss
Weak abdominal musculature

Heart and Heart-Lung Transplants

Delayed heart rate response to exercise-deprived hearts
   (requires at least 5 min for circulating catecholamines to
   increase heart rate; requires at least 10 min to resorb and
   return to resting heart rate after cessation of exercise)
Two heart beats (in heterotopic transplants)
Decreased shoulder range of motion
Muscle weakness
Pulmonary congestion
Loss of endurance

Bone Marrow Transplants

Pancytopenia
Sensitive skin (from graft or host disease)
Nausea

16

FOR MORE INFORMATION

Dimsdale, JE, et al: Postexercise peril: Plasma catecholamines and
   exercise. JAMA, 251:630, 1984.
Kavanaugh, T, et al: Cardiorespiratory responses to exercise training
   after orthotopic cardiac transplantation. Circulation 77:162;
   1988.
Smith, SL (ed): Tissue and Organ Transplantation, St. Louis, Mosby,
   1990.

HYPERTHYROIDISM AND HYPOTHYROIDISM

PRIMARY SYMPTOMS OF HYPERTHYROIDISM AND HYPOTHYROIDISM

Hyperthyroidism	Hypothyroidism
Nervousness	Lethargy/slow cerebration
Weight loss	Weight gain (in adult hypothyroidism)
Diarrhea	Constipation
Tachycardia	Bradycardia
Insomnia	Sleepiness
Increased appetite	Anorexia
Heat intolerance	Cold intolerance
Oligomenorrhea	Menorrhagia
Muscle wasting	Weakness
Goiter	Dry, coarse skin
Exophthalmos	Facial edema

Based on Kuhn, MA: Thyroid and Parathyroid Glands. In Kuhn, MA (ed): Pharmacotherapeutics: A Nursing Process Approach, ed 3. FA Davis, Philadelphia, p 981, 1994.

PRIMARY TYPES OF HYPERTHYROIDISM AND HYPOTHYROIDISM

Hyperthyroidism (Thyrotoxicosis)	Hypothyroidism (Hypothyroxinemia)

Primary hyperthyroidism
  Graves' disease
  Thyroid adenoma/carcinoma
	Primary hypothyroidism
	  Genetic deficiency of enzymes that synthesize thyroid hormones

Secondary hyperthyroidism
  Hyperthyroidism induced by excessive hypothalamic or pituitary stimulation
	Secondary hypothyroidism
	  Hypothyroidism induced by hypothalamic or pituitary deficiencies
	  Cretinism (childhood hypothyroidism)
	  Myxedema (adult hypothyroidism)
	Other forms of hypothyroidism
	  Hypothyroidism induced by peripheral insensitivity to thyroid hormones, inadequate hormone transport, etc.

From Ciccone, CD: Pharmacology in Rehabilitation, ed 2. FA Davis, Philadelphia, 1996, p 465, with permission.

17

Material in this chapter is taken from Ciccone, CD: Pharmacology in Rehabilitation, ed 2. FA Davis, Philadelphia, 1996, with permission (with the exception of pages 1049 and 1054–1060).

Elsewhere in the book material on pharmacology also comes from this source. Readers interested in understanding pharmacology and its relationship to rehabilitation are urged to examine this text. The authors wish to thank Dr. Ciccone for the use of his material and for his assistance.

CONTROLLED SUBSTANCES

In 1970, federal legislation was enacted to help control the abuse of legal and illegal drugs. The Comprehensive Drug Abuse Prevention and Control Act (or Controlled Substances Act, as it is also known) placed drugs into specific categories, or "schedules," according to their potential for abuse. Descriptions of these schedules for controlled drugs follow.

Schedule I: These drugs are regarded as having the highest potential for abuse, and the legal use of agents in this category is restricted to approved research studies or therapeutic use in a very limited number of patients (e.g., use of marijuana as an antiemetic). Examples of schedule I drugs include heroin, lysergic acid diethylamide (LSD), psilocybin, mescaline, peyote, marijuana, tetrahydrocannabinols, and several other hallucinogens.

Schedule II: Drugs in this category are approved for specific therapeutic purposes but still have a high potential for abuse and possible addiction. Examples include opioids such as morphine and meperidine, barbiturates such as pentobarbital and secobarbital, and drugs containing amphetamines.

Schedule III: Although these drugs have a lower abuse potential than those in schedules I and II, there is still the possibility of developing mild to moderate physical dependence or strong psychologic dependence, or both. Drugs in schedule III include opioids (e.g., codeine, hydrocodone) that are combined in a limited dosage with other nonopioid drugs. Other drugs in this category are certain barbiturates and amphetamines that are not included in schedule II.

17

FOR MORE INFORMATION

Kuhn, MA and Moraca-Sawicki, AM: Pharmacology and the nurse's role. In Kuhn, MA (ed): Pharmacotherapeutics: A Nursing Process Approach, ed 3. FA Davis, Philadelphia, 1994.

United States Pharmacopeia XXII National Formulary XVII. United States Pharmacopeia Convention, Inc., Rockville, MD, 1990, pp 1629–1665.

COMMON DRUG SUFFIXES

Drug Class	Suffix	Common Examples	Primary Indication or Desired Effect
Angiotensin-converting enzyme (ACE) inhibitors	-pril	Captopril, enalapril	Antihypertensive, congestive heart failure
Barbiturates	-barbital	Phenobarbital, secobarbital	Sedative-hypnotic, antiseizure
Benzodiazepines	-epam or -olam	Diazepam, temazepam, alprazolam, triazolam	Sedative-hypnotic, antianxiety, antiseizure
β-Blockers	-olol	Metoprolol, propranolol	Antihypertensive, antianginal, antiarrhythmic
Bronchodilators (adrenergic)	-erol	Albuterol, pirbuterol	Bronchodilation
Bronchodilators (xanthine derivatives)	-phylline	Theophylline, aminophylline	Bronchodilation
Calcium channel blockers (dihydropyridine group)	-ipine	Nifedipine, nicardipine	Antihypertensive, antianginal

	-sone or -olone*	Cortisone, dexamethasone, prednisone, prednisolone, triamcinolone	Anti-inflammatory, immunosuppressants
Glucocorticoids			
Histamine H$_2$-receptor blockers	-idine	Cimetidine, ranitidine	Gastric ulcers
Local anesthetics	-caine	Lidocaine, bupivicaine	Local anesthetic, antiarrhythmics
Oral hypoglycemics	-amide	Chlorpropamide, tolbutamide	Antidiabetic (type II diabetes mellitus)
Penicillin antibiotics	-cillin	Penicillin, ampicillin, amoxicillin	Bacterial infections
Tetracycline antibiotics	-cycline	Tetracycline, doxycycline	Bacterial infections
Various other antibacterials	-micin or -mycin†	Streptomycin, gentamicin, erythromycin	Bacterial infections

*Some anabolic steroids also end with -olone, e.g., nandrolone, oxymetholone.
†Some antibiotics ending with "-mycin" or "rubicin" are used as antineoplastics.
From Ciccone, CD: Pharmacology in Rehabilitation, ed 2. FA Davis, Philadelphia, p 609, with permission.

17

ROUTES OF DRUG ADMINISTRATION

Route	Advantages	Disadvantages	Examples
		ENTERAL	
Oral	Easy, safe, convenient	Limited or erratic absorption of some drugs; chance of first-pass inactivation in liver.	Analgesics, sedative-hypnotics, many others
Sublingual	Rapid onset; not subject to first-pass inactivation	Drug must be easily absorbed from oral mucosa.	Nitroglycerin
Rectal	Alternative to oral route; local effect on rectal tissues	Poor or incomplete absorption; chance of rectal irritation.	Laxatives, suppository forms of other drugs
		PARENTERAL	
Inhalation	Rapid onset; direct application for respiratory disorders; large sur-face area for systemic absorption	Chance of tissue irritation; patient compliance sometimes a problem.	General anesthetics, anti-asthmatic agents
Injection	Provides more direct administra-tion to target tissues; rapid onset	Chance of infection if sterility is not maintained.	Insulin, antibiotics, anticancer drugs, narcotic analgesics
Topical	Local effects on surface of skin	Only effective in treating outer layers of skin.	Antibiotic ointments, creams used to treat minor skin irritation and injury

ROUTES OF DRUG ADMINISTRATION (Continued)

Route	Advantages	Disadvantages	Examples
Transdermal	Introduces drug into body without breaking the skin	Drug must be able to pass through dermal layers intact.	Nitroglycerin, motion sickness medications, drugs used with phonophoresis and iontophoresis

From Ciccone, CD: Pharmacology in Rehabilitation, ed 2. FA Davis, Philadelphia, 1996, p 16, with permission.

SIGNS AND SYMPTOMS OF DRUG ABUSE

17

ABSTINENCE SYNDROMES: SYMPTOMS OF NARCOTIC WITHDRAWAL

Body aches	Runny nose
Diarrhea	Shivering
Fever	Sneezing
Gooseflesh	Stomach cramps
Insomnia	Sweating
Irritability	Tachycardia
Loss of appetite	Uncontrollable yawning
Nausea/vomiting	Weakness/fatigue

From Ciccone, CD: Pharmacology in Rehabilitation, ed 2. FA Davis, Philadelphia, 1996, p 189, with permission.

SIGNS OF DRUG INTERACTIONS, OVERDOSE, AND WITHDRAWAL

Drug	Acute Intoxication[a] and Overdose	Withdrawal Syndrome
CNS Stimulants: Cocaine, amphetamine, dextroamphetamine, methylphenidate, phenmetrazine, phenylpropanolamine, STP[b], MDMA[c], Bromo-DMA[d], diethylpropion, most amphetamine-like antiobesity drugs	*Vital signs:* temperature elevated; heart rate increased; respirations shallow; BP elevated. *Mental status:* sensorium hyperacute or confused; paranoid ideation; hallucinations; delirium; impulsivity; agitation; hyperactivity; stereotypy. *Physical Exam:* pupils dilated and reactive; tendon reflexes hyperactive; cardiac dysrhythmias; dry mouth; sweating; tremors; convulsions; coma; stroke.	Muscular aches; abdominal pain; chills, tremors, voracious hunger; anxiety; prolonged sleep; lack of energy; profound depression, sometimes suicidal; exhaustion

Drug	Signs and symptoms of overdose	Withdrawal syndrome
Opioids: heroin, morphine, codeine, meperidine, methadone, hydromorphone, opium, pentazocine, propoxyphene, fentanyl, sufentanil	*Vital signs:* temperature decreased; respiration depressed; BP decreased, sometimes shock. *Mental status:* euphoria; stupor. *Physical exam:* pupils constricted (may be dilated with meperidine or extreme hypoxia); reflexes diminished to absent; pulmonary edema; constipation; convulsions with propoxyphene or meperidine; cardiac dysrhythmias with propoxyphene; coma.	Pupils dilated; pulse rapid; gooseflesh; lacrimation; abdominal cramps; muscle jerks; "flu" syndrome; vomiting; diarrhea; temulousness; yawning; anxiety
CNS depressants: barbiturates, benzodiazepines, glutethimide, meprobamate, methaqualone, ethchlorvynol, chloral hydrate, methyprylon, paraldehyde	*Vital signs:* respiration depressed; BP decreased, sometimes shock. *Mental status:* drowsiness or coma; confusion; delirium. *Physical exam:* pupils dilated with glutethimide or in severe poisoning; tendon reflexes depressed; ataxia; slurred speech; nystagmus; convulsions or hyperirritability with methaqualone; signs of anticholinergic poisoning with glutethimide; cardiac dysrhythmias with chloral hydrate.	Tremulousness; insomnia; sweating; fever; clonic blink reflex; anxiety; cardiovascular collapse; agitation; delirium; hallucinations; disorientation; convulsions; shock

Continued on following page

17

Drug	Acute Intoxication[a] and Overdose	Withdrawal Syndrome
Hallucinogens: LSD[e], psilocybin, mescaline, PCP[l]	*Vital signs:* temperature elevated; heart rate increased; BP elevated. *Mental status:* euphoria; anxiety or panic; paranoia; sensorium often clear; affect inappropriate; illusions; time and visual distortions; visual hallucinations; depersonalization; with PCP hypertensive encephalopathy. *Physical exam:* pupils dilated (normal or small with PCP); tendon reflexes hyperactive; with PCP cyclic coma or extreme hyperactivity, drooling, blank stare, mutism, amnesia, analgesia, nystagmus (sometimes vertical), gait ataxia, muscle rigidity, impulsive or violent behavior; violent, scatological, pressured speech.	None

Cannabis group: marijuana, hashish, THC^g, hash oil, sinsemilla

Vital signs: heart rate increased; BP decreased on standing. *Mental status*: anorexia, then increased appetite; euphoria; anxiety; sensorium often clear; dreamy, fantasy state; time-space distortions; hallucinations may be rare. *Physical exam*: pupils unchanged; conjunctiva injected; tachycardia, ataxia, and pallor in children.

Nonspecific symptoms including anorexia, nausea, insomnia, restlessness, irritability, anxiety, depression

Continued on following page

17

SIGNS OF DRUG INTERACTIONS, OVERDOSES, AND WITHDRAWAL (Continued)

Drug	Acute Intoxication[a] and Overdose	Withdrawal Syndrome
Anticholinergics: atropine, belladonna, henbane, scopolamine, trihexyphenidyl, benztropine mesylate, procyclidine, propantheline bromide; jimson weed seed	*Vital signs:* temperature elevated; heart rate increased; possibly decreased BP. *Mental status:* drowsiness or coma; sensorium clouded; amnesia; disorientation; visual hallucinations; body image alterations; confusion; with propantheline restlessness, excitement. *Physical exam:* pupils dilated and fixed; decreased bowel sounds; flushed, dry skin and mucous membranes; violent behavior, convulsions; with propantheline circulatory failure, respiratory failure, paralysis, coma.	Gastrointestinal and musculoskeletal symptoms

[a]Mixed intoxications produce complex combinations of signs and symptoms.
[b]STP (2,5-dimethoxy-4-methylamphetamine)
[c]MDMA (3,4-methylenedioxymethamphetamine)
[d]Bromo-DMA (4-bromo-2,5-dimethoxyamphetamine)
[e]LSD (D-lysergic acid diethylamide)
[f]PCP (phencyclidine)
[g]THC (γ-9-tetrahydrocannabinol)
BP = blood pressure.
Reprinted with permission from the Medical Letter Vol 29, September 11, 1987.

COMMONLY PRESCRIBED DRUGS

DRUGS AND DOSES USED FOR PREOPERATIVE PREMEDICATION

Classification	Drug	Typical Adult Dose (mg)	Route of Administration (Oral, IM)
Barbiturates	Secobarbital	50–150	Oral, IM
	Pentobarbital	50–150	Oral, IM
Opioids	Morphine	5–15	IM
	Meperidine	50–100	IM
Benzodiazepines	Diazepam	5–10	Oral
	Lorazepam	2–4	Oral, IM
Antihistamines	Diphenhydramine	25–75	Oral, IM
	Promethazine	25–50	IM
	Hydroxyzine	50–100	IM
Anticholinergics	Atropine	0.3–0.6	IM
	Scopolamine	0.3–0.6	IM
	Glycopyrrolate	0.1–0.3	IM
Antacids	Particulate	15–30 ml	Oral
	Nonparticulate	15–30 ml	Oral

IM = intramuscular.
Based on Stoelting, RK: Psychological preparation and preoperative medication. In Stoelting, RK and Miller, RD (eds): Basics of Anesthesia. Churchill Livingstone, New York, NY, 1984, p 381.

17

NEUROMUSCULAR JUNCTION BLOCKERS: NONDEPOLARIZING AND DEPOLARIZING FORMS

Drug	Onset of Initial Action* (min)	Time to Peak Effects (min)	Duration of Peak Effect (min)
Nondepolarizing blockers			
Atracurium	Within 2	3–5	20–35
Gallamine	1–2	3–5	15–30
Metocurine	1–4	1.5–10	35–60
Pancuronium	Within 0.75	4.5	35–45
Tubocurarine	Within 1	2–5	20–40
Vecuronium	1	3–5	25–30
Depolarizing blockers			
Succinylcholine	0.5–1	1–2	4–10

*Reflects usual adult intravenous dosage.

CHOLINERGIC STIMULANTS: DIRECT-ACTING AND INDIRECT-ACTING FORMS

Generic Name	Trade Name(s)	Primary Clinical Use(s)*
DIRECT-ACTING (CHOLINERGIC AGONISTS)		
Bethanechol	Duvoid, Urecholine, others	Postoperative gastrointestinal and urinary atony
Carbachol	Isopto Carbachol, Miostat	Glaucoma
Methacholine	Provocholine	Diagnosis of asthma
Pilocarpine	Pilocar, Adsorbocarpine, many other	Glaucoma
INDIRECT-ACTING (CHOLINESTERASE INHIBITORS)		
Ambenonium	Mytelase	Myasthenia gravis
Demecarium	Humorsol	Glaucoma
Echothiophate	Phospholine Iodide	Glaucoma
Edrophonium	Reversol, Tensiolon	Myasthenia gravis, reversal of neuro-muscular blocking drugs
Isoflurophate	Floropryl	Glaucoma
Neostigmine	Prostigmin	Postoperative gastro-intestinal and urinary atony, myasthenia gravis, reversal of neuromuscular blocking drugs
Physostigmine	Isopto Eserine, Antilirium	Glaucoma, reversal of CNS toxicity caused by anticholinergic drugs
Pyridostigmine	Mestinon, Regonol	Myasthenia gravis, reversal of neuro-muscular blocking drugs

*Agents used to treat glaucoma are administered topically, that is, directly to the eye. Agents used for other problems are given systemically by oral administration or injection.

CNS = central nervous system.

From Ciccone, CD: Pharmacology in Rehabilitation, ed 2. FA Davis, Philadelphia, 1996, p 262, with permission.

COMMON ANTICHOLINERGIC DRUGS

Generic Name	Trade Name(s)	Primary Clinical Use(s)*
Anisotropine	Valpin	Peptic ulcer
Atropine	Dey-Dose, others	Peptic ulcer, irritable bowel syndrome, neurogenic bladder, bronchospasm, preoperative antisecretory agent, cardiac dysrhythmias (e.g., symptomatic bradycardia, postmyocardial infarction, asystole)
Belladonna	Generic	Peptic ulcer, irritable bowel syndrome, dysmenorrhea, nocturnal enuresis
Clidinium	Quarzan	Peptic ulcer, irritable bowel syndrome
Cyclopentolate	Pentolate, Cyclogyl, others	Induces mydriasis for ophthalmologic procedures
Dicyclomine	Bentyle, others	Irritable bowel syndrome
Glycopyrrolate	Robinul	Peptic ulcer, preoperative antisecretory agent
Homotropine	Homapin	Peptic ulcer, irritable bowel syndrome
Hyoscyamine	Cystospaz, Levsin, others	Peptic ulcer, irritable bowel syndrome, urinary bladder hypermotility, preoperative antisecretory agent
Ipratropium	Altrovent	Antiasthmatic
Isopropamide	Darbid	Peptic ulcer, irritable bowel syndrome
Mepenzolate	Cantil	Peptic ulcer
Methantheline	Banthine	Peptic ulcer, neurogenic bladder
Methscopolamine	Pamine	Peptic ulcer
Oxybutynin	Ditropan	Neurogenic bladder

COMMON ANTICHOLINERGIC DRUGS (Continued)		
Generic Name	**Trade Name(s)**	**Primary Clinical Use(s)***
Oxyphencyclimine	Daricon	Peptic ulcer
Propantheline	Pro-Banthine, Norpanth, others	Peptic ulcer, irritable bowel syndrome
Scopolamine	Transderm Scop	Motion sickness, preoperative antisecretory agent
Tridihexethyl	Pathilon	Peptic ulcer, irritable bowel syndrome

From Ciccone, CD: Pharmacology in Rehabilitation, ed 2. FA Davis, Philadelphia, 1996, p 267, with permission.

THERAPEUTIC GLUCOCORTICOIDS

Generic Name	Common Trade Name(s)	Type of Preparation Available					
		Systemic	Topical	Inhalation	Ophthalmic	Otic	Nasal
Alclometasone	Aclovate		X				
Amcinonide	Cyclocort		X				
Beclomethasone	Beclovent, Vanceril			X			X
Betamethasone	Celestone, Uticort	X	X		X	X	
Clobetasol	Dermovate, Temovate		X				
Clocortolone	Cloderm		X				
Cortisone	Cortone	X					
Desonide	DesOwen, Tridesilon		X				
Desoximetasone	Topicort		X				
Dexamethasone	Decadron, Dexasone	X	X	X	X	X	X
Diflorasone	Florone, Maxiflor		X				

Generic Name	Trade Name(s)					
Flumethasone	Locacorten					X
Flunisolide	AeroBid, Nasalide			X		X
Fluocinolone	Fluonid, Flurosyn			X		
Fluocinonide	Lidex					
Fluorometholone	FML, S.O.P., Fluor-Op		X			
Flurandrenolide	Cordran			X		
Fluticasone	Cultivate			X		
Halcinonide	Halog			X		
Halobetasol	Ultravate			X		
Hydrocortisone	Cortaid, Hydrocortone	X		X	X	X
Medrysone	HMS Liquifilm			X		
Methylprednisolone	Medrol	X		X		
Mometasone	Elocon			X		
Paramethasone	Haldrone	X				
Prednisolone	Hydeltrasol, Prelone	X				
Prednisone	Deltasone, Meticorten	X				X
Triamcinolone	Azmacort, Aristocort	X	X	X		

From Ciccone, CD: Pharmacology in Rehabilitation, ed 2. FA Davis, Philadelphia, 1996, p 427, with permission.

17

NONENDOCRINE DISORDERS TREATED WITH GLUCOCORTICOIDS

General Indication	Principal Desired Effect of Glucocorticoids	Examples of Specific Disorders
Allergic disorders	Decreased inflammation	Anaphylactic reactions, drug-induced allergic reactions, severe hay fever, serum sickness
Collagen disorders	Immunosuppression	Acute rheumatic carditis, dermatomyositis, systemic lupus erythematosus
Dermatologic disorders	Decreased inflammation	Alopecia areata, dermatitis (various forms), keloids, lichens, mycosis fungoides, pemphigus, psoriasis
Gastrointestinal disorders	Decreased inflammation	Inflammatory bowel disease, Crohn's disease, ulcerative proctosigmoiditis
Hematologic disorders	Immunosuppression	Autoimmune hemolytic anemia, congenital hypoplastic anemia, erythroblastopenia, thrombocytopenia

Nonrheumatic inflammation	Decreased inflammation	Bursitis, tenosynovitis
Neoplastic disease	Immunosuppression	Leukemias, lymphomas, nasal polyps, cystic tumors
Neurologic disease	Decreased inflammation and immunosuppression	Tuberculous meningitis, multiple sclerosis, myasthenia gravis
Neurotrauma	Decreased edema*	Brain surgery, closed head injury, certain brain tumors
Ophthalmic disorders	Decreased inflammation	Chorioretinitis, conjunctivitis, herpes zoster, iridocyclitis, keratitis, optic neuritis
Respiratory disorders	Decreased inflammation	Bronchial asthma, berylliosis, aspiration pneumonitis, symptomatic sarcoidosis, pulmonary tuberculosis
Rheumatic disorders	Decreased inflammation and immunosuppression	Ankylosing spondylitis, psoriatic arthritis, rheumatoid arthritis, gouty arthritis, osteoarthritis

*Efficacy of glucocorticoid use in decreasing cerebral edema has not been conclusively proved.
From Ciccone, CD: Pharmacology in Rehabilitation, ed 2. FA Davis, Philadelphia, 1996, p 429, with permission.

17

CLINICAL USES OF ANDROGENS

Generic Name	Trade Name(s)	Primary Indication(s)	Routes of Administration
Fluoxymesterone	Halotestin	Androgen replacement, breast cancer, delayed puberty in males, anemia	Oral
Methyltestosterone	Android, Oreton, Testred, Virilon	Androgen replacement, breast cancer, delayed puberty in males	Oral
Nandrolone	Andralone, Durabolin	Anemia, breast cancer	Intramuscular
Oxandrolone	Anavar	Catabolic states	Oral
Oxymetholone	Anadrol	Anemia, angioedema	Oral
Stanozolol	Winstrol	Angioedema	Oral
Testosterone*	Histerone, Testaqua, Andro-Cyp, Depotest, Testex, others	Anemia, androgen replacement, delayed puberty in males, breast cancer	Intramuscular

*Testosterone is available as testosterone sterile suspension, testosterone cypionate, testosterone enanthate, and testosterone propionate; specific trade names and indications depend on the specific form of testosterone administered.
From Ciccone, CD: Pharmacology in Rehabilitation, ed 2. FA Davis, Philadelphia, 1996, p 443, with permission.

EXAMPLES OF ANABOLIC ANDROGENS THAT ARE ABUSED BY ATHLETES

Generic Name	Trade Name
Orally active androgens	
Ethylestrenol	Maxibolin
Fluoxymesterone	Android-F; Halotestin
Methandrostenolone	Dianabol
Oxandrolone	Anavar
Oxymetholone	Anadrol-50
Stanozolol	Winstrol
Androgens administered by intramuscular injection	
Nandrolone phenpropionate	Durabolin
Nandrolone decanoate	Deca-Durabolin
Testosterone cypionate	Depo-Testosterone
Testosterone enanthate	Delatestryl

From Ciccone, CD: Pharmacology in Rehabilitation, ed 2. FA Davis, Philadelphia, 1996, p 445, with permission.

DRUGS USED TO TREAT OVERACTIVE CLOTTING

Drug Category	Primary Effect and Indication
Anticoagulants	Inhibit synthesis and function of clotting factors; used primarily to prevent and treat venous thromboembolism
Heparin (Calciparine; Liquaemin)	
Oral anticoagulants	
Anisindione (Miradon)	
Dicumarol (generic)	
Warfarin (Coumadin, Panwarfin)	
Antithrombotics	Inhibit platelet aggregation and platelet-induced clotting; used primarily to prevent arterial thrombus formation
Aspirin	
Dipyridamole (Dipridacot, Persantine)	
Sulfinpyrazone (Anturane)	
Thrombolytics	Facilitate clot dissolution; used to reopen occluded vessels in arterial and venous thrombosis
Anistreplase (Eminase)	
Streptokinase (Kabikinase, Streptase)	
Tissue-plasminogen activator (t-PA)	
Urokinase (Abbokinase)	

From Ciccone, CD: Pharmacology in Rehabilitation, ed 2. FA Davis, Philadelphia, 1996, p 351, with permission.

DRUGS USED TO TREAT HYPERLIPIDEMIA

Generic Name	Trade Name(s)	Dosage*	Primary Effect
Cholestyramine	Cholybar, Questran	4 g 1–6 times each day before meals and at bedtime	Decreases plasma LDL-cholesterol levels
Clofibrate	Abitrate, Atromid-S	1.5–2.0 g each day in 2–4 divided doses	Lowers plasma triglycerides by decreasing LDL and IDL levels
Gemfibrozil	Lopid	1.2 g each day in 2 divided doses 30 min before morning and evening meal	Similar to clofibrate
Lovastatin	Mevacor	20–80 mg each day as a single dose or in divided doses with meals	Decreases plasma LDL-cholesterol levels; may also decrease triglycerides and increase HDL somewhat
Niacin	Niacor, Nicobid, others	1–2 g 3 times each day	Lowers plasma triglycerides by decreasing VLDL levels
Pravastatin	Pravachol	10–40 mg once each day at bedtime	Similar to lovastatin
Probucol	Lorelco	500 mg 2 times each day with morning and evening meal	Decreases LDL and HDL cholesterol; may also inhibit deposition of fat into arterial wall
Simvastatin	Zocor	5–40 mg once each day in the evening	Similar to lovastatin

*Doses represent typical adult oral maintenance dose.

HDL = high-density lipoproteins; IDL = intermediate-density lipoproteins; LDL = low-density lipoproteins; VLDL = very low density lipoproteins.

From Ciccone, CD: Pharmacology in Rehabilitation, ed 2. FA Davis, Philadelphia, 1996, p 359, with permission.

ANTIDIARRHEAL AGENTS

Generic Name	Trade Names	Dosage
Adsorbents		
Kaolin	Kaopectate,	60–120-ml regular-
Pectin	Kao-tin,	strength suspension
	Kapectolin*	after each loose bowel
		movement
Bismuth salicylate	Pepto-Bismol	525 mg every ½–1 h or 1050 mg every hour if needed
Opioid derivatives		
Diphenoxylate	Diphenatol, Lomotil, others†	2.5–5 mg 3 or 4 times daily
Loperamide	Imodium	4 mg initially, 2 mg after each unformed stool
Opium tincture	—	0.3–1.0 ml 1–4 times daily
Paregoric	—	5–10 ml 1–4 times daily

*Commercial products typically contain both kaolin and pectin.
†Commercial products often combine diphenoxylate (an opioid) with atropine (an anticholinergic).
From Ciccone, CD: Pharmacology in Rehabilitation, ed 2. FA Davis, Philadelphia, 1996, p 394, with permission.

17

Acquired Immunodeficiency Syndrome (AIDS)

18

ESTIMATES OF RISK OF ACQUIRING HIV INFECTION BY PORTALS OF ENTRY

Entry Site	Type of Risk	Risk Virus Gets to Entry Site	Risk Virus Enters	Risk Inoculated
Conjunctiva	Random	Moderate	Moderate	Very low*
Oral mucosa	Random	Moderate	Moderate	Low*
Nasal mucosa	Random	Low	Low	Very low*
Lower respiratory	Low	Very low	Very low	Very low
Anus	High	Very high	Very high	Very high
Skin, intact	Low	Very low	Very low	Very low
Skin, broken	High	Low	High	High
Sexual:				
Vagina	Choice	Low	Low	Medium
Penis	Choice	High	Low	Low
Ulcers (STD)	Choice	High	High	Very high

Blood:				
Products	Choice	High	High	High
Shared needles	Choice	High	High	Very high
Accidental needle	Accident	Low	High	Low
Traumatic wound	Accident	Modest	High	High
Perinatal	Accident	High	High	High

STD = sexually transmitted disease.

*Based on data summarized in Recommendations for prevention of HIV transmission in health-care settings. MMWR 36:3S, August 21, 1987; and Update: Universal precautions for prevention of transmission of HIV, hepatitis B virus, and other bloodborne pathogens in health-care settings. MMWR 37:377, June 24, 1988. Adapted from Hopp, JW and Rogers, EA: AIDS and the Allied Health Professions. FA Davis, Philadelphia, 1989, p 68.

Portal of Exit	Virus Content	Potential for Spread	Chance to Be Inoculated
Respiratory nasal:			
Sputum	Very low	Efficient	Very low
Saliva	Very low	Efficient	Very low
Tears	Very low	Inefficient	Very low
GI:	Low	Dependent	Very low
Vomitus	Very low	Dependent	Very low
Stool	Very low	Dependent	Very low
Urine	Very low	Inefficient	Very low
Sweat	Very low	Inefficient	Very low
Skin fomites	Very low	Inefficient	Very low
Intact skin	Very low	Dependent	Low
Broken skin	Low	Dependent	Med-high
Bleeding wound	High	Efficient	Very high
Sexual:			
Ejaculate	Very high	Efficient	Low-mod
Vaginal secretions	Moderate	Efficient	Very high
Purulent	Very high	Efficient	Very high

ESTIMATES OF RISK OF ACQUIRING HIV INFECTION BY PORTALS OF EXIT

Blood:			
Transfusion	Very high	Efficient	Very high
Shared needles	High	Efficient	Low
Accidental needle	Low	Inefficient	Very low
Body fluids (usually blood tinged):			
Cerebrospinal fluid	Low	Inefficient	Very low
Synovial fluid	Low	Inefficient	Very low
Pleural fluid	Very low	Inefficient	Very low
Peritoneal fluid	Very low	Inefficient	Very low
Pericardial fluid	Very low	Inefficient	Very low
Amniotic fluid	Low	Efficient	Very high
Perinatal:	High	Dependent	Low
Breast milk	Low	Unknown	Low

GI = gastrointestinal.
Based on data summarized in Recommendations for prevention of HIV transmission in health-care settings. MMWR 36:3S, August 21, 1987; and Update: Universal precautions for prevention of transmission of HIV, hepatitis B virus, and other bloodborne pathogens in health-care settings. MMWR 37:377, June 24, 1988. Adapted from Hopp, JW and Rogers, EA: AIDS and the Allied Health Professions. FA Davis, Philadelphia, 1989, p 66.

18

WALTER REED STAGING CLASSIFICATION FOR HIV INFECTION

Stage	HIV Antibody or Virus Isolation	Chronic Lymphadenopathy	T helper Cells/mm^3	Delayed Hypersensitivity
0	−	−	>400	None
1	+	−	>400	None
2	+	+	>400	None
3	+	+/−	<400	None
4	+	+/−	<400	Partial
5	+	+/−	<400	Total cutaneous
6	+	+/−	<400	Partial total cutaneous

+ = present; − = absent.

Based on Hart, M and Rogers, EA: Acquired Immunodeficiency Syndrome. In Fletcher, GF, et al (eds): Contemporary Clinical Perspectives. Lea & Febiger, Philadelphia, 1992, pp 335–366; and Volberding, PA and Cohen, PT: Clinical Spectrum of HIV Infection. In Cohen, PT, Sande, MA, and Volberding, PA (eds): The AIDS Knowledge Base. Medical Publishing Group, Waltham, 1990.

CLASSIFICATION OF HIV INFECTION PROGRESSION BY GROUP DESIGNATION

Group I   Acute infection
Group II   Asymptomatic infection
Group III Persistent generalized
              lymphadenopathy
Group IV Appearance of other disease
             A. Constitutional
             B. Neurologic
             C. Secondary infection
                 1. Infectious diseases
                 2. Other specified diseases
             D. Secondary cancers
             E. Other conditions

BASED ON

Hart, M and Rogers, EA: Acquired Immunodeficiency Syndrome. In Fletcher, GF, et al (eds): Contemporary Clinical Perspectives. Lea & Febiger, Philadelphia, 1992, p 336.

SIGNS AND SYMPTOMS OF AIDS DEMENTIA COMPLEX

Early Signs of Dementia

Impaired cognition (mild to moderate)
Leg monoparesis
Leg paraparesis
Motor-verbal slowness
Normal mental status
Pyramidal tract signs
Tremor

Late Signs of Dementia

Ataxia
Dementia (moderate to severe)
Hemiparesis
Hypertonia
Incontinence
Mutism
Myoclonus
Organic psychosis (persistent and nonpersistent)
Paraparesis
Quadraparesis
Seizures

BASED ON

Hart, M and Rogers, EA: Acquired Immunodeficiency Syndrome. In Fletcher, GF, et al (eds): Contemporary Clinical Perspectives. Lea & Febiger, Philadelphia, 1992, p 345.

UNIVERSAL PRECAUTIONS*

OSHA Bloodborne Pathogens Standard

Who Is Covered?

The Occupational Safety and Health Administration (OSHA) standard protects employees who may be occupationally exposed to blood and other potential infectious materials, which includes but is not limited to physicians, nurses, phlebotomists, emergency medical personnel, operating room personnel, therapists, orderlies, laundry workers, and other health care workers.

Blood means human blood, blood products, or blood components. Other potentially infectious materials include human body fluids such as saliva in dental procedures, semen, vaginal secretions; cerebrospinal, synovial, pleural, pericardial, peritoneal, and amniotic fluids; body fluids visibly contaminated with blood; unfixed human tissues or organs; HIV-containing cell or tissue cultures; and HIV- or HBV-containing culture mediums or other solutions.

Occupational exposure means a "reasonably anticipated skin, eye, mucous membrane, or parenteral contact with blood or other potentially infectious materials that may result from the performance of the employee's duties."

Federal OSHA authority extends to all private sector employers with one or more employees, as well as federal civilian employees. In addition, many states administer their own occupational safety and health programs through plans approved under section 18(b) of the OSH Act. These plans must adopt standards and enforce requirements that are at least as effective as federal requirements. Of the current 25 state plan states and territories, 23 cover the private and public (state and local governments) sectors and 2 cover the public sector only.

Determining occupational exposure and instituting control methods and work practices appropriate for specific job assignments are key requirements of the standard. The required written exposure control plan and methods of compliance show how employee exposure can be minimized or eliminated.

The Exposure Control Plan

A written exposure control plan is necessary for the safety and health of workers. At a minimum, the plan must include the following:

- Identify job classifications where there is exposure to blood or other potentially infectious materials.
- Explain the protective measures currently in effect in the acute care facility and/or a schedule and methods of compliance to be implemented, including hepatitis B vaccination and post-exposure follow-up procedures; how hazards are communicated to employees; personal protective equipment; housekeeping; and recordkeeping.
- Establish procedures for evaluating the circumstances of an exposure incident.

The schedule of how and when the provisions of the standard will

---

* As appearing in Thomas, CL (ed): Taber's Cyclopedic Medical Dictionary, ed 18. FA Davis, Philadelphia, 1997, pp 2137–2143.

be implemented may be a simple calendar with brief notations describing the compliance methods, an annotated copy of the standard, or a part of another document, such as the infection control plan.

The written exposure control plan must be available to workers and OSHA representatives and updated at least annually or whenever changes in procedures create new occupational exposures.

Who Has Occupational Exposure?

The exposure determination must be based on the definition of occupational exposure **without regard to personal protective clothing and equipment.** Exposure determination begins by reviewing job classifications of employees within the work environment and then making a list divided into two groups: job classifications in which **all** of the employees have occupational exposure, and those classifications in which **some** of the employees have occupational exposure.

Where **all** employees are occupationally exposed, it is not necessary to list specific work tasks. Some examples include phlebotomists, lab technicians, physicians, nurses, nurse's aides, surgical technicians, and emergency room personnel.

Where only **some** of the employees have exposure, specific tasks and procedures causing exposure must be listed. Examples include ward clerks or secretaries who occasionally handle blood or infectious specimens, and housekeeping staff who may be exposed to contaminated objects and/or environments some of the time.

When employees with occupational exposure have been identified, the next step is to communicate the hazards of the exposure to the employees.

Communicating Hazards to Employees

The initial training for current employees must be scheduled within 90 days of the effective date of the bloodborne pathogens standard, at no cost to the employee, and during working hours.[1] Training also is required for new workers at the time of their initial assignment to tasks with occupational exposure or when job tasks change, causing occupational exposure, and annually thereafter.

Training sessions must be comprehensive in nature, including information on bloodborne pathogens as well as on OSHA regulations and the employer's exposure control plan. The person conducting the training must be knowledgeable in the subject matter as it relates to acute care facilities.

Specifically, the training program must do the following:

1. Explain the regulatory text and make a copy of the regulatory text accessible.
2. Explain the epidemiology and symptoms of bloodborne diseases.
3. Explain the modes of transmission of bloodborne pathogens.
4. Explain the employer's written exposure control plan.
5. Describe the methods to control transmission of HBV and HIV.

18

---

[1]Employees who received training in the year preceding the effective date of the standard need only receive training pertaining to any provisions not already included.

Continued on following page

6. Explain how to recognize occupational exposure.
7. Inform workers about the availability of free hepatitis B vaccinations, vaccine efficacy, safety, benefits, and administration.
8. Explain the emergency procedures for and reporting of exposure incidents.
9. Inform workers of the post-exposure evaluation and follow-up available from health care professionals.
10. Describe how to select, use, remove, handle, decontaminate, and dispose of personal protective clothing and equipment.
11. Explain the use and limitations of safe work practices, engineering controls, and personal protective equipment.
12. Explain the use of labels, signs, and color coding required by the standard.
13. Provide a question-and-answer session on training.

In addition to communicating hazards to employees and providing training to identify and control hazards, other preventive measures also must be taken to ensure employee protection.

Preventive Measures

Preventive measures such as hepatitis B vaccination, universal precautions, engineering controls, safe work practices, personal protective equipment, and housekeeping measures help reduce the risks of occupational exposure.

Hepatitis B Vaccination

The hepatitis B vaccination series must be made available within 10 working days of initial assignment to every employee who has occupatioinal exposure. The hepatitis B vaccination must be made available without cost to the employee, at a reasonable time and place for the employee, by a licensed health care professional,[2] and according to recommendations of the U.S. Public Health Service, including routine booster doses.[3]

The health care professional designated by the employer to implement this part of the standard must be provided with a copy of the bloodborne pathogens standard. The health care professional must provide the employer with a written opinion stating whether the hepatitis B vaccination is indicated for the employee and whether the employee has received such vaccination.

Employers are not required to offer hepatitis B vaccination (a) to employees who have previously completed the hepatitis B vaccination series, (b) when immunity is confirmed through antibody testing, or (c) if vaccine is contraindicated for medical reasons. Participation in a prescreening program is not a prerequisite for receiving

---

[2]Licensed health care professional is a person whose legally permitted scope of practice allows him or her to perform independently the activities required under paragraph (f) of the standard regarding hepatitis B vaccination and post-exposure and follow-up.

[3]Health care professionals can call the Centers for Disease Control disease information hotline (404) 332-4555, extension 234, for updated information on hepatitis B vaccination.

hepatitis B vaccination. Employees who decline the vaccination may request and obtain it at a later date, if they continue to be exposed. Employees who decline to accept the hepatitis B vaccination must sign a declination form, indicating that they were offered the vaccination but refused it.

Universal Precautions

The single most important measure to control transmission of HBV and HIV is to treat all human blood and other potentially infectious materials AS IF THEY WERE infectious for HBV and HIV. Application of this approach is referred to as "universal precautions." *Blood and certain body fluids from all acute care patients should be considered as potentially infectious materials.*[4] These fluids cause *contamination,* defined in the standard as "the presence or the reasonably anticipated presence of blood or other potentially infectious materials on an item or surface."

Methods of Control

Engineering and Work Practice Controls

Engineering and work practice controls are the primary methods used to control the transmission of HBV and HIV in acute care facilities. Engineering controls isolate or remove the hazard from employees and are used in conjunction with work practices. Personal protective equipment also shall be used when occupational exposure to bloodborne pathogens remains even after instituting these controls. Engineering controls must be examined and maintained, or replaced, on a scheduled basis. Some engineering controls that apply to acute care facilities and are required by the standard include the following:

1. Use puncture-resistant, leak-proof containers, color-coded red or labeled, according to the standard to discard contaminated items like needles, broken glass, scalpels, or other items that could cause a cut or puncture wound.
2. Use puncture-resistant, leak-proof containers, color-coded red or labeled to store contaminated reusable sharps until they are properly reprocessed.
3. Store and process reusable contaminated sharps in a way that ensures safe handling. For example, use a mechanical device to retrieve used instruments from soaking pans in decontamination areas.
4. Use puncture-resistant, leak-proof containers to collect, handle, process, store, transport, or ship blood specimens and potentially infectious materials. Label these specimens if shipped outside the facility. Labeling is not required when specimens are handled by employees trained to use universal precautions with all specimens and when these specimens are kept within the facility.

Similarly, work practice controls reduce the likelihood of exposure by altering the manner in which the task is performed. All pro-

18

---

[4]SEE ALSO: "Recommendations for Prevention of HIV Transmission in Health-Care Settings," *MMWR* (36) 2S: August 21, 1987.

Continued on following page

cedures shall minimize splashing, spraying, splattering, and generation of droplets. Work practice requirements include the following:

1. Wash hands when gloves are removed and as soon as possible after contact with blood or other potentially infectious materials.
2. Provide and make available a mechanism for immediate eye irrigation, in the event of an exposure incident.
3. Do not bend, recap, or remove contaminated needles unless required to do so by specific medical procedures or the employer can demonstrate that no alternative is feasible. In these instances, use mechanical means such as forceps, or a one-handed technique to recap or remove contaminated needles.
4. Do not shear or break contaminated needles.
5. Discard contaminated needles and sharp instruments in puncture-resistant, leak-proof, red or biohazard-labeled containers[5] that are accessible, maintained upright, and not allowed to be overfilled.
6. Do not eat, drink, smoke, apply cosmetics, or handle contact lenses in areas of potential occupational exposure. (Note: use of hand lotions is acceptable.)
7. Do not store food or drink in refrigerators or on shelves where blood or potentially infectious materials are present.
8. Use red, or affix biohazard labels to, containers to store, transport, or ship blood or other potentially infectious materials, such as lab specimens. (See figure below.)
9. Do not use mouth pipetting to suction blood or other potentially infectious materials; **it is prohibited.**

Personal Protective Equipment

In addition to instituting engineering and work practice controls, the standard requires that appropriate personal protective equip-

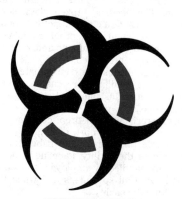

BIOHAZARD SYMBOL

---

[5]Biohazard labeling requires a fluorescent orange or orange-red label with the biological hazard symbol as well as the word **Biohazard** in contrasting color affixed to the bag or container.

ment be used to reduce worker risk of exposure. Personal protective equipment is specialized clothing or equipment used by employees to protect against direct exposure to blood or other potentially infectious materials. Protective equipment must not allow blood or other potentially infectious materials to pass through to workers' clothing, skin, or mucous membranes. Such equipment includes, but is not limited to, gloves, gowns, laboratory coats, face shields or masks, and eye protection.

The employer is responsible for providing, maintaining, laundering, disposing, replacing, and assuring the proper use of personal protective equipment. The employer is responsible for ensuring that workers have access to the protective equipment, at no cost, including proper sizes and types that take allergic conditions into consideration.

An employee may temporarily and briefly decline to wear personal protective equipment **under rare and extraordinary circumstances** and when, in the employee's professional judgment, it prevents the delivery of health care or public safety services or poses an increased or life-threatening hazard to employees. In general, **appropriate personal protective equipment is expected to be used whenever occupational exposure may occur.**

The employer also must ensure that employees observe the following precautions for safely handling and using personal protective equipment.

1. Remove all personal protective equipment immediately following contamination and upon leaving the work area, and place in an appropriately designated area or container for storing, washing, decontaminating, or discarding.
2. Wear appropriate gloves when contact with blood, mucous membranes, non-intact skin, or potentially infectious materials is anticipated; when performing vascular access procedures;[6] and when handling or touching contaminated items or surfaces.
3. Provide hypoallergenic gloves, liners, or powderless gloves or other alternatives to employees who need them.
4. Replace disposable, single-use gloves as soon as possible when contaminated, or if torn, punctured, or barrier function is compromised.
5. Do not reuse disposable (single-use) gloves.
6. Decontaminate reusable (utility) gloves after each use and discard if they show signs of cracking, peeling, tearing, puncturing, deteriorating, or failing to provide a protective barrier.
7. Use full face shields or face masks with eye protection, goggles, or eyeglasses with side shields when splashes of blood and other bodily fluids may occur and when contamination of the eyes, nose, or mouth can be anticipated (e.g., during invasive and surgical procedures).
8. Also wear surgical caps or hoods and/or shoe covers or boots when gross contamination may occur, such as during surgery and autopsy procedures.

18

---

[6]Phlebotomists in volunteer blood donation centers are exempt in certain circumstances. See section (d)(3)(ix)(D) of the standard for specific details.

Continued on following page

Remember: The selection of appropriate personal protective equipment depends on the quantity and type of exposure expected.

Housekeeping Procedures

EQUIPMENT

The employer must ensure a clean and sanitary workplace. Contaminated work surfaces must be decontaminated with a disinfectant upon completion of procedures or when contaminated by splashes, spills, or contact with blood, other potentially infectious materials, and at the end of the work shift. Surfaces and equipment protected with plastic wrap, foil, or other nonabsorbent materials must be inspected frequently for contamination; and these protective coverings must be changed when found to be contaminated.

Waste cans and pails must be inspected and decontaminated on a regularly scheduled basis. Broken glass should be cleaned up with a brush or tongs; never pick up broken glass with hands, even when wearing gloves.

WASTE

Waste removed from the facility is regulated by local and state laws. Special precautions are necessary when disposing of contaminated sharps and other contaminated waste, and include the following:

1. Dispose of contaminated sharps in closable, puncture-resistant, leak-proof, red or biohazard-labeled containers.
2. Place other regulated waste[7] in closable, leak-proof, red or biohazard-labeled bags or containers. If outside contamination of the regulated waste container occurs, place it in a second container that is closable, leak-proof, and appropriately labeled.

LAUNDRY

Laundering contaminated articles, including employee lab coats and uniforms meant to function as personal protective equipment, is the responsibility of the employer. Contaminated laundry shall be handled as little as possible with minimum agitation. This can be accomplished through the use of a washer and dryer in a designated area on-site, or the contaminated items can be sent to a commercial laundry. The following requirements should be met with respect to contaminated laundry:

1. Bag contaminated laundry as soon as it is removed and store in a designated area or container.
2. Use red laundry bags or those marked with the biohazard symbol unless universal precautions are in effect in the facility and all employees recognize the bags as contaminated and have been trained in handling the bags.

---

[7]Liquid or semiliquid blood or other potentially infectious materials; items contaminated with these fluids and materials, which could release these substances in a liquid or semiliquid state, if compressed; items caked with dried blood or other potentially infectious materials that are capable of releasing these materials during handling; contaminated sharps; and pathological and microbiological wastes containing blood or other potentially infectious materials.

3. Clearly mark laundry sent off-site for cleaning, by placing it in red bags or bags clearly marked witht he orange biohazard symbol; and use leak-proof bags to prevent soak-through.
4. Wear gloves or other protective equipment when handling contaminated laundry.

What to Do if an Exposure Incident Occurs

An exposure incident is the specific eye, mouth or other mucous membrane, non-intact skin, parenteral contact with blood or other potentially infectious materials that results from the performance of an employee's duties. An example of an exposure incident would be a puncture from a contaminated sharp.

The employer is responsible for establishing the procedure for evaluating exposure incidents.

When evaluating an exposure incident, immediate assessment and confidentiality are critical issues. Employees should immediately report exposure incidents to enable timely medical evaluation and follow-up by a health care professional as well as a prompt request by the employer for testing of the source individual's blood for HIV and HBV. The "source individual" is any patient whose blood or body fluids are the source of an exposure incident to the employee.

At the time of the exposure incident, the exposed employee must be directed to a health care professional. The employer must provide the health care professional with a copy of the bloodborne pathogens standard; a description of the employee's job duties as they relate to the incident; a report of the specific exposure, including route of exposure; relevant employee medical records, including hepatitis B vaccination status; and results of the source individual's blood tests, if available. At that time, a baseline blood sample should be drawn from the employee, if he/she consents. If the employee elects to delay HIV testing of the sample, the health care professional must preserve the employee's blood sample for at least 90 days.[8]

Testing the source individual's blood does not need to be repeated if the source individual is known to be infectious for HIV or HBV; and testing cannot be done in most states without written consent.[9] The results of the source individual's blood tests are confidential. As soon as possible, however, the test results of the source individual's blood must be made available to the exposed employee through consultation with the health care professional.

Following post-exposure evaluation, the health care professional will provide a written opinion to the employer. This opinion is limited to a statement that the employee has been informed of the results of the evaluation and told of the need, if any, for any further evaluation or treatment. The employer must provide a copy of the

18

---

[8]If, during this time, the employee elects to have the baseline sample tested, testing shall be performed as soon as feasible.

[9]If consent is not obtained, the employer must show that legally required consent could not be obtained. Where consent is not required by law, the source individual's blood, if available, should be tested and the results documented.

Continued on following page

written opinion to the employee within 15 days. This is the only information shared with the employer following an exposure incident; all other employee medical records are confidential.

All evaluations and follow-up must be available at no cost to the employee and at a reasonable time and place, performed by or under the supervision of a licensed physician or another licensed health care professional, such as a nurse practitioner, and according to recommendations of the U.S. Public Health Service guidelines current at the time of the evaluation and procedure. In addition, all laboratory tests must be conducted by an accredited laboratory and at no cost to the employee.

Recordkeeping

There are two types of records required by the bloodborne pathogens standard: medical and training.

A medical record must be established for each employee with occupational exposure. **This record is confidential and separate from other personnel records.** This record may be kept on-site or may be retained by the health care professional who provides services to employees. The medical record contains the employee's name, social security number, hepatitis B vaccination status, including the dates of vaccination and the written opinion of the health care professional regarding the hepatitis B vaccination. If an occupational exposure occurs, reports are added to the medical record to document the incident and the results of testing following the incident. The post-evaluation written opinion of the health care professional is also part of the medical record. The medical record also must document what information has been provided to the health care provider. Medical records must be maintained 30 years past the last date of employment of the employee.

Emphasis is on confidentiality of medical records. No medical record or part of a medical record should be disclosed without direct, written consent of the employee or as required by law.

Training records document each training session and are to be kept for 3 years. Training records must include the date, content outline, trainer's name and qualifications, and names and job titles of all persons attending the training sessions.

If the employer ceases to do business, medical and training records are transferred to the successor employer. If there is no successor employer, the employer must notify the Director of the National Institute for Occupational Safety and Health, U.S. Department of Health and Human Services, for specific directions regarding disposition of the records at least 3 months prior to disposal.

Upon request, both medical and training records must be made available to the Assistant Secretary of Labor of Occupational Safety and Health. Training records must be available to employees upon request. Medical records can be obtained by the employee or anyone having the employee's written consent.

Additional recordkeeping is required for employers with 11 or more employees (see OSHA's "Recordkeeping Guidelines for Occupational Injuries and Illnesses" for more information).

Other Sources of OSHA Assistance

CONSULTATION PROGRAMS

Consultation assistance is available to employers who want help in establishing and maintaining a safe and healthful workplace. Largely funded by OSHA, the service is provided at no cost to the employer. Primarily developed for smaller employers with more hazardous operations, the consultation service is delivered by state government agencies or universities employing professional safety consultants and health consultants. Comprehensive assistance includes an appraisal of all mechanical, physical work practice, and environmental hazards of the workplace and all aspects of the employer's present job safety and health program. No penalties are proposed or citations issued for hazards identified by the consultant.

VOLUNTARY PROTECTION PROGRAMS .

Voluntary protection programs (VPPs) and on-site consultation services, when coupled with an effective enforcement program, expand worker protection to help meet the goals of the OSH Act. The three VPPs—Star, Merit, and Demonstration—are designed to recognize outstanding achievement by companies that have successfully incorporated comprehensive safety and health programs into their total management system. They motivate others to achieve excellent safety and health results in the same outstanding way, and they establish a cooperative relationship between employers, employees, and OSHA.

TRAINING AND EDUCATION

OSHA's area offices offer a variety of informational services, such as publications, audiovisual aids, technical advice, and speakers for special engagements. Each regional office has a bloodborne pathogens coordinator to assist employers.

OSHA's Training Institute in Des Plaines, IL, provides basic and advanced courses in safety and health for federal and state compliance officers, state consultants, federal agency personnel, and private sector employers, employees, and their representatives.

OSHA also provides funds to nonprofit organizations, through grants, to conduct workplace training and education in subjects where OSHA believes there is a lack of workplace training. Current grant subjects include agricultural safety and health, hazard communication programs, and HIV and HBV. Grants are awarded annually, with a 1-year renewal possible. Grant recipients are expected to contribute 20 percent of the total grant cost.

For more information on grants, and training and education, contact the OSHA Training Institute, Office of Training and Education, 1555 Time Drive, Des Plaines, IL 60018, (708) 297-4810.

For more information on AIDS, contact the Centers for Disease Control National AIDS Clearinghouse, (800) 458-5231.

FROM

Thomas, CL (ed): Taber's Cyclopedic Medical Dictionary, ed 18. FA Davis, Philadelphia, 1997, pp 2137–2143. Source: Bloodborne Pathogens and Acute Care Facilities (OSHA 3128), Occupational Safety and Health Administration, Washington, DC, 1992.

DRUG TREATMENT OF OPPORTUNISTIC INFECTIONS IN PATIENTS WITH AIDS

Organism	Type of Infection	Drug Treatment*
Viral infections		
Cytomegalovirus	Pneumonia; hepatitis; chorioretinitis; involvement of many other organs	Foscarnet, ganciclovir
Herpes simplex	Unusually severe vesicular and necrotizing lesions of mucocutaneous areas and GI tract	Acyclovir
HIV	Infections of CNS and peripheral nerves; immune thrombocytopenic purpura; lymphadenopathy; other infections	Zidovudine, zalcitabine, didanosine
Varicella-zoster	Painful, vesicular eruption of skin according to dermatomal boundaries (shingles)	Acyclovir, vidarabine
Bacterial infections		
Mycobacterium avium complex	Involvement of bone marrow, reticuloendothelial tissues	Combination therapy using isoniazid, ethambutol, clofazimine, clarithromycin, and other antibacterials

Mycobacterium tuberculosis	Tuberculosis	Combination therapy using isoniazid, rifampin, and other drugs
Fungal infections		
Candida	Oral candidiasis; esophagitis; systemic infections	Clotrimazole, fluconazole, ketoconazole, nystatin
Cryptococcus	Meningoencephalitis	Amphotericin B, fluconazole
Protozoal infections		
Pneumocystis carinii	Pneumonia	Trimethoprim-sulfamethoxazole, pentamidine
Toxoplasma	CNS infections (cerebral degeneration meningoencephalitis)	Pyrimethamine and sulfadiazine

CNS = central nervous system.

*Choice of specific drugs varies according to disease status, presence of other infections, and so forth. Pharmacotherapeutic rationale is also changing constantly as new agents are developed and tested.

From Ciccone, CD: Pharmacology in Rehabilitation, ed 2. FA Davis, Philadelphia, 1996, p 542, with permission.

18

HIV AND AIDS GLOSSARY

acquired immunodeficiency syndrome (AIDS): The most severe manifestation of infection with the human immunodeficiency virus (HIV). The Centers for Disease Control and Prevention (CDC) list numerous opportunistic infections and neoplasms (cancers) that, in the presence of HIV infection, constitute an AIDS diagnosis. In addition, a CD4+ T-cell count below 200/mm³ in the presence of HIV infection constitutes an AIDS diagnosis. The period between infection with HIV and the onset of AIDS averages 10 y in the United States. People with AIDS often suffer infections of the lungs, brain, eyes, and other organs, and frequently suffer debilitating weight loss, diarrhea, and a type of cancer called Kaposi's sarcoma. Even with treatment, most people with AIDS die within 2 y of developing infections or cancers that take advantage of their weakened immune systems.

acute HIV infection: As related to HIV infection: Once the virus enters the body, HIV infects a large number of CD4+ T cells and replicates rapidly. During this acute or primary phase of infection, the blood contains many viral particles that spread throughout the body, seeding themselves in various organs, particularly the lymphoid tissues.

acute retroviral syndrome: The acute or primary HIV infection often passes unrecognized, but may be present as a mononucleosis-like syndrome within 3 mo of the infection. The diagnosis is made by demonstrating HIV antibody seroconversion.

affected community: This includes HIV-positive people, persons living with AIDS and other individuals, including their families, friends, and advocates, directly impacted by HIV infection and its physical, psychologic, and sociologic ramifications.

AIDS bibliography: The National Library of Medicine (NLM) publishes the monthly *AIDS Bibliography,* which includes all citations from the AIDSLINE database. The *AIDS Bibliography* is available from the Superintendent of Documents (Phone: 202-783-3238).

AIDS clinical trials group (ACTG): The ACTG is composed of a number of U.S. medical centers that evaluate treatment for HIV and HIV-associated infections. ACTG studies are sponsored by the National Institute of Allergy and Infectious Diseases (NIAID).

AIDS dementia complex: About half the people infected with HIV, the virus that causes AIDS, develop infections or other problems involving the brain or spinal cord. These neurologic complications may include inflammation of the brain (encephalitis), or of the membrane surrounding the brain (meningitis), infections of the brain, brain or spinal cord tumors, nerve damage, difficulties in thinking and behavioral changes (i.e., AIDS dementia complex), and stroke.

AIDSDRUGS: An online database service administered by the NLM, with references to drugs undergoing testing against AIDS, AIDS-related complex, and related opportunistic infections.

AIDS education and training centers (AETC): The Health Resources and Services Administration supports a network of 15 regional centers that serve as resources for educating health professionals in prevention, diagnosis, and care of HIV-infected patients. The centers train primary caregivers to incorporate HIV prevention strategies into their clinical priorities, along with diagnosis, counseling, and care of HIV-infected persons and their families.

AIDSKNOWLEDGE base: Full-text electronic database on AIDS, available in print as well as in electronic form, produced and maintained by physicians and other health-care professionals. The database is edited by P. T. Cohen (San Francisco General Hospital), Merle Sande, and Paul Volberding.

AIDSLINE: An online database service administered by the NLM, with citations and abstracts covering the published scientific and medical literature on AIDS and related topics.

AIDS-related cancers: Several cancers are more common or more aggressive in people infected with HIV, the virus that causes AIDS. These malignancies include certain types of immune system cancers known as lymphomas, Kaposi's sarcoma, and anogenital cancers primarily affecting the cervix and the anus. HIV, or the immune suppression it induces, appears to play a role in the development of these cancers.

AIDS-related complex (ARC): (1) A term, not officially defined or recognized by the CDC, that has been used to describe a variety of symptoms and signs found in some persons infected with HIV. These may include recurrent fevers, unexplained weight loss, swollen lymph nodes, and/or fungus infection of the mouth and throat. Also commonly described as symptomatic HIV infection. (2) Symptoms that appear to be related to infection by the HIV virus. They include an unexplained, chronic deficiency of white blood cells (leukopenia) or a poorly functioning lymphatic system with swelling of the lymph nodes (lymphadenopathy) lasting for more than 3 mo without the opportunistic infections required for a diagnosis of AIDS.

AIDS research advisory committee: Board that advises and makes recommendations to the Director, NIAID, on all aspects of HIV-related research, vaccine development, pathogenesis, and epidemiology.

AIDS service organization (ASO): A health association, support agency, or other service active in the prevention and treatment of AIDS.

AIDSTRIALS: An online database service administered by the NLM, with information about clinical trials of agents under evaluation against HIV infection, AIDS, and related opportunistic infections.

alternative therapy: In Western countries, alternative therapy refers to any type of medicine that supplements or is used in lieu of biomedicine (i.e., conventional medicine) or allopathic medicine. In other parts of the world, where traditional medicine predominates, the term may refer to biomedicine itself.

anergy: (1) The loss or weakening of the body's immunity to an irritating agent, or antigen. The strength of the body's immune response is often quantitatively measured by means of a skin test where a solution containing an antigen known to cause a response, such as mumps or candidae infection, is injected immediately under the skin. The lack of a reaction to these common antigens indicates anergy. (2) Researchers in cell culture have shown that CD4+ T cells can be

Continued on following page

turned off by a signal from HIV that leaves them unable to respond to further immune system stimulation. This inactivated state is known as anergy.

antibodies: Molecules in the blood or secretory fluids that tag, destroy, or neutralize bacteria, viruses, or other harmful toxins. They are members of a class of proteins known as immunoglobulins, which are produced and secreted by B lymphocytes in response to stimulation by antigens. An antibody is specific to an antigen.

antibody-dependent cell-mediated cytotoxicity (ADCC): An immune response in which antibodies bind to target cells, identifying them for attack by the immune system.

antigen: A substance that, when introduced into the body, is capable of inducing the production of a specific antibody.

assembly and budding: Names for a portion of the processes by which new HIV virus is formed in infected host cells. Viral core proteins, enzymes, and RNA gather just inside the cell's membrane, while the viral envelope proteins aggregate within the membrane. An immature viral particle is formed and then pinches off from the cell, acquiring an envelope and the cellular and HIV proteins from the cell membrane. The immature viral particle then undergoes processing by an HIV enzyme called protease to become an infectious virus.

asymptomatic: Without symptoms. Usually used in AIDS literature to describe a person who has a positive reaction to one of several tests for HIV antibodies, but who shows no clinical symptoms of the disease.

attenuated: Weakened or decreased. For example, an attenuated virus can no longer produce disease, but might be used to produce a vaccine.

autoantibody: (1) An antibody that is active against some of the tissues of the organism that produced it. (2) An antibody directed against the body's own tissue.

AZT: Azidothymidine (also called zidovudine or ZDV; the Burroughs-Wellcome trade name is Retrovir). One of the first drugs used against HIV infection, AZT is a nucleoside analogue that suppresses replication of HIV.

B lymphocytes (B cells): One of the two major classes of lymphocytes. During infections, these cells are transformed into plasma cells that produce large quantities of antibody directed at specific pathogens. This transformation occurs through interactions with various types of T cells and other components of the immune system. In persons with AIDS, the functional ability of both the B and the T lymphocytes is damaged, with the T lymphocytes being the principal site of infection by the HIV virus. See T cells.

body fluids: Any fluid in the human body, such as blood, urine, saliva, sputum (spit), tears, semen, mother's milk, or vaginal secretions. Only blood, semen, mother's milk, and vaginal secretions have been linked directly to the transmission of the HIV virus.

breakthrough infection: An infection, caused by the infectious agent the vaccine is designed to protect against, that occurs during the course of a vaccine trial. These infections may be caused by exposure to the infectious agent before the vaccine has taken effect, or before all doses of the vaccine have been given. Breakthrough infections also occur in trial participants receiving placebos.

CD4 (T4) or CD4+ cells: (1) White blood cells killed or disabled during HIV infection. These cells normally orchestrate the immune response, signaling other cells in the immune system to perform their special functions. Also known as helper T cells. (2) HIV's preferred targets are cells that have a docking molecule called cluster designation 4 (CD4) on their surfaces. Cells with this molecule are known as CD4-positive (or CD4+) cells. Destruction of CD4+ lymphocytes is the major cause of the immunodeficiency observed in AIDS, and decreasing CD4+ lymphocyte levels appear to be the best indicator of morbidity in these patients. Although CD4 counts fall, the total T-cell level remains fairly constant through the course of HIV disease, due to a concomitant increase in the CD8+ cells. The ratio of CD4+ to CD8+ cells is therefore an important measure of disease progression.

CD8 (T8) cells: A protein embedded in the cell surface of suppressor T lymphocytes. Also called cytotoxic T cells.

CD nomenclature: This nomenclature was developed to standardize and compare monoclonal antibodies from different sources. Antibodies with similar reactivity patterns are assigned to CD groups representing "clusters of differentiation." T lymphocytes are CD3+ and can be separated into the CD4+ helper T cells and the CD8+ cytotoxic/suppressor cells. Although CD4+ cells are predominantly T lymphocytes, some monocytes are also CD4+.

CDC National AIDS Clearinghouse (CDC NAC): The CDC's comprehensive reference, referral and publication distribution service for HIV and AIDS information. The clearinghouse works in partnership with national, regional, state, and local organizations that develop and deliver HIV prevention programs and services.

cell lines: Specific cell types artificially maintained in the laboratory (i.e., in vitro) for scientific purposes.

cell-mediated immunity (CMI): The branch of the immune system in which the reaction to foreign material is performed by specific defense cells (i.e., killer cells, macrophages, and other white blood cells) rather than antibodies.

Centers for Disease Control and Prevention (CDC): A Public Health Service agency responsible (among others) for assessing the status and characteristics of the AIDS epidemic and the prevalence of HIV infections. CDC supports the design, implementation, and evaluation of prevention activities and maintains various HIV and AIDS information services, such as the CDC NAC.

central nervous system (CNS): Composed of the brain, spinal cord, and its coverings (meninges).

CNS damage: (By HIV infection). Although monocytes and macrophages can be infected by HIV, they appear to be relatively resistant to killing. However, these cells travel throughout the body and carry HIV to various organs, especially the lungs and the brain. People infected with HIV often experience abnormalities in the CNS.

Continued on following page

Investigators have hypothesized that an accumulation of HIV in brain and nerve cells or the inappropriate relase of cytokines or toxic byproducts by these cells may be to blame for the neurologic manifestations of HIV disease.

clinical latency: The state or period of an infectious agent, such as a virus or bacterium, living or developing in a host without producing clinical symptoms. As related to HIV infection: Although infected individuals usually exhibit a period of clinical latency with little evidence of disease, the virus is never truly latent. Even early in the disease, HIV is active within lymphoid organs where large amounts of virus become trapped in the FDC network. Surrounding germinal centers are areas rich in CD4+ T cells. These cells increasingly become infected and viral particles accumulate both in infected cells and as free virus.

compassionate use: A method of providing experimental drugs to very sick patients who have no other treatment options. Often, case-by-case approval must be obtained from the Food and Drug Administration (FDA) for "compassionate use" of a drug.

contagious: Any infectious disease capable of being transmitted by casual contact from one person to another. Casual contact can be defined as normal day-to-day contact between people at home, school, work, or in the community. A contagious infection (e.g., a common cold) can be communicable by casual contact; an infectious infection, on the other hand, is communicable by intimate contact such as sex. AIDS is infectious, not contagious.

core protein: As related to HIV: An integral protein of the HIV virus composed of three units, p24, p15, and p18.

DDC: Dideoxycytidine (zalcitabine, HIVID), a nucleoside analogue drug that inhibits the replication of HIV.

DDI: Dideoxyinosine (didanosine, Videx), a nucleoside analogue drug that inhibits the replication of HIV.

d4T: (Also known as Stavudine and Zerit). d4T is a dideoxynucleoside pyrimidine analogue (2'3'-didehydro-3'-deoxythymidine). Like other nucleoside analogues, d4T inhibits HIV replication by inducing premature viral DNA chain termination. d4T has been approved for patients with advanced HIV infection intolerant to or failing other antiretroviral drugs.

deoxyribonucleic acid (DNA): 1) The molecular chain found in genes within the nucleus of each cell, which carries the genetic information that enables cells to reproduce. 2) DNA is the principal constituent of chromosomes, the structures that transmit hereditary characteristics. The amount of DNA is constant for all typical cells of any given species of plant or animal (including humans), regardless of the size or function of that cell. Each DNA molecule is a long, two-stranded chain made up of subunits, called nucleotides, containing a sugar (deoxyribose), a phosphate group, and one of four nitrogenous bases: adenine (A), guanine (G), thymine (T), and cytosine (C). In 1953 J. D. Watson and F. H. Crick proposed that the strands, connected by hydrogen bonds between the bases, were coiled in a double helix. Adenine bonds only with thymine (A—T or T—A) and guanine only with cytosine (G—C or C—G). The complementarity of this bonding ensures that DNA can be replicated (i.e., that identical copies can be made in order to transmit genetic information to the next generation).

ELISA: (Enzyme-Linked Immunosorbent Assay). A laboratory test to determine the presence of antibodies to HIV in the blood. A positive ELISA test generally is confirmed by the Western Blot test.

epidemic: A disease that spreads rapidly through a demographic segment of the human population, such as everyone in a given geographic area, a military base, or similar population unit, or everyone of a certain age or sex, such as the children or women of a region. Epidemic diseases can be spread from person to person or from a contaminated source such as food or water.

GP41: Glycoprotein 41, a protein embedded in the outer envelope of HIV. Plays a key role in HIV's infection of CD4+ T cells by facilitating the fusion of the viral and the cell membranes.

GP120: Glycoprotein 120, a protein that protrudes from the surface of HIV and binds to CD4+ T cells.

GP160: Glycoprotein 160, a precursor of HIV envelope proteins gp41 and gp120.

helper T cells: See *CD4 (T4) or CD4+ cells.*

hemophilia: An inherited disease that prevents the normal clotting of blood.

hepatitis: An inflammation of the liver caused by certain viruses and other factors such as alcohol abuse, some medications, and trauma. Although many cases of hepatitis are not a serious threat to health, the disease can become chronic and can sometimes lead to liver failure and death. There are four major types of viral hepatitis: (a) *hepatitis A,* caused by infection with the hepatitis A virus; (b) *hepatitis B,* caused by infection with the hepatitis B virus (HBV), which is most commonly passed on to a partner during intercourse, especially during anal sex, as well as through sharing drug needles; (c) *non-A, non-B hepatitis,* caused by the hepatitis C virus, which appears to be spread through sexual contact as well as through sharing drug needles (another type of non-A, non-B hepatitis is caused by the hepatitis E virus, principally spread through contaminated water); (d) *delta hepatitis* occurs only in people who are already infected with HBV and is caused by the HDV virus; most cases of delta hepatitis occur among people who are frequently exposed to blood and blood products such as people with hemophilia.

18

HIV disease: An infectious disease characterized by a gradual deterioration of immune function. During the course of infection, crucial immune cells called CD4+ T cells are disabled and killed, and their numbers progressively decline. CD4+ T cells play a crucial role in the immune response, signaling other cells in the immune system to perform their special functions.

human immunodeficiency virus type 1 (HIV-1): (1) The retrovirus isolated and recognized as the etiologic (i.e., causing or contributing to the cause of a disease) agent of AIDS. HIV-1 is classified as a lentivirus in a subgroup of retroviruses. See also *lentivirus; retrovirus.* (2) Most viruses and all bacteria, plants, and animals have genetic

Continued on following page

codes made up of DNA, which uses RNA to build specific proteins. The genetic material of a retrovirus such as HIV is the RNA itself. HIV inserts its own RNA into the host cell's DNA, preventing the host cell from carrying out its natural functions and turning it into an HIV virus factory.

human immunodeficiency virus type 2 (HIV-2): A virus closely related to HIV-1 that has been found to cause immune suppression. Most common in Africa.

human leukocyte antigens (HLA): Markers that identify cells as "self" and prevent the immune system from attacking them.

human papillomavirus (HPV): A virus that is the cause of warts of the hands and feet, as well as lesions of the mucous membranes of the oral, anal, and genital cavities. More than 50 types of HPV have been identified, some of which are associated with cancerous and precancerous conditions. The virus can be transmitted through sexual contact and is a precursor to cancer of the cervix. There is no specific cure for an HPV infection, but the virus often can be controlled by podophyllin (medicine derived from the roots of the plant *Podophyllum peltatum*) or interferon, and the warts can be removed by cryosurgery, laser treatment, or conventional surgery.

immune complex: Clusters formed when antigens and antibodies bind together.

immune deficiency: A breakdown or inability of certain parts of the immune system to function, thus making a person susceptible to certain diseases that they would not ordinarily develop.

immune system: The complex functions of the body that recognize foreign agents or substances, neutralize them, and recall the response later when confronted with the same challenge.

immune thrombocytopenic purpura (ITP): Also idiopathic immune thrombocytopenic purpura. A condition in which the body produces antibodies against the platelets in the blood, which are cells responsible for blood clotting. ITP is very common in HIV-infected people.

immunity: A natural or acquired resistance to a specific disease. Immunity may be partial or complete, long lasting or temporary.

immunocompetent: 1) Capable of developing an immune response. 2) Possessing a normal immune system.

immunodeficiency: A deficiency of immune response or a disorder characterized by deficient immune response; classified as antibody (B cell), cellular (T cell), combined deficiency, or phagocytic dysfunction disorders.

immunogen: A substance, also called an antigen, capable of provoking an immune response.

immunogenicity: The ability of an antigen or vaccine to stimulate an immune response.

immunomodulator: Any substance that influences the immune system.

immunostimulant: Any agent or substance that triggers or enhances the body's defense; also called immunopotentiators.

immunosuppression: A state of the body in which the immune system is damaged and does not perform its normal functions. Immunosuppression may be induced by drugs or result from certain disease processes, such as HIV infection.

immunotherapy: Treatment aimed at reconstituting an impaired immune system.

immunotoxin: A plant or animal toxin (i.e., poison) that is attached to a monoclonal antibody and used to destroy a specific target cell.

interferon: A general term used to describe a family of 20–25 proteins that cause a cell to become resistant to a wide variety of viruses. They are produced by cells infected by almost any virus.

interleukin-2 (IL-2): One of a family of molecules that control the growth and function of many types of lymphocytes. IL-2 is an immune system protein produced in the body by T cells. It has potent effects on the proliferation, differentiation, and activity of a number of immune system cells, including T cells, B cells, and natural killer cells. Commercially, IL-2 is produced by recombinant DNA technology and is approved by the FDA for the treatment of metastatic renal (i.e., kidney) cell cancer. Studies have shown that in the test tube, addition of IL-2 can improve some of the immunologic functions that are abnormal in HIV-infected patients. In addition, IL-2 is a growth factor for T cells, causing them to increase in number. In a clinical study with IL-2, it was found that in a small number of HIV-infected patients, IL-2 boosted levels of CD4+ T cells (i.e., the infection-fighting white blood cells normally destroyed during HIV infection) for more than 2 years, a far longer time than typically seen with currently available anti-HIV drugs.

investigational new drug (IND): The status of an experimental drug after the FDA agrees that it can be tested in people.

Kaposi's sarcoma: (1) A previously uncommon form of cancer that attacks the connective tissue, bones, cartilage, and muscles of the body. The cancer may spread and also attack the eyes. If the cancerous area is near the surface of the skin, lesions inches in length may develop. This disease was initially seen only in elderly men and natives of Central Africa. Experimental work has shown that the AIDS-related Kaposi's sarcoma and the Central African variety respond differently to some types of medications. Radiotherapy and chemotherapy are usually recommended. (2) A type of cancer characterized by abnormal growths of blood vessels that develop into purplish or brown lesions. It is suspected that the cause of Kaposi's sarcoma is a newly found herpesvirus.

lentivirus: "Slow" virus characterized by a long interval between infection and the onset of symptoms. HIV is a lentivirus as is the simian immunodeficiency virus (SIV), which infects nonhuman primates.

long-term nonprogressors: Individuals who are HIV-infected for 7 or more years, have stable CD4+ T-cell counts of 600 or more cells per cubic millimeter of blood, no HIV-related diseases, and no previous antiretroviral therapy. Data suggest that this phenomenon is associated with the maintenance of the integrity of the lymphoid tissues

Continued on following page

18

and with less virus-trapping in the lymph nodes than seen in other individuals infected with HIV.

long terminal repeat sequence (LTR): A component of the AIDS genome.

lymphadenopathy syndrome (LAS): Swollen, firm, and possibly tender lymph nodes. The cause may range from an infection such as HIV, the flu, mononucleosis, or lymphoma (cancer of the lymph nodes).

lymphocyte: A white blood cell. Present in the blood, lymph, and lymphoid tissue.

mutation: In biology, a sudden change in a gene or unit of hereditary material that results in a new inheritable characteristic. In higher animals and many higher plants, a mutation may be transmitted to future generations only if it occurs in germ—or sex cell—tissue; body cell mutations cannot be inherited. Changes within the chemical structure of single genes may be induced by exposure to radiation, temperature extremes, and certain chemicals. The term mutation may also be used to include losses or rearrangements of segments of chromosomes, the long strands of genes. Drugs such as colchicine double the normal number of chromosomes in a cell by interfering with cell division. Mutation, which can establish new traits in a population, is important in evolution. As related to HIV: HIV mutates rapidly. During the course of HIV disease, viral strains may emerge in an infected individual that differ widely in their ability to infect and kill different cell types, as well as in their rate of replication. Strains of HIV from patients with advanced disease appear to be more virulent and infect more cell types than strains obtained earlier from the same individual.

mycobacterium: Any bacterium of the genus *Mycobacterium* or a closely related genus.

***Mycobacterium avium* complex (MAC):** (1) A common opportunistic infection caused by two very similar mycobacterial organisms, *Mycobacterium avium* and *Mycobacterium intracellulare*. (2) A bacterial infection that can be localized (limited to a specific organ or area of the body) or disseminated throughout the body. It is a life-threatening disease, although new therapies offer promise for both prevention and treatment. MAC disease is extremely rare in people who are not infected with HIV.

mycoplasma: (1) Smallest free-living organisms known to infect humans. Mycoplasma cause a variety of illnesses, especially of the lungs and sexual organs. (2) Any microorganism of the genus *Mycoplasma,* also called *pleuropneumonia-like* organism.

natural killer cells: (NK cells). A type of lymphocyte that does not carry the markers to be B cells or T cells. Like cytotoxic T cells, they attack and kill tumor cells and protect against a wide variety of infectious microbes. They are "natural" killers because they do not need additional stimulation or need to recognize a specific antigen in order to attack and kill. Persons with immunodeficiencies such as those caused by HIV infection have a decrease in NK cell activity.

nef: One of the regulatory genes of the HIV virus. Three HIV regulatory genes—tat, rev, and nef—and three so-called auxiliary genes—

vif, vpr, and vpu—contain information necessary for the production of proteins that control the virus's ability to infect a cell, produce new copies of the virus or cause disease.

null cell: A lymphocyte that develops in the bone marrow and lacks the characteristic surface markers of the B and T lymphocytes. Null cells represent a small proportion of the lymphocyte population. Stimulated by the presence of antibody, null cells can attack certain cellular targets directly and are known as "natural killer" or NK cells.

opportunistic infection: (1) An illness caused by an organism that usually does not cause disease in a person with a normal immune system. People with advanced HIV infection suffer opportunistic infections of the lungs, brain, eyes, and other organs. (2) Opportunistic infections common in AIDS patients include *Pneumocystis carinii* pneumonia (PCP); Kaposi's sarcoma; shigellosis; histoplasmosis; and other parasitic, viral, and fungal infections, and some types of cancers.

p24: (1) Within the envelope of the HIV virus is a bullet-shaped core made of another protein, p24, that surrounds the viral RNA. (2) The p24 antigen test looks for the presence of this protein in a patient's blood. (3) A positive result for the p24 antigen suggests active HIV replication. p24 found in the peripheral blood is thought to also correlate with the amount of virus in the peripheral blood. It is believed that there are measurable levels of p24 when first infected with the virus after which there is a strong antibody response to p24 in early disease. Low or unmeasurable levels of p24 may indicate that the virus is in a dormant stage. Spikes in p24 levels may indicate that HIV has begun active replication.

pandemic: A disease prevalent throughout an entire country, continent, or the whole world.

pentamidine: An approved antiprotozoal drug used for the treatment and prevention of PCP infection. It can be delivered intravenously or intramuscularly or inhaled as an aerosol. Aerosolized pentamidine is approved for the prophylaxis of PCP in HIV-positive individuals with CD4+ counts below $200/mm^3$ or for those with prior episodes of PCP. The drug is also known under the names Pentam and NebuPent.

Pneumocystis carinii **pneumonia (PCP):** (1) A protozoal infection of the lungs. (2) A life-threatening lung infection that can affect people with weakened immune systems, such as those infected with HIV. More than three quarters of all people with HIV disease will develop PCP if they do not receive treatment to prevent it. The standard treatment for people with PCP is either a combination of trimethoprim and sulfamethoxazole (TMP/SMX, also called Bactrim or Septra) or pentamidine.

protease inhibitors: HIV protease is an aspartyl enzyme essential to the replicative life cycle of HIV. The three-dimensional molecular structure of the HIV protease has been fully determined. Pharmaceutical developers are therefore able to rationally design compounds to inhibit it and thus interfere with replication of the virus. In the United States, five peptide-based protease inhibitors (saquinavir, Roche; A–80987, ABT–538, Abbott Laboratories; L735,524, Merck;

Continued on following page

KNI–272, NCI) are in clinical development. All compounds inhibit HIV-1 in vitro in nanomolar concentrations. In Europe, two peptide-based compounds (ABT–987, Abbott Laboratories; AG–1343, Agouron Pharmaceuticals, Inc.) are currently in development.

regulatory genes: As related to HIV: Three regulatory HIV genes— tat, rev, and nef—and three so-called auxiliary genes—vif, vpr, and vpu—contain information for the production of proteins that control (i.e., regulate) the virus's ability to infect a cell, produce new copies of the virus, or cause disease.

regulatory T cells: T cells that direct other immune cells to perform special functions. The chief regulatory cell, the CD4+ T cell or helper T cell, is HIV's chief target.

remissions: The lessening of the severity or duration of outbreaks of a disease, or the abatement (diminution in degree or intensity) of symptoms altogether over a period of time.

retrovirus: HIV and other viruses that carry their genetic material in the form of RNA and that have the enzyme reverse transcriptase. Like all viruses, HIV can replicate only inside cells, commandeering the cell's machinery to reproduce. Like other retroviruses, HIV uses the enzyme called reverse transcriptase to convert its RNA into DNA, which is then integrated into the host cell DNA.

rev: One of the regulatory genes of the HIV virus. Three HIV regulatory genes—tat, rev, and nef—and three so-called auxiliary genes— vif, vpr, and vpu—contain information necessary for the production of proteins that control the virus's ability to infect a cell, produce new copies of the virus, or cause disease.

reverse transcriptase: This enzyme of the HIV virus (and other retroviruses) converts the single-stranded viral RNA into DNA, the form in which the cell carries its genes. The antiviral drugs approved in the United States for the treatment of HIV infection—AZT, ddC, and ddI—all work by interfering with this stage of the viral life cycle.

ribonucleic acid (RNA): 1) A nucleic acid, found mostly in the cytoplasm of cells, that is important in the synthesis of proteins. The amount of RNA varies from cell to cell. RNA, like the structurally similar DNA, is a chain made up of subunits called nucleotides. In protein synthesis, messenger RNA (mRNA) replicates the DNA code for a protein and moves to sites in the cell called ribosomes. There, transfer RNA (tRNA) assembles amino acids to form the protein specified by the messenger RNA. Most forms of RNA (including messenger and transfer RNA) consist of a single nucleotide strand, but a few forms of viral RNA that function as carriers of genetic information (instead of DNA) are double-stranded. 2) A nucleic acid associated with the control of chemical activities inside a cell. One type of RNA transfers information from the cell's DNA to the protein-forming system of a cell outside the nucleus. Some viruses (e.g., HIV) carry RNA instead of the more usual genetic material DNA.

Ryan White CARE Act: The Ryan White Comprehensive AIDS Resources Emergency (CARE) Act of 1990 represents the largest dollar investment made by Congress to date specifically for the provision of services for people with HIV infection. The purpose of the act is "to improve the quality and availability of care for individuals and families with HIV disease."

seroconversion: The development of antibodies to a particular antigen. When people develop antibodies to HIV or an experimental HIV vaccine, they "seroconvert" from antibody-negative to antibody-positive.

simian immunodeficiency virus (SIV): An HIV-like virus that infects monkeys, chimpanzees, and other nonhuman primates.

superantigen: Investigators have proposed that a molecule known as a superantigen, made either by HIV or by an unrelated agent, may stimulate massive quantities of CD4+ T cells at once, rendering them highly susceptible to HIV infection and subsequent cell death.

suppressor T cells: (T8, CD8). Subset of T cells that halt antibody production and other immune responses.

surrogate marker: A substitute; a person or thing that replaces another. In HIV disease, the number of CD4+ T cells and CD8+ cells is a surrogate immunologic marker of disease progression.

T cells: (T lymphocytes). A thymus-derived white blood cell that participates in a variety of cell-mediated immune reactions. Three fundamentally different types of T cells are recognized: helper, killer, and suppressor (each has many subdivisions). T lymphocytes are CD3+ and can be separated into the CD4+ T helper cells and the CD8+ cytotoxic/suppressor cells.

tat: One of the regulatory genes of the HIV virus. Three HIV regulatory genes—tat, rev, and nef—and three so-called auxiliary genes—vif, vpr, and vpu—contain information necessary for the production of proteins that control the virus's ability to infect a cell, produce new copies of the virus or cause disease. The tat gene is thought to enhance virus replication.

3TC: Also known as Lamivudine, 3TC is composed of the (—) enantiomer of the racemic mixture 2′-deoxy-3′-thiacytidine. Like other nucleoside analogues, 3TC inhibits HIV replication through viral DNA chain termination. It has been used in clinical trials in combination with AZT.

transmission: In the context of HIV disease: HIV is spread most commonly by sexual contact with an infected partner. The virus can enter the body through the mucosal lining of the vagina, vulva, penis, rectum, or, very rarely, the mouth during sex. The likelihood of transmission is increased by factors that may damage these linings, especially other sexually transmitted diseases that cause ulcers or inflammation. Studies of SIV infection of the genital membranes of nonhuman primates suggest that the sentinel cells known as mucosal dendritic cells may be the first cells infected. Infected dendritic cells may migrate to lymph nodes and infect other cells. HIV also is spread through contact with infected blood, most often by the sharing of drug needles or syringes contaminated with minute quantities of blood containing the virus. Children can contract HIV from their infected mothers either during pregnancy or birth, or postnatally, via breastfeeding. Current research indicates that the AIDS virus may be 100–1000 times more con-

Continued on following page

18

tagious during the first 2 mo of infection, when routine AIDS tests are unable to tell whether people are infected.

tuberculosis (TB): A bacterial infection caused by *Mycobacterium tuberculosis*. TB bacteria are spread by airborne droplets expelled from the lungs when a person with active TB coughs, sneezes, or speaks. Repeated exposure to these droplets can lead to infection in the air sacs of the lungs. The immune defenses of healthy people usually prevent TB infection from spreading beyond a very small area of the lungs. If the body's immune system is impaired because of infection with HIV, aging, malnutrition, or other factors, the TB bacterium may begin to spread more widely in the lungs or to other tissues.

viral burden: (Viral Load). The amount of HIV virus in the circulating blood. Monitoring a person's viral burden is important because of the apparent correlation between the amount of virus in the blood and the severity of the disease: sicker patients generally have more virus than those with less advanced disease. A new, sensitive, rapid test—called the branched DNA assay for HIV-1 infection—can be used to monitor the HIV viral burden. In the future, this procedure may help clinicians to decide when to give anti-HIV therapy. It may also help investigators determine more quickly if experimental HIV therapies are effective.

viral core: (1) Typically a virus contains an RNA or DNA core of genetic material surrounded by a protein coat. See also deoxyribonucleic acid; ribonucleic acid. (2) As related to HIV: Within HIV's envelope is a bullet-shaped core made of another protein, p24, that surrounds the viral RNA. Each strand of HIV RNA contains the virus's nine genes. Three of these—gag, pol, and env—are structural genes that contain information needed to make structural proteins. The env gene, for example, codes for gp160, a protein that is later broken down to gp120 and gp41.

viral envelope: As related to HIV: HIV is spherical in shape with a diameter of 1/10,000 of a millimeter. The outer coat, or envelope, is composed of two layers of fatlike molecules called lipids, taken from the membranes of human cells. Embedded in the envelope are numerous cellular proteins, as well as mushroom-shaped HIV proteins that protrude from the surface. Each mushroom is thought to consist of a cap made of four glycoprotein molecules called gp120, and a stem consisting of four gp41 molecules embedded in the envelope. The virus uses these proteins to attach to and infect cells.

virus: Organism composed mainly of nucleic acid within a protein coat, ranging in size from 100–2000 Å (unit of length; 1 Å is equal to 10^{-10} m); they can be seen only with an electron microscope. During the stage of their life cycle when they are free and infectious, viruses do not carry out the usual functions of living cells, such as respiration and growth; however, when they enter a living plant, animal, or bacterial cell, they make use of the host cell's chemical energy and protein- and nucleic acid–synthesizing ability to replicate themselves. Viral nucleic acids are single- or double-stranded and may be DNA or RNA. After viral components are made by the infected host cell, virus particles are released; the host cell is often dissolved. Some viruses do not kill cells but transform them into a cancerous state; some cause illness and then seem to disappear, while remaining latent and later causing another, sometimes much more severe, form of disease. Viruses, known to cause cancer in animals, are suspected of causing cancer in humans. Viruses also cause measles, mumps, yellow fever, poliomyelitis, influenza, and the common cold. Some viral infections can be treated with drugs.

wasting syndrome: The HIV wasting syndrome involves involuntary weight loss of 10% of baseline body weight plus either chronic diarrhea (two loose stools per day for more than 30 days) or chronic weakness and documented fever (for 30 days or more, intermittent or constant) in the absence of a concurrent illness or condition other than HIV infection that would explain the findings.

BASED ON

CDC RT National AIDS Clearinghouse: Glossary of HIV/AIDS-Related Terms, Publication #B037, June 1995. CDC National AIDS Clearinghouse publications can be obtained by contacting the CDC National AIDS Clearinghouse at (800)458-5231.

AIDS RESOURCES

Organizations and Hotlines

These organizations have been active with AIDS-related issues and may be helpful in locating local programs, materials, and general or specific information on AIDS.

CDC National AIDS Hotline
English: (800)342-AIDS (2437)
Spanish: (800)344-SIDA (7432)
TDD Service for the Deaf: (800)243-7889

National AIDS Clearinghouse
(800)458-5231

HIV/AIDS Treatment Information Service
(800)448-0440

Sexually Transmitted Disease Hotline
(800)227-8922

AIDS Clinical Trials Information Service
(800)874-2572
Clinical trials conducted by the NIH or FDA-approved trials.

American Foundation for AIDS Research (AmFAR)
(800)392-6237

HIV/AIDS Teen Hotline
(800)440-8336

National Minority AIDS Council
(800)559-4145

National Women's Health Network
(202)347-1140

Pediatric HIV Resource Center
(201)268-8251

18

Continued on following page

HIV and AIDS-Related Internet Sites
How to Read an Internet Address

The addresses in this guide are given as URLs. URL stands for Uniform Resource Locator, and is the format an Internet address takes when used by the World Wide Web. URLs are a fairly standard, widely recognized way to present addresses, which can be broken down into three basic parts: the type of tool or resource, the address of the site, and the location of the file on the site. URLs look like this:

> http://www.cdc.gov
> gopher://gopher.cdcnac.aspensys.com:72/00/2/sep95/ads3617
> telnet://locis.loc.gov

Uniform Resource Locators are read from left to right. The first section, the part which ends with ://, tells the Web browser (and you) what type of tool you will be looking at. This is a list of the major tool types:

> http://   = World Wide Web site
> gopher:// = Gopher
> ftp://   = FTP site
> telnet://   = Telnet connection

The section between the tool type and the first single slash (/) is the address of the site. In our examples, these are the addresses:

> www.cdc.gov
> gopher.cdcnac.aspensys.com:72
> locis.loc.gov

Anything after the first single slash indicates the directory path through which you go to get to the file. In our examples, "00/2/sep95/" is the directory path and "ads3617" is the filename.

Canadian HIV Trials Network (CTN)

URL: http://www.hivnet.ubc.ca
                ftp://hivnet.ubc.ca

Listserv: health@hivnet.ubc.ca

Contact: Fortin@hivnet.ubc.ca

Description: *The CTN is a partnership committed to developing treatments, vaccines, and a cure for HIV and AIDS by conducting scientifically sound and ethical clinical trials. The home page includes descriptions of network projects, network publications, ongoing clinical trials, and contact information and links to other organizations.*

CDC NAC

URL: http://www.cdcnac.org
                ftp://198.77.70.84

Listserv: aidsnews@cdcnac.aspensys.com

Contact: aidsinfo@cdcnac.aspensys.com

Description: *The CDC NAC provides current information on HIV and AIDS. The clearinghouse Web site contains information about clearinghouse services, allows users to read and/or download the current* AIDS Daily Summary *and search a database of back issues, and to link to other AIDS-related Web and Gopher sites. Included in the FTP and Gopher sites are fact sheets, FAQs, brochures, AIDS-related* Morbidity and Mortality Weekly Reports *(MMWRs), and documents from the Standard Search Series. The read-only listserv distributes the* AIDS Daily Summary *as well as AIDS-related MMWRs and press releases and publications from other government agencies.*

Department of Health and Human Services (DHHS)

URL: http://www.os.dhhs.gov
gopher://gopher.os.dhhs.gov

Contact: Bob Cooley, bcooley@os.dhhs.gov

Description: *The Gopher and Web sites for the Office of the Secretary, U.S. DHHS provides a centralized point of access to DHHS data available on the Internet, including the FDA, Public Health Service, NIH, and Social Security Administration.*

FEDIX

URL: http://web.fie.com/htdoc/fed/all/any/any/menu/any/index.htm

Contact: webmaster@fedix.fie.com

Description: *The Federal Information Exchange provides Web sites for several federal agencies, including the NIAID. Some agencies provide comprehensive information about all opportunities and activities within their area of responsibility, including selected research programs, minority program information, employment opportunities, and procurements, grants, and assistance. Other agencies offer minority information exclusively.*

18

FedWorld BBS

URL: http://www.fedworld.gov
ftp://ftp.fedworld.gov
telnet://fedworld.gov

Contact: FedWorld Help Desk, (703) 487-4608

Description: *Provided by the U.S. Technology and Information Agency, this system provides access to more than 100 federal BBSs. Provided on the FedWorld system itself are full-text versions of U.S. government publications,*
Continued on following page

statistical files, federal job lists, satellite images, and more. The FTP site contains full text versions of selected documents. The telnet site may be difficult to access owing to limited number of available phone lines.

FDA

URL:	http://www.fda.gov
Contact:	FDA Press Office, 5600 Fishers Lane, Rockville, MD 20857, (301) 443-3285
Description:	*The FDA Web site contains information about FDA activities in the areas of animal drugs, biologics, cosmetics, human drugs, foods, toxicology, medical devices and radiologic health, and inspection and imports. Also included are the full texts of FDA news releases, enforcement reports, import alerts, drug and product approval lists, Federal Register summaries, agency publications, and articles from* FDA Consumer.

Medscape

URL:	http://www.medscape.com/Home/Medscape-AIDS/Medscape-AIDS.html
Contact:	webmaster@scp.com
Description:	*This web site provides access to the full texts of research articles and columns relating to many aspects of HIV and AIDS. The articles are free, but you must be a registered user to access the full text. Abstracts of selected articles are available to nonregistered users.*

MEDWEB - Emory University

URL:	http://www.cc.emory.edu/WHSCL/medweb.html
Contact:	Steve Foote, libsf@web.cc.emory.edu
Description:	*This is a comprehensive listing of AIDS-related Internet sites, including databases, electronic newsletters, and information on the 1996 International Conference on AIDS.*

National Centre in HIV Social Research

URL:	http://www.bhs.mq.edu.au/nchsr.html
Contact:	nat.centre.hiv@mq.edu.au.
Description:	*The Australian National Centre in HIV Social Research consists of several National Priority Programs. This site provides details of current research activities of the National Priority Program, Macquarie University, Sydney, Australia, focusing on education and prevention for gay and homosexually active men.*

NIAID (National Institute of Allergy and Infectious Disease)

URL: http://www.niaid.nih.gov
             gopher://gopher.niaid.nih.gov:70/
             gopher://odie.niaid.nih.gov

Contact: Brent Sessions, (301) 402-0980 x424; sessions@gopher.
             niaid.nih.gov

Description: *The NIAID Web site contains AIDS-related press releases and publications and grant and contract information. This Gopher site provides a wide variety of information, targeted both to researchers and administrators. Information contained on this gopher site includes the* AIDS Daily Summary, *NIAID news releases, and* AIDS Treatment News *and other newsletters, as well as links to research and reference tools.*

NIH (National Institutes of Health)

URL: http://www.nih.gov
             gopher://gopher.nih.gov

Contact: gopher@gopher.nih.gov

Description: *These sites distribute information for and about the NIH. They provide access to information about NIH health and clinical issues, NIH-funded grants and research projects, and a variety of research resources in support of NIH intramural scientists.*

NLM (National Library of Medicine)

URL: http://www.nlm.nih.gov
             gopher://gopher.nlm.nih.gov
             ftp://nlmpubs.nlm.nih.gov
             telnet://medlars.nlm.nih.gov

Contact: MEDLARS Help Desk, (800) 638-8480
             hyperdoc@nlm.nih.gov
             admin@gopher.nih.gov

Description: *The NLM's Internet sites contain information about the library and selected reference materials. Access is provided to Locator, NLM's online catalog system, and to MEDLARS and TOXNET (for those with access codes). Publications available include NLM Current Bibliographies in Medicine, AIDS Bibliographies, UMLS documentation, chapters of the Online Services Reference Manual, and NLM fact sheets. The World Wide Web site also contains images and movies of the NIH campus.*

Continued on following page

World Health Organization (WHO)

URL: http://www.who.ch
                   http://gpawww.who.ch
                   gopher://gopher.who.ch
                   gopher://gpagopher.who.ch

Contact: gopher@who.ch
                   akazawa@who.ch

Description: *The WHO offers its bibliographic databases, WHOLIS and WHODOC, via Internet. WHOLIS is the bibliographic database of all WHO publications (also articles in several WHO periodicals and final reports and technical discussions of the World Health Assembly, Executive Board, and Regional Committees) and unpublished technical documents of the headquarters and regional offices, and the Pan American Health Organization. Publications of the International Agency for Research on Cancer, Lyon, and the Council for International Organizations on Medical Sciences, Geneva, are also included. WHODOC is a bimonthly update to WHOLIS.*

The addresses gpagopher.who.ch and gpawww.who.ch are sites devoted to WHO's General Programme on AIDS (now the Joint United Nations Programme on HIV/AIDS). The sites contain information such as the current global situation of the HIV and AIDS epidemic, information on EPI (Expanded Programme on Information) Info and EPI Map software, the GPA (General Programme on AIDS) Docbase, Paris AIDS Summit—Reports of Preparatory Strategic Meetings, as well as access to several other Internet-based AIDS resources.

YAHOO

URL: http://akebono.stanford.pedu/yahoo/Health/Medicine/
AIDS-HIV
http://www.yahoo.com/Health/Diseases_and_Condi-
tions/AIDS_HIV

Contact: admin@yahoo.com

Description: *Yahoo is a popular resource service that is used to
search for sites and that lists Internet sites by subject.
Sites linked to the AIDS-HIV section include conference
listings, organizations, and usenet news groups, as well
as gopher and Web sites.*

BASED ON

CDC National AIDS Clearinghouse: Guide to Selected HIV/AIDS-Re-
lated Internet Resources, #B322, June 1995. CDC National AIDS
Clearinghouse publications can be obtained by contacting the
CDC National Aids Clearinghouse at (800) 458-5231.

18

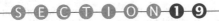

Burns

19

BURN CLASSIFICATIONS

The Nature of the Burn Wound

Based on cellular events, a typical burn wound that is more severe than a superficial burn can be said to have three zones. In the zone of coagulation, there is cell death. In the zone of stasis, cells are injured and will usually die within 24–48 h unless there is adequate treatment. In the zone of hyperemia, there is minimal cell damage. The extent of each wound is dependent on the intensity and duration of the heat source, skin thickness, vascularity, age, and pigmentation.

Classification of Burn Injury

Most medical literature now classifies burn injuries by the depth of the skin tissue destroyed rather than by the previously used classification of first-, second-, and third-degree burns. The following figures identify the extent of the burn wound for each classification and include a brief description of general clinical signs and symptoms.

Superficial Burn

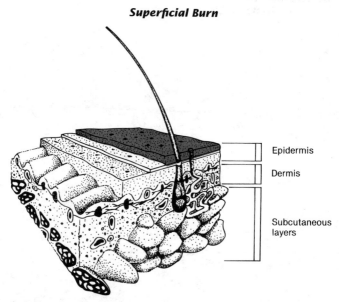

Epidermis

Dermis

Subcutaneous layers

As indicated by the colored area in the figure, cell damage is limited to the outer epidermis. The skin appears red or erythematous and the skin surface is dry. Blisters are typically absent but slight edema may be present. Pain and tenderness are delayed and skin healing occurs without scarring.

Superficial Partial-Thickness Burn

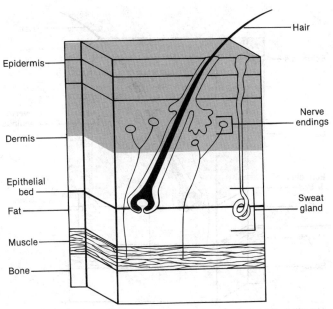

As indicated by the colored area in the figure, the epidermis is damaged, as is the upper part of the dermis. This type of wound is characterized by intact blisters and severe pain. Healing occurs with minimal or no scarring.

19

Deep Partial-Thickness Burn

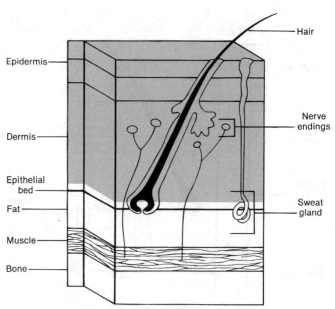

As indicated by the colored area in the figure, there is complete destruction of the epidermis and severe damage to the dermal layer. This type of wound appears as a mixed red or waxy white color with broken blisters and moderate edema. The pain may be less severe than with a superficial partial thickness burn because some nerve endings are destroyed by the burn. Healing occurs with hypertrophic scars and keloids.

Full-Thickness Burn

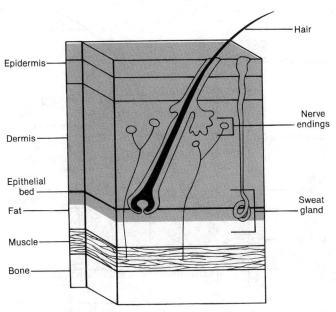

Epidermis—

Dermis—

Epithelial bed—

Fat—

Muscle—

Bone—

Hair

Nerve endings

Sweat gland

As indicated by the colored area in the figure, there is complete destruction of the epidermis and dermis. In addition, some of the subcutaneous fat layer may be damaged. This type of wound is characterized by a hard, parchment-like eschar formation and little pain. Infection is common with this type of burn. Grafts are necessary because new tissue can be regenerated only from the edges of the burn, and this is insufficient for coverage.

19

Subdermal Burn

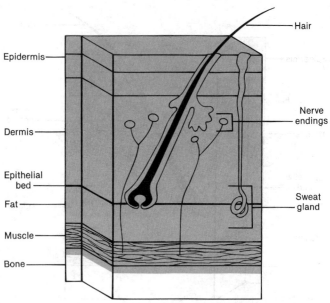

Epidermis

Dermis

Epithelial bed

Fat

Muscle

Bone

Hair

Nerve endings

Sweat gland

As indicated by the colored area in the figure, there is complete destruction of all tissue from the epidermis down to and including the subcutaneous tissue. Damage may extend to muscle and bone. This type of wound usually occurs as a result of prolonged contact with flame, hot liquid, or electricity. Extensive surgery is usually necessary to remove necrotic tissue, including the possibility of limb amputation.

FOR MORE INFORMATION

Richard, R and Staley, M (eds): Burn Care and Rehabilitation: Principles and Practice, FA Davis, Philadelphia, 1993.

ESTIMATING BURN AREA

Rule of Nines for Estimating Burn Area

The rule of nines is used to estimate the percentage of body area burned. Body areas are said to constitute either 9% of the area or some number divisible by 9. The head and each upper extremity are 9% (4.5% on each surface). The posterior surface of the trunk (the back) is 18%, as is the anterior surface of the trunk. The genital area is 1%, and each lower extremity is 18% (9% on each surface). Although the rule of nines is very practical, it provides only gross estimates of the areas and has been supplanted for exact estimates by use of Lund-Browder charts (pages 1120–1121).

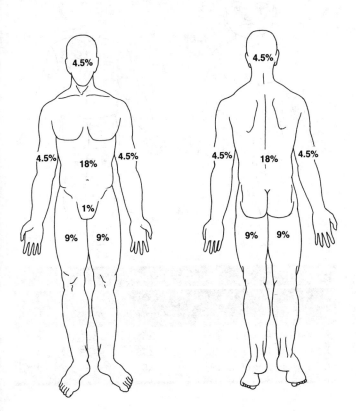

Lund-Browder Charts for Estimating Body Areas

The rule of nines is widely used to estimate body surface area, (see previous page), but more accurate estimates of areas are thought to be obtainable by use of Lund-Browder Charts. These take into account changes that occur during normal growth.

Young Children

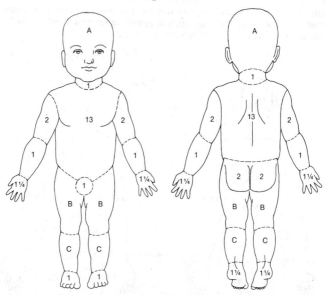

YOUNG CHILDREN			
		Age in Years	
Area	0	1	5
A Each surface of the head	9.5	8.5	6.5
B Each surface of the thigh	2.75	3.25	4.0
C Each surface of the leg	2.5	2.5	2.75

Children and Adults

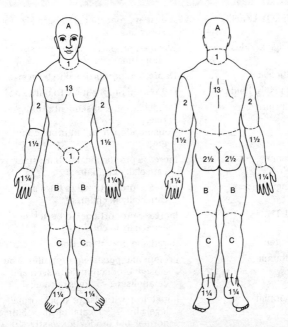

	CHILDREN AND ADULTS			
		Age in Years		
	Area	*10–14*	*15*	*Adult*
A	Each surface of the head	5.5	4.5	3.5
B	Each surface of the thigh	4.25	4.5	4.75
C	Each surface of the leg	3.0	3.25	3.5

19

BASED ON

Lund, CC and Browder, NC: Estimation of area of burns. Surg Gynecol Obstet 79:352, 1955.

FOR MORE INFORMATION

Richard, R and Staley, M (eds): Burn Care and Rehabilitation: Principles and Practice. FA Davis, Philadelphia, 1993.

BIOLOGIC EVENTS IN RESPONSE TO BURN INJURIES

Free fatty acids	Elevated proportional to burn size for short time.
Triglycerides	Elevated proportional to burn size for short time.
Cholesterol	Depressed proportional to burn size.
Phospholipids	Depressed proportional to burn size.
Fibrinogen	Initial fall with subsequent prolonged rise. Consumption great but production greater.
Renin	Increase proportional to burn size, especially in children.
Angiotensin	Increase proportional to burn size, especially in children.
ACTH	Increase proportional to burn size, especially in children.
Protein	Rapid and persistent drop.
Albumin	Prompt and persistent drop until wound closed; production depressed and catabolism 2–3 times normal.
Globulin	Initial drop with rise to supranormal levels by 5–7 d; catabolism 2–3 times normal, but production vastly increased.
IgG	Immediate depression followed by slow rise.
IgM	Altered little by burn in adults but in children follows pattern of IgG.
IgA	Altered little by burn in adults but in children follows pattern of IgG.
Red blood cells	Immediate loss proportional to burn size and depth. Life span 30% of normal due to plasma factor.
White blood cells	Initial and prolonged rise. May drop with sepsis.
Cardiac output	Precipitous drop to 20%–40% of normal with slow spontaneous recovery in 24–36 h. Myocardial depressant factor demonstrated.
Blood viscosity	Sharp rise proportional to hematocrit.

Carboxyhemoglobin	Not significant after 72 h ($<2\%$). Most prominent with inhalation injury (80%). Exists with or without surface burns.
BSP	Retention proportional to burn size with rapid rise and persistence for several weeks.
Cortisol	Prompt rise to 2–4 times normal.
Aldosterone	Usually returns to normal by end of first week but may remain elevated for long periods. Varied response to ACTH often nil in early period.
Peripheral resistance	Rises sharply—slow fall.
Pulmonary vascular resistance	Rises sharply—slow fall.
Pulmonary artery pressure	Prompt rise and slow return.
Left aterial pressure	Normal or low. High with failure.
Po_2	Low with delay or inadequate therapy.
pH	Prompt response to therapy.
Pco_2	Initial alkalosis or hyperventilation promptly resolves.
Blood lactate	May rise to high levels with hyperventilation or poor perfusion.
Excess lactate	Mild elevations characteristic but may rise to high levels with inadequate or delayed resuscitation.
ALT AST Alk phos	Prompt rise with peak at 2–3 d and persistence for several weeks owing to liver damage, not release of skin enzymes.
Renal function	Renal plasma flow depressed more than glomerular filtration rates. Free water clearances down. All values promptly return to normal with adequate resuscitation.
Evaporative water loss	Donor sites and partial-thickness burns have intermediate loss rates. Full-thickness burns lose at same rate as open pan of water.

19

Continued on following page

	Estimate $(25 + \%$ burn$) \times M^2$ body surface.
	Fifteen to 20 times normal skin rates.
Pulmonary function (in absence of pneumonia)	Proportional to magnitude of burn; independent of inhalation injury.
	Minute ventilation (V_e) increased up to 500%; peak at 5 d.
	Static compliance (CSTAT) usually normal but may change with onset pneumonia.
	Lung clearance index (LCI) normal until terminal.
	Oxygen consumption greatly increased.
	Forced vital capacity (FVC) normal even with V_e increase; may drop with pneumonia.

ACTH = adrenocorticotropic hormone; AlK phos = alkaline phosphatase; ALT = alanine transaminase; AST = aspartate transaminase; BSP = bromsulphalein.

From O'Sullivan, SB and Schmitz, TJ: Physical Rehabilitation: Assessment and Treatment, ed 3. FA Davis, Philadelphia, 1994, p 518, with permission.

MEDICATIONS

TOPICAL MEDICATIONS FREQUENTLY USED IN THE TREATMENT OF BURNS

Medication	Description	Method of Application
Furacin (nitrofurazone)	Antibacterial cream used in less severe burns; indicated to decrease bacteria growth; may be used to prepare wound for graft and/or used prophylactically	Applied directly; may be in rolled form or applied as gauze pad
Garamycin (gentamycin)	Antibiotic used against gram-negative organism and staphyloccal and streptococcal bacteria	Cream or ointment applied with sterile glove and covered with gauze

TOPICAL MEDICATIONS FREQUENTLY USED IN THE TREATMENT OF BURNS (Continued)

Medication	Description	Method of Application
Silver sulfadiazine	Topical antibacterial agent effective against *Pseudomonas* infections; may delay eschar separation	Cream applied with sterile glove in a film 2–4 mm thick; may be left uncovered
Sulfamylon (mafenide acetate)	Topical antibacterial agent effective against gram-negative and gram-positive organisms; diffuses easily through eschar; may prevent conversion of burns	Cream applied directly to wound in thin 1–2-mm layer BID; may be left undressed or used with thin layer of gauze; must be completely removed before reapplied or may cause bacterial growth
Silver nitrate	Caustic antiseptic germicide and astringent; penetrates only 1–2 mm of eschar; used only for surface bacteria; stains black	Small sticks used to cauterize small areas; dressings or soaks also used every 2 h; not used with full thickness burns
Travase/Elase	Enzyme debrider has no bacterial control action; used with silver sulfadiazine	Applied to eschar and covered with moist occlusive dressing

From O'Sullivan, SB and Schmitz, TJ: Physical Rehabilitation: Assessment and Treatment, ed 3. FA Davis, Philadelphia, 1994, p 521, with permission.

19

SKIN GRAFTS AND FLAPS USED IN
THE TREATMENT OF BURNS

advancement flap: A local flap in which skin adjacent to a defect is moved to cover the defect without detachment of the flap from its original site.

allograft (homograft, cadaver): A graft taken from donor who is a member of the same species but who is not genetically identical to the recipient.

autograft: A graft taken from the recipient's body.

delayed graft: A graft that is partially elevated and then replaced so that it can be moved to another site.

free flap: Skin tissue (includes blood vessels) which is moved to a distant site where vascular reconnection is made.

full-thickness graft: A graft that contains all layers of the skin but no subcutaneous fat.

heterograft (xenograft): A graft taken from a member of another species.

isologous: Donor and recipient are genetically identical.

local flap: Movement of skin to an adjacent site with part of the flap remaining attached to retain its blood supply.

mesh graft: The donor's skin is cut to form a mesh so that it can be expanded to cover a larger area.

myocutaneous flap: A flap composed of muscle, subcutaneous fat, skin, and patent blood vessels.

pedicle flap: One end is left attached until the free end is viable through its own blood supply.

rotational flap: Local flap where a section of skin tissue is incised on three sides and pivoted to cover an adjacent defect (the z-plasty is a simple form of the rotational flap).

sheet graft: A graft where the donor skin is applied without alteration to the recipient's site.

split-thickness graft: A graft that contains only superficial dermal layers.

z-plasty: See rotational flap.

S E C T I O N 2 0

Reference Tables and Conversion Charts

20

TEMPERATURE CONVERSIONS

TO CONVERT CENTIGRADE TO FAHRENHEIT

Degrees Fahrenheit = (Degrees Centigrade $\times \frac{9}{5}$) + 32

TO CONVERT FAHRENHEIT TO CENTRIGRADE

Degrees Centigrade = (Degrees Fahrenheit − 32) $\times \frac{5}{9}$

TO CONVERT CENTIGRADE TO ABSOLUTE (KELVIN)

Degrees Kelvin = Degrees Centigrade − 273

TO CONVERT ABSOLUTE (KELVIN) TO CENTIGRADE

Degrees Centigrade = Degrees Kelvin + 273

COMMON EQUIVALENT TEMPERATURES	
Fahrenheit	*Centigrade*
− 19.4	12.04
32	0
98.6	37
100	37.7
212	100
0	− 17.8

GAS LAWS

Charles's Law (Gay-Lussac's Law): All gases expand equally upon being heated (they increase their volume 1/273.16 at 0° centigrade for every degree centigrade they are heated).

Boyle's Law (Mariotte's Law): For a gas held at a constant temperature, the volume varies inversely with the pressure.

METRIC PREFIXES

Quantity	Multiples/Submultiples	Prefix	Symbol
1,000,000,000,000	10^{12}	tera	T
1,000,000,000	10^9	giga	G
1,000,000	10^6	mega	M
1,000	10^3	kilo	k
100	10^2	hecto	h
10	10^1	deka	da
0.1	10^{-1}	deci	d
0.01	10^{-2}	centi	c
0.001	10^{-3}	milli	m
0.000 001	10^{-6}	micro	μ
0.000 000 001	10^{-9}	nano	n
0.000 000 000 01	10^{-12}	pico	p
0.000 000 000 000 001	10^{-15}	femto	f
0.000 000 000 000 000 001	10^{-18}	atto	a

ENGLISH-TO-METRIC CONVERSIONS

To convert an English measurement to a metric measurement, multiply by the factor shown. To convert a metric measurement into an English measurement, divide by the factor shown in the tables.

Area

To obtain square meters, multiply:

Sq inches	× 6.4516^{-4}
Sq feet	× 0.092903
Sq yards	× 0.8361274
Sq miles	× 2,589,988
Acres	× 4,046.856
Sq millimeters	× 1.0^{-6}
Sq centimeters	× 1.0^{-4}
Sq meters	× 1.0
Sq kilometers	× 1,000,000
Hectares	× 10,000

20

Length

To obtain meters, multiply:

Inches	×	0.0254
Feet	×	0.3048
Statute miles	×	1609.344
Nautical miles	×	1852
Millimeters	×	0.001
Centimeters	×	0.01
Meters	×	1.0
Kilometers	×	1000

Pressure

To obtain pascals (N/m^2), multiply:

Inches Hg at 0°C	×	3,386.389
Feet H_2O 4°C	×	2,988,98
Pounds per sq inch	×	6,894.757
Pounds per sq foot	×	47.88026
Short tons per sq foot	×	95,760.52
Atmospheres at 760 mm Hg	×	101,325
Centimeters Hg at 0°C	×	1,333.22
Meters H_2O at 4°C	×	9,806.38
Kilograms per sq centimeters	×	98,066.5
Pascals (N/m^2)	×	1.0

Speed and Velocity

To obtain meters per seconds, multiply:

Inches per minute	×	4.2333^{-4}
Feet per second	×	0.3048
Feet per minute	×	0.00508
Miles per second	×	1609.344
Miles per hour	×	0.44704
Knots	×	0.5144444
Centimeters per minute	×	1.6667^{-4}
Meters per second	×	1.0
Meters per minute	×	0.0166667
Kilometers per hour	×	0.2777778

Volume and Capacity

To obtain cubic meters, multiply:

Cubic inches	×	1.6387^{-5}
Cubic feet	×	0.0283168
Cubic yards	×	0.7645549
Ounces	×	2.9574^{-5}
Quarts	×	9.4634^{-4}
U.S. gallons	×	0.0037854
Imperial gallons	×	0.0045461
Cubic centimeters	×	1.0^{-6}
Cubic meters	×	1.0
Liters	×	0.001

Weight, Mass, and Force

To obtain kilograms, multiply:

Grains	$\times$	6.4799^{-5}
Ounces (avdp)	$\times$	0.0283495
Pounds (avdp)	$\times$	0.4535924
Short tons	$\times$	907.1847
Long tons	$\times$	1,016.047
Milligrams	$\times$	1.0^{-6}
Grams	$\times$	0.001
Metric tons	$\times$	1,000,000
Newtons	$\times$	.1019716

To obtain newtons, multiply:

Grains	$\times$	6.3546^{-4}
Ounces (avdp)	$\times$	0.2780139
Pounds (avdp)	$\times$	4.448222
Short tons	$\times$	8896.443
Tons	$\times$	9964.016
Milligrams	$\times$	9.8067^{-6}
Grams	$\times$	0.0098067
Kilograms	$\times$	9.80665
Metric tons	$\times$	9806.65
Newtons	$\times$	1.0

Work, Energy, and Power

To obtain joules (watt-sec), multiply:

Foot-pounds	$\times$	1.355818
Btu (IT)	$\times$	1055.056
Btu (mean)	$\times$	1055.87
Btu (TC)	$\times$	1054.350
Meter-kilograms	$\times$	9.80665
Kilocalories (IT)	$\times$	4186.8
Kilocalories (mean)	$\times$	4190.02
Kilocalories (TC)	$\times$	4184.0
Joules (watt-second)	$\times$	1.0
Watt-hours	$\times$	3600

To obtain watts, multiply:

Foot-pounds per second	$\times$	1.355818
Foot-pounds per minute	$\times$	0.0225970
Btu (IT) per hour	$\times$	0.2930711
Btu (TC) per minute	$\times$	17.57250
Horsepower (550 fpps)	$\times$	745.6999
Horsepower (electric)	$\times$	746
Horsepower (metric)	$\times$	735.4988
Kilocalories (TC) per second	$\times$	4184
Watts	$\times$	1.0
Kilowatts	$\times$	1000

20

SYMBOLS

♏	Minim
℈	Scruple
℥	Dram
℥	Fluidram
℥	Ounce
℥	Fluidounce
O	Pint
lb	Pound
℞	Recipe (L. take)
M	Misce (L. mix)
$\overline{aa}$	Of each
A, Å	angstrom unit
C-1, C-2, etc.	Complement
c, $\overline{c}$	cum (L. with)
△	Change; heat
E_0	Electroaffinity
F_1	First filial generation
F_2	Second filial generation
$m\mu$	Millimicron, nanometer
μg	Microgram
mEq	Milliequivalent
mg	Milligram
mg%	Milligrams percent; milligrams per 100 ml
Q_{O_2}	Oxygen consumption
m-	Meta-
o-	Ortho-
p-	Para-
$\overline{p}$	After
P_{O_2}	Partial pressure of oxygen
P_{CO_2}	Partial pressure of carbon dioxide
$\overline{s}$	Without
$\overline{ss}$, ss	[L. *semis*]. One-half
μm	Micrometer
μ	Micron (former term for micrometer)
$\mu\mu$	Micromicron
+	Plus; excess; acid reaction; positive
−	Minus; deficiency; alkaline reaction; negative
±	Plus or minus; either positive or negative; indefinite
#	Number; following a number, pounds
÷	Divided by
×	Multiplied by; magnification
/	Divided by
=	Equals
≈	Approximately equal

>	Greater than; from which is derived
<	Less than; derived from
≮	Not less than
≯	Not greater than
≤	Equal to or less than
≥	Equal to or greater than
≠	Not equal to
√	Root; square root; radical
∛	Square root
∛	Cube root
∞	Infinity
:	Ratio; "is to"
::	Equality between ratios; "as"
∴	Therefore
°	Degree
%	Percent
π	3.1416—ratio of circumference of a circle to its diameter
□, ♂	Male
○, ♀	Female
⇌	Denotes a reversible reaction
n	Subscripted n indicates the number of the molecules can vary from two or greater

A

a	before
abs feb	while the fever is absent
ac	before meals
ad lib	as desired
ADL	activities of daily living
adv	against
aeg	the patient
alt	alternate
alt die	alternate days
alt hor	every other hour
alt noc	every other night
AMA	against medical advice
ante	before
aq	water
aq ferv	hot water
aq frig	cold water
aq tep	tepid water

B

b	bath
bal	bath
bib	drink
bid	twice a day
bin	twice a night
bis	twice
bol	pill
BR	bedrest
BRP	bathroom privileges

C

c, c̄	with
C/O	complains of
cc	chief complaint
CCW	counterclockwise
cf	compare, refer to
cib	food
CM	tomorrow morning
cms	to be taken tomorrow morning
CN	tomorrow night
cns	to be taken tomorrow night
cont	continue
CV	tomorrow evening
CW	clockwise

D

d	day

D	dose, duration, give, let it be given, right
D/C	discharge
da	give
dc, D/C	discontinue
de d in d	from day to day
decr	decrease
decub	lying down
det	let it be given
dieb alt	on alternate days
dieb tert	every third day
dil	dilute
DISC	discontinue
disch	discharge
div	divide
DP	with proper direction
dur dolor	while the pain lasts

E

ead	the same
EMP	as directed
et	and
eval	evaluation

F

feb dur	while the fever lasts
FLD	fluid
freq	frequent

G

GRAD	gradually, by degrees

H

Hd	at bedtime
HOB	head of bed
hor decub	at bedtime
hor interm	at intermediate hours
hor som	at bedtime
hor un spatio	at the end of an hour
hs	at bedtime

I

id	the same
in d	daily
Incr	increase

L

L	left
LIQ	liquid
loc dol	to the painful spot
lt	left

Continued on following page

20

M

M&R	measure and record
mit	send
mor dict	as directed
mor sol	in the usual way
mp	as directed

N

NB	note well
NBM	nothing by mouth
noc	night
noct	at night
non rep	do not repeat
NOS	not otherwise specified
NPO	nothing by mouth
NPO/HS	nothing by mouth at bedtime
NR	do not repead

O

Occ	occasional
OD	once daily
om	every morning
om quar hor	every quarter of an hour
omn bih	every two hours
omn hor	every hour
omn noct	every night
on	every night
OOB	out of bed

P

P	after, position
par aff	the part affected
PC, p.c.	after meals
per	by, for each, through
PO	postoperative
PO, po	by mouth
POD	postoperative day
pp	postpartum, postprandial
prn	as the occasion
pta	prior to admission

Q

q	each, every
q2h	every two hours
q3h	every three hours
q4h	every four hours
qam	every morning
qd	every day
qh	every hour
qhs	every bedtime
qid	four times a day

ql	as much as desired
qm	every morning
qn	every night
qns	quantity not sufficient
qod	every other day
qoh	every other hour
qp	at will
qqh	every four hours
qqhor	every hour
quotid	daily
qv	as much as you like

R

R	right
REP	let it be repeated
RO/R/O	rule out
ROM	range of motion
ROS	review of systems
Rot	rotate
RT	right
RX, Rx	prescription, take, treatment

S

s, $\bar{s}$	without
S	label, left, sign, without
S/P	status post
si op sit	if it is necessary
simul	at the same time
SOS	if it is necessary, when necessary
stat	immediately
std	let it stand

T

Tab	tablet
tds	take three times a day
tid	three times a day
TLC	tender loving care
TO	telephone order

U, V, W

UNK	unknown
ut dict	as directed
VIZ	namely
VO, vo, V/O	verbal order
WNL	within normal limits

20

MANUAL ALPHABET

A		H		O		V	
B		I		P		W	
C		J		Q		X	
D		K		R		Y	
E		L		S		Z	
F		M		T			
G		N		U			

BRAILLE ALPHABET AND NUMBERS

DESIRABLE HEIGHTS AND WEIGHTS ACCORDING TO FRAME TYPE

	Men						Women		
Height (in Shoes)*		Weight in Pounds (in Indoor Clothing)†			Height (in Shoes)*		Weight in Pounds (in Indoor Clothing)†		
ft	in	Small Frame	Medium Frame	Large Frame	ft	in	Small Frame	Medium Frame	Large Frame
5	2	128–134	131–141	138–150	4	10	102–111	109–121	118–131
5	3	130–136	133–143	140–153	4	11	103–113	111–123	120–134
5	4	132–138	135–145	142–156	5	0	104–115	113–126	122–137
5	5	134–140	137–148	144–160	5	1	106–118	115–129	125–140
5	6	136–142	139–151	146–164	5	2	108–121	118–132	128–143
5	7	138–145	142–154	149–168	5	3	111–124	121–135	131–147
5	8	140–148	145–157	152–172	5	4	114–127	124–138	134–151
5	9	142–151	148–160	155–176	5	5	117–130	127–141	137–155
5	10	144–154	151–163	158–180	5	6	120–133	130–144	140–159
5	11	146–157	154–166	161–184	5	7	123–136	133–147	143–163
6	0	149–160	157–170	164–188	5	8	126–139	136–150	146–167
6	1	152–164	160–174	168–192	5	9	129–142	139–153	149–170
6	2	155–168	164–178	172–197	5	10	132–145	142–156	152–173
6	3	158–172	167–182	176–202	5	11	135–148	145–159	155–176
6	4	162–176	171–187	181–207	6	0	138–151	148–162	158–179

*Shoes with 1-in heels.
†Indoor clothing weighing 5 lb for men and 3 lb for women.
Source of basic data: Build Study, 1979, Society of Actuaries and Association of Life Insurance Medical Directors of America, 1980. Copyright 1983 Metropolitan Life Insurance Company. Based on Taber's Cyclopedic Medical Dictionary, ed 16. FA Davis, Philadelphia, 1989, p 2017.

Body Mass Index

Body Mass Index (BMI) Nomogram

Instructions for use: Place a straightedge across the scales for weight and height. BMI is found where the straightedge crosses the middle scale.

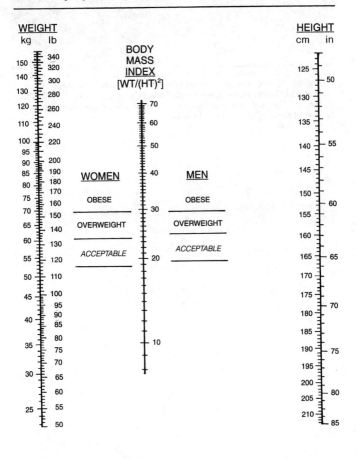

DESIRABLE BODY MASS INDEX IN RELATION TO AGE

Age Group, y	BMI (kg/m^2)
19–24	19–24
25–34	20–25
35–44	21–26
45–54	22–27
55–65	23–28
>65	24–29

From National Academy of Sciences, Committee on Diet and Health, Food and Nutrition Board, Commission on Life Sciences, National Research Council: Diet and Health: Implications for Reducing Chronic Disease Risk. Washington, DC: National Academy Press, 1989, pp 564–565. Reproduced by permission of the publisher; copyright © 1989.

MEDICAL WORD ELEMENTS:
PREFIXES, ROOT WORDS, AND SUFFIXES

ENGLISH MEANINGS OF MEDICAL WORD ELEMENTS

Medical Word Element	Pronunciation	Meaning
a-	ăh	without, not, lack of
ab-	ăb	from, away from
-ac	ăk	pertaining to
acr/o-	ăk-rō	extremity
acromi/o	ă-krō-mē-ō	acromion, projection of scapula
ad-	ăd	to, toward, near
aden/o	ăd-ē-nō	gland
adenoid/o	ăd-ē-noid-ō	adenoid
adip/o	ăd-ĭ-pō	fat
adren/o	ăd-rē-nō	adrenal glands
adrenal/o	ă-drĕn-ăl-ō	adrenal glands
agranul/o	ă-grăn-ū-lō	without granules
-al	ăl	pertaining to
albumin/o	ăl-bū-mĭn-ō	white protein, albumin
-algesia	ăl-gē-sē-ah	pain
-algia	ăl-jē-ah	pain
alveol/o	ăl-vē-ŏl-ō	alveolus (pl. alveoli)
ambi-	ăm-bĭ	both, both sides
ambly/o	ăm-blē-ō	dull, dim
amphi-	ăm-fĭ	on both sides
an-	ăn	without, not, lack of
an/o	ă-nō	anus, opening of the rectum
andr/o	ăn-drō	male
angi/o	ăn-jē-ō	vessel
ankly/o	ăng-kĭ-lō	stiff joint, fusion or growing together of parts
ante-	ăn-tē	before, in front of
anter/o	ăn-tĕr-ō	before, in front of, anterior
anthrac/o	ăn-thrah-kō	coal
anti-	ăn-tī	against
aort/o	ă-ŏr-tō	aorta
aque/o	ă-kwē-ŏ	water
ar-	ăr	without, not, lack of
-ar	ĕr	pertaining to
-arche	ăr-kē	beginning
arteriol/o	ăr-tĕr-ĭ-ŏl-ō	little artery, arteriole
arthr/o	ăr-thrō	joint

Continued on following page

Medical Word Element	*Pronunciation*	*Meaning*
-ary	ĕr-ē	pertaining to
-asthenia	ăs-thē-nē-ăh	without strength
atel/o	ăt-ē-lō	incomplete, imperfect
ather/o	ăth-ĕr-ō	fatty deposit, fatty degeneration
atri/o	ā-trē-ō	atrium
audi/o	aw-dē-ō	hearing
bacteri/o	băk-tē-rē-ō	bacteria
balan/o	bah-lăn-ō	glans penis
bas/o	bā-sō	basic or alkaline
bi-	bī	two
bil/i	bīl-ē	biliary system
-blast	blăst	germ cell, embryonic, primitive
blast/o	blăs-tō	embryonic, primitive, germ cell
blephar/o	blĕf-ah-rō	eyelid
brachi/o	brăk-ē-ō	arm
brady-	brăd-ē	slow
bronch/o	brŏng-kō	bronchus (pl. bronchi)
bronchi/o	brŏng-kē-ō	bronchus (pl. bronchi)
bucc/o	bŭk-ō	cheek
calc/o	kăl-kō	calcium
calcane/o	kal-kā-nē-ō	calcaneum, heel bone
-capnia	kăp-nē-ah	carbon dioxide, CO_2
carcin/o	kăr-sĭn-ō	cancer
cardi/o	kăr-dē-ō	heart
carp/o	kăr-pō	wrist, carpus
-cele	sĕl	hernia, swelling
celi/o	sē-lē-ō	belly, abdomen
-centesis	sĕn-tē-sĭs	surgical puncture
cephal/o	sĕf-ăl-ō	head
cerebell/o	sĕr-ē-bĕl-lō	cerebellum
cerebr/o	sĕr-ē-brō	cerebrum
cervic/o	sĕr-vĭ-kō	neck, cervix
cheil/o	kī-lō	lip
chem/o	kē-mō	chemical, drug
chlor/o	klŏr-ō	green
-chlorhydria	klŏr-hī-drē-ah	hydrochloric acid
chol/e	kō-lē	bile, gall
cholangi/o	kō-lăn-jē-ō	bile vessel
cholecyst/o	kō-lē-sĭs-tō	gallbladder
choledoch/o	kō-lē-dō-kō	bile duct
chondr/o	kŏn-drō	cartilage

Medical Word Element	Pronunciation	Meaning
choroid/o	kō-roid-ō	choroid
chrom/o	krōm-ō	color
-chrome	krōm	color
circum-	sĕr-kŭm	around
cirrh/o	sĭr-rō	yellow, tawny
-clasis	klăh-sĭs	a breaking (of), refracture
-clast	klăst	to break
col/o	kō-lō	colon
colp/o	kŏl-pō	vagina
condyl/o	kŏn-dĭ-lō	condyle
coni/o	kō-nē-ō	dust
contra-	kŏn-trah	against
cor/e	kō-rē	pupil
core/o	kō-rē-ō	pupil
corne/o	kŏr-nē-ō	cornea
coron/o	kŏr-ō-nō	heart
cost/o	kŏs-tō	ribs
crani/o	krā-nē-ō	skull bones, cranium, skull
-crine	krĭn or krīn	to secrete
cry/o	krī-o	cold
crypt/o	krĭp-tō	hidden
-cusis	kū-sĭs	hearing
cutane/o	kū-tă-nē-ō	skin
cyan/o	sī-ăn-ō	blue
cycl/o	sī-klō	ciliary body
-cyesis	sī-ē-sĭs	pregnancy
cyst/o	sĭs-tō	bladder, sac of fluid
cyt/o	sī-tō	cell
dacry/o	dăk-rē-ō	tear
dacryoaden/o	dăk-rē-ō-ăd-ĕn-ō	tear gland
dactyl/o	dăk-tĭ-lō	digit (finger or toe)
dent/o	dĕnt-ō	tooth
derm/o	dĕr-mō	skin
dermat/o	dĕr-mah-tō	skin
-desis	dē-sĭs	binding, stabilization, fusion
dextr/o	dĕks-trō	to the right of
di-	dī	two
dia-	dē-ah	through, across
diplo-	dĭp-lō	double
-dipsia	dĭp-sē-ăh	thirst

Continued on following page

20

Medical Word Element	Pronunciation	Meaning
dist/o	dĭs-tō	distant
dors/o	dĭor-sō	back
duoden/o	dū-ĭod-ē-nō	duodenum
-dynia	dĭn-ē-ĭah	pain
dys-	dĭs	bad, painful, difficult
ec-	ĭek	out, out from
-ectasis	ĭek-tĭah-sĭs	dilation, expansion
ecto-	ĭek-tō	outside
-ectomy	ĭek-tĭo-mē	excision, removal
embol/o	ĭem-bŏl-ō	embolus, plug
-emesis	ē-mĭe-sĭs	vomit
-emia	ē-mē-ĭah	blood condition (of)
emmetr/o	ĭem-ē-trō	correct measure
encephal/o	ĭen-sĭef-ah-lō	brain
endo-	ĭen-dō	in, within
enter/o	ĭen-tĭer-ō	intestines
eosin/o	ē-ō-sĭn-ō	red, rosy, dawn colored
epi-	ĭep-ĭ	upon, over, in addition to
epididym/o	ĭep-ĭ-dĭd-ĭ-mō	epididymis
epiglott/o	ĭep-ĭ-glĭot-ō	epiglottis
episi/o	ē-pĭz-ē-ō	vulva
-er	ĭer	one who
erythem/o	ĭer-ĭ-thē-mō	red
erythr/o	ē-rĭth-rō	red
erythrocyt/o	ē-rĭth-rō-sī-tō	red cell
esophag/o	ē-zĭof-ah-gō	esophagus
-esthesia	ĭes-thē-zē-ah	feeling, sensation
eu-	ū	good, easy
ex-	ĭeks	out, out from
exo-	ĭeks-ō	outside
extern/o	ĭeks-tĭern-ō	outside
extra-	ĭeks-trah	outside
femor/o	fĭem-ō-rō	femur, thigh bone
fibul/o	fĭb-ū-lō	fibula
galact/o	gĭa-lĭak-tō	milk
gangli/o	gĭang-glē-ō	ganglion (knot)
ganglion/o	gĭang-glē-ĭon-ō	ganglion (knot)
gastr/o	gĭas-trō	stomach
-gen	jĭen	to produce
-genesis	jĭen-ē-sĭs	origin, beginning process
gingiv/o	jĭn-jĭ-vō	gum
glauc/o	glaw-kō	gray

Medical Word Element	Pronunciation	Meaning
gli/o	glī-ō	glue
-globin	glō-bĭn	protein
glomerul/o	glō-mĕr-ū-lō	glomerulus
gloss/o	glĭos-ō	tongue
gluc/o	gloo-kō	sugar, sweetness
glucos/o	gloo-kō-sō	sugar
glyc/o	glī-kō	sugar, sweetness
gonad/o	gō-nĭad-ō	sex glands
-gram	grĭam	a writing, record
granul/o	grĭan-ū-lō	granule
-graph	grĭaf	instrument used for recording
-graphy	grĭa-fē	process of recording
-gravida	grĭav-ĭ-dah	pregnancy
gynec/o	jĭn-ē-kō-gĭ-nē-kō	woman, female
hem/o	hēm-o	blood
hemangi/o	hē-mĭan-jē-ō	blood vessel
hemat/o	hĭem-ah-tō	blood
hemi-	hĭem-ē	half, partial
hepat/o	hĭep-ah-tō	liver
heter/o	hĭet-ĭer-ō	different
hidr/o	hī-drō	sweat
hist/o	hĭs-tō	tissue
home/o	hō-mē-ō	likeness, resemblance
homo-	hō-mō	same
humer/o	hū-mĭer-ō	humerus
hydr/o	hī-drō	water
hyper-	hī-pĭer	over, above, excessive, beyond
hypo-	hī-pō	under, below, beneath, less
hyster/o	hĭs-tĭer-ō	uterus, womb
-ia	ē-ah	condition (of), process
-iasis	ī-ā-sĭs	abnormal condition, formation of, presence of
-ic	ĭk	pertaining to
-ical	ĭk-ĭal	pertaining to
ichthy/o	ĭk-thē-ō	dry, scaly
-icle	ĭk-ĭal	small, little, minute
ile/o	ĭl-ē-ō	ileum
ili/o	ĭl-ē-ō	ilium
im-	ĭm	not
immun/o	ĭm-ū-nō	safe, protected

Continued on following page

Medical Word Element	Pronunciation	Meaning
in-	ĭn	not
infra-	ĭn-frah	under, below, beneath, after
inter-	ĭn-tĭer	between
intra-	ĭn-trah	in, within
ir/o	ĭr-ō	iris
irid/o	ĭr-ĭ-dō	iris
-is	ĭs	forms noun from root
is/o	ĭ-sō	equal
ischi/o	ĭs-kē-ō	ischium
-ism	ĭzm	condition, state of being
-ist	ĭst	one who specializes
-itis	ĭ-tĭs	inflammation
jejun/o	jĭe-joo-nō	jejunum
kary/o	kĭar-ē-ō	nucleus
kerat/o	kĭer-ĭah-tō	cornea; hornlike; hard; horny substance
kinesi/o	kĭ-nē-sē-ō	movement
-kinesia	kĭ-nē-zē-ĭah	movement
labi/o	lā-bē-ō	lip
labyrinth/o	lĭab-ĭ-rĭn-thō	labyrinth, inner ear, maze
lacrim/o	lĭak-rĭ-mō	tear
lact/o	lĭak-tō	milk
lamin/o	lĭam-ĭ-nō	lamina
lapar/o	lĭap-ĭar-ō	abdominal wall, abdomen
laryng/o	lah-rĭng-ō	larynx
later/o	lat-er-ō	side
leiomy/o	lī-ō-mī-ō	smooth (visceral) muscle
-lepsy	lĭep-sē	seizure
leuc/o-	loo-kō	white
leuk/o	loo-kō	white
leukocyt/o	loo-kō-sī-tō	white cell
lingu/o	lĭng/gwō	tongue
lip/o	lĭ-pō	fat
-lith	lĭth	stone, calculus
-lithiasis	lĭth-ī-ah-sĭs	presence, condition, or formation of calculi
lob/o	lō-bō	lobe
-logy	lō-jē	study of
lumb/o	lĭum-bō	loins
lymph/o	lĭm-fō	lymph, lymph tissue

Medical Word Element	Pronunciation	Meaning
-lysis	lĭ-sĭs	separate, destroy, break down
macro-	mĭak-rō	large
mal-	mĭal	ill, bad, poor
-malacia	mĭah-lā-shē-ĭah	softening
mamm/o	mĭa-mō	breast
-manometer	mĭan-ĭom-ĭet-ĭer	instrument to measure pressure
mast/o	mĭas-tō	breast
mastoid/o	mĭas-toi-dō	mastoid process
medi-	mē-dē	middle
medull/o	mĭed-ū-lō	medulla
-megaly	meg-ĭah-lē	enlargement
melan/o	mĭel-ah-nō	black
men/o	mĭen-ō	menses, menstruation
mening/o	mĭe-nĭng-gō	meninges, brain covering
meningi/o	mĭe-nĭn-jē-ō	meninges, brain covering
mes/o	mĭes-ō	middle
meta	mĭet-ah	after, beyond, over, change
metacarp/o	mĭet-ah-kĭar-pō	metacarpus, bones of the hand
-meter	mē-tĭer	measure, instrument for measuring
metr/o	mĭe-trō	uterus, womb
-metry	mĭet-rē	act of measuring, to measure
micro-	mī-krō	small
mid-	mĭd	middle
mono-	mĭon-ō	one
morph/o	mĭor-fō	shape
multi-	mĭul-tē	many, much
my/o	mī-ō	muscle
myc/o	mī-kō	fungus
-mycosis	mī-kō-sĭs	fungal infection
myel/o	mī-e-lō	bone marrow, spinal cord
myring/o	mĭe-rĭng-gō	tympanic membrane, eardrum
narc/o	nĭar-kō	sleep
nas/o	nā-zō	nose
nat/a	nā-tĭa	birth

Continued on following page

20

Medical Word Element	Pronunciation	Meaning
ne/o	nē-ō	new
nephr/o	nĭef-rō	kidney
neur/o	nū-rō	nerve, neuron
neutr/o	nū-trō	neutral dye
noct/o	nĭok-tō	night
nucle/o	nū-klē-ō	nucleus
ocul/o	ĭok-ū-lō	eye
odont/o	ō-dĭon-tō	tooth
-oid	oid	resemble
-ole	ĭol	small, little, minute
olig/o	ō-lĭ-gō	scanty
-oma	ō-mĭah	tumor
onc/o	ĭong-kō	tumor, mass
onych/o	ĭon-ĭ-kō	nail
oo/o	ō-ō	egg, ovum
oophor/o	ō ĭof-ō-rō	ovary
ophthalm/o	ĭof-thĭal-mō	eye
-opia	ōpē-ah	vision
-opsia	ĭop-sē-ah	vision
opt/o	ĭop-tō	eye
or/o	ĭor-ō	mouth
orch/o	ĭor-kō	testes
orchi/o	ĭor-kē-ō	testes
orchid/o	ĭor-kĭ-dō	testes
orth/o	ĭor-thō	straight
-ory	ĭor-ē	pertaining to
-osis	ō-sĭs	abnormal condition, increase
-osmia	ĭoz-mē-ah	smell
oste/o	ĭos-tē-ō	bone
ot/o	ō-tō	ear
-ous	ĭus	pertaining to
ovari/o	ō-vĭar-ē-ō	ovary
ox/o	ĭoks-ō	oxygen, O_2
oxy/o	ĭok-sĭ-ō	oxygen, O_2
pachy/o	pĭak-ē-ō	thick, heavy
pan-	pĭan	all
pancreat/o	pĭan-krē-ĭa-tō	pancreas
papill/o	pĭap-ĭ-lō	nipplelike protuberance or elevation
para-	pĭar-ah	near, beside, beyond, abnormal

Medical Word Element	Pronunciation	Meaning
-para	pĭar-ah	to bear
parathyroid/o	pĭar-ah-thī-roi-dō	parathyroid glands
-paresis	pah-rē-sĭs	partial or incomplete paralysis
patell/o	pah-tĭel-ō	patella, kneecap
-pathy	pĭah-thē	disease
pector/o	pĭek-tō-rō	chest
ped/i	pĭed-ē	foot
pelv/i	pĭel-vē	pelvis
-penia	pē-nē-ĭah	decrease, deficiency, lack of
peri-	pĭer-ĭ	around
perine/o	pĭer-ĭ-nē-ō	perineum
peritone/o	pĭer-ĭ-tō-nē-ō	peritoneum
-pexy	pĭek-sē	fixation, suspension
phag/o	fĭag-ō	swallow, eat
-phagia	fă-jē-ah	eating, ingesting, swallowing
phak/o	fā-kō	lens
phalang/o	fĭal-ĭan-jō	phalanges, bones of fingers and toes
pharyng/o	fah-rĭng-gō	pharnyx, throat
-phasia	fā-zē-ah	speech
-phil	fĭl	to love, attraction for
-philia	fĭl-ē-ĭah	attraction for, to love
phleb/o	flĭeb-ō	vein
-phobia	fō-bē-ĭah	fear
-phonia	fō-nē-ah	voice
-phoresis	fō-rē-sĭs	borne, carried
phren/o	frĭen-ō	diaphragm, mind
-phylaxis	fĭ-lĭak-sĭs	protection
-physis	fĭ-sĭs	growth, to grow
pil/o	pī-lō	hair
-plakia	plĭak-ē-ĭah	plate
-plasia	plā-zē-ĭah	formation, development, growth
-plasm	plāzm	formation, growth, development
-plasty	plĭas-tē	formation, plastic repair, surgical repair
-plegia	plē-jē-ĭah	paralysis, stroke
pleur/o	ploo-rō	pleura
-pnea	nē-ah	breathing
pneum/o	nū-mō	lung, air
pneumat/o	nū-mah-tō	air, breath

20

Continued on following page

Medical Word Element	Pronunciation	Meaning
pneumon/o	nū-mī on-ō	lung, air
pod/o	pō-dō	foot
-poiesis	poi-ē-sĭs	formation, production
poikil/o	poi-kĭ-lō	varied, irregular
polio-	pō-lē-ō	gray
poly-	pĭol-ē	many, much
-porosis	pō-rō-sĭs	pores or cavities
post-	pōst	after, backward, behind
poster/o-	pōs-tĭer-ō	after, backward, back, behind, posterior
-prandial	prĭan-dē-ĭal	pertaining to a meal
pre-	prē	before, in front of
presby/o	prĭes-bē-ō	old age, elderly
primi-	prĭ-mĭ	first
pro-	prō	before, in front of
proct/o	prĭok-tō	anus, rectum
prostat/o	prĭos-tah-tō	prostate
proxim/o	prĭok-sĭm-ō	near
pseudo-	soo-dō	false
-ptosis	tō-sĭs	prolapse, falling, dropping
-ptysis	tĭ-sĭs	spitting
pub/o	pū-bō	pubis anterior
pulmon/o	pĭul-mĭon-ō	lung
pupill/o	pū-pĭ-lō	pupil
purpur/o	pĭur-pū-rō	purple
py/o	pī-ō	pus
pyel/o	pī-ē-lĭo	renal pelvis
pylor/o	pī-lō-rō	pylorus
-pyorrhea	pī-ō-rē-ah	discharge of pus, purulent discharge
quad-	kwŏd	four
quadri-	kwŏd-rĭ	four
rach/o	rāk-ō	vertebrae, spinal column
rachi/o	răk-ē-ō	vertebrae, spinal column
rect/o	rĕk-tō	rectum
ren/o	rē-nō	kidney
reticul/o	rē-tĭk-ū-lō	net, mesh (immature red blood cell)
retin/o	rĕt-ĭ-nō	retina

Medical Word Element	Pronunciation	Meaning
retro-	rĕt-rō	after, backward, behind
rhabd/o	răb-dō	rod
rhabdomy/o	răb-dō-mī-ō	striated (skeletal) muscle
rhin/o	rī-nō	nose
-rrhage	rĭj	burst forth (of)
-rrhagia	rā-jē-ăh	burst forth (of)
-rrhaphy	ră-fē	suture
-rrhea	rē-ăh	discharge, flow
-rrhexis	rek-sĭs	rupture
rube/o	roo-bē-ō	red
salping/o	săl-pĭn-gō/săl-pĭn-jō	fallopian tubes, oviducts, uterine tubes, eustachian tube
-salpinx	săl-pĭnks	fallopian tubes, oviducts, uterine tubes
sarc/o	săr-kō	flesh
scirrh/o	skĭr-rō	hard
scler/o	sklē-rō	sclera, hard
-sclerosis	sklē-rō-sĭs	abnormal condition (of) hardening
-scope	skōp	instrument to view or examine
-scopy	skō-pē	visual examination
seb/o	sĕb-ō	sebum
semi-	sĕm-ē	half, partial
sial/o	sī-ăh-lō	saliva, salivary gland
sider/o	sĭd-ĕr-ō	iron
sigmoid/o	sĭg-moi-dō	sigmoid colon
sinistr/o	sĭn-ĭs-trō	left
sinus/o	sī-nŭs-ō	sinus, cavity
somat/o	sō-măt-ō	body
-spasm	spăzm	involuntary contraction, twitching
spermat/o	spĕr-mah-tō	sperm
spher/o	sfē-rō	globe, round
sphincter/o	sfĭngk-tĕr-ō	sphincter
sphygm/o	sfĭg-mō	pulse
spir/o	spī-rō	breathe
splen/o	splē-nō	spleen
spondyl/o	spŏn-dĭ-lō	vertebrae, backbone
squam/o	skwā-mō	scale

Continued on following page

20

Medical Word Element	Pronunciation	Meaning
staped/o	stā-pē-dō	stapes
-stasis	stā-sĭs	standing still, control, stop
steat/o	stē-ă-tō	fat, fatty
-stenosis	stĕ-nō-sĭs	constriction, narrowing
stern/o	stĕr-nō	sternum, breastbone
steth/o	stĕth-ō	chest
stomat/o	stō-mah-tō	mouth
-stomy	stō-mē	mouth, forming a new opening
sub-	sŭb	under, beneath, below
super-	soo-pĕr	above
supra-	soo-prah	above
sym-	sĭm	union, together
syn-	sĭn	union, together
tachy-	tăk-ē	rapid
-taxia	tăk-sē-ah	muscular coordination
ten/o	tĕn-ō	tendon
tend/o	tĕnd-ō	tendon
tendin/o	tĕn-dĭn-ō	tendon
-tension	tĕn-shŭn	pressure
test/o	tĕs-tō	testes
thalam/o	thăl-ăh-mō	thalamus, chamber
thel/o	thē-lō	nipple
-therapy	thĕr-ăh-pē	treatment
therm/o	thĕr-mō	heat
thorac/o	thō-rah-kō	chest
-thorax	thō-răks	chest
thromb/o	thrŏm-bō	clot
thrombocyt/o	thrŏm-bō-sī-tō	platelet, thrombocyte
thym/o	thī-mō	thymus
thyr/o	thī-rō	thyroid
thyroid/o	thī-roī-dō	thyroid
tibi/o	tĭb-ē-ō	tibia
-tic	tĭk	pertaining to
-tocia	tō-sē-ah	childbirth, labor
-tome	tōm	instrument to cut
-tomy	tō-mē	incision, cut into
ton/o	tŏn-ō	tone
tonsill/o	tŏn-sĭ-lō	tonsil
tox/o	tŏks-ō	poison
-toxic	tŏks-ĭk	poison
trache/o	trā-kē-ō	trachea
trans-	trănz	through, across

Medical Word Element	Pronunciation	Meaning
tri-	trī	three
trich/o	trĭk-ō	hair
-tripsy	trĭp-sē	crush
-trophy	trō-fē	nourishment, development
-tropia	trō-pē-ah	turning
-tropin	trō-pĭn	stimulate
tympan/o	tĭm-pah-nō	tympanic membrane, eardrum
-ula	ūlā	small, little, minute
-ule	yool	small, little, minute
ultra-	ul-trah	beyond, excess
ungu/o	ŭng-gwō	nail
uni-	yoo-nē	one
ur/o	ū-rō	urine
ureter/o	ū-rē-tĕr-ō	ureter
urethr/o	ū-rē-thrō	urethra
-uria	ū-rē-ah	urine
uter/o	ū-tĕr-ō	uterus, womb
vagin/o	vă-jĭn-ō	vagina
vas/o	vah-sō	vas deferens, vessel
ven/o	vē-nō	vein
ventr/o	vĕn-trō	belly, belly-side
ventricul/o	vĕn-trĭk-ū-lō	ventricles, little belly
venul/o	vĕn-ū-lō	venule
vertebr/o	vĕr-tē-brō	vertebrae, backbone
vesic/o	vĕs-ĭ-kō	bladder
vesicul/o	vĕ-sĭk-ū-lō	seminal vesicle
viscer/o	vĭs-ĕr-ō	organ
vulv/o	vŭl-vō	vulva
xanth/o	zăn-thō	yellow
xer/o	zē-rō	dry
-y	ē	condition, process

20

From Gylys, BA and Wedding, ME: Medical Terminology: A Systems Approach, ed 3. FA Davis, Philadelphia, 1995, pp 391–400.

GLOSSARY OF TERMS USED TO
DESCRIBE INSTRUMENTS
in alphabetical order

AAMI: Association for Advancement of Medical Instrumentation.

address buss: The conductors within a computer that pass power or data back and forth.

address code: A numerical code used to describe a location within a computer memory where a unit of information is stored.

ASCII: American Standard Code for Information Interchange. A code standardizing control commands and alphanumeric data units in computers.

assembly language: A system of computer programming codes characteristic to a given class of computers (determined by the type of microprocessor used in the computer).

astable multivibrator: A form of square wave or rectangular wave generator that yields a continuous output when power is applied. It is used to provide timing pulses in all types of devices, particularly transcutaneous electrical nerve stimulation units and other stimulators.

bandwidth: The range of frequencies within which performance (in respect to a specific characteristic) falls within specified limits.

barrier layer cell: An optical sensor that is sometimes used in colorimeters (also called *photovoltaic cell*).

BASIC: A computer programming language (Beginners All purpoSe Instructional Code).

baud rate: The units describing the rate at which data are transmitted by a computer (usually by a modem or a serial communications device).

binary code: A term used to describe a computer's machine-level programming language. The language consists of ones and zeroes.

bit: The smallest unit of information or data handled by a computer.

bode plot: A graph used to describe the frequency-gain characteristic of an electronic amplifier.

boolean algebra: The basis for the laws governing the design of computer logic circuits.

bridge amplifier: A specialized type of amplifier that is often used to amplify the difference between two signals, where one signal usually serves as the reference (a form of differential amplifier).

bridge circuit: A term used most often to describe a Wheatstone bridge measuring circuit or a bridge amplifier; often used as part of the circuitry of a strain gauge.

bridge rectifier: An electronic rectifier using four diodes in a bridge design to convert AC current into DC current.

buss: A general term in electronics used to describe a common conductor that connects parts of a device.

byte: The term used to describe the number of bits of data that defines a given computer's word size. A byte can be 4, 8, 16, 32, or 64 bits in length. (Note that an 8-bit byte can encode up to 256 different characters.)

common mode rejection ratio (CMRR): The ability of an amplifier to amplify a signal in the presence of electrical noise; the higher the number, the less the noise amplification.

computer interface: A term that describes a circuit or part that is used to connect a computer to an external device such as a printer or modem.

decibel: A unit of audio power that is also used to describe the gain or attenuation of an electronic circuit by the following formulae:

Power in dB = 20 log (V out/V in)

Power in dB = 10 log (P out/P in)

A gain of 100 in an amplifier is equivalent to a gain of 40 dB.

detector (optical): A sensor that yields an output voltage or current that is proportional to the intensity of the light striking it. It may be a light-sensitive resistor, a photodiode, or a photomultiplier tube.

differential amplifier: A specialized type of amplifier that is used to amplify the difference between two signals. One signal usually serves as the reference. A bridge amplifier is a form of differential amplifier.

digital computer: A computer that processes information in the form of discrete digits or units.

digital-to-analog convertor: Converts digital data into analog data (the opposite of an analog-to-ditigal converter, or ADC).

distortion: A term used to describe variations in the amplitude or frequency of a signal brought about by overdriving an amplifier.

electrode (surface): Usually a metal element that detects bioelectrical (chemoelectrical) activity; surface electrodes, which are placed on the skin, are usually silver or silver chloride (Ag/AgCl).

file: A term used to describe data stored as a single unit by a computer.

filter: A circuit that allows only a single frequency or band (range) of frequencies to pass.

flip-flop: A computer circuit that yields as an output one of two possible conditions: either high (1) or low (10). These are used in memory circuits and counters (also called *biostable multivibrator*).

full-wave rectifier: An electronic circuit found in most instrument power supplies; converts AC voltage into DC voltage.

gain: The term used in electronics to describe the amplification factor of a given circuit (the ratio of voltage in to voltage out); also used to describe the sensitivity of the amplifier setting.

gate: A term used to describe the smallest possible decision-making (logic) circuit in a computer.

hexidecimal: A numbering system in computers that uses base eight, rather than base two (binary) or base ten (decimal).

Continued on following page

inductor: An electronic component used in filter circuits and transformers that employs electromagnetic induction.

integrator: An electronic circuit that yields as an output the mathematical integral (total) of the input signal.

interface: A device or part of a computer that allows two normally incompatible circuits or parts to function together so as to pass data back and forth.

modem (modulator-demodulator): A device that allows computers to transmit and receive data in a serial fashion over phone lines.

modulation: An electronics term that describes the manner in which a signal is used to vary either the amplitude, frequency, or phase of a normally constant carrier signal. It is a method of coding information onto a carrier.

multiplexor: A circuit used in computers and instruments that allows a single processor to sample multiple channels by sequencing them.

multivibrator: A class of electronic circuits that provides a square wave output. They may be free running or may require a trigger.

noise: An unwanted signal or distortion of a signal due to electromagnetic or thermal effects.

null: A condition in which a measuring circuit is balanced and yields zero output.

offset voltage: The term used to describe the unwanted DC voltage at the input end of a signal-processing circuit. This voltage must be "offset" before the output yields zero reference (i.e., a true zero). An offset voltage is most often encountered when using a transducer that cannot be zeroed.

one shot: A circuit that yields a single preset pulse when triggered (also called a *monostable multivibrator*).

open circuit: A circuit in which the normal path for current has been broken. No current may flow in an open circuit.

oscillator: A circuit used to generate a continuous output signal in the form of a sine wave, or, in the case of relaxation oscillators, a rectangular or square wave.

parallel circuit: A circuit in which there is more than one path in which current may flow.

peak detector: A circuit that detects the maximum value of a signal, even though that signal may vary continuously.

peak-to-peak amplitude: The amplitude of a signal voltage from the most positive point to the most negative.

potentiometer (POT): A variable resistor most often used as an operator-adjustable control on instruments.

potentiometry: The measurement of a half-cell potential at zero current; the basis upon which many chemical sensors (electrodes) operate.

power: In electronics it is the product of the current times voltage. It is a measure of the amount of energy dissipated by a circuit (measured in units of watts).

random access memory (RAM): The portion of a computer's memory that holds temporary information (a program or data). This information is lost when the computer loses power.

range: A measure of the frequency range of an amplifier; the range of voltages that can be read by a voltimeter.

read only memory (ROM): The portion of a computer's memory that contains permanent information that cannot be changed by the user through programming. This information is stored in a way that it remains even if the computer loses power.

resonance: A condition in which an electrical circuit exhibits zero reactance and is therefore capable of filtering a given frequency, or in the case of an amplifier is capable of being driven into oscillation if positive feedback is present.

silicon-controlled rectifier (SCR): A triggered rectifier used to control large amounts of current; used in motors.

semiconductor: The term used to describe electronic components that are manufactured from a silicon chip, such as transistors, diodes, and integrated circuits.

sensitivity: The ability of a device to detect a small amount of voltage; usually given in ohms per volt when describing a voltmeter. The greater the ratio of ohms per volt, the better the sensitivity.

sensor: That part of a measurement instrument that senses activity to be measured; usually they are in the form of transducers.

series circuit: A circuit in which the current can follow only one path.

short circuit: A circuit in which the normal path for current flow has been passed (replaced) by a path of lower resistance. This results in excess circuit current, and often the device containing the circuit is damaged.

signal-to-noise ratio: The ratio of signal voltage to noise voltage. It is used to describe the sensitivity of an amplifier or measuring device; the greater the signal-to-noise ratio, the better.

span (chart recorder): The voltage required by a recorder to cause the pen to deflect fully across the chart paper.

strain gauge: A transducer that employs a resistive element to change an applied force into a resistance change and into a voltage (used in force measuring devices).

thermistor: A thermally sensitive resistor often used as the active element in some temperature-monitoring applications.

Continued on following page

transducer: A device that transforms energy of one form into energy of another form. A light bulb, a photodiode, a car, and a stereo speaker are all transducers.

zener diode: A two-element device in the form of diode that functions, when reversed biased, as a simple voltage regulator. It is most often used to provide small reference voltages.

FOR MORE INFORMATION

Bushsbaum, WH: Bushsbaum's Complete Handbook of Practical Electronic Reference Data, ed 3. Prentice Hall, Englewood Cliffs, NJ, 1987.

Institute of Electrical and Electronics Engineers: The New IEEE Dictionary of Electrical and Electronics Terms, ed 5. New York, Institute of Electrical and Electronics Engineers, 1993.

Translations:
Useful Expressions

21

ENGLISH

Hello. I want to help you. I do not speak (English) but will use this book to ask you some questions. I will not be able to understand your spoken answers. Please respond by shaking your head or raising one finger to indicate "no"; nod your head or raise two fingers to indicate "yes."

Translation	Phonetic
SPANISH	

Saludos. Quiero ayudarlo. Yo no hablo español, pero voy a usar este libro para hacerle algunas preguntas. No voy a poder entender sus respuestas; por eso haga el favor de contestar, negando con la cabeza o levantando un dedo para indicar "no" y afirmando con la cabeza o levantando dos dedos para indicar "sí."

Sah-loo'dohs. Ki-air'oh ah-joo-dar'loh. Joh noh ah'bloh es'pan-yohl, pair'oh voy ah oo-sawr' es'tay lee'broh pahr'ah ah-sair'lay ahl-goo'nahs pray-goon'tahs. Noh voy ah poh-dair' en-ten-dair' soos res-poo-es'tahs; pore es-soh ah'gah el fah-vohr' day kohn-tes-tahr', nay-gahn'doh kohn lah kah-bay'thah oh lay-vahn-tahn'doh oon day'doh pahr'ah een-dee-kahr' noh ee ah-feer-manh'doh kohn lah kah-bay'thah oh lay-vahn-tahn'doh dohs day'dohs pahr'a een-dee-kahr' see.

ITALIAN	

Buon giorno. La voglio aiutare. Io non parlo italiano, ma userò questro libro per farle qualche domanda. Non potrò comprendere le sue domande. Per favore risponda con un cenno di testa. Alzi un dito per indi-care 'no'; muova la sua testa su e giù o alzi due dita per indicare 'sì.'

Bwon jih-or'noh. Lah vol'yoh ah-yoo-tar'ay. Ee'oh nohn par'loh ee-towl-ee-ah'noh mah oo-say'roh kwes'tro lee'broh pehr fahr'lay kwall'kay doh-mahn'dah. Non poh'throh kohm-prehn'deh-ray lay soo'ee doh-mahn'day. Pehr fah-vohr'ay ree-spohn'dah kohn oon chay'noh dee tes'tah. Ahlt'zih oon dee'toh pehr in-dee-kar'ay noh; moo-eh'vah lah soo'ah tes'tah soo eh joo oh alht'zih doo'ay dee'tay pehr in-dee-kar'ay see.

Bonjour. Je veux bien vous aider. Je ne parle pas français mais tout en me servant de ce livre je vais vous poser des questions. Je ne comprendrai pas ce que vous dites en français. Je vous en prie, pour répondre: pour indiquer "non", secouez la tête ou levez un seul doigt; pour indiquer "oui", faites un signe de tête ou levez deux doigts.

Bon-zhoor'. Zheh vuh bih-ehn' voo ay-day'. Zheh neh parl pah frahn-say' may too ahn meh sehr-vahn' d' seh lee'vrah zheh vay voo poh-say' day kehs-tih-on'. Zheh neh kahm-prahn'dray pah seh keh voo deet ahn frahn-say'. Zheh voo ahn pree, poor ray-pahn'drah; poor ahn-dee-kay' nohn, seh-kway' lah teht oo leh-vay' oon sool dwoit; poor ahn-dee-kay' wee', fayt oon seen deh teht oo leh-vay' duh dwoit.

Hallo! Ich möchte Ihnen helfen. Ich spreche kein Deutsch, aber ich werde dieses Buch benützten um Sie einiges zu fragen. Ich werde Ihre Antworten nicht verstehen. Deshalb antworten Sie mir indem Sie Ihren Kopf schütteln oder heben Sie Ihren Finger um "nein" auszudrücken; nicken Sie mit dem Kopf oder heben Sie zwei Finger um "ja" auszudrücken.

Ha-loh! Ich möhh'tuh ee'nuhn hel'fuhn. Ich shpre'huh kīn doitsh, ah'buhr ich ver'duh dee'zuhs bookh bā-nüt'zuhn um zee ī'ni-guhs tsoo frah'guhn. Ich ver'duh ee'ruh ant'vor-tuhn nihht fershtay'uhn. Dās-halb' ant'vor-tuhn zee meer in-dām' zee ee'ruhn kopf shü'tln ō'der hāb'uhn zee ee'ruhn fing'uhr um nīn ows'tsoo-drük-uhn; nick'uhn zee mit dām kopf ō'der hāb'uhn zee tsvī fing'uhr um ya ows'tsoo-drük-uhn.

COMMON PHYSICAL THERAPY DIRECTIONS

English	Spanish	Italian	French	German
Good morning/afternoon/evening.	Buenos días/Buenas tardes/Buenas noches.	Buon giorno/Buon pomeriggio/Buona sera.	Bonjour/Bon soir.	Guten Morgen/Nachmittag/Abend.
I am a physical therapist; my name is . . .	Soy la terapista; me llamo . . .	Sono un fisioterapista, mi chiamo . . .	Je suis physio-thérapeute; mon nom est . . .	Ich bin Physiotherapeut; ich heisse . . .
Answer only . . .	Conteste solamente . . .	Risponda solamente . . .	Répondez seulement . . .	Antworten Sie nur
Yes.	Sí.	Sì.	Oui.	Ja.
No.	No.	No.	Non.	Nein.
Speak slower.	Hable más despacio.	Parli più adaggio.	Parlez plus lentement.	Sprechen Sie langsamer.
Say it once again.	Repítalo, por favor.	Lo dica ancora una volta.	Répétez ça.	Wiederholen Sie das.
Please wait; I will be right back.	Espere usted, por favor; regresaré pronto.	Per favore aspetti, ritorno subito.	Attendez s'il vous plaît; je reviens tout de suite.	Warten Sie bitte; ich bin gleich zurück.
Don't be afraid.	No tenga miedo.	Non abbia paura.	N'ayez pas peur.	Haben Sie keine Angst.
Try to remember.	Trate de recordar.	Cerchi di ricordarsi.	Cherchez à vous en rappeler.	Versuchen Sie sich zu erinnern.
Pay attention.	Preste atención.	Faccia attenzione.	Prêtez attention.	Aufpassen.
Come to my office.	Venga a mi oficina.	Venga nel mio ufficio.	Venez à mon bureau.	Kommen Sie in mein Sprechzimmer.
Show me . . .	Muéstreme . . .	Mi faccia vedere . . .	Montrez-moi . . .	Ziegen Sie mir . . .
Right.	Derecha.	A destra.	A droit.	Rechts.

English	Spanish	Italian	French	German
Left.	Izquierda.	A sinistra.	A gauche.	Links.
Here.	Aquí.	Qui.	Ici.	Hier.
There.	Allí. OR Allá.	Qua.	Là.	Da.
Good.	Bien (adv.); Bueno(a) (adj.).	Bene.	Bien.	Gut.
Bad.	Mal. OR Malo(a).	Male.	Mal.	Schlecht.
More or less.	Más o menos.	Più o meno.	Plus ou moins.	Mehr oder weniger.
That is correct.	Es correcto(a).	È giusto.	C'est juste.	Das stimmt.
Not much.	No mucho.	Non molto.	Pas beaucoup.	Nicht viel.
Never.	Nunca.	Mai.	Jamais.	Niemals.
Never mind.	Olvídelo.	Non importa.	Ça ne fait rien.	Lassen Sie es gut sein.
That will do.	Es suficiente.	Basta così.	Ça suffit.	Das ist genug.
You must be very careful.	Tiene que tener mucho cuidado.	Deve usare molte precauzioni.	Vous devez prendre garde.	Sie müssen sehr vorsichtig sein.
Please listen.	Escuche, por favor.	Per favore ascolti.	Écoutez s'il vous plaît.	Bitte hören Sie zu.
It is important to be safe.	Es importante tener cuidado.	È importante essere sicuri.	C'est important d'être sauf.	Es ist wichtig, vorsichtig zu sein.
Keep very quiet.	No haga ningún ruido. OR Quédese quieto(a).	Stia tranquillo.	Restez tranquille.	Verhalten Sie sich sehr ruhig.
You must not speak.	No tiene que hablar.	Non deve parlare.	Vous ne devez pas parler.	Sie dürfen nicht sprechen.

QUESTIONS USED IN HISTORY TAKING

English	Spanish	Italian	French	German
What is your name?	¿Como se llama usted?	Come si chiama?	Quel est votre nom?	Wie heissen Sie?
How old are you?	¿Cuántos años tiene usted?	Quanti anni ha?	Quel âge avez-vous?	Wie alt sind Sie?
Do you understand me?	¿Me entiende? OR ¿Me comprende?	Mi capisce?	Me comprenez-vous?	Verstehen Sie mich?
What did you say?	¿Qué dijó usted?	Che cosa ha detto?	Qu'est-ce que vous avez dit?	Wie bitte?
Are you married?	¿Está usted casado(a)?	È sposato(a)?	Êtes-vous marié?	Sind Sie verheiratet?
Do you have children?	¿Tiene usted hijos OR niños?	Ha bambini?	Avez-vous des enfants?	Haben Sie Kinder?
What are your children's ages?	¿Cuántos años tienen sus niños OR hijos?	Che età hanno i suoi bambini?	Quel âge ont vos enfants?	Wie alt sind Ihre Kinder?
Do you have any sisters/brothers?	¿Tiene usted hermanas/hermanos?	Ha sorelle/fratelli?	Avez-vous des soeurs/frères?	Haben Sie Schwestern/Brüder?
Is your mother/father alive?	¿Vive su madre/padre?	Sua madre/padre è ancora viva(o)?	Est-ce que votre mère/père est en vie?	Lebt Ihre Mutter/Ihr Vater noch?
Of what did your mother die? And your father?	¿De qué murió su madre? ¿Y su padre?	Di che cosa è morta sua mamma? E suo padre?	De quoi est morte votre mère? Et votre père?	Woran ist Ihre Mutter gestorben? Und Ihr Vater?
Where were you born?	¿Dónde nació usted?	Dov'è nato?	Où êtes-vous né?	Wo sind Sie geboren?

1166

Can you read?	¿Puede usted leer?	Sa leggere?	Pouvez-vous lire?	Können Sie lesen?
Can you write?	¿Puede usted escribir?	Sa scrivere?	Pouvez-vous écrire?	Können Sie schreiben?
Are you nervous?	¿Está usted nervioso(a)?	È nervoso(a)?	Êtes-vous nerveux (nerveuse)?	Sind Sie nervös?
Can you remember?	¿Puede usted recordar?	Riesce a ricordare?	Pouvez-vous vous rappeler?	Können Sie sich erinnern?
Is it possible?	¿Es posible?	È possibile?	Est-ce possible?	Ist es möglich?
Is it necessary?	¿Es necesario?	È necessario?	Est-ce nécessaire?	Ist es notwendig?
Which side?	¿A qué lado?	Quale lato?	Quel côté?	Welche Seite?
Since when?	¿Desde cuándo?	Da quando?	Depuis quand?	Seit wann?
How long?	¿Cuánto tiempo?	Da quanto?	Combien de temps?	Wie lange?
How often?	¿Cuántas veces? OR ¿Con cuánta frequencia?	Ogni quanto?	Combien de fois?	Wie oft?
Why?	¿Por qué?	Perchè?	Pourquoi?	Warum?
When?	¿Cuándo?	Quando?	Quand?	Wann?
About how much?	¿Cuánto?	Circa quanto?	A peu près combien?	Wieviel?
Do you have any questions?	¿Tiene usted algunas preguntas?	Ha delle domande?	Est-ce que vous avez des questions?	Haben Sie Fragen?
Why are you here?	¿Por qué está usted aquí?	Perchè è qui?	Pourquoi êtes-vous ici?	Warum sind Sie hier?

Continued on following page

21

QUESTIONS USED IN HISTORY TAKING (Continued)

English	Spanish	Italian	French	German
How do you feel?	¿Cómo está usted? OR ¿Cómo se siente usted?	Come si sente?	Comment vous sentez-vous?	Wie geht es Ihnen?
When did you first become sick?	¿Cuándo se enfermó usted al principio?	Quando si é ammalato la prima volta?	Quand êtes-vous tombé malade pour la première fois?	Wann sind Sie krank geworden?
How long have you felt like this?	¿Cuánto tiempo se ha sentido así?	Da quanto si sente cosi?	Depuis combien de temps vous sentez-vous ainsi?	Wie lange fühlen Sie sich schon so?
How did this illness begin?	¿Cómo empezó esta enfermedad?	Come è cominciata la malattia?	Comment cette maladie a-t-elle commencée?	Wie hat die Krankheit angefangen?
What happened?	¿Qué ocurrió? OR ¿Qué pasó?	Che cosa è successo?	Qu'est-ce qu'il s'est passé?	Was ist passiert?
Did you have an accident?	¿Había un accidente? OR ¿Tuvo un accidente?	Ha avuto un incidente?	Avez-vous eu un accident?	Hatten Sie einen Unfall?
Did it begin gradually?	¿Empezó gradualmente?	È cominciato gradualmente?	Est-ce que cela a commencé progressivement?	Hat es langsam angefangen?
Did you take anything for it?	¿Tomó usted algo para esto?	Prende qualcosa per questo?	Avez-vous pris quelque chose pour cela?	Haben Sie etwas dafür genommen?

English	Spanish	Italian	French	German
Do you feel like you are falling?	¿Le parece que se va a caer?	Si sente come se dovesse cadere?	Vous sentez-vous comme si vous allez tomber?	Ist es Ihnen als ob Sie fallen werden?
Do you feel dizzy?	¿Tiene usted vértigo?	Ha delle vertigini?	Avez-vous le vertige?	Ist Ihnen schwindlig?
Have you any difficulty in breathing?	¿Tiene dificultad de respirar?	Ha difficoltà di respirare?	C'est difficile à respirer?	Fällt Ihnen das Atemholen schwer?
Have you lost weight?	¿Ha perdido usted peso?	É dimagrito?	Avez-vous maigri?	Haben Sie abgenommen?
Are you warm?	¿Tiene usted calor?	Ha caldo?	Avez-vous chaud?	Ist Ihnen heiss?
Are you cold?	¿Tiene usted frío?	Ha freddo?	Avez-vous froid?	Ist Ihnen kalt?
Can you eat?	¿Puede usted comer?	Può mangiare?	Pouvez-vous manger?	Können Sie essen?
Do you have a good appetite?	¿Tiene usted buen apetito?	Ha buon appetito?	Avez-vous un bon appétit?	Haben Sie guten Appetit?
Are you thirsty?	¿Tiene usted sed?	Ha sete?	Avez-vous soif?	Haben Sie Durst?
Do you still feel very weak?	¿Se siente muy débil todavía?	Si sente ancora molto debole?	Vous sentez-vous encore très faible?	Fühlen Sie sich noch sehr schwach?
Had you been drinking an alcoholic beverage?	Había tomado usted alguna bebida alcohólica?	Ha bevuto?	Est-ce que vous-aviez bu quelque chose d'alcoolique?	Waren Sie angetrunken?
Do you drink alcohol?	¿Bebe usted alcohol?	Beve alcolici?	Buvez-vous de l'alcool?	Trinken Sie Alkohol?
Do you smoke cigarettes?	¿Fuma usted cigarillos?	Fuma?	Fumez-vous?	Rauchen Sie Zigaretten?

Continued on following page

21

1169

QUESTIONS USED IN HISTORY TAKING (Continued)

English	Spanish	Italian	French	German
Have you had any surgeries?	¿Ha tenido usted algunas operaciones?	È mai stato sottoposto a interventi chirurgici?	Avez-vous déjà eu des opérations?	Hatten Sie irgendwelche Operationen?
Does your (body part) feel paralyzed?	¿Se siente (parte del cuerpo) paralizado(a)?	Sente il/la (parte del corpo) paralizzato(a)?	Est-ce que votre (partie du corps) est paralysé(e)?	Fühlt sich Ihr (Körperteil) gelähmt an?
Are you tired?	¿Está usted cansado(a)?	È stanco(a)?	Êtes-vous fatigué(e)?	Sind Sie müde?
Have you slept well?	¿Ha dormido bien usted?	Ha dormito bene?	Avez-vous bien dormi?	Haben Sie gut geschlafen?
In what position do you sleep?	¿En qué posición duerme usted?	In che posizione dorme?	Dans quelle position dormez-vous?	In welcher Position schlafen Sie?
How long do you sleep at night?	¿Cuántas horas duerme usted por la noche?	Quanto dorme per notte?	Combien de temps dormez-vous la nuit?	Wie lange schlafen Sie in der Nacht?
How many times do you wake up during the night?	¿Cuántas veces se despierta usted durante la noche?	Quante volte si sveglia durante la notte?	Combien de fois vous réveillez-vous la nuit?	Wie oft wachen Sie nachts auf?
How many times do you get up to use the bathroom?	¿Cuántas veces se levanta usted para usar el baño?	Quante volte si alza per andare in bagno?	Combien de fois vous levez-vous la nuit pour aller aux toilettes?	Wie oft stehen Sie nachts auf, um die Toilette zu benutzen?

QUESTIONS USED TO ASSESS PAIN

English	Spanish	Italian	French	German
Have you any pain?	¿Tiene dolor?	Ha dolori?	Avez-vous du mal?	Haben Sie Schmerzen?
Where does it hurt?	¿Dónde le duele?	Dove le fa male?	Où avez-vous mal?	Wo haben Sie Schmerzen?
Point to where it hurts.	Muéstreme dónde le duele.	Indichi dove le fa male.	Montrez-moi où vous avez mal.	Zeigen Sie wo es weh tut.
When does it hurt?	¿Cuándo le duele?	Quando le fa male?	Quand cela vous fait-il mal?	Wann tut es weh?
Do you have pain here?	¿Le duele aquí?	Ha dolori qui?	Avez-vous mal ici?	Haben Sie Schmerzen hier?
Do you have a pain in your chest?	¿Le duele el pecho?	Ha dolori al torace?	Avez-vous une douleur à la poitrine?	Haben Sie Schmerzen in der Brust.
Does it hurt you to breathe?	¿Le duele respirar?	Le fa male respirare?	Avez-vous mal lorsque vous respirez?	Tut es Ihnen weh zu atmen?
Did you feel much pain at the time?	¿Sintió mucho dolor entonces? OR ¿Le dolia mucho?	Avete sentito molto dolore allora?	Est-ce que ça vous a fait beaucoup de mal alors?	Haben Sie gleich damals arge Schmerzen gespürt?
Is it better/worse now?	¿Está mejor/peor ahora?	Va meglio/peggio ora?	Est-ce que c'est mieux/pire maintenant?	Ist es jetzt besser/schlechter?

Continued on following page

QUESTIONS USED TO ASSESS PAIN (Continued)

English	Spanish	Italian	French	German
Does it still hurt you?	¿Todavía le duele?	Le fa ancora male?	Est-ce que cela vous fait toujours mal?	Tut es immer noch weh?
Is your pain a shooting pain?	¿El dolor es un dolor punzante?	È un dolore lancinante?	Est-ce que la douleur est soudaine?	Ist es ein stechender Schmerz?
Is your pain an aching pain?	¿El dolor es un latido doloroso?	È un dolore persistente?	Est-ce que la douleur est continue?	Ist es ein anhaltender Schmerz?
Is your pain a burning pain?	¿El dolor es un dolor que quema?	È un bruciore?	Est-ce que la douleur vous brule?	Ist es ein brennender Schmerz?
Is your pain as if one were pricking you with pins?	¿El dolor es como pinchar a uno?	È come se qualcuno la stesse pungendo con spilli?	Est-ce que la douleur est comme si on vous piquait avec des épingles?	Ist der Schmerz als ob man Sie mit Nadeln stechen würde?
Does it feel the same as the other side?	¿Se siente lo mismo al otro lado?	Sente lo stesso che dall'altra parte?	Ressentez-vous la même chose de l'autre côté?	Fühlt es sich auf der anderen Seite gleich an?
Does your (body part) feel like "pins and needles"?	¿Está (parte del cuerpo) en brazas?	Sente un formicolio al/alla (parte del corpo)?	Ressentez-vous des picotements dans la (partie du corps)?	Fühlen Sie ein Kribbeln in Ihrem (Körperteil)?

1172

English	Spanish	Italian	French	German
What are your goals?	¿Cuáles son sus objetivos?	Quali sono i suoi obiettivi?	Quels sont vos objectifs?	Was sind Ihre Ziele?
What are you unable to do because of your condition?	¿Cuáles son las cosas que no puede usted hacer a causa de esta condición?	Che cosa è incapace di fare a causa della sua condizione?	Qu'est-ce que vous êtes incapable de faire à cause de votre condition?	Was können Sie nicht tun wegen Ihres Zustandes?
What would you like to do? to be able to do?	¿Qué quisiera hacer?	Che cosa vorrebbe poter fare?	Qu'aimeriez-vous être capable de faire?	Was würden Sie gerne tun?
What could we help you do better?	¿Qué podremos hacer para ayudarle a usted?	Che cosa possiamo aiutarla a fare meglio?	Qu'est-ce que nous pourrions vous aider à faire mieux?	Was können wir Ihnen helfen besser zu erledigen?
Are you able to dress yourself?	¿Puede usted vestirse?	È in grado di vestirsi da sè?	Êtes-vous capable de vous habiller seul(e)?	Können Sie sich selbst anziehen?
Are you able to bathe yourself?	¿Puede usted bañarse?	È in grado di farsi il bagno da sè?	Êtes-vous capable de vous laver seul(e)?	Können Sie sich selbst waschen?
Are you able to drink from a glass?	¿Puede usted beber de un vaso?	È in grado di bere dal bicchiere?	Êtes-vous capable de boire dans un verre?	Können Sie aus einem Glas trinken?
Are you able to feed yourself?	¿Puede usted comer por sí solo/sola?	È in grado di mangiare da solo(a)?	Êtes-vous capable de vous alimenter?	Können Sie selbständig essen?

Continued on following page

21

1173

QUESTIONS USED TO ASSESS FUNCTION (Continued)

English	Spanish	Italian	French	German
Are you able to use the toilet?	¿Puede usted irse al baño?	È in grado di andare al gabinetto?	Êtes-vous capable d'aller aux toilettes?	Können Sie selbständig die Toilette benutzen?
Are you able to use the telephone?	¿Puede usted usar el teléfono?	È in grado di usare il telefono?	Êtes-vous capable d'utiliser le téléphone?	Können Sie das Telefon benutzen?
Does anyone help you?	¿Hay alguien que le ayuda?	Qualcuno l'aiuta?	Est-ce que quelqu'un vous aide?	Hilft Ihnen jemand?
Who do you live with: Mother/father? Husband/wife?	¿Vive usted con: Su madre/padre? Su esposo/ esposa?	Con chi vive: Madre/padre? Marito/moglie?	Vivez-vous avec: Votre mère/père? Votre mari/femme?	Mit wem leben Sie: Mutter/Vater? Mann/Frau?
Children? Alone? Aunt/uncle? Grandmother/ grandfather? Friend(s)?	Sus niños? Por sí solo/sola? Su tía/tío? Su abuela/ abuelo? Su amiga(o)/ amigas (amigos)?	Figli? Solo(a)? Zia/zio? Nonna/nonno? Amico(i)?	Vos enfants? Seul? Seule? Votre tante/oncle? Votre grand'mère/ grand-père? Votre ami (Vos amis)?	Kinder? Alleine? Tante/Onkel? Grossmutter/ Grossvater? Freund(e)?
Where do you live?	¿Dónde vive usted?	Dove vive?	Où vivez-vous?	Wo leben Sie?

Do you have to go up/down stairs?	¿Tiene usted que pasearse en las escaleras o arriba o abajo?	Deve salire/scendere le scale?	Avez-vous des escaliers à monter/ ou à descendre?	Müssen Sie Treppen hinauf/herab steigen?
Do you have stairs in your house?	¿Hay escaleras en casa?	Ci sono scale a casa sua?	Avez-vous des escaliers dans votre maison?	Haben Sie Treppen in Ihrem Haus?
Do you have stairs outside?	¿Hay escaleras afuera?	Ci sono scale fuori?	Avez-vous des escaliers à l'extérieur?	Haben Sie draussen Treppen?
Is there a handrail?	¿Hay pasamano?	C'è il corrimano?	Y a-t-il une rampe?	Gibt es ein Geländer?
Do you have an elevator?	¿Hay ascensor?	Ha l'ascensore?	Avez-vous un ascenseur?	Haben Sie einen Aufzug?
Do you use a walker?	¿Usa usted un walker?	Usa il girello?	Vous servez-vous d'un marcheur?	Benutzen Sie eine Gehhilfe?
Do you use a cane?	¿Usa usted un bastón?	Usa il bastone?	Vous servez-vous d'une canne?	Benutzen Sie einen Stock?
Do you use crutches?	¿Usa usted muletas?	Usa le stampelle?	Vous servez-vous de béquilles?	Benutzen Sie Krüken?
Do you use a brace?	¿Usa usted una abrazadera?	Usa il busto ortopedico?	Vous servez-vous d'une attache?	Benutzen Sie eine Stütze?
Do you play any sports?	¿Juega usted a los deportes?	Fa sport?	Faites-vous du sport?	Betreiben Sie Sport?

21

1175

QUESTIONS USED TO ASSESS WORK				
English	**Spanish**	**Italian**	**French**	**German**
Are you working?	¿Trabaja usted?	Lavora?	Est-ce vous travaillez?	Arbeiten Sie?
What work do you do?	¿Cuál es su ocupación?	Che lavoro fa?	Quelle est votre profession?	Was ist Ihr Beruf?
Is it heavy physical work?	¿Es un trabajo corporal pesado?	È un pesante lavoro manuale?	Est-ce que c'est un travail physiquement fatigant?	Ist es eine schwere körperliche Arbeit?
What work have you done?	¿Qué trabajo ha hecho?	Che lavoro ha fatto?	A quoi avez-vous travaillé?	Welche Arbeit haben Sie getan?

EXPRESSIONS RELATED TO MEDICATIONS

English	Spanish	Italian	French	German
Are you taking any medications?	¿Toma usted medicina?	Sta assumendo medicinali?	Prenez-vous des médicaments?	Nehmen Sie Medikamente?
What medications do you take?	¿Cuáles son las medicinas que toma?	Che medicine prende?	Quels médicaments prenez-vous?	Welche Medikamente nehmen Sie?
Have you taken the medicine?	¿Ha tomado usted la medicina?	Ha preso la medicina?	Avez-vous pris le médicament?	Haben Sie die Medizin genommen?
Bring in your pill bottle.	Traiga consigo la botella de píldoras.	Porti la confezione dei medicinali.	Amenez votre boîte de cachets.	Bringen Sie Ihre Pillenschachtel.
Bring in a list of the names of the medications you are taking.	Traiga consigo una lista de las medicinas que toma.	Porti una lista con i nomi dei medicinali che sta assumendo.	Amenez la liste de médicaments que vous prenez.	Bringen Sie eine Liste der Medikamente, die Sie nehmen.

21

TERMS USED TO DESCRIBE DISEASES AND MEDICAL CONDITIONS

English	Spanish	Italian	French	German
What diseases/ medical problems have you had?	¿Cuáles son las enfermedades o problemas que usted ha tenido?	Che malattie/ problemi medici ha avuto?	Quelles maladies/quels problèmes médicaux avez-vous eu?	Welche Krankheiten/ medizinische Probleme haben Sie bisher gehabt?
Arthritis.	Artritis.	Artrite.	L'arthrite.	Arthritis.
Bleeding.	Flujo de sangre.	Emorraggia.	Un saignement.	Blutung.
Burn.	Quemadura.	Ustione.	Une brûlure.	Verbrennung.
Cancer.	Cáncer.	Cancro.	Le cancer.	Krebs.
Chickenpox.	Varicela.	Varicella.	La varicelle.	Windpocken.
Diabetes.	Diabetes.	Diabete.	Le diabète.	Zuckerkrankheit.
Diphtheria.	Difteria.	Difterite.	La diphthérie.	Diphtherie.
Ear infections.	Dolores de oido.	Infezioni alle orecchie.	Une infection des oreilles.	Ohrentzündung.
Fracture.	Fracturas.	Frattura.	Une fracture.	Bruch.
German measles.	Rubéola.	Rosolia.	Rubéole.	Röteln.
Gonorrhea.	Gonorrea.	Gonorrea.	La gonorrhée.	Gonorrhöe, Tripper.
Head injury.	Daño de cabeza.	Trauma cranico.	Une blessure à la tête.	Kopfverletzung.
Headaches.	Dolores de cabeza.	Mal di testa.	Des maux de tête.	Kopfschmerzen.

Heart disease.	Enfermedad del corazón.	Malattie cardiache.	Une maladie de coeur.	Herzkrankheit.
High blood pressure.	Tensión sanguínea elevada.	Pressione alta del sangue.	La tension arterielle trop élevée.	Hohen Blutdruck.
High fevers.	Fiebres elevadas.	Febbri alte.	Des fortes fièvres.	Hohes Fieber.
HIV.	HIV.	HIV.	Le virus du sida.	HIV.
Influenza.	Gripe (influenza).	Influenza.	La grippe.	Grippe.
Measles.	Sarampión.	Morbillo.	La rougeole.	Die Masern.
Mental disease.	Enfermedad mental.	Malattie mentale.	Une maladie mentale.	Geisteskrankheit.
Mumps.	Paperas.	Orecchioni.	Les oreillons.	Mumps.
Nervous disease.	Enfermedad nerviosa.	Malattie nervosa.	Une maladie nerveuse.	Nervenkrankheit.
Pleurisy.	Pleuresía.	Pleurite.	La pleurésie.	Rippenfellentzündung.
Pneumonia.	Pulmonía.	Polmonite.	Pneumonie.	Die Lungenentzündung.
Polio	Poliomielitis. OR Parálisis infantil.	Poliomelite.	La polio.	Polio.
Rheumatic fever.	Fiebre reumática.	Febbre reumatica.	La fièvre rhumatismale.	Rheumatisches Fieber.
Rheumatoid arthritis.	Artritis reumatoidea.	Artrite reumatoide.	L'arthrite rhumatismale.	Rheumatische Arthritis.

Continued on following page

21

TERMS USED TO DESCRIBE DISEASES AND MEDICAL CONDITIONS (Continued)

English	Spanish	Italian	French	German
Scarlet fever.	Escarlatina.	Scarlattina.	La fièvre scarlatine.	Das Scharlachfieber.
Seizures.	Ataques.	Crisi epilettiche.	Une attaque.	Anfälle.
Smallpox.	Viruela.	Variolo.	La variole.	Pocken.
Sprain.	Torcedura.	Distorsione.	Une entorse.	Verstauchung.
Stroke.	Ataque fulminante.	Ictus.	Une congestion cérébrale.	Schlaganfall.
Syphilis.	Sífilis.	Sifilide (lue).	La syphilis.	Syphilis.
Tuberculosis.	Tuberculosis.	Tuberculosi.	Tuberculose.	Die Tuberkulose.
Typhoid fever.	Fiebre tifoidea.	Febbre tifoide.	La fièvre typhoide.	Der Typhus.
Ulcer.	Úlcera.	Ulcera.	Un ulcère.	Geschwür.

EXAMINATION: GENERAL INSTRUCTIONS

English	Spanish	Italian	French	German
Please.	Por favor.	Per favore.	S'il vous plaît.	Bitte.
Thank you.	Gracias.	Grazie.	Merci.	Danke.
You are welcome.	De nada.	Prego.	De rien.	Bitte.
Please remove your	Por favor quítese.	Per favore si tolga	S'il vous plaît enlevez	Bitte legen Sie
Dress.	El vestido.	Il vestito.	Votre robe.	Ihr Kleid.
Pants.	Los pantalones.	I pantaloni.	Votre pantalon.	Ihre Hosen.
Shirt.	La camisa.	La camicia.	Votre jupe.	Ihr Hemd.
Shoes.	Los zapatos.	Le scarpe.	Vos chaussures.	Ihre Schuhe.
Socks.	Las calcetines.	Le calze.	Vos chausettes.	Ihre Socken ab.
Let me see . . .	Déjeme ver . . .	Mi lasci vedere . . .	Permettez-moi de voir	Lassen Sie mich sehen . . .
Let me feel your pulse.	Déjeme tomarle el pulso.	Mi lasci sentire il polso.	Permettez-moi de vous tâter le pouls.	Lassen Sie mich Ihren Puls fühlen.
Show me your right/left (body part).	Muéstreme (parte del cuerpo) derecho(a)/izquierdo(a).	Mi faccia vedere il/la (parte del corpo) destra/sinistra.	Montrez-moi votre (partie du corps) droit/gauche.	Zeigen Sie mir Ihren rechten/linken (Körperteil).
Look straight ahead.	Mire usted hacia delante.	Guardi diritto davanti a sé.	Regardez devant.	Geradeaus sehen.

Continued on following page

21

1181

EXAMINATION: GENERAL INSTRUCTIONS (Continued)

English	Spanish	Italian	French	German
You are not going to fall.	Usted no se va a caer.	Non cadrà.	Vous n'allez pas tomber.	Sie werden nicht fallen.
This will not hurt.	Ésto no le va a doler.	Questo non farà male.	Ceci ne va pas faire mal.	Es wird nicht weh tun.
Tell me when it starts to hurt.	Dígame cuándo empieza a doler.	Mi dica quando incomincia a farle male.	Dites-moi quand ça commence à faire mal.	Sagen Sie mir wenn es weh tut.
You are okay.	Usted está bien.	Lei è a posto.	Vous allez bien.	Sie sind OK.
Don't cry.	No llore.	Non pianga.	Ne pleurez pas.	Nicht weinen.
Don't worry.	No se preocupe.	Non tema.	Ne vous inquiétez pas.	Machen Sie sich keine Sorgen.
Sit up.	Siéntese.	Si metta a sedere.	Asseyez-vous.	Aufsitzen.
Sit down.	Siéntese.	Si sieda.	Asseyez-vous.	Setzen Sie sich.
Stand.	Levántese.	Si alzi.	Levez-vous.	Aufstehen.
Walk.	Ande.	Cammini.	Marchez.	Gehen.
Roll over.	Vuelva.	Si giri.	Tournez-vous.	Umdrehen.
Lie on your stomach on the table (face down).	Acuéstese en la mesa con boca abajo.	Si metta prono sul lettino (faccia in giù).	Allongez-vous sur le ventre sur la table.	Legen Sie sich auf Ihren Bauch auf den Tisch.

English	Spanish	Italian	French	German
Lie on your back on the table (face up).	Acuéstese en la mesa con boca arriba.	Si metta supino sul lettino (faccia in su).	Couchez-vous sur le dos sur la table.	Legen Sie sich auf den Rücken.
Lie on your side.	Acuéstese de lado.	Si corichi sul fianco.	Couchez-vous sur le côté.	Legen Sie sich auf die Seite.
Lie on your other side.	Acuéstese al otro lado.	Si corichi sull'altro fianco.	Couchez-vous sur l'autre côté.	Legen Sie sich auf die andere Seite.
Squat.	Agáchese usted.	Si accovacci.	Accroupissez-vous.	Hocken Sie sich hin.
Kneel.	Arrodíllese usted.	Si inginocchi.	Mettez-vous à genoux.	Knien Sie sich nieder.
Raise.	Levante.	Si alzi.	Levez.	Höher.
Lower.	Baje.	Si abbassi.	Abaissez.	Tiefer.
This way.	Por aca.	Così.	Ainsi.	Hierhin.
Again.	Otra vez.	Di nuovo.	Encore.	Noch einmal.
Hold it.	Sosténgalo.	Lo tenga.	Restez ainsi.	Halten.
Push against me.	Empuje contra mí.	Spinga contro di me.	Poussez contre moi.	Drücken Sie gegen mich.
Push down with your hands to lift your body.	Empuje con las manos para levantar el cuerpo.	Faccia forza sulle mani al fine di alzare il corpo.	Appuyez vous sur les mains et soulevez votre corps.	Stemmen Sie mit den Händen.
Push as hard as you can.	Empuje con la fuerza que sea posible.	Spinga più forte che può.	Poussez tant que vous pouvez.	Drücken Sie so stark Sie können.

Continued on following page

21

1183

	EXAMINATION: GENERAL INSTRUCTIONS (Continued)			
English	**Spanish**	**Italian**	**French**	**German**
Is that the best you can do?	¿Es lo mejor que puede usted hacer?	È questo il meglio che può fare?	Est-ce le mieux que vous puissiez faire?	Können Sie nicht stärker?
Relax.	Cálmese.	Si rilassi.	Detendez-vous.	Entspannen Sie sich.
Slowly.	Lentamente.	Adagio.	Lentement.	Langsam.
Not so fast.	No tan rápido.	Non così in fretta.	Pas si vite.	Nicht so schnell.
Rest.	Descánse.	Si riposi.	Reposez-vous.	Ausruhen.
Stay there.	Quédese allí.	Stia là.	Restez là.	Bleiben Sie hier.
Move your (body part) like this.	Mueve su (parte del cuerpo) así.	Muova il/la (parte del corpo) così.	Bougez votre (partie du corps) comme ceci.	Bewegen Sie Ihre (Körperteil) so.
Now with your other (body part).	Ahora con el otro/la otra (parte del cuerpo).	Ora con l'altro/a (parte del corpo).	Maintenant avec votre autre (partie du corps).	Nun mit dem anderen (Körperteil).

EXPRESSIONS USED WHEN EXAMINING THE FACE AND NECK

English	Spanish	Italian	French	German
Lift your head.	Levante la cabeza.	Alzi la testa.	Levez la tête.	Kopf heben.
Open your mouth.	Abra la boca.	Apra la bocca.	Ouvrez la bouche.	Mund öffnen.
Close your mouth.	Cierre la boca.	Chiuda la bocca.	Fermez la bouche.	Mund schliessen.
Open your eyes.	Abra los ojos.	Apra gli occhi.	Ouvrez les yeux.	Augen öffnen.
Close your eyes.	Cierre los ojos.	Chiuda gli occhi.	Fermez les yeux.	Augen schliessen.
Wrinkle your nose.	Arruga la nariz.	Corrughi il naso.	Plissez le nez.	Nase runzeln.
Smile.	Sonréase.	Sorrida.	Souriez.	Lächeln.
Bend your head toward your chest.	Incline la cabeza hacia el pecho.	Pieghi la testa verso il torace.	Inclinez la tête vers votre poitrine.	Beugen Sie Ihren Kopf vorwärts.
Bend your head backward.	Incline la cabeza hacia atrás.	Pieghi la testa indietro.	Inclinez la tête en arrière.	Beugen Sie Ihren Kopf zurück.
Turn your head to look behind you.	Vuelva la cabeza para mirar atrás.	Giri la testa di lato e guardi dietro di sé.	Tournez la tête pour regarder derrière vous.	Drehen Sie Ihren Kopf nach hinten.
Bend your neck so that your ear moves toward your shoulder.	Incline la cabeza para que su oído se mueva hacia el hombro.	Pieghi la testa portando l'orecchio verso la spalla.	Inclinez votre nuque de façon à ce que votre oreille aille vers votre épaule.	Beugen Sie Ihren Hals, sodass Ihr Ohr sich gegen die Schulter bewegt.

21

		EXPRESSIONS USED WHEN EXAMINING HEARING		
English	Spanish	Italian	French	German
Do you have ringing in the ears?	¿Le pitan los oídos?	Le ronzano le orecchie?	Avez-vous des bourdonnements d'oreilles?	Haben Sie Ohrenbrausen?
Do you have discharge from the ears?	¿Sale flúido de los oídos?	Le esce materia dalle orecchie?	Est-ce que vous avez un écoulement des oreilles?	Eitern Ihre Ohren?
Do you have difficulty hearing?	¿Tiene dificultad para oír?	Ha problemi di udito?	Avez-vous des difficultés pour entendre?	Hören Sie schwer?
Do you wear a hearing aid?	¿Lleva usted auxilio para oír?	Porta l'apparecchio acustico?	Portez-vous un appareil pour entendre?	Benutzen Sie eine Gehörhilfe?

EXPRESSIONS USED WHEN EXAMINING VISION

English	Spanish	Italian	French	German
Look up.	Mire usted hacia el cielo.	Guardi su.	Regardez en haut.	Schauen Sie hinauf.
Look down.	Mire usted hacia el suelo.	Guardi giù.	Regardez en bas.	Schauen Sie hinunter.
Look toward your nose.	Mire usted hacia la nariz.	Si guardi il naso.	Regardez votre nez.	Schauen Sie auf Ihre Nase.
Look at me.	Míreme.	Mi guardi.	Regardez-moi.	Sehen Sie mich an.
Can you see what is on the wall?	¿Puede usted ver lo que está en la pared?	Può vedere cosa c'e sui muro?	Pouvez-vous voir ce qu'il y a contre le mur?	Können Sie sehen, was hier an der Wand ist?
Can you see it now?	¿Puede usted verlo ahora?	Può vederlo adesso?	Le voyez-vous maintenant?	Können Sie es jetzt sehen?
What is it?	¿Qué es ésto?	Che cosa è?	Qu'est-ce que c'est?	Was ist es?
Tell me what number it is.	Dígame qué número es.	Mi dica che numero è.	Dites-moi quel est le numéro.	Sagen Sie mir welche Nummer es ist.
Tell me what letter it is.	Dígame qué letra es.	Mi dica che lettera è.	Dites-moi quelle est la lettre.	Nennen Sir mir diesen Buchstaben.
Can you see clearly?	¿Puede ver claramente?	Può vedere chiaro?	Pouvez-vous voir clairement?	Sehen Sie deutlich?

Continued on following page

21

English	Spanish	Italian	French	German
		EXPRESSIONS USED WHEN EXAMINING VISION (Continued)		
Can you see better at a distance?	¿Puede usted ver mejor a la distancia?	Vede meglio da lontano?	Voyez-vous mieux à la distance?	Sehen Sie in die Entfernung besser?
Do your eyes water?	¿Derraman lágrimas los ojos?	Le lacrimano gli occhi?	Est-ce que les yeux vous coulent?	Tränen Ihre Augen?
Can you open your eyes?	¿Puede usted abrir los ojos?	Può aprire gli occhi?	Pouvez-vous ouvrir vos yeux?	Können Sie Ihre Augen aufmachen?
Did anything get into your eye?	¿Hay algo en el ojo?	Le è entrata qualche cosa nell'occhio?	Est-ce que quelque chose est entrée dans l'oeil?	Ist Ihnen etwas ins Auge geflogen?
Do you sometimes see things double?	¿Ve usted las cosas doble algunas veces?	Vede qualche volta le cose doppie?	Est-ce que la vue est double parfois?	Sehen Sie manchmal doppelt?
Do you wear glasses?	¿Lleva usted anteojos?	Porta gli occhiali?	Portez-vous des lunettes?	Tragen Sie eine Brille?
Has your vision changed?	¿Ha cambiado la visión?	È cambiata la sua vista?	Votre vue a-t-elle changée?	Ist Ihre Sicht verändert?
Do your eyes hurt?	¿Le duelen los ojos?	Le fanno male gli occhi?	Vos yeux vous font-ils mal?	Tuen Ihre Augen weh?

English	Spanish	Italian	French	German
Raise your arm.	Levante el brazo.	Alzi il braccio.	Levez le bras.	Arm heben.
Move your arm out to the side.	Mueve el brazo arriba al lado.	Muova il braccio di lato.	Ecartez le bras du corps.	Arm zur Seite bewegen.
Move your arm back to your side.	Mueve el brazo a su lado.	Muova il braccio verso il fianco.	Ramenez le bras vers le corps.	Arm anlegen.
Bend your elbow.	Doble el codo.	Pieghi il gomito.	Pliez le coude.	Ellbogen bewegen.
Straighten your elbow.	Enderece el codo.	Distenda il gomito.	Redressez le coude.	Ellbogen strecken.
Turn your hand over.	Revuelva la mano.	Giri la mano.	Retournez la main.	Hand drehen.
Bend your fingers.	Doble los dedos.	Pieghi le dita.	Pliez les doigts.	Finger bewegen.
Straighten your fingers.	Enderece los dedos.	Distenda le dita.	Redressez les doigts.	Finger strecken.
Bend your wrist (flexion).	Doble la muñeca.	Pieghi il polso.	Pliez le poignet.	Handgelenk beugen.
Lift your wrist (extension).	Levante la muñeca.	Alzi il polso.	Relevez le poignet.	Hand strecken.
Pull your shoulders back.	Mueve los hombros hacia atrás.	Tiri indietro le spalle.	Mettez vos épaules en arrière.	Ziehen Sie Ihre Schultern zurück.
Circle your shoulder.	Haga círculo con el hombro.	Faccia roteare le spalle.	Faites tourner votre épaule.	Kreisen Sie Ihre Schultern.

Continued on following page

21

EXPRESSIONS USED WHEN EXAMINING THE UPPER EXTREMITY (Continued)

English	Spanish	Italian	French	German
Let me see your hand.	Muéstreme la mano.	Mi faccia vedere la sua mano.	Montrez-moi la main.	Zeigen Sie mir Ihre Hand.
Squeeze my hand.	Apriete mi mano.	Stringa forte la mia mano.	Serrez ma main.	Drücken Sie meine Hand.
Take this from me.	Tome éste.	Prenda questo da me.	Prenez-moi ceci.	Nehmen Sie das von mir.
When did you notice weakness in your arms?	¿Cuándo notó usted la debilidad de los brazos?	Quando si è accorto che le sue braccia erano deboli?	Quand avez-vous remarqué une faiblesse dans vos bras?	Seit wann ist Ihr Arm schwach?
Had you been sleeping on your arm?	¿Había usted dormido encima del brazo?	Ha dormito col braccio sotto la testa?	Vous êtes-vous endormi sur le bras?	Sind Sie auf Ihrem Arm eingeschlafen?
Can you move your arm at all?	¿Puede usted mover el brazo?	Non può movere il braccio per niente?	Pouvez-vous bouger votre bras?	Können Sie Ihren Arm bewegen?

EXPRESSIONS USED WHEN EXAMINING THE LOWER EXTREMITY

English	Spanish	Italian	French	German
Bend your hip.	Doble la cadera.	Pieghi l'anca.	Pliez la hanche.	Hüfte beugen.
Lift your leg.	Levante la pierna.	Alzi la gamba.	Levez la jambe.	Bein anheben.
Bend your knee.	Doble la rodilla.	Pieghi il ginocchio.	Pliez le genou.	Knie beugen.
Straighten your knee.	Enderece la rodilla.	Distenda il ginocchio.	Redressez le genou.	Knie strecken.
Roll your leg in.	Mueva la pierna hacia el interior.	Giri la gamba in dentro.	Faites tourner la jambe en-dedans.	Bein einwärts drehen.
Roll your leg out.	Mueva la pierna hacia el exterior.	Giri la gamba in fuori.	Faites tourner la jambe en-dehors.	Bein auswärts drehen.
Lift your foot.	Levante el pie.	Alzi il piede.	Levez le pied.	Fuss hoch heben.
Push your foot down.	Empuje el pie para abajo.	Spinga il piede in giù.	Poussez le pied contre en-bas.	Fuss herunterdrehen.
Lift your toes.	Levante los dedos de pie.	Alzi le dita del piede.	Levez les orteils.	Zehen strecken.
Bend your toes.	Doble los dedos de pie.	Pieghi le dita del piede.	Pliez les orteils.	Zehen beugen.
Pull your foot in.	Mueva el pie para adentro.	Muova il piede in dentro.	Tournez le pied en-dedans.	Fuss nach innen ziehen.
Pull your foot out.	Mueva el pie para afuera.	Muova il piede in fuori.	Tournez le pied en-dehors.	Fuss nach aussen ziehen.

	EXPRESSIONS USED WHEN EXAMINING THE BACK			
English	**Spanish**	**Italian**	**French**	**German**
Bend forward.	Doble hacia adelante.	Si pieghi in avanti.	Penchez-vous en avant.	Beugen Sie sich vorwärts.
Bend backward.	Doble hacia atrás.	Si pieghi in dietro.	Penchez-vous en arrière.	Beugen Sie sich hinunter.
Bend sideways.	Doble al lado.	Si pieghi di lato.	Penchez-vous sur le côté.	Beugen Sie sich seitwärts.
Keep your knees straight/bent.	Mantenga las rodillas directas/dobladas.	Tenga il ginocchio diritto/piegato.	Gardez vos genoux droits/pliés.	Lassen Sie Ihre Knie gestreckt/gebogen.
Lift this way.	Levante así.	Sollevi in questo modo.	Levez de cette façon.	Heben Sie es so hoch.
Keep things close to your body.	Mantenga cosas cerca del cuerpo.	Tenga le cose vicino al corpo.	Gardez les choses près de votre corps.	Behalten Sie alles nahe an Ihrem Körper.

EXPRESSIONS USED WHEN EXAMINING THE RESPIRATORY SYSTEM

English	Spanish	Italian	French	German
Cough.	Tosa.	Tossisca.	Toussez.	Husten Sie.
Cough again.	Tosa otra vez.	Tossisca ancora.	Toussez encore une fois.	Husten Sie noch einmal.
Open your mouth.	Abra la boca.	Apra la bocca.	Ouvrez la bouche.	Öffnen Sie den Mund.
Does it hurt you to open your mouth?	¿Le duele abrir la boca?	Le fa male aprir la bocca?	Vous fait-il mal d'ouvrir la bouche?	Spüren Sie Schmerzen, wenn Sie den Mund öffnen?
When did you first start coughing?	¿Cuándo empezó usted toser?	Quando ha cominciato a tossire la prima volta?	Quand avez-vous commencé à tousser?	Wann fingen Sie zu husten an?
Do you cough a lot?	¿Tose mucho?	Tossisce molto?	Toussez-vous beaucoup?	Husten Sie viel?
I will now listen to your lungs.	Ahora voy a escuchar los pulmones.	Ora le sentirò i polmoni.	Maintenant, je vais écouter vos poumons.	Jetzt höre ich auf Ihre Lungen.
Take a deep breath.	Respire profundamente.	Faccia un respiro profondo.	Respirez profondement.	Atmen Sie tief.
Exhale.	Espire.	Espiri.	Expirez.	Atmen Sie aus.

Continued on following page

21

EXPRESSIONS USED WHEN EXAMINING THE RESPIRATORY SYSTEM (Continued)

English	Spanish	Italian	French	German
Do you cough up fluid?	¿Cuando tosa, esputa flema?	Espelle liquidi tossendo?	Toussez-vous des crachats?	Husten Sie Flüssigkeit aus?
What is the color of what you cough up?	¿De qué color es la flema?	Che colore ha ciò che espelle?	Quelle est la couleur de ce que vous crachez?	Welche Farbe hat das, was Sie ausspucken?
Does your tongue feel swollen?	¿Siente usted hinchada la lengua?	Ha la lingua gonfia?	Est-ce que la langue vous paraît gonflée?	Fühlt sich Ihre Zunge wie geschwollen an?
Do you have a sore throat?	¿Le duele la garganta?	Ha mal di gola?	Avez-vous mal à la gorge?	Haben Sie Halsschmerzen?
Does it hurt to swallow?	¿Le duele tragar?	Quando deglutisce le fa male?	Ça vous fait mal d'avaler?	Spüren Sie Schmerzen beim Schlucken?

English	Spanish	Italian	French	German
Do you have stomach cramps?	¿Tiene usted calambres en el estómago?	Ha dei dolori acuti allo stomaco?	Avez-vous des crampes d'estomac?	Haben Sie Magenkrämpfe?
Do you have pain in your stomach?	¿Le duele el estómago?	Ha dolori allo stomaco?	Avez-vous une douleur à l'estomac?	Haben Sie Bauchschmerzen?
Are you nauseated?	¿Está mareado(a)?	Ha nausea?	Avez-vous la nausée?	Ist Ihnen schlecht?
Does eating make you vomit?	¿Cuando come, tiene que vomitar?	Vomita dopo aver mangiato?	Vomissez-vous ce que vous mangez?	Erbrechen Sie nachdem Sie gegessen haben?
Have you vomited? Do you still vomit?	¿Ha usted vomitado? ¿Vomita todavía?	Ha vomitato? Vomita ancora?	Avez-vous vomi? Vomissez-vous encore?	Haben Sie erbrochen? Erbrechen Sie noch immer?
Is it of a dark or bright red color?	¿Es de color rojo oscuro o claro?	É di colore rosso chiaro o rosso scuro?	La couleur est elle rouge foncé ou clair?	Ist es dunkel oder hellrot?
Are any of your limbs swollen?	¿Están hinchados alguno miembros?	Si sente gonfio in qualche parte?	Avez-vous des membres gonflés?	Ist irgendeines Ihrer Glieder geschwollen?
How long have they been swollen like this?	¿Desde cuándo estan hinchados asi?	Da quanto tempo che li ha cosi gonfi?	Depuis quand sont-ils gonflés comme ça?	Seit wann sind Sie so angeschwollen?

Continued on following page

21

EXPRESSIONS USED WHEN EXAMINING THE GASTROINTESTINAL SYSTEM (Continued)

English	Spanish	Italian	French	German
Were they ever swollen before?	¿Han estado hinchados alguna vez antes?	Sono stati mai gonfi prima?	Ont-ils jamais été gonflés autrefois?	Sind Sie je früher so angeschwollen gewesen?
How long has your tongue been that color?	¿Cuánto tiempo hace que la lengua está de ese color?	Da quanto tempo ha la lingua di quel colore?	Depuis combien de temps votre langue a-t-elle cette couleur?	Wie lange hat Ihre Zunge schon diese Farbe?
How are your stools?	¿Cómo son las defecaciones?	Come va di corpo?	Comment allez-vous à la selle?	Wie ist der Stuhlgang?
Are they regular?	¿Son regulares?	Va regolarmente?	Allez-vous à la selle régulièrement?	Ist er regelmässig?
Have you noticed their color?	¿Se ha fijado usted en el color?	Si è accorto di che colore?	Avez-vous remarqué la couleur de vos selles?	Haben Sie auf die Farbe geachtet?
Are you constipated?	¿Está usted estreñido?	È stitico?	Êtes-vous constipé?	Leiden Sie an Verstopfung?
Do you have diarrhea?	¿Tiene diarrea?	Ha diarrea?	Avez-vous la diarrhée?	Haben Sie Durchfall?
Do you pass any blood?	¿Hay sangre en las defecaciones?	Passa sangue?	Y'a-t-il du sang?	Ist Blut im Stuhl?
Have you any difficulty urinating?	¿Tiene usted dificultad en orinar?	Ha della difficoltà nell' urinare?	Avez-vous de la difficulté uriner?	Haben Sie Schwierigkeiten?
Do you urinate involuntarily?	¿Orina usted sin querer?	Urina involontariamente?	Urinez-vous involontairement?	Lassen Sie den Harn ohne es zu wollen?

English	Spanish	Italian	French	German
EXPRESSIONS USED WHEN EXAMINING THE CENTRAL NERVOUS SYSTEM				
How does your head feel?	¿Cómo e siente la cabeza?	Come si sente la testa?	Comment va votre tête?	Wie geht es Ihrem Kopf?
Do you have a good memory?	¿Tiene usted buena memoria?	Ha buona memoria?	Avez-vous une bonne mémoire?	Haben Sie ein gutes Gedächtnis?
Do you have any pain in the head?	¿Le duele usted la cabeza?	Ha dolor di testa?	Avez-vous mal à la tête?	Haben Sie Kopfschmerzen?
Did you fall?	¿Se cayó usted?	È caduto?	Êtes-vous tombé?	Sind Sie gefallen?
How did you fall?	¿Cómo se cayó?	Come è caduto?	Comment êtes-vous tombé?	Wie sind Sie gefallen?
Did you faint?	¿Se desmayó?	È svenuto?	Vous êtes-vous évanoui?	Sind Sie ohnmächtig geworden?
Have you ever had fainting spells?	¿Se desmayó usted alguna vez?	È mai svenuto regolarmente?	Avez-vous jamais eu des évanouissements?	Haben Sie jemals Ohnmachtsanfälle gehabt?
Do you get headaches?	¿Tiene usted dolores de cabeza?	Le viene mal di testa?	Avez-vous des maux de tête?	Haben Sie Kopfschmerzen?
Did you become unconscious?	¿Estuvo inconsciente?	Ha perso conoscenza?	Avez-vous perdu conscience?	Wurden Sie bewusstlos?

Continued on following page

21

EXPRESSIONS USED WHEN EXAMINING THE CENTRAL NERVOUS SYSTEM (Continued)

English	Spanish	Italian	French	German
Do people have difficulty understanding you?	¿Tiene la gente dificultad de entenderle?	La gente ha difficoltà a capirla?	Les gens ont-ils des difficultés pour vous comprendre?	Haben Leute Schwierigkeiten Sie zu verstehen?
Do you have difficulty understanding what people say to you?	¿Tiene usted dificultad de entender lo que le dice la gente?	Ha difficoltà a capire cosa le dice la gente?	Avez-vous des difficultés pour comprendre les gens?	Haben Sie Schwierigkeiten zu verstehen was Leute zu Ihnen sagen?
What is the date?	¿Cuál es la fecha de hoy?	Quanti ne abbiamo?	Quelle est la date?	Welches Datum ist heute?
What month is it?	¿En qué mes estamos?	Che mese è?	Quel mois est-ce?	Welcher Monat ist jetzt?
What day is it?	¿Qué día es hoy?	Che giorno è?	Quel jour est-ce?	Welcher Tag ist heute?
What year is it?	¿En qué año estamos?	Che anno è?	Quelle année est-ce?	Welches Jahr ist jetzt?

What do you use this for?	¿Para qué se usa esto?	Per che cosa usa questo?	Que faites-vous avec cela?	Wozu benutzen Sie das?
Follow the moving pencil with your eyes.	Siga el movimiento del lápiz con los ojos.	Segua il movimento della matita con gli occhi.	Suivez le crayon avec vos yeux.	Folgen Sie dem Bleistift mit Ihren Augen.
Copy this.	Copie esto.	Copi questo.	Copiez ceci.	Kopieren Sie das.
Tell me when you see it.	Dígame cuando lo vea.	Mi dica quando lo vede.	Dites-moi quand vous le voyez.	Sagen Sie mir, wenn Sie es Sehen.
Do not move your head.	No mueva la cabeza.	Non muova la testa.	Ne bougez pas votre tête.	Nicht den Kopf drehen.
Draw a circle.	Dibuje un círculo.	Disegni un cerchio.	Dessinez un rond.	Zeichnen Sie einen Kreis.
Draw a triangle.	Dibuje un triángulo.	Disegni un triangolo.	Dessinez un triangle.	Zeichnen Sie ein Dreieck.
Draw a cross.	Dibuje una cruz.	Disegni una croce.	Dessinez une croix.	Zeichnen Sie ein Kreuz.
Draw a house.	Dibuje una casa.	Disegni una casa.	Dessinez une maison.	Zeichnen Sie ein Haus.
Pick the one that is different.	Escoja el(la) que es diferente.	Scelga quello diverso.	Prenez celui(celle) qui est différent.	Wählen Sie dasjenige, das anders aussieht.

Continued on following page

21

	EXPRESSIONS USED WHEN EXAMINING THE CENTRAL NERVOUS SYSTEM (Continued)			
English	Spanish	Italian	French	German
Pick the one that is the same.	Escoja el(la) que es igual.	Scelga quello uguale.	Prenez celui(celle) qui est pareil.	Wählen Sie dasjenige, das gleich aussieht.
Connect these dots.	Conecte estos puntos.	Unisca questi punti.	Reliez ces points.	Verbinden Sie diese Punkte.
Draw a person.	Dibuje una persona.	Disegni una persona.	Dessinez une personne.	Zeichnen Sie eine Person.
Put this . . .	Ponga esto . . .	Metta questo . . .	Mettez ça . . .	Stellen Sie das . . .
Under.	Debajo.	Sotto.	Dessous.	Unter.
Behind.	Detrás.	Dietro.	Derrière.	Hinter.
In front.	Enfrente.	Davanti.	Devant.	Vor.

English	Spanish	Italian	French	German
EXPRESSIONS USED FOR SENSORY TESTING				
Close your eyes.	Cierre los ojos.	Chiuda gli occhi.	Fermez vos yeux.	Schliessen Sie ihre Augen.
Point to where I touch you.	Apunte adonde yo le toco a usted.	Indichi dove la sto toccando.	Montrez-moi où je vous touche.	Deuten Sie dahin wo ich Sie anfasse.
Say "yes" when I touch you.	Dígame "sí" cuando yo le toco a usted.	Dica "sì" quando la tocco.	Dites "oui" quand je vous touche.	Sagen Sie "ja" wenn ich Sie anfasse.
Tell me if you feel:	Dígame si se siente:	Mi dica se sente:	Dites-moi si vous sentez:	Sagen Sie mir ob Sie fühlen:
Hot or cold.	Calor o frío.	Caldo o freddo.	Chaud ou froid.	Heiss oder kalt.
Sharp or dull.	Punteagudo o sin punta.	Affilato o smussato.	Aigüe ou émoussé.	Spitz oder stumpf.
Tell me what is in your hand without looking:	Dígame lo que tiene en la mano sin mirar:	Mi dica che cosa ha in mano senza guardare:	Dites-moi ce qu'il y a dans votre main sans regarder:	Sagen Sie mir was Sie in der Hand haben ohne hinzu sehen:
Coin.	Moneta.	Moneta.	Une pièce (de monnaie).	Münze.
Cotton.	Algodón.	Cotone.	Coton.	Baumwolle.
Key.	Llave.	Chiave.	Une clef.	Schlüssel.
Pencil.	Lápiz.	Matita.	Un crayon.	Bleistift.
Safety pin.	Imperdible.	Spilla da balia.	Une épingle de sûreté.	Sicherheitsnadel.

21

PATIENT INSTRUCTIONS

English	Spanish	Italian	French	German
Follow these instructions.	Siga usted estas instrucciones.	Segua queste istruzioni.	Suivez les instructions.	Folgen Sie den Anweisungen.
Do exactly as I tell you.	Haga exactamente lo que le digo.	Faccia esattamente come le dico.	Faites exactement ce que je vous dis.	Machen Sie genau was ich sage.
Do like this.	Hágalo así.	Lo faccia così.	Faites-le comme ça.	Machen Sie so.
I will demonstrate.	Demostraré.	Le farò vedere.	Je vais montrer.	Ich zeige es Ihnen.
Watch how I do the exercise.	Mire cómo hago yo el ejercicio.	Guardi come faccio l'esercizio.	Regardez comment je fais l'exercice.	Schauen Sie wie ich die Übung mache.
Do this at home.	Hágalo en casa.	Faccia questo a casa.	Faites-ça à la maison.	Machen Sie das zu Hause.
Do it ___ times each day.	Hágalo ___ veces cada día.	Lo faccia ___ volte al giorno.	Faites-le ___ fois chaque jour.	Machen Sie es ___ mal jeden Tag.
Let me do the movement for you.	Permítame hacer el movimiento para usted.	Mi faccia fare il movimento per lei.	Laissez-moi vous montrer le movement.	Lassen Sie mich die Bewegung vormachen.
It is nothing serious.	No es nada grave.	Non è nulla.	Ce n'est rien de grave.	Es ist nichts ernstliches.
You will get better.	Usted se mejorará.	Si sentirà meglio.	Vous vous remettrez.	Es wird besser werden.

English	Spanish	Italian	French	German
Soak your (body part) in hot/cold water.	Tiene que empaparse el/la (parte del cuerpo) en agua caliente/fría.	Lavi il/la (parte del corpo) in acqua calda/fredda.	Trempez votre (partie du corps) dans l'eau chaude/froide.	Weichen Sie (Körperteil) in heisses/kaltes Wasser ein.
Do it for ___ minutes.	Hágalo por ___ minutos.	Lo faccia per ___ minuti.	Faites ça pendant ___ minutes.	Machen Sie es ___ Minuten.
I will use electricity.	Usaré la electricidad.	Userò dell'elettricità.	Je ferai un traitment a électricité.	Ich werde elektrischen Strom anwenden.
You will feel a tingling sensation.	Se sentirá la sensasión de brasas.	Sentirà un formicolio.	Vous allez sentir un fourmillement.	Sie werden ein prickelndes Gefühl haben.
Tell me if it hurts too much.	Digame si le duele demasiado.	Mi dica se fa troppo male.	Dites-moi si cela fait trop mal.	Sagen Sie wenn es zu arg weh tut.
Apply bandage to . . .	Ponga un vendaje a . . .	Si metta una fasciatura . . .	Mettez un bandage à . . .	Verbinden Sie . . .
Apply ointment.	Ponga ungüento.	Applichi un unguento.	Appliquez un onguent.	Verwenden Sie Salbe.
Heat.	Calor.	Caldo.	Chaleur.	Hitze.
Cold.	Frío.	Freddo.	Froid.	Kälte.
Ultrasound.	Ultrasonido.	Ultrasuono.	Ultrason.	Ultraschall.
Use a ___ pound weight.	Use una pesa de ___ libra(s).	Usi un peso di ___ libbra(e).	Utilisez un poids de ___ livre(s).	Benutzen Sie ein ___ Pfundgewicht.

Continued on following page

21

PATIENT INSTRUCTIONS (Continued)

English	Spanish	Italian	French	German
Repeat this exercise ___ times without stopping	Repita este ejercicio ___ veces sin parar.	Ripeta questo esercizio ___ volte senza fermarsi.	Refaites cet exercice ___ fois sans vous arrêter.	Wiederholen Sie diese Übung ___ mal ohne Pause.
Take a break between exercises.	Pause entre los ejercicios.	Faccia una pausa tra un esercizio e l'altro.	Prenez une pause entre les exercices.	Machen Sie eine Pause zwischen den Übungen.
Do these exercises ___ times a day every day.	Haga usted estos ejercicios ___ veces por día, cada día.	Faccia questi esercizi ___ volte al giorno ogni giorno.	Faites ces exercices ___ fois par jour chaque jour.	Machen Sie diese Bewegungen ___ mal pro Tag jeden Tag.
Stop the exercise if your pain increases.	Si crece la pena, páre de hacer el ejercicio.	Sospenda l'esercizio se il dolore aumenta.	Arrêtez l'exercice si la douleur augmente.	Unterbrechen Sie die Bewegungen wenn Ihre Schmerzen stärker werden.

English	Spanish	Italian	French	German
Sit with your back straight.	Siéntese con la espalda erecta.	Si sieda con la schiena diritta.	Asseyez-vous droit.	Sitzen Sie aufrecht.
Place your heel on the ground first.	Ponga primero el talón en el piso.	Appoggi il tallone a terra per primo.	Posez d'abord votre talon sur le sol.	Stellen Sie Ihre Ferse zuerst auf den Boden.
Place your foot flat on the ground.	Ponga el pie de plano en el piso.	Appoggi l'intera pianta del piede a terra.	Posez votre pied à plat sur le sol.	Stellen Sie Ihren Fuss flach auf den Boden.
Take a step with your right/left leg.	Camine primero con la pierna derecha/izquierda.	Faccia un passo con la gamba destra/sinistra.	Faites un pas avec votre jambe droite/gauche.	Machen Sie einen Schritt mit Ihrem rechten/linken Fuss.
Your next appointment is on ___.	Su próxima cita es el ___.	Il suo prossimo appuntamento è il ___.	Votre prochain rendez-vous est le ___.	Ihr nächster Termin ist am ___.

ANATOMICAL NAMES

English	Spanish	Italian	French	German
Head.	La cabeza.	La testa.	La tête.	Der Kopf.
Forehead.	La frente.	La fronte.	Le front.	Die Stirn.
Neck.	El cuello.	Il collo.	Le cou.	Der Hals.
Face.	La cara.	La faccia.	Le visage.	Das Gesicht.
Ear.	El oído.	L'orecchio.	L'oreille.	Das Ohr.
Nose.	La nariz.	Il naso.	Le nez.	Die Nase.
Mouth.	La boca.	La bocca.	La bouche.	Der Mund.
Eyes	Los ojos.	Gli occhi.	Les yeux.	Die Augen.
Chest.	El pecho.	Il torace.	La poitrine.	Die Brust.
Back.	La espalda.	La schiena.	Le dos.	Der Rücken.
Spine.	La espina dorsa.	La spina dorsale.	L'épine dorsale.	Das Rückgrad.
Abdomen.	El abdomen.	Il addome.	L'abdomen.	Der Leib.
Arm.	El brazo.	Il braccio.	Le bras.	Der Arm.
Shoulder.	El hombro.	La spalla.	L'épaule.	Die Schulter.
Elbow.	El codo.	Il gomito.	Le coude.	Der Elbogen.
Wrist.	La muñeca.	Il polso.	Le poignet.	Das Gelenk.
Hand.	La mano.	La mano.	La main.	Die Hand.

English	Spanish	Italian	French	German
Fingers.	Los dedos.	Le dita.	Les doigts.	Die Fingern.
Thumb.	El dedo grande.	Il pollice.	Le pouce.	Die Daumen.
Leg.	La pierna.	La gamba.	La jambe.	Das Bein.
Hip.	La cadera.	L'anca.	La hanche.	Die Hüfte.
Buttocks.	Las nalgas.	Le natiche.	Les fesses.	Der Popo.
Knee.	La rodilla.	Il ginocchio.	Le genou.	Das Knie.
Ankle.	El tobillo.	La caviglia.	La cheville.	Der Knöchel.
Foot.	El pie.	Il piede.	Le pied.	Der Fuss.
Heel.	El talón	Il tallone.	Le talon.	Der Absatz.
Toes.	Los dedos de pie.	Le dita dei piedi.	Les orteils.	Die Zehen.
Side.	El lado.	Parte.	Le côté.	Die Seite.
Top of . . .	Encima de; el pico.	Parte superiore di . . .	Le haut du . . .	Oberer Teil . . .
Bottom of . . .	Al fondo de; el fondo.	Parte inferiore di . . .	Le bas du . . .	Die Unterseite . . .

21

English	Spanish	Italian	French	German
One.	Uno.	Uno.	Un.	Eins.
Two.	Dos.	Due.	Deux.	Zwei.
Three.	Tres.	Tre.	Trois.	Drei.
Four.	Cuatro.	Quattro.	Quatre.	Vier.
Five.	Cinco.	Cinque.	Cinq.	Fünf.
Six.	Seis.	Sei.	Six.	Sechs.
Seven.	Siete.	Sette.	Sept.	Sieben.
Eight.	Ocho.	Otto.	Huit.	Acht.
Nine.	Nueve.	Nove.	Neuf.	Neun.
Ten.	Diez.	Dieci.	Dix.	Zehn.
Twenty.	Veinte.	Venti.	Vingt.	Zwanzig.
Thirty.	Treinta.	Trenta.	Trente.	Dreissig.
Forty.	Cuarenta.	Quaranta.	Quarante.	Vierzig.
Fifty.	Cincuenta.	Cinquanta.	Cinquante.	Fünfzig.
Sixty.	Sesenta.	Sessanta.	Soixante.	Sechzig.
Seventy.	Setenta.	Settanta.	Soixante-dix.	Siebzig.
Eighty.	Ochenta.	Ottanta.	Quatre-vingt.	Achtzig.

English	Spanish	Italian	French	German
Ninety.	Noventa.	Novanta.	Quatre-vingt-dix.	Neunzig.
One hundred.	Cien (by itself); ciento(a,os,as) (otherwise).	Cento.	Cent.	Hundert.
At 10:00.	A las diez.	Alle dieci.	A dix heures.	Um zehn Uhr.
At 2:30.	A las dos y media.	Alle due e mezzo.	A deux heures et demi.	Um halb drei.
Early in the morning.	Temprano por la mañana.	Di buon mattino.	De bonne heure du matin.	Frühmorgens.
In the daytime.	Durante el día.	Durante il giorno.	Pendant la journée.	Bei Tag.
At noon.	A mediodía.	A mezzo giorno.	A midi.	Mittags.
At bedtime.	Al acostarse.	All' ora di coricarsi.	A l'heure de se coucher.	Vor dem Schlafengehen.
At night.	Por la noche.	Alla sera.	Le soir.	Abends.
Before meals.	Antes de comer.	Prima dei pasti.	Avant les repas.	Vor den Mahlzeiten.
After meals.	Después de comer.	Dopo dei pasti.	Après les repas.	Nach den Mahlzeiten.
Today.	Hoy.	Oggi.	Aujourd'hui.	Heute.
Tomorrow.	Mañana.	Domani.	Demain.	Morgen.
Every day.	Todos los días; OR cada día.	Ogni giorno.	Chaque jour.	Jeden Tag.
Every hour.	Cada hora.	Ogni ora.	Chaque heure.	Jede Stunde.

21

SEASONS

English	Spanish	Italian	French	German
Summer.	El verano.	L' estate.	Été.	Sommer.
Autumn.	El otoño.	L' autunno.	Automne.	Herbst.
Winter.	El invierno.	L' inverno.	Hiver.	Winter.
Spring.	La primavera.	La primavera.	Printemps.	Frühjahr.

MONTHS

English	Spanish	Italian	French	German
January.	enero.	gennaio.	janvier.	Januar.
February.	febrero.	febbraio.	février.	Februar.
March.	marzo.	marzo.	mars.	März.
April.	abril.	aprile.	avril.	April.
May.	mayo.	maggio.	mai.	Mai.
June.	junio.	giugno.	juin.	Juni.
July.	julio.	luglio.	juillet.	Juli.
August.	agosto.	agosto.	août.	August.
September.	septiembre.	settembre.	septembre.	September.
October.	octubre.	ottobre.	octobre.	Oktober.
November.	noviembre.	novembre.	novembre.	November.
December.	diciembre.	dicembre.	décembre.	Dezember.

21

DAYS OF WEEK

English	Spanish	Italian	French	German
Sunday.	domingo.	domenica.	dimanche.	Sonntag.
Monday.	lunes.	lunedì.	lundi.	Montag.
Tuesday.	martes.	martedì.	mardi.	Dienstag.
Wednesday.	miércoles.	mercoledì.	mercredi.	Mittwoch.
Thursday.	jueves.	giovedì.	jeudi.	Donnerstag.
Friday.	viernes.	venerdì.	vendredi.	Freitag.
Saturday.	sábado.	sabato.	samedi.	Samstag.

	COLORS			
English	**Spanish**	**Italian**	**French**	**German**
Black.	Negro(a, os, as).	Nero.	Noir.	Schwartz.
Blue.	Azul.	Blu.	Bleu.	Blau.
Green.	Verde.	Verde.	Vert.	Grün.
Pink.	Rosado(a, os, as).	Rosa.	Rose.	Rosa.
Red.	Rojo(a, os, as).	Rosso.	Rouge.	Rot.
White.	Blanco(a, os, as).	Bianco.	Blanc.	Weiss.
Yellow.	Amarillo(a, os, as).	Giallo.	Jaune.	Gelb.

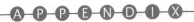

First Aid

HEIMLICH MANEUVER

Techniques

The Heimlich sign is used to indicate when a person is choking. The choking victim grabs the throat with the thumb on one side of the neck and the index finger on the other side.

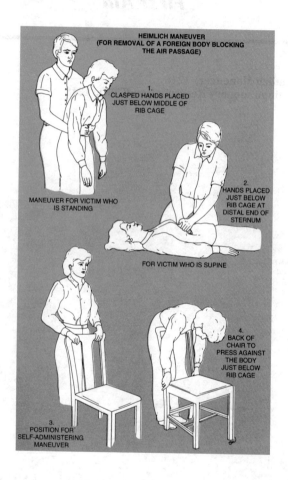

HEIMLICH MANEUVER
(FOR REMOVAL OF A FOREIGN BODY BLOCKING
THE AIR PASSAGE)

1.
CLASPED HANDS PLACED
JUST BELOW MIDDLE OF
RIB CAGE

MANEUVER FOR VICTIM WHO
IS STANDING

2.
HANDS PLACED
JUST BELOW
RIB CAGE AT
DISTAL END OF
STERNUM

FOR VICTIM WHO IS SUPINE

3.
POSITION FOR
SELF-ADMINISTERING
MANEUVER

4.
BACK OF
CHAIR TO
PRESS AGAINST
THE BODY
JUST BELOW
RIB CAGE

HEIMLICH MANEUVER

Anatomic Correlates

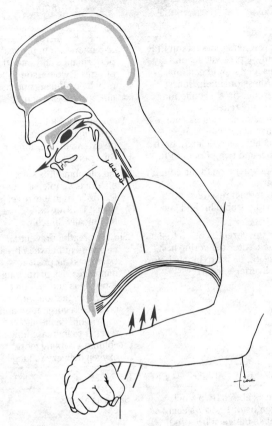

This illustration shows the proper hand placement for performing the Heimlich maneuver on a standing victim. The rescuer forms a fist with one hand and places it below the sternum. The rescuer then grasps the wrist of the hand forming the fist. The hands are then rapidly brought inward and upward.

BASIC CARDIAC LIFE SUPPORT STANDARDS

Present Standard	*Rationale*
TRAINING OF RESCUERS	
Lay rescuers: one-person CPR only. If present, second lay rescuer should call for professional help. If first rescuer tires, second may provide relief.	One-person CPR improves performance and retention of skills. Two-person CPR may be confusing and has not been used often.
Professional rescuers (nurses, physicians, emergency medical technicians): both one- and two-person CPR.	Two-person CPR is less fatiguing; performance may be extended over longer time periods.
Lay rescuers: head tilt/chin lift only. Professional rescuers: both head tilt/chin lift and jaw thrust.	Head tilt/chin lift is safe, effective, simple, and easy to learn. Though effective, jaw thrust is tiring and technically difficult.
Two slow breaths of 1.5 to 2 s each. After delivering first breath, pause to inhale before delivering second.	Slower breaths prevent air entrapment between breaths. Decreased air pressure minimizes risk of opening the esophagus and creating gastric distention with possible regurgitation and aspiration. Pause allows rescuer to increase lung volume, enabling more oxygen delivery to lungs.
AFTER ESTABLISHING BREATHLESSNESS (INFANT VICTIM)	
Same as above (two slow breaths of 1.5 to 2 s each; pause between breaths).	Same as above.
AFTER ESTABLISHING COMPLETE AIRWAY OBSTRUCTION	
The abdominal thrust is the only recommended technique for removal of a foreign body causing airway obstruction in victims over 1 year of age. The chest thrust remains the approved technique for obese persons and women in late pregnancy. Due to risk of abdominal injury, the combination of chest	Exclusive use of abdominal thrusts is more effective and safer than back blows alone or back blows in combination with abdominal thrusts.

Continued on following page

Present Standard	Rationale
thrusts and back blows remains accepted protocol in infant victims under 1 year of age.	

NEAR-DROWNING VICTIMS

Rescue breathing is started as soon as possible. Perform abdominal thrusts only if a foreign object appears to be obstructing the airway or if victim does not respond to mouth-to-mouth ventilation. If necessary, start CPR after abdominal thrusts have been performed.	The necessity of clearing lower airway of aspirated water has not been proved. Attempts to remove water from airway by nonsuctioning techniques are unnecessary and may be dangerous by causing ejection of gastric contents and subsequent aspiration.

AFTER ESTABLISHING LACK OF PULSE (INFANT VICTIM)

Victim's sternum is compressed one fingerwidth below nipple line with two or three fingers.	Recent studies demonstrate that an infant's heart lies lower in the chest (in relation to external landmarks) than previously believed.

EXTERNAL CHEST COMPRESSION, ONE-PERSON CPR

80–100 External chest compressions per minute	Rapid chest compressions increase blood flow from the heart. Increase in intrathoracic pressure promotes blood flow from the thoracic cavity to the brain and heart.

DELIVERING BREATHS, ONE-PERSON CPR

Two breaths (1.5 to 2 s each) after each cycle of 15 cardiac compressions.	One-person CPR allows for 12–15 breaths/min.

DELIVERING BREATHS, TWO-PERSON CPR

One breath of 1–1½ seconds *during a pause* after every fifth chest compression. Pause may be shorter.	Slower breaths minimize risk of gastric distension, regurgitation, and aspiration.

CPR = cardiopulmonary resuscitation.
Based on Thomas, CL (ed): Taber's Cyclopedic Medical Dictionary, ed 18. FA Davis, Philadelphia, 1997, pp 317–318; and The Merck Manual, ed 16. Merck & Co, Rahway, NJ, 1992, pp 524–531.

Illustration on following page

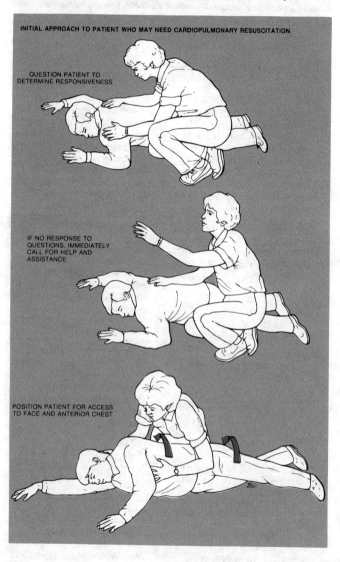

INITIAL APPROACH TO PATIENT WHO MAY NEED CARDIOPULMONARY RESUSCITATION

QUESTION PATIENT TO DETERMINE RESPONSIVENESS

IF NO RESPONSE TO QUESTIONS, IMMEDIATELY CALL FOR HELP AND ASSISTANCE

POSITION PATIENT FOR ACCESS TO FACE AND ANTERIOR CHEST

CARDIOPULMONARY RESUSCITATION

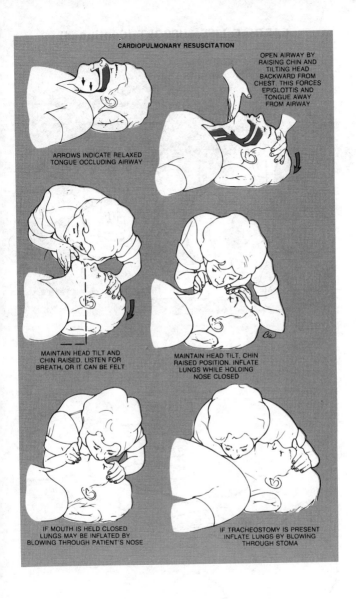

OPEN AIRWAY BY RAISING CHIN AND TILTING HEAD BACKWARD FROM CHEST. THIS FORCES EPIGLOTTIS AND TONGUE AWAY FROM AIRWAY

ARROWS INDICATE RELAXED TONGUE OCCLUDING AIRWAY

MAINTAIN HEAD TILT AND CHIN RAISED. LISTEN FOR BREATH, OR IT CAN BE FELT

MAINTAIN HEAD TILT, CHIN RAISED POSITION. INFLATE LUNGS WHILE HOLDING NOSE CLOSED

IF MOUTH IS HELD CLOSED LUNGS MAY BE INFLATED BY BLOWING THROUGH PATIENT'S NOSE

IF TRACHEOSTOMY IS PRESENT INFLATE LUNGS BY BLOWING THROUGH STOMA

Continued on following page

CARDIAC LIFE SUPPORT (Continued)

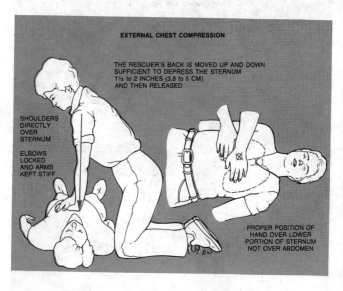

EXTERNAL CHEST COMPRESSION

THE RESCUER'S BACK IS MOVED UP AND DOWN
SUFFICIENT TO DEPRESS THE STERNUM
1½ to 2 INCHES (3.8 to 5 CM)
AND THEN RELEASED

SHOULDERS
DIRECTLY
OVER
STERNUM

ELBOWS
LOCKED
AND ARMS
KEPT STIFF

PROPER POSITION OF
HAND OVER LOWER
PORTION OF STERNUM
NOT OVER ABDOMEN

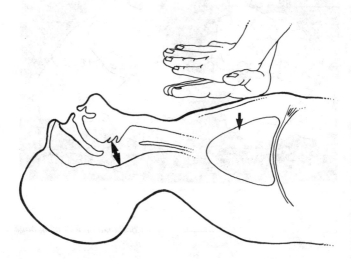

Note the overlapping of the hands and their placement over the lower sternum.

Index

An "f" following a page number indicates a figure;
a "t" following a page number indicates a table.

Illustration Credits

Americans with Disabilities Act Handbook. US Equal Employment Opportunity Commission and the US Department of Justice. Washington, DC, 1992 (pp 14–47).

Bard, CR: Department of Professional and Clinical Education Services, USCI Division: A Patient's Guide to PTC, Billerica, Massachusetts, 1985 (p 643).

Berkow, R (ed): The Merck Manual of Diagnosis and Therapy, ed 13. Merck & Co., Rahway, NJ, 1977 (pp 418).

Berkow, R (ed): The Merck Manual of Diagnosis and Therapy, ed 16. Merck & Co., Rahway, NJ, 1992 (pp 504–507).

Brown, RK and Jacobson, S: Mastering Dysrhythmias: A Problem-Solving Guide. FA Davis, Philadelphia, 1988 (pp 608–616).

Carpenter, W and Rudo, A: Tardive dyskinesia. Behavorial Medicine 6:35, 1979 (p 880).

Choosing a wheelchair system. Journal of Rehabilitation Research and Development. Clinical Supplement #2, 1990. US Department of Veterans Affairs, Washington, DC (pp 60, 61).

Fairbank, JCT, et al: The Oswestry Low Back Disability Questionnaire. Physiotherapy 66:271, 1980 (pp 206, 207).

Froelicher, VF, et al: Exercise and the Heart: Clinical Concepts, ed 3. Mosby–Year Book, Inc., St. Louis, 1993 (p 682).

Gilman, S and Newman, SW: Manter and Gatz's Clinical Neuroanatomy and Neurophysiology, ed 9. FA Davis, Philadelphia, 1996 (pp 234–237, 239–258, 275, and 433).

Gustilo, RB: The Fracture Classification Manual. Mosby-Year Book, St. Louis, 1991 (pp 98–101).

Hall, CB, Brooks, MD, and Dennis, JF: Congenital skeletal deficiencies of the extremities: Classification and fundamentals of treatment. JAMA 181:591, 1962 (p 822).

Haymaker, W and Woodhall, B: Peripheral Nerve Injuries, ed 2. WB Saunders, Philadelphia, 1953 (pp 303, 307, 309, 312, 314, 316, 320, 326, 331, 335, 337, 339, 342, 347, 349, 359, and 361).

Materials that originally appeared in the same form elsewhere are acknowledged throughout the book by the word "from".

Kendall, FP, McCreary, EK, and Provance, PG: Muscles: Testing and Function, ed 4. Williams & Wilkins, Baltimore, 1993 (pp 116, 117).

Keogh, J and Sugden, D: Movement Skill Development. Macmillan, New York, 1985 (pp 693–695).

Kimura, J: Electrodiagnosis in Diseases of Nerve and Muscle: Principles and Practice, ed 2. FA Davis, Philadelphia, 1989 (p 384).

Malick, MH and Carr, JA: Manual on Management of the Burn Patient. Harmarville Rehabilitation Center, Pittsburgh, PA 1982 (pp 1115–1118).

Nashner, L: A Systems Approach to Understanding and Assessing Orientation and Balance. Neurocom International, Clackamas, OR, 1987 (p 458).

National Academy of Sciences, Committee on Diet and Health, Food and Nutrition Board, Commission on Life Sciences, National Research Council. Diet and Health: Implications for Chronic Disease Risk. Washington, DC: National Academy Press, 1989, pp 564–565. Reproduced by permission of the publisher, copyright 1989 (p 1141).

Nurse's Clinical Library: Cardiovascular Disorders. Springhouse Corporation, Springhouse, PA, 1984. Used with permission from Cardiovascular Disorders/Nurse's Clinical Library. © 1984 Springhouse Corporation. All rights reserved (pp 628–631, 646–653).

O'Sullivan, SB and Schmitz, TJ: Physical Rehabilitation: Assessment and Treatment, ed 3. FA Davis, Philadelphia, 1994 (pp 58, 59, 1114, 1119–1121).

Perry, J: Gait Analysis: Normal and Pathologic Function. Slack, Thorofare, NJ, 1992 (pp 793–795).

Price, SA and Wilson, LM: Pathophysiology: Clinical Concepts of Disease Processes, ed 5. Mosby–Year Book, Inc., St. Louis, 1997, p 481 (p 641).

Robinson, AJ and Snyder-Mackler, L (eds): Clinical Electrophysiology: Electrotherapy and Electrophysiologic Testing, ed 2. Williams & Wilkins, Baltimore, 1995 (pp 909–914, 917, and 919).

Roland, M and Morris, R: A study of the natural history of back pain, Part I: The development of a reliable and sensitive measure of disability in low back pain. Spine 8:141, 1983 (pp 204, 205).

Reprinted from Physical Therapy, Rothstein, JM and Echternach, JC: Hypothesis-oriented algorithm for clinicians: A method for evaluation and treatment planning. Phys Ther 66:1388, 1986 with the permission of the APTA (pp 775, 776).

Salters, RB: Textbook of Disorders and Injuries of the Musculoskeletal System, ed 2. Williams & Wilkins, Baltimore, 1983 (pp 213–216).

Scanlon, V and Sanders, T: Essentials of Anatomy. FA Davis, Philadelphia, 1991 (p 488).

Scanlon, V and Sanders, T: Essentials of Anatomy, ed 2. FA Davis, Philadelphia, 1994 (pp 238, 259, 263, 264, 280-282, 489, 492, 546, 576, 601, 602, 604, 686, and 1217).

Schaumburg, HH, et al: Disorders of Peripheral Nerves, ed 2. FA Davis, Philadelphia, 1992 (pp 296–298).

Thomas, CL (ed): Taber's Cyclopedic Medical Dictionary, ed 17. FA Davis, Philadelphia, 1993 (p 1139).

Thomas, CL (ed): Taber's Cyclopedic Medical Dictionary, ed 18. FA Davis, Philadelphia, 1997 (pp 1020, 2242).

Thomas, CL (ed): Taber's Cyclopedic Medical Dictionary, ed 18. FA Davis, Philadelphia, 1997, Beth Anne Willert, M.S., Dictionary Illustrator (pp 544, 1216, and 1220–1222).

Thomson, A, Skinner, A, and Piercy, J: Tidy's Physiotherapy, ed 12. Butterworth-Heineman, Boston (p 823).

Von Lanz, T and Mayet, A: Die gelenkorper des menschlichen hufgelenkes in der progredienten phase inherer umweigigen ausformung. Z Anat 117:317, 1953. As appearing in Hensinger, RN: Standards in Pediatric Orthopedics: Tables, Charts, and Graphs Illustrating Growth. Raven Press, New York, 1986 (pp 686, 687).

Warren and Lewis: Diagnostic Procedures in Cardiology. Yearbook Publications, Chicago, 1987 (p 633).